COMPUTATIONAL INTELLIGENCE IN ELECTROMYOGRAPHY ANALYSIS – A PERSPECTIVE ON CURRENT APPLICATIONS AND FUTURE CHALLENGES

Edited by **Ganesh R. Naik**

Computational Intelligence in Electromyography Analysis –
A Perspective on Current Applications and Future Challenges
http://dx.doi.org/10.5772/3315
Edited by Ganesh R. Naik

Contributors

Javier Rodriguez-Falces, Javier Navallas, Armando Malanda, Penka A. Atanassova, Nedka T. Chalakova, Borislav D. Dimitrov, Runer Augusto Marson, Begoña Gavilanes-Miranda, Juan J. Goiriena De Gandarias, Gonzalo A. Garcia, Leandro Ricardo Altimari, José Luiz Dantas, Marcelo Bigliassi, Thiago Ferreira Dias Kanthack, Antonio Carlos de Moraes, Taufik Abrão, Min Lei, Guang Meng, Mark Halaki, Karen Ginn, Angkoon Phinyomark, Sirinee Thongpanja, Huosheng Hu, Pornchai Phukpattaranont, Chusak Limsakul, Saara M. Rissanen, Markku Kankaanpää, Mika P. Tarvainen, Pasi A. Karjalainen, Chiharu Ishii, Adriano O. Andrade, Alcimar B. Soares, Slawomir J. Nasuto, Peter J. Kyberd, Ryuji Sakakibara, Tomoyuki Uchiyama, Tatsuya Yamamoto, Fuyuki Tateno, Tomonori Yamanishi, Masahiko Kishi, Yohei Tsuyusaki, Takeshi Tsujimura, Sho Yamamoto, Kiyotaka Izumi, Gabriela Winkler Favieiro, Alexandre Balbinot, R.K. Jain, S. Datta, S. Majumder, César Ferreira Amorim, Runer Augusto Marson, Alcimar Barbosa Soares, Edgard Afonso Lamounier Júnior, Adriano de Oliveira Andrade, Alexandre Cardoso, Muhammad Zahak Jamal

Published by InTech

Janeza Trdine 9, 51000 Rijeka, Croatia

Copyright © 2012 InTech

Notice

Publishing Process Manager Sandra Bakic
Technical Editor InTech DTP team
Cover InTech Design team

Additional hard copies can be obtained from orders@intechopen.com

Computational Intelligence in Electromyography Analysis –
A Perspective on Current Applications and Future Challenges, Edited by Ganesh R. Naik
p. cm.
ISBN 978-953-51-0805-4

For EU product safety concerns:
IN TECH d.o.o., Prolaz Marije Krucifikse Kozulić 3, 51000 Rijeka, Croatia,
info@intechopen.com or visit our website at intechopen.com.

Meet the editor

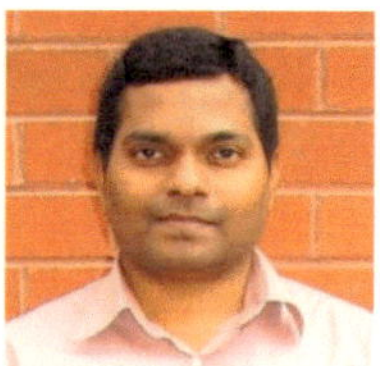

Ganesh R. Naik received B.E. degree in Electronics and Communication Engineering from the University of Mysore, India, in 1997. M.E. degree in Communication and Information Engineering from Griffith University, Brisbane, Australia, in 2002, and a PhD degree in the area of Electronics Engineering from RMIT University, Melbourne, Australia, in 2009. He is currently an academician and researcher at RMIT University. As an early career researcher, he has edited 6 books, authored more than 75 papers in peer reviewed journals, conferences, and book chapters over the last five years. He was a recipient of the Baden–Württemberg Scholarship from the University of Berufsakademie, Stuttgart, Germany (2006–2007). In 2010, Dr. Naik was awarded with ISSI overseas fellowship from skilled Institute Victoria, Australia.

Contents

Preface

Electromyography (EMG) is a technique for evaluating and recording the electrical activity produced by skeletal muscles. Since the contracting skeletal muscles are greatly responsible for loading of the bones and joints, information about the muscle EMG is important to gain knowledge about muscular-skeletal biomechanics. Myoelectric signals can also demonstrate the development of loading imbalance and asymmetry, which in turn relates to physical disability. EMG may be used clinically for the diagnosis of neuromuscular problems and for assessing biomechanical and motor control deficits and other functional disorders. Furthermore, it can be used as a control signal for interfacing with orthotic and/or prosthetic devices or other rehabilitation assists and – aside from muscular activity - EMG can be used to indicate and quantify the development of muscle fatigue.

A great challenge in biomedical engineering is to non-invasively assess the physiological changes occurring in different internal organs of the human body. These variations can be modeled and measured often as biomedical source signals that indicate the function or malfunction of various physiological systems. To extract the relevant information for diagnosis and therapy, expert knowledge in medicine and engineering is required. Biomedical source signals, especially EMG, are usually weak, stationary signals and distorted by noise and interference. Moreover, they are usually mutually superimposed. Besides classical signal analysis tools (such as adaptive supervised filtering, parametric or non-parametric spectral estimation, time frequency analysis, and higher order statistics), Intelligent Signal Processing techniques are used for pre-processing, noise and artefact reduction, enhancement, detection and estimation of EMG signals by taking into account their spatio-temporal correlation and mutual statistical dependence.

This book is aimed to provide a self-contained introduction to the subject as well as offering a set of invited contributions, which we see as lying at the cutting edge of both empirical and computational aspects of EMG research. This book was born from discussions with researchers in the EMG community and aims to provide a snapshot of some current trends and future challenges in EMG research.

Book presents an updated overview of signal processing applications and recent developments in EMG from a number of diverse aspects and various applications in clinical and experimental research. It will provide readers with a detailed introduction to EMG signal processing techniques and applications, while presenting several new results and explanation of existing algorithms. Furthermore, the research results previously scattered in many scientific journals and conference papers worldwide, are methodically collected and presented in the book in a unified form. The book is likely to be of interest to graduate and postgraduate students, neurologists, engineers and scientists - in the field of neural signal processing and biomedical engineering. This book is organized into 18 chapters, covering the current theoretical and practical approaches of EMG research. Although these chapters can be read almost independently, they share the same notations and the same subject index. Moreover, numerous cross- references link the chapters to each other.

As an Editor and also an Author in this field, I am privileged to be editing a book with such fascinating topics, written by a selected group of gifted researchers. I would like to extend my gratitude to the authors, who have committed so much effort to the publication of this book.

Dr. Ganesh R. Naik
RMIT University,
Melbourne,
Australia

Section 1

EMG Modelling

Chapter 1

EMG Modeling

Javier Rodriguez-Falces, Javier Navallas and Armando Malanda

Additional information is available at the end of the chapter

http://dx.doi.org/10.5772/50304

1. Introduction

The aim of this chapter is to describe the approaches used for modelling electromyographic (EMG) signals as well as the principles of electrical conduction within the muscle. Sections are organized into a progressive, step-by-step EMG modeling of structures of increasing complexity. First, the basis of the electrical conduction that allows for the propagation of the EMG signals within the muscle is presented. Second, the models used for describing the electrical activity generated by a single fibre described. The third section is devoted to modeling the organization of the motor unit and the generation of motor unit potentials. Based on models of the architectural organization of motor units and their activation and firing mechanisms, the last section focuses on modeling the electrical activity of a complete muscle as recorded at the surface.

A mathematical model of a system describes the relations between a number of physical variables involved in the system. A mathematical model is a set of equations that can be implemented on a computer to study and to simulate the behaviour (response) of the system under specific conditions. EMG models presented in this chapter are structure based or structural, which means that they describe elements of the real biological structure and characterize them in a reductional way in order to represent the system's elements, behaviours or mechanism that are of importance. In the EMG models outlined here, the input variables or parameters are those that describe the anatomical, physiological, and functional properties of the biological structure under study (single fibre, motor unit, or entire muscle), whereas the output parameters are typically the extracellular generated potentials and/or specific quantitative measurements of these potentials.

Models of EMG activity are useful to address the "forward problem", that is, how specific mechanism and phenomena influence the generated potentials, as well as the "inverse problem", that is, how the extracellular potentials provide information about the underlying mechanism and phenomena. Accordingly, a desirable feature of an EMG model is that it allows studying the effect of the model's (input) parameters on the waveform of the potential, providing insight into the relationships between the anatomical and/or physiological properties of the fibre and the shape of the potential.

2. Modeling electrical conduction in skeletal muscle

Striated muscle is composed of a large number of striated muscle cells, also called muscle fibers. These elongated, cylindrical cells are arranged parallel to one another, and each one is surrounded by a plasma membrane called the sarcolemma. Muscle contraction is created via the repeated activation of several groups of muscle fibers, each of which is governed by a single motorneuron through its axon (Lieber, 2010). Figure 1(a) shows a portion of a muscle fiber that is attached, at the neuromuscular junction, to the terminal branch of its axon.

2.1. Depolarization and repolarization of a muscle fiber membrane

A muscle cell (fiber) is activated by electrical impulses coming from the motorneuron, which brings about the fiber's depolarization and the generation of a transmembrane voltage (normally defined as the extracellular electrical potential minus the intracellular one). Under normal conditions, the extracellular potential is practically zero, and so the transmembrane voltage can be considered to be practically the same as the intracellular action potential (IAP) (Burke, 1981; Plonsey and Barr, 2000). Membrane depolarization starts at the neuromuscular junction and extends along the muscle fiber towards both ends of the cell. As a result, two IAPs propagate without attenuation and with constant velocity v along the muscle fiber towards the tendons, where they extinguish (Lieber, 2010).

The plasma membrane of a muscle fiber has the well-studied property of actively maintaining a nearly constant potential difference between the intracellular and extracellular environment. This voltage is normally referred to as the resting potential and has a value of about -80 mV [Fig. 1(b)]. The negative sign indicates that the interior is more negative than the exterior (negative polarization). In Fig. 1(a) the polarization of the fiber membrane is represented by a number of layers of negative signs. When the fiber is at rest, the number of negative layers remains unchanged. After fiber activation, two potential profiles (one at each side of the neuromuscular junction) arise along the fiber membrane. These profiles are normally referred to as waves of excitation, excitation sources or simply IAPs [Fig. 1(a)]. In Fig. 1(a) it can be seen that, along the spatial profile of the IAP, the number of negative-signed layers changes progressively with axial distance (the x-axis in Fig. 1). This reflects the fact that the IAP profile has gradual depolarization and repolarization transitions, as shown in Fig. 1(b).

2.2. The electric volume conduction

Knowledge of muscle fiber excitability and IAP propagation would be clinically useless if the electromyographist had to penetrate muscle fibers to obtain information about membrane processes. Moreover, recording of the IAP *in situ* from human muscle fibers has not yet proved feasible in EMG studies (Ludin, 1973). All electromyography (EMG) techniques are based on the fact that local electrophysiological processes result in a detectable flow of the transmembrane current at a certain distance from the active sources (i.e., muscle fibers). This flow of current in the tissue (i.e., the volume conduction), allows EMG measurements to be made at a distance from the sources.

The so-called *Principle of Volume Conduction* can be considered as a three-dimensional version of Ohm's law, which establishes that an electric current I, flowing between two points connected through a resistance R, generates a potential difference V between these points: $V = I{\cdot}R$. In the case of living tissue, the electrical impedance is the inverse of the electrical conductivity σ. So, the potential recorded at a point P_0 (x_0, y_0, z_0) within an infinite volume with uniform conductivity σ_i produced by a current I_s injected in the same volume at a point P (x, y, z) can be calculated as

$$V_{P_0} = \frac{1}{4\pi\sigma_i}\frac{I_s}{r_i} \quad (1)$$

where r_i is the shortest distance between the points P_0 and P.

From inspection of (1), two main conclusions can be drawn. First, the potential recorded at a certain point is proportional to the strength of the current source, a feature highly desirable for electrodiagnostic medicine. Second, both r_i and σ_i are in the denominator of the equation (1). Thus, assuming a constant transmembrane current, the potential decreases with increasing radial distance and with increasing conductivity.

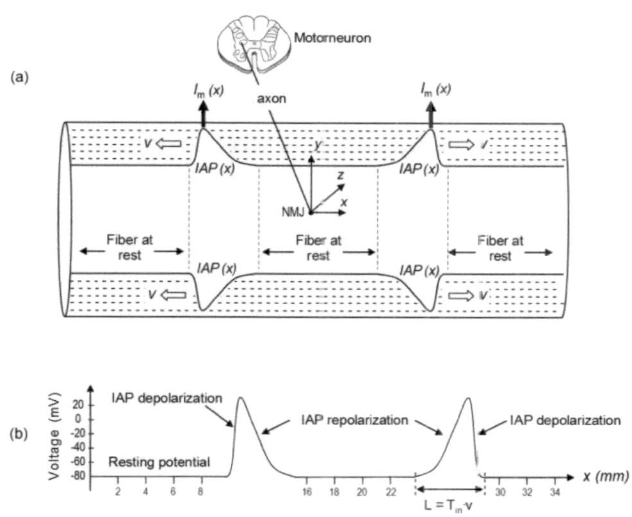

Figure 1. (a) Schematic representation of a portion of muscle fiber in which two excitation sources [IAP(x)] are propagating with velocity v from the neuromuscular junction (NMJ) to the fiber ends. The polarization of the fiber membrane is represented by several layers of negative signs. The number of negative-signed layers within the fiber region delimited by the intracellular action potential (IAP) changes gradually with axial distance, but it is constant within the regions where the fiber is at rest. The transmembrane ionic electric current, $I_m(z)$, is also indicated. (b) Spatial profile of the IAP with its depolarization and repolarization phases. L and T_{in} are the spatial extension and temporal duration of the IAP, respectively.

The principle of volume conduction is valid only as an intuitive approach to an understanding of the generation of an extracellular potential within a muscle. The simplicity of equation (1) hides important aspects that need to be clarified. First, the bioelectrical source cannot be described as a single injected current at a certain point, but it is rather a compound of multiple sources (see Section 3.1.2). Second, muscle fibers are of finite length, which implies that the assumption of an infinitely large volume conductor is never satisfied in practice. This will have important consequences: it will give rise to non-propagating components (see Section 2.2). Third, as muscle fibers can often be considered parallel to each other, conductivity of the muscle tissue in the longitudinal direction (σ_x) is higher than in the transversal (σ_r), i.e., the volume conductor is anisotropic with anisotropy ratio $K_{an} = \sigma_x/\sigma_r$.

3. Modeling the electrical activity of the single muscle fiber

In the last half of the 20th century EMG studies have directed attention to the calculation of single fiber action potentials (SFAPs) produced by excitable fibers and especially by fibers of finite length. The development of SFAP models was possible only after the principles of volume conductivity had been determined and the modelling of bioelectrical sources was well established.

3.1. Modeling the bioelectrical sources of muscle fibers

3.1.1. The principles of bioelectricity

The principle of the electromotive surface proposed by Helmholtz in 1853 provided the basis for the electrical potential theory of volume conductors. In addition, he introduced the concept of an electrical double layer into the theory of electricity and suggested its use for the solution of certain boundary problems in electrical potential theory. The concept of the double layer (or dipole) source, however, went unused for about 30 years until Wilson et al. (1933) demonstrated its appropriateness for modelling the excitation source of a single circular cylindrical fiber. After Wilson, it was not until 1974 that Plonsey definitively clarified the underlying electrostatic principles of the single and double layer sources and related them to the concepts of monopole and dipole, respectively.

Traditionally, two kinds of sources (generators) have been considered in the literature (Lorente de No, 1947; Plonsey, 1974), namely, the "monopole" and the "dipole". A monopole is a single (point) source or sink of current within a conducting medium. It is quite rare that problems in bioelectricity involve monopoles, since all bioelectric generators involve at least source and sink combinations (Plonsey, 1974).

3.1.2. A distributed presentation of the excitation source (excitation function)

Because of its propagation along the fiber, an IAP does not merely exist as a function of time: it also spreads out along the fiber as a function of space. The length of the IAP profile along the fiber, L, is defined by the product of the IAP duration, T_{in}, and the propagation velocity v [Fig. 1(b)]. In fact, the formation of an electrical field around a fiber depends on the spatial extension of the IAP along the fiber (Dimitrova and Dimitrov, 2006; Rodriguez et al., 2011). In addition, the spatial profile of the IAP is smooth [Fig. 1(a)], implying that the electric properties of the fiber membrane affected by the IAP change gradually with axial distance. Accordingly, a correct presentation of the excitation function consists of a sequence of cylinders (fiber portions) of equally-infinitesimal length *dx*, each cylinder containing a density of sources, as represented in Figs. 2(b) and (c). If these sources are considered dipoles, then each of these cylinders should be represented by a double-layer disk [Fig. 2(b)], whereas if the sources are regarded as monopoles, then cylinders should be modeled as single-layer disks.

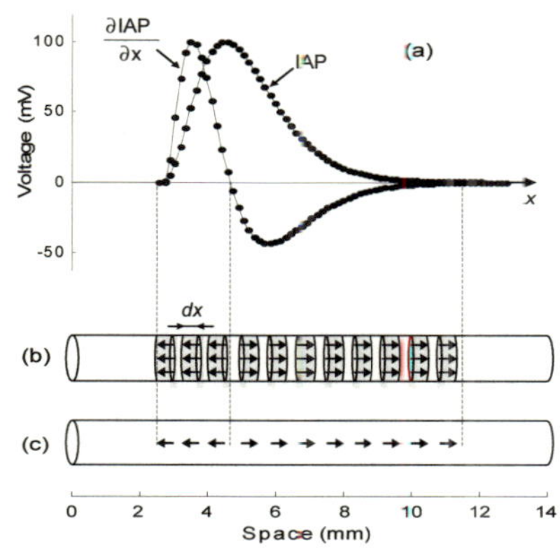

Figure 2. (a) Representation of the IAP spatial profile and its first spatial derivative, ∂IAP/∂x. Schematic representations of the IAP as a sequence of double layer disks (b) (each disk comprising a density of dipoles), and as a sequence of lumped (point) dipoles (c) lying along the axis of the fiber.

From the above it follows that the calculation of the extracellular potential generated by a single excited fiber, Φ_e, can be reduced to the sum of the potentials produced by a sequence of double (or single) layer disks distributed along the IAP spatial course (Dimitrova and Dimitrov, 2006). The specific mathematical derivation by which the extracellular potential is expressed in terms of double layer disks is presented below.

3.1.3. Calculation of the extracellular potential on the basis of dipoles

The dipole-based presentation of the source was first introduced by Wilson et al. (1933) and subsequently developed by Plonsey (1974). It is based on the hypothesis that the variation of the membrane electrical potential across an infinitesimal portion of the fiber membrane produces, in the extracellular medium, an electrical field that can be assumed to be equivalent to that produced by a lumped dipole (Wilson et al., 1933). So, the potentials produced by a double layer disk and a point dipole whose moment is proportional to the disk area are almost identical. This provides the basis for representing the portion of the fiber affected by the IAP as a sequence of dipoles distributed equidistantly along the IAP spatial profile (Dimitrova and Dimitrov, 2006; Rodriguez et al., 2011), as shown in Fig. 2(c). The strength of each of the dipoles (or dipole moment) is determined by the spatial derivative of the potential profile along the fiber ∂IAP(x)/∂x. Orientation of the dipoles is determined by the sign of ∂IAP(x)/∂x.

Let us consider a fiber element of infinitesimal length *dx* of Fig. 2(b) lying within the region occupied by the action potential. A current emerges from this differential fiber element into the extracellular region. If we assume that all the current is concentrated along the fiber axis, then this current can be expressed as $\overline{p} \cdot dx$, where $\overline{p}$ is the dipole current per unit length. Since this current emerges essentially from a point into an unbounded space, it behaves like a point source of current (dipole generator) that lies in an extensive conducting medium. Then, the contribution to the extracellular potential generated from this component can be expressed as

$$d\Phi_e = \frac{1}{4\pi\sigma_e} \cdot \frac{d(1/r)}{dx} \cdot \overline{p}(x,t)dx \tag{2}$$

where σ_e is the conductivity of the extracellular medium and r is the distance from excitation source to the recording point, P_0 [see Fig. 3(e)]. If the element $\overline{p}\ dx$ is located at the coordinate (x, y, z) and P_0 is located at (x_0, y_0, z_0) then

$$r = \left[(x - x_0)^2 + (y - y_0)^2 + (z - z_0)^2 \right]^{1/2} \tag{3}$$

Normally, the coordinate origin is placed on the fiber axis, whereupon $y = z = 0$. The total field produced in the extracellular medium by the propagation of a single dipole along the fiber is found simply by integrating with respect to x (i.e., summing up the contributions to the potential from the propagation of this single dipole current element). The result is

$$\Phi_e(x_0, y_0, z_0, t) = \int_{x=-\infty}^{x=\infty} \frac{\overline{p}(x,t)}{4\pi\sigma_e \cdot \left[(x - x_0)^2 + y_0^2 + z_0^2 \right]^{3/2}} dx \tag{4}$$

At this point, we should remember that the source of excitation is actually a "distributed source", which means that we do not have just one dipole but a sequence of dipoles distributed equidistantly along the IAP profile. The distribution of the dipole moments (strengths) along the fiber axis is determined by the function ∂IAP(x)/∂x. Thus, to be strictly correct, the actual source of excitation is a linear axial dipole source density

$$\overline{p} = -\pi a^2 \sigma_i \cdot \frac{\partial IAP}{\partial x} \cdot \overline{a}_x \tag{5}$$

where σ_i is the intracellular conductivity and a is the fiber radius. If we now substitute (5) into (4), we obtain the dipole-based expression for the extracellular potential

$$\Phi_e(t) = -\frac{a^2 \cdot \sigma_i}{4 \cdot \sigma_e} \cdot \int_{-\infty}^{+\infty} \frac{\partial IAP(x,t)}{\partial x} \cdot \overline{a}_x \cdot \frac{\partial}{\partial x}\left(\frac{1}{r(x)} \right) dx \tag{6}$$

In (6) it can be seen that the term $\partial(1/r)/\partial x$ represents the scalar potential generated by a propagating dipole and the term $\partial IAP/\partial x$ corresponds to the distribution of moments of the collection of dipoles that form the excitation function.

Calculation of the extracellular potential on the basis of monopoles can also be derived following the steps outlined above, as shown in Plonsey and Barr (2000).

3.2. Models of the extracellular potential generated by a single muscle fiber

3.2.1. The first SFAP models

Lorente de Nó (1947) was the first to obtain an expression for the potential of the external field of a nerve in a volume conductor as a function of an action potential. However, he did not provide a physical interpretation for the concepts of double and single layer sources. Nevertheless, his contribution to the understanding and modelling of the extracellular fields produced by an excitable fiber in a volume conductor was essential for subsequent researchers.

In 1968, Clark and Plonsey proposed a SFAP approximation based on formal solutions of Poisson's or Laplace's equation with the corresponding boundary conditions using a method of separation of variables. The solution was based on the Fourier transform technique and modified Bessel functions. The formal solution, however, gave no opportunity for transparent physical interpretations (Andreassen and Rosenfalck, 1981). In addition, the mathematical expressions describing SFAPs using the volume conductor theory were quite complex, computationally time consuming and, therefore, somewhat unsuitable for simulating motor unit potentials (MUPs). In response to these limitations, simplified models were presented. The dipole and tripole models approximated the transmembrane current by two and three point sources, respectively. These models, however, presented important shortcomings. The dipole model was not able to describe the effects of the excitation origin and extinction correctly (George, 1970; Boyd et al., 1978; Griep et al., 1978). The tripole models failed to correctly describe SFAPs close to fibers (Griep et al., 1978; Andreassen and Rosenfalck, 1981).

3.2.2. Assumptions of the core-conductor model and the line-source model: the first approach to convolutional models

Clark and Plonsey (1966, 1968) and then Andreassen and Rosenfalck (1981), provided thorough compilations of the approaches that relate intracellular and extracellular potentials. Both works stressed the necessity of finding the conditions to simplify existing SFAP models. These conditions are summarized in the assumptions of the core-conductor:

a. Axial symmetry is assumed. That is $\partial/\partial\varphi=0$ (where ϕ is the azimuth angle) so that, at most, all field quantities are functions of the cylindrical coordinates only. In fact, transmembrane currents as well as intra- and extra-cellular potentials are considered to be functions only of x (i.e., the core-conductor is linear).

b. For a fiber in an extracellular medium of considerable extent, it is assumed that the resistance of the extracellular medium is practically 0, and so the influence of the medium surrounding the active fiber is neglected.
c. The excitation source is assumed to be distributed along the axis of the fiber. Since in general fiber radius is many times smaller than fiber length, this approximation is normally justified.

On the basis of the volume conductor theory, Plonsey (1974) was the first to show that a SFAP can be expressed as a convolution of an excitation source and a weight function. An important step towards the simplification of this model was made by Andreassen and Rosenfalck (1981) who assumed that the transmembrane current was distributed and concentrated along the axis of the fiber (a line-source model). In addition, the authors theorized that the error caused by such a source simplification would be less than 5% provided the radial distance was 5 fiber radii or greater from the fiber axis. However, both the approach of Clark and Plonsey and that of Andreassen and Rosenfalck were still far from being simple and intuitive as they included an intricate mathematical formulation.

3.2.3. Towards an easy formulation of the SFAP convolutional model

After the key contributions of Clark and Plonsey and then Andreassen and Rosenfalck, great effort was directed towards including in SFAP models the effects of the finite size (Gootzen et al., 1991), inhomogeneity (Dimitrova and Dimitrov, 2001), and frequency dependency (Albers et al., 1988) of the volume conductor. All of these authors were more interested in improving the accuracy of the SFAP model at the expense of reducing the physical transparency and the time efficiency of their approximations. However, these latter two considerations were precisely two features that scientists in other areas of EMG research and practice were increasingly demanding from SFAP models.

The key step towards an easy and intuitive presentation of the SFAP convolutional model was made by Nandedkar and Stalberg in 1983. The authors substituted the complex weight function used by Andreassen and Rosenfalck (that involved Bessel functions) for the simpler expression of a potential generated by a point current source (i.e., a monopole) that propagates along the fiber axis from the neuromuscular junction towards the tendons.

Although the Nandedkar and Stalberg model was found computationally more efficient and more accurate than the dipole and tripole models, it still lacked a suitable approach for dealing with the excitation onset and extinction. To overcome this problem, the excitation wave should be represented with two stacks of double-layer disks distributed equidistantly along the fiber axis. Following this idea, Dimitrov and Dimitrova (1998) replaced the stacks of distributed current dipoles by dipoles lumped along the axis of the fiber (line source model). The weight function was computed as the potential produced by two lumped current dipoles propagating in opposite directions from the endplate toward the fiber ends.

Let us assume that a unit dipole originates at time zero at the neuromuscular junction and propagates along a fiber with a constant velocity v. The potential produced by this unit dipole at the electrode is $IR(\mathrm{t})$ [Fig. 3(a)]. However, the source of excitation is actually a sequence of n

dipoles distributed equidistantly along the IAP profile, whose strengths (moments) are given by the function ∂IAP(x,t)/∂t. The first dipole originates at time zero, and each subsequent dipole at an interval Δt. Let the amplitude of these dipoles be $a_1, a_2, \ldots, a_n$ [Fig. 3(b)]. The first dipole originates at time zero, propagates towards the tendons, generating a potential $a_1 \cdot IR(t)$. The second dipole originates at time Δt, propagates towards the tendons, generating a potential $a_2 \cdot IR(t-\Delta t)$ [Fig. 3(c)]. Hence the total potential recorded by the electrode is

$$SFAP(t) = a_1 IR(t) + a_2 IR(t-\Delta t) + \ldots + a_n IR(t-(n-1)\Delta t) \tag{7}$$

As Δt tends to zero and n tends to infinity, the total potential produced at the point P_0 by the propagating excitation function represents the convolution of $dIAP(x,t)/dt$ and $IR(t)$:

$$SFAP(t) = \frac{dIAP(t)}{dt} * IR(t) \tag{8}$$

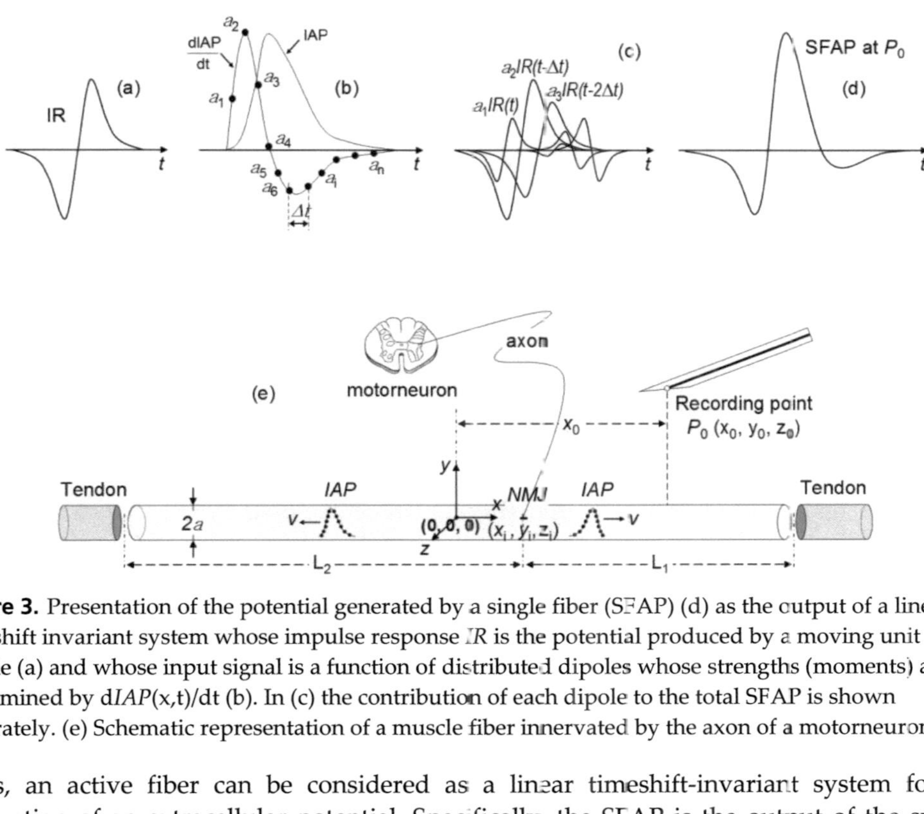

Figure 3. Presentation of the potential generated by a single fiber (SFAP) (d) as the output of a linear timeshift invariant system whose impulse response *IR* is the potential produced by a moving unit dipole (a) and whose input signal is a function of distributed dipoles whose strengths (moments) are determined by $dIAP(x,t)/dt$ (b). In (c) the contribution of each dipole to the total SFAP is shown separately. (e) Schematic representation of a muscle fiber innervated by the axon of a motorneuron.

Thus, an active fiber can be considered as a linear timeshift-invariant system for the generation of an extracellular potential. Specifically, the SFAP is the output of the system with the impulse response $IR(t)$ [Fig. 3(d)] and input signal $dIAP(x,t)/dt$. Since the activation of a skeletal muscle fiber gives rise to two oppositely-directed propagating IAPs, $IR(t)$ is the sum of potentials generated at the observation point by two dipoles moving in opposite directions from the neuromuscular junction to the fiber ends, where they disappear (McGill et al., 2001; Dimitrov and Dimitrova, 1998). This sum of potentials can be described as

$$SFAP(t) = K \cdot \int_0^t \frac{dIAP(\tau)}{d\tau} \cdot \frac{1}{v} \cdot \left[IR_1(t-\tau) + IR_2(t-\tau) \right] \cdot d\tau = K \cdot \frac{1}{v} \cdot \frac{dIAP(t)}{dt} * IR(t) \quad (9)$$

where * means convolution and $IR = IR_1 + IR_2$, $0 \le t \le t_{max}$. Constant K is equal to $(a^2 \cdot \sigma_i)/(4 \cdot \sigma_e)$. The expressions for IR_1 and IR_2 and can be found in Dimitrov and Dimitrova (1998).

3.3. Models of electrodes for recording single-fibre potentials

The advent of single fiber electromyography (SFEMG) allowed investigators to analyze the shape peculiarities of the SFAP. The routine single fibre (SF) electrode consists of a montage of a 25-μm recording port (leading-off surface) referenced to the cannula (Ekstedt, 1964; Stålberg and Trontelj, 1979). When modelling SF electrodes, the leading-off surface is normally considered as a detection point, whereas the cannula is simulated through a plate electrode (Stalberg and Trontelj, 1992). As established by Ekstedt (1964), the conditions for recording an SFAP in a voluntarily activated muscle using an SF electrode are: (1) that the fibre is close to the electrode and thus gives rise to a potential with a short peak-to-peak interval (rise-time, RT), and (2) that any other fibres in the same motor unit that have coincident action potentials are sufficiently remote from the electrode that their contribution to the recorded signal is small.

4.1. Anatomy and physiology of the motor unit

4.1.1. Motoneuron, motor unit fibers, and motor unit territory

The motor unit is the entity that serves as a functional building block for the production of force and movement, both in reflex and voluntary contractions. Sherrington defined the motor unit as the set comprising a single motoneuron axon and the many muscle fibers to which that axon runs and which are hence innervated by it. The motor unit fibers (MUFs) are the different muscle fibers innervated by a single motoneuron. The numbers of muscle fibers supplied by a single motor neuron, through branching of its axons, is often referred to as the motor unit size or innervation ratio, and we will refer to this number as the motor unit fiber number (MUFN). In addition, we can consider the extent of the muscle cross-section that these fibers occupy, which is the motor unit territory (MUT), and the spatial distribution of these fibers within the motor unit territory area (MUTA). Subsequently, the motor unit can be characterization in terms of the motor unit fiber density (MUFD), measured as the number of MUFs per unit of area of its territory.

The MUFN varies greatly from one muscle to another and from one motor unit to another within the same muscle. The glycogen-depletion technique allows identification of the MUFs of a single motor unit within a muscle cross-section. Studies using this technique have demonstrated the large range of variation in MUFN (Burke and Tsairis, 1973), which extends from just a few fibers per motor unit in some muscles to thousands in others. Studies also show great variation within a single muscle: up to 100-fold from the smallest to the largest motor units.

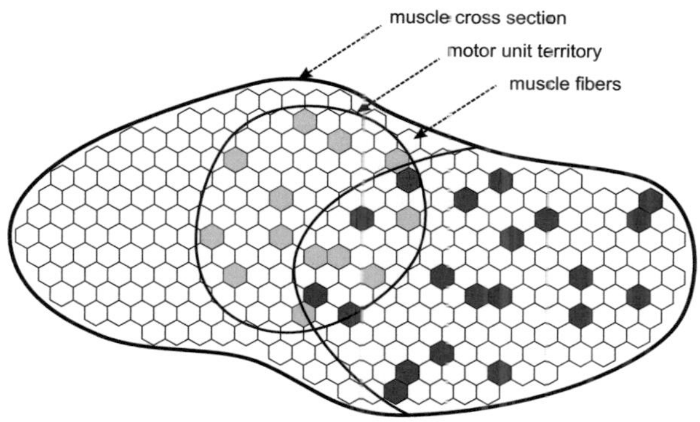

Figure 4. A schematic representation of the motor unit cross-section showing the MUFs of two motor units and delineating their MUTs which may overlap and may occupy only a fraction of the muscle cross-section.

By delineating the boundary enclosing the MUFs, we obtain a picture of the MUT. MUTs have been shown to be distributed over a localized region of a muscle's volume, with an approximately elliptical shape in cross-section [4] (see Fig. 4). That is, in terms of the muscle cross-section, only a fraction of its area is occupied by each motor unit (Bodine et al, 1988). This spatial feature was confirmed in humans using multilead-electrode-EMG, and using scanning-EMG (Stålberg and Antoni, 1980), with typical cross-sectional corridors between 5 and 10 mm long. Research based on glycogen-depletion techniques demonstrates that motor unit fibers of different motor units are intermingled, hence motor unit territories overlap within the muscle cross-section.

Defining the MUFD as the ratio of the MUFN to the MUTA, it is found that the ranges for MUFD are independent of the MUFN, while MUTA is strongly correlated with MUFN (Kanda and Hashizume, 1992). In reconstructions of the three-dimensional structure of motor units, MUFD is almost constant within a single motor unit when comparing the values obtained over the different cross-sections of the unit along the longitudinal axis of the muscle.

4.1.2. Spatial distribution of motor unit fibers

Another important feature related to motor unit fibers is their spatial distribution within the motor unit territory. Quantitative statistical studies in glycogen-depleted motor units by means of Monte Carlo simulation analysis (Bodine et al, 1988), suggest that MUFs are not homogeneously distributed: there are alternating regions of high and low MUF density within the MUT. High-density MUF areas are not usually located in the center of the MUT, as had been previously assumed. The various studies indicate that MUFs are arranged in small subclusters separated by holes with relatively few fibers, and researchers have suggested that if any clustering is present, it should be related to the axonal branching pattern established during development. The scanning EMG has confirmed the presence of silent areas within motor units of human muscles (Stålberg and Antoni, 1980), which most likely correspond to the holes observed in glycogen-depletion studies. Hence these results seem to agree with the long-range distribution findings in non-human vertebrates by the glycogen-depletion technique.

4.1.3. Motor end-plate zone, fiber diameter, and initiation of depolarization

Electrophysiologically, the motor end-plate is the region where the motor end-plate potential is generated, hence where the intracellular action potential of the muscle fiber starts. Thus, the relative longitudinal position of the motor end-plates of the set of muscle fibers belonging to a single motor unit is determinant in the synchronization of the single fiber action potentials. In addition, there will be different times for the initiation of the depolarization of the different motor end-plates, depending on the length of the axonal sprout innervating it. Besides, SFAPs will propagate at different conduction velocities through the muscle fiber, mainly dependent on muscle fiber diameter. All these factors (spatial configuration of end-plates, initiation of depolarization, and muscle fiber conduction velocity) affect synchronization of the SFAPs contributing to the MUP, and ultimately this will affect the shape, amplitude, and duration of recorded MUPs.

Neuromuscular junctions tend to reside in the middle part of muscle fibers, as the connection is established while a muscle fiber is still growing in both directions. The three-dimensional reconstruction of the motor end-plate zones leads to a two-dimensional membrane lying in the muscle volume. Measurements show that the width of this membrane, which corresponds to the variability in the longitudinal position of the individual motor end-plates, ranges between 6 and 10 mm in the *biceps brachii* (Aquilonious et al, 1984).

Muscle fiber conduction velocities can be measured *in situ* (Stålberg, 1966) and have a normal distribution of values for the whole of a given muscle. It is assumed that conduction velocity is directly proportional to fiber diameter, with histological analyses also showing a normal distribution for the diameters of muscle fibers.

Finally, a delay in the initiation of depolarization is caused by two factors: the axonal propagation delay, which is clearly dependent on the length of the axonal terminal branch and its propagation velocity; and the neuromuscular junction transmission delay, which has an average value, but also some variability (the "jitter").

4.2. Models for the motor unit cross section

The first computational muscle architecture models found in the literature were restricted to the simulation of a single motor unit. In essence, if individual motor units are modeled, of the triad: MUFN, MUTA, and MUFD, two quantities can be arbitrarily fixed, while the third will be a subsidiary quantity. After considering the dimensions and number of fibers of the motor unit, the models must deal with the placement of the individual MUFs within the MUT, in order to follow a certain spatial distribution.

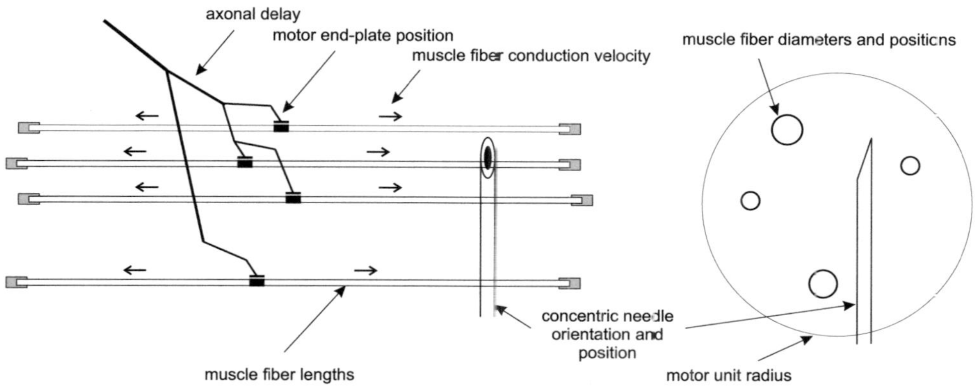

Figure 5. Representation of a simulated motor unit including the most relevant anatomical and physiological factor to reproduce the architecture and physiology of the motor unit.

The first motor unit model (Griep et al, 1978) was proposed in order to study the properties of the motor unit potential (MUP) by means of computer simulation. Other researchers, (Miller-Larsson, 1980; Gath and Stålberg, 1982; Hilton-Brown et al, 1985), were concerned with the modeling of fiber density and spatial distribution of muscle fibers of a single motor unit, in order to determine the influence of architectural changes produced by neuromuscular disease on clinical electrophysiological recordings. Other single motor unit models have been developed more recently. Other studies (Nandedkar et al, 1988; Stålberg and Karlsson, 2001) proposed a muscle model to study the correlation between anatomical parameters and MUP signals by means of simulations, allowing the study of the MUP variations under different pathological conditions such as denervation and re-innervation.

Two main approaches are used to model the spatial distribution of MUFs: random location and random selection from a muscle fiber grid. In the first approach, a number of MUFs are placed following a given spatial distribution, usually normal or uniform. In the second approach, a predefined grid of evenly distributed muscle fibers is created, and a number of them are selected to be innervated by the motor unit under simulation.

4.3. Models of the physiological parameters affecting the temporal dispersion of a MUAP

In all the above-mentioned models, muscle fiber conduction velocity, delay of initiation of depolarization, and longitudinal position of the motor end-plate are modeled as random variables from statistical distributions. It is important to note that, as individual motor units are being modeled, simulated distributions refer to the MUFs and not to all the fibers of the muscle bundle.

Muscle fiber diameter is modeled as a normally distributed variable with mean and standard deviation fixed to match corresponding values observed in real counterparts of the simulated muscle. Muscle fiber conduction velocity (MFCV) is modeled as a normally distributed variable, obtained from a linear transformation of the muscle fiber diameter. The most widely used relationship between fiber diameter and conduction velocity (Nandedkar and Stålberg, 1983) is:

$$v = 3.7 + 0.05\,(\,d - 55\,) \tag{10}$$

With v being the MFCV in m/s and d the muscle fiber diameter in μm. This equation assumes a linear relationship between both quantities, and a MFCV of 3.7 m/s for a muscle fiber diameter of 55 μm. Both these values are the central values of the corresponding distributions for the human *biceps brachii* muscle.

The delay in initiation of depolarization is usually modeled as a normal or uniform random variable, although in some cases its influence on simulation outcomes is assumed to be negligible and consequently it is not modeled and set to zero for all the muscle fibers.

Finally, the longitudinal position of the motor end-plates is modeled as a normal or uniform random variable, emulating the narrow width that the motor end-plate zone occupies within the longitudinal section of the muscle. Uniform distributions usually lead to overly complex MUPs, which seems to call for normal distributions. However, a specific model accounting for the motor unit fractions observed in scanning-EMG recordings, modeled the motor end-plates of small groups of motor unit fibers as narrower normal distributions with the mean of the distributions again distributed uniformly (Navallas and Stålberg, 2009). This model allows for a motor end-plate zone that is wider, whilst keeping the dispersion, and hence the MUP complexity, locally low.

4.4. Models of recording electrodes for intramuscular EMG

Point recording models, which are accurate enough for the simulation of single fiber EMG recordings, must be extended in order to simulate other needle electrodes where electrode poles are not small enough to be considered as points. Two main approaches are available. One is the analytical approach, which requires calculation of the integrals in order to simplify the calculations (Nandedkar and Stålberg, 1983; Dimitrov and Dimitrova, 1998). The other is the discrete elements approach, where the poles are modeled as grids of points where the potentials are calculated individually, and lately averaged to give the potential of the pole. In the case of concentric needle EMG, two poles must be modeled: the core, which represents the active recording region; and the cannula, used as the reference potential. The core, which is a small plane elliptical region, can be directly modeled using either approach. The cannula, a cylindrical region, which averages the potential over a much broader region than the core, can be simplified as a one dimensional cable structure coincident with the needle axis. In the case of macro EMG recordings, the active area is the cannula itself, and the electrode may be modeled accordingly.

There are other effects related to the needle insertion procedure that can also be modeled. Whenever the needle electrode is inserted, fibers in the way of insertion can be displaced by the needle shaft. This effect, named "fiber ploughing", calls for an update in the fiber positions according to the displacement suffered. The electrode manipulation typically performed by an electromyographist while recording concentric needle EMG can also be modeled. The electromyographist tries to bring the core closer to active fibers, producing sharp spikes in MUPs. In the corresponding model, the electrode is allowed to move 1 mm around the original insertion point in the longitudinal direction of the needle, and the position with the shortest distance to an active fiber is selected (Nandedkar et al, 1988; Hamilton-Wright and Stashuk, 2005).

5. Modeling electrical activity of skeletal muscle

In this section, the modeling of the electrical activity of a complete and functional muscle is described. After summarizing the principal anatomical and physiological characteristics of skeletal muscle, the different elements for building a model of a surface EMG signal generated by such a muscle are presented. Together with models of motor unit activity, discussed in the previous section, these elements comprise models for the architecture and geometric organization of the motor units within the muscle, models for the motor neuron pool activity, and models for the potentials recorded at the skin surface.

5.1. Physiological aspects concerning muscle EMG

In order to better understand the anatomical and physiological scenario which the models should recreate, an overview of the arrangement of MUs within the muscle and of the organization and strategies of the motor control is first provided.

5.1.1. Anatomical and architectural organization of the motor units in skeletal muscle

When trying to analyze a muscle's cross-section as a whole, overall statistics for the MUFN, MUTA and MUFD must be provided. We can think of the muscle cross-section as a tightly packed set of muscle fibers that are innervated by a smaller set of motoneurons. The innervation process, which determines the actual set of muscle fibers innervated by each motoneuron, defines the number and spatial distribution of the MUFs, hence the MUFN and the MUTA, and, subsequently, the MUFD.

The MUFNs of the motor units in a muscle tend to distribute exponentially, with fewer motor units with lower MUFN and less motor units with higher MUFN. Indirectly, MUFN can be studied on the basis of the mechanical response of the muscle. Studies of the mechanical response of skeletal muscle support the idea that many factors influence the force production of a single motor unit, including the MUFN, the cross-sectional area of motor unit fibers, and the specific tension output for the different muscle fiber types. However, within motor units of a single type, the main factor determining force production is shown to be the MUFN (Bodine et al, 1987). This makes it reasonable to assume that MUFN is proportional to motor unit maximum tetanic tension (Fuglevand et al, 1993). All these findings support the use of maximum tetanic force estimation techniques in order to investigate the MUFN in humans, where glycogen-depletion techniques obviously cannot be applied. The relative MUFNs can be assessed by measuring the sizes of the electrical and mechanical responses of individual motor units when motor axons are excited by threshold stimuli. Such a strategy involves determining the range of tetanic forces, and estimating the number of muscle fibers required to achieve these forces. These two parameters can be related by linear regression, which enables the estimation of MUFNs in human muscles.

Large ranges of variation of motor unit twitch force are found within single muscles, and the statistical distributions are shown to be highly skewed, with higher number of motor units with small motor unit twitch force, and lower number of motor units with large motor unit twitch force. Fuglevand et al. modeled the distribution of motor unit twitch forces by an exponential function (Fuglevand et al, 1993) that agrees highly with the experimental data (Kernell et al, 1983). Due to the high correlation found between MUFN and motor unit twitch tension, it can be assumed that an exponential function also governs the distribution of MUFN within motor units of a given pool.

The number of overlapping motor units at a given point of the muscle cross-section has been shown to range from 10 to 25 units in some human muscles (McIntosh, 2006). Glycogen-depletion studies have shown that the average MUTA differs for different motor unit types, in the order S<FR<FF, hence showing the same ordering as observed for MUFN. A strong positive correlation ($\varrho = 0.97$) between MUTA and the maximum tension and a strong correlation between MUFN and motor unit maximum tension ($\varrho = 0.94$) can be observed (Bodine et al, 1987). It is also found that the ranges for MUFD are different for each motor unit type and independent of the MUFN within each motor unit type, while MUTA is strongly correlated with MUFN within each motor unit (Kanda and Hashizume, 1992).

5.1.2. Hierarchical organization of motor control

Control of motor function is organized in three levels that act hierarchically and in parallel: the spinal cord, the brain stem and the motor areas of the cortex (Kandel, 1995). Each of these levels receives relevant sensory information from afferent pathways. This organization allows higher centres to give general commands, whilst leaving the control of detailed motor actions to lower level centres. The spinal cord is the lowest level of the hierarchy and contains neuronal circuits responsible for automatic motor patterns and reflexes. It contains a central region of grey matter that is occupied by millions of cell bodies of neurons of two types: interneurons and motor neurons (Guyton, 1994). Interneurons have many interconnections among themselves and with motor neurons, which form interneuronal circuits responsible for integration and feedback-based motor control functions. Motor neurons provide direct control of muscle activity by being directly innervated to muscle fibers. The MNs that innervate individual muscles are arranged in longitudinal columns forming what is known as the 'motor unit pool' (Kandel, 1995). The input to the motor neuron pool is the afferent information from peripheral receptors (muscle spindle, Golgi organs, Renshaw cells, etc.) and the efferent information (drive) from higher centres. The output of the motor unit pool consists on the firings of the different motoneurons in response to the different synaptic inputs they receive in the pool. Smooth coordinated movement relies on the subtle interplay of the command orders coming from the higher brain centers and the feedback information obtained by the peripheral receptors. Four interrelated mechanisms constitute the modulators of muscle activity: (1) MU recruitment, (2) motoneuron firing frequency (rate coding), (3) synchronization between pairs of MUs, and (4) the so-called 'common drive'. The first two are the principal gears of force modulation; while the other two are only secondary mechanisms for control of muscle force output.

5.1.3. Motor unit activation and firing strategies

5.1.3.1. Motor unit recruitment

Motor unit recruitment refers to the way in which the central nervous system selects the specific motor units to come into action as muscle force is required. Henemann and colleagues, in experiments on cats, observed an orderly recruitment of the motor neurons in the pool as the stimuli increased (Henneman, 1965). Specifically, smaller motor neurons were recruited before larger motor neurons. They refer to this behaviour as the 'size principle'. Many other works have reinforced the 'size principle', extending it to other species, different muscles and contraction tasks (Basmajian, 1985). Amplitude and conduction velocity of the MN impulses have been used as indirect indicators of motor neuron size. Twitch tension and MUAP amplitude have also shown strong positive correlation with recruitment order and spike amplitude (Merletti, 2004; Basmajian, 1985). As twitch tension and MUAP amplitude are known to be related to MU size, the 'size principle' indirectly links the order of the recruited MUs and their sizes.

The way recruitment is performed varies among muscles. In powerful muscles, such as the *biceps brachii* or deltoid, recruitment has been observed at least up to 80% maximal voluntary contraction (MVC) (Basmajian, 1985). On the other hand, in small muscles, as those of the hand, the pool of MUs is completely recruited for only 50% MVC. It has also been observed that when the voluntary force decreases, decruitment (deactivation of motor units) is performed in the opposite order to recruitment, in both isometric (De Luca, 1982) and dynamic contractions (Kossev, 1998).

5.1.3.2. Rate coding

Together with recruitment, rate coding is the most important mechanisms to modulate muscle force; the higher the discharge firing rate of a MU in a given task, the higher the force exerted by that MU. However different muscles and different contraction modalities exhibit different characteristics with respect to minimal and maximal firing frequencies and excitation-firing frequency curves (Basmajian, 85). Much of the current knowledge about recruitment and rate coding has been obtained thanks to the availability of reliable techniques for decomposition of MUAP trains from intramuscular EMG signals. One of these techniques is the so-called 'Precision Decomposition' technique, which was developed by De Luca and co-workers and included a recording system based on a quadrifilar needle electrode and programs to isolate several MUAP trains from the recorded signals (De Luca, 1993). With this system the researchers were able to track the evolution of several motor units in exercise protocols where force output was intended to follow a trajectory based on a linear increment, a constant level and a linear decrement. Various important paradigms of motor control could be formulated from the results of these experiments: (a) Lower threshold MUs tend to have lower initial firing rates than higher threshold MUs. (b) Earlier recruited MUs have higher firing rates than later recruited MUs. This occurs throughout the duration of the contraction, which gives rise to the typical 'onion skin' curves (Fig 6). (c) During sustained contractions the firing rates of MUs tend to decrease (De Luca 82) (Erim, 1996) (Fig 6). (d) The firing rate at decruitment is lower than at recruitment (Erim, 1996) (Fig. 6). (e) The firing rates of MUs with different thresholds tend to converge at maximum contractions (100% MVC).

All these findings indicate a hierarchy of MUs in the pool, which determines the recruitment order and the firing rates of MUs as a function of the required force (Erim, 1996).

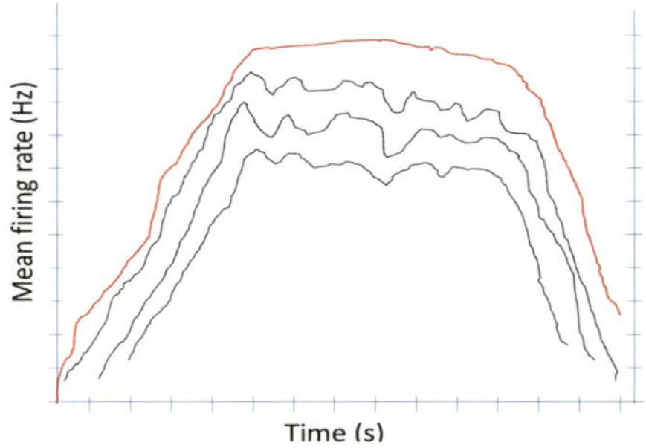

Figure 6. Schematic representation of the output force (red) and MUs mean firing rate evolution (Black) in an increasing ramp-sustained level decreasing ramp exercise.

Even in sustained contractions, the spikes of a MUAP train do not appear with an exact periodicity. The so-called interspike interval (ISI) variability is also an important aspect of rate coding (Merletti, 2004). When a MU is recruited, the ISI variability is relatively high and gets smaller as the firing rate increases (Basmajian, 1985).

5.1.3.3. Synchronization

MN synchronization refers to the "time-locked" spike trains delivered by two MNs in the pool over a certain time interval during a voluntary contraction. The "time-locked" (synchronous) pair of MUAP trains may be simultaneous or have a fixed lag, with a dispersion of a few milliseconds around the average lag (for example, of ±3ms (Sears, 1976) or ±5 ms (Datta, 1990). The number of synchronous spike pairs is more than what would be expected if the two MNs were discharging independently. Synchronization may have different neurological origins, but the most accepted one is the excitatory pre-synaptic potentials coming from brain stem descending neurons that branch into different motor neurons in the pool (Sears, 1976; Datta, 1990).

Using the cross-correlogram technique (Sears, 1976), Datta et. al. analyzed the synchronization of the first dorsal *interosseous* (FDI) muscle in isometric contractions and observed that the level of synchronization of two MU trains decreased as the difference between the recruitment thresholds of the two MUs increased (Datta, 1990). Kim *et. al.*

studied synchronization in four muscles under the conditions of slight isometric contraction and by means of two simultaneous intramuscular recordings (Kim, 2001). The selection of muscles for study was made in order to investigate proximal-distal and upper-lower dichotomies. Results showed synchronization in the four muscles, with higher degrees in distal relative to proximal muscles, and in muscles of the upper extremity relative to the lower. Analysis of synchronization in the frequency domain with the use of the coherence spectrum revealed coherence peaks in the 1-5 and 25-30 Hz bands, which indicated a common rhythmic input to the MN pool, probably related to oscillating activity in the brain and corticospinal projections (Kim, 2001).

5.1.3.4. Common drive

The tendency of the firing rates of different MU trains to fluctuate together in a low frequency range (1-2 Hz) over the course of contractions was first described by De Luca and his team (De Luca, 1982). They observed this common behaviour of MUs on FDI and deltoid muscles during sustained, linearly increasing and linearly decreasing contractions, and called it 'common drive'. They pointed to common excitatory inputs to several MUs in the pool as the probable origin of the phenomenon. Several subsequent studies evidenced similar effects in different muscles, with different exercises and in subjects of different ages (De Luca, 2002). Common drive has also been observed in muscles acting simultaneously in a certain task, either synergistically (De Luca, 2002) or in agonist-antagonist pairs (De Luca, 1987).

An interesting question is whether the phenomena of synchronization and common drive share a common origin. Semmler et al. recorded SEMG data from two separate fine-wire electrodes inserted into FDI muscles during slight isometric abduction. A low statistical correlation (<10%) between the indices that measured the extent of these processes was obtained (Semmler, 1997). Using simulated data, Jiang et. al. also studied the relationship between synchronization and common drive (Jiang, 2006). They found no correlation between the phenomena and a relationship of each of them to a different parameter in the proposed model (see Section 5.3.4, below). As Semmler et al., these authors concluded that synchronization and common drive must have a different physiological origin.

5.2. Models for muscle cross section

Several muscle architecture models have been proposed for EMG modeling. One of the objectives of these models is to reproduce the MUFN, MUTA, and MUFD distributions observed in real muscles. This implies modeling of the layout of the muscle fibers that form the muscle volume, sizing and placement of motor unit territories, and recreation of innervation patterns.

All models follow, to some degree, a common simulation scheme, depicted in Fig. 7. In order to compare the different models, we provide a classification of them based on the two components that most significantly affect the resulting properties of the models: the model of the motor unit territory placement, and the model of the innervation pattern. The different solutions proposed for each of the two components are identified. In addition, the parts which are common to most of the approaches are exposed.

The general procedure in all these models follows three main steps: (1) determination of the intended motor unit distributions (MUFN, MUFD, and MUTA); (2) placement of the MUTs; and (3) recreation of the innervation process by identifying the MUFs belonging to each of the motor units. In the following sections we will detail the different approaches available in these three steps.

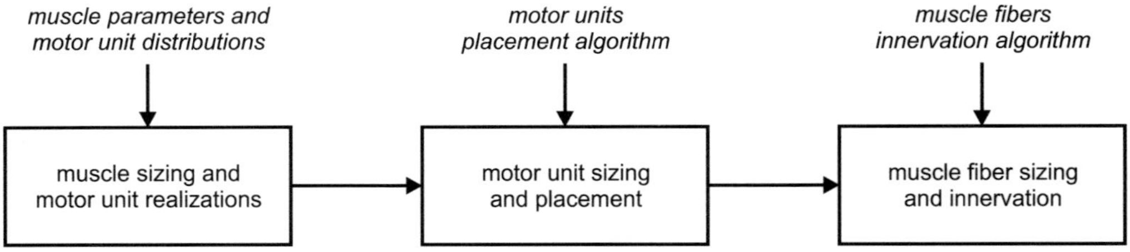

Figure 7. A general muscle cross-section model includes three steps in the simulation.

5.2.1. Determination of the motor unit distributions

Several parts of muscle architecture models tend to be common to all the available models. The geometry of the muscle is modeled by a cylinder with cross-sectional radius RMCS. Within the muscle cross-section, muscle fibers are assumed to be densely packed with a constant fiber density. Motor unit territories are modeled as circles on the muscle cross-section. Muscle fibers of different motor units are assumed to be intermingled, hence motor unit territories are allowed to overlap to a variable extent. To explain variation in maximum tetanic forces of motor units, physiological studies indicate a non-uniform distribution, which can be modeled by an exponential distribution (Fuglevand et al, 1993). If we accept that the number of muscle fibers within a motor unit is the main factor affecting the tetanic force variation (Bodine et al, 1997), we can assume, as well, an exponential distribution for the MUFN. A strong positive correlation between the MUFN and the MUTA has also been observed (Bodine et al, 1997). This seems to be consistent with a uniform value of the MUFD over the muscle cross-section. However, there is also evidence to suggest that MUFD distribution can depend on the motor unit type (Kanda and Hashizume, 1992). Hence, we should consider the assumption of constant MUFD as an approximation of the real properties of the entire motor unit pool. Accordingly, MUFD is usually assumed to be constant (20 fibers/mm^2, taking the value reported in (Burke et al, 1971)), and MUFN is assumed to follow an exponential curve:

$$n_i = \alpha \exp(\beta\ (i\text{-}1)) \quad ; i = 1, \ldots, N \tag{11}$$

where i is the motor unit index that ranks the motor units of a muscle from smaller to larger when sorted by the so called "size principle"; n_i is the MUFN of the i-th motor unit; and α and β are calculated to satisfy the MUFN range determined by n_{min} and n_{max} (the number of fibers in the smaller and larger motor units, respectively). The former equation is consistent both with the exponential distribution observed for the maximum tetanic forces of motor units, and with the linear relationship observed between the maximum titanic force and fiber number of motor units.

Finally, motor unit territory areas are usually calculated to fit both MUFN and MUFD, defined as MUFN/MUFD. In this way, as long as MUFD is assumed to be constant, MUTAs follow an exponential curve (Stashuk, 1993),

$$a_i = \alpha\, d_{MUF} \exp(\beta\, (i-1)) \quad ; i = 1, \ldots, N \tag{12}$$

where a_i is the MUTA of the i-th motor unit, d_{MUF} is the MUFD, and the rest of quantities are as given in (11). As MUTs are modeled as circles, (12) provides the means to calculate their radii.

5.2.2. MUT location: uniform, optimized, and developmental models

For motor unit territory placement, there are different approaches. The first three are based on independent uniform placement of territory centers within the muscle cross-section. Some authors (Fuglevand et al, 1993; Stashuk, 1993; Duchêne and Hogrel, 2000; Dimitrov et al, 2008) propose a uniform distribution of the territory centers within the muscle cross-section but with the restriction that the territories must lie completely inside the muscle cross-section. Other approach (Shenhav and Gath, 1986; Farina et al 2002; Keenan et al, 2006) is to consider a uniform distribution of the territory centers within the muscle cross-section, allowing the territories to partially exceed the muscle boundary and then cutting off the outlying part. A slight modification (Keenan and Valero-Cuevas, 2007) consists on assuming a uniform distribution of the territory centers within the muscle cross-section, allowing the territories to partially exceed the muscle boundary, cutting off the outlying part as in the previous model, and augmenting the territory radius until the inside region equals the original territory area. In general, these models tend to suffer from severe edge-effects, which lead to much higher MUT overlapping toward the center of the muscle cross-section than toward the edge (Navallas et al, 2009a; b). When the MUTs are cut-off, an additional effect of MUT area loss is present, leading to an increase of the MUFD beyond that intended (Navallas et al, 2009a; b). Although usually neglected, these effects severely affect the desired properties of the simulated muscle, and have to be taken into account.

Another approach, (Hamilton-Wright and Stashuk, 2005), is based on a seed-scattering algorithm. In this model, a grid of possible positions for the motor unit territory centers is created. The MUT center is placed at a seed position which is selected at random from this grid without replacement, and perturbed according to a bivariate normal distribution. When all the seed points have been used, the grid is replaced and the procedure of selecting the seed points without replacement begins again for the remaining MUTs. The resulting positions are refined during the innervation process such that they are the mean of the positions (center of mass) of the currently innervated muscle fibers. Similarly, the MUT radii are recalculated at the end of the innervation process.

The last approach considered here, (Schnetzer et al, 2001), consists in applying optimization algorithms to place the motor unit territories in such a disposition that the final muscle fiber density is as constant as possible. The authors presented two different algorithms. The first one places the motor unit territories at positions where the spatial variance of the muscle fiber density is minimized, and this algorithm can be used either with radius augmentation or without it. The second algorithm places the motor unit territories at positions where the muscle fiber density is minimal, and this approach can also be used with or without radius augmentation. These approaches ensure a uniform overlapping of the MUTs throughout the muscle cross-section, and a uniform muscle fiber density (Navallas et al, 2009b; 2010), which are desired properties for any muscle architecture model. As with the uniform models, cutting-off the MUTs leads to a loss of MUT area with negative effects on the simulation of the MUFD (Navallas et al, 2009b). Therefore, cut-off should be avoided in favor of the "augmented radius" versions of the algorithms.

5.2.3. MUF innervation: scatter, random, and weighted models

In the literature, some models explicitly state the algorithm used to model the innervation process. In these models, prior to innervation, a square or hexagonal grid of muscle fibers is created within the muscle cross-section. Then, for each of the muscle fibers, an innervating motor unit is selected from the set of units whose territories cover the fiber position. This assignment can be done in a completely random manner (Stashuk, 1993) or by weighting the innervation probabilities. The idea behind such assignments is to model non-homogeneous distributions of muscle fibers within the motor unit territory (Cohen et al, 1987; Hamilton-Wright and Stashuk, 2005; Navallas, 2010), or to control the number of innervated fibers (Hamilton-Wright and Stashuk, 2005). A further refineed algorithm (Navallas, 2010) uses an analytical expression of the probability distributions of the outcomes (MUFN, MUFD, and MUTA) to determine the innervation probabilities in order to satisfy certain target distributions.

Other approaches simply state that muscle fibers of a given motor unit are scattered within the motor unit territory (Duchêne and Hogrel, 2000; Stålberg and Karlsson, 2001; Farina et al, 2002; Dimitrov et al, 2008; Keenan et al 2006) with no prior grid of muscle fibers within the muscle cross-section. Often, papers describing scatter models do not provide the algorithms used for the placement of the motor unit fibers within the motor unit territory. The reader might guess that one of two possible approaches have been used: we can assume that the exact number of motor unit fibers is assigned to each motor unit, or that the number of motor unit fibers assigned to each motor unit is calculated to satisfy the expected MUFD. Note that, as long as MUTA remains unchanged, both approaches would be equivalent. In both cases, the final motor unit fiber positions can be obtained at random from a uniform distribution over the motor unit territory. This approach should imply the use of a particular mechanism to avoid collisions between muscle fibers, solving the so called "fiber packing problem".

All of these models are adequate as long as optimized-augmented MUT placement has been carried out previously (Navallas et al, 2009b). However, only the inverse-model for weighted innervation ensures that exactly the intended MUFN, MUFD, and MUTA distributions will be obtained for the simulated muscle (Navallas et al, 2010).

5.2.4. Motor unit temporal dispersion parameters

If whole-muscle distribution characteristics are used in modeling the distributions of muscle fiber conduction velocities and motor end-plate locations of the motor unit, the result is usually overly complex MUPs. Muscle fiber diameters can be modeled to follow a normal distribution within individual motor units but with an increasing mean and standard deviation as a function of the motor unit index (Hamilton-Wright and Stashuk, 2005). The rationale behind this approach lies in the differences in diameters of fibers of different types. With this approach, the variability in muscle fiber conduction velocities within individual motor units is narrower, leading to more accurate levels of MUP complexity, while the overall distribution for the whole muscle follows a wider and almost normal distribution, as expected.

Generally, the approach to modeling end-plate locations is the same as that used for individual motor units, hence drawing the locations from normal or uniform distributions as described in section 3.3. Thus, end-plate locations are assumed to be uncorrelated between different motor units. However, more complex approaches (Navallas and Stålberg, 2009) can also be used to ensure further realism in the degree of complexity of the simulated MUPs, although end-plate locations are always independent from one motor unit to another.

Axonal delays and the mean neuromuscular transmission delay, as in the case of single motor units, are usually neglected and left unmodeled. However, in more accurate models (Hamilton-Wright and Stashuk, 2005), the neuromuscular junction transmission delay variability is accommodated. This model of "jitter" values, in which individual transmission delay variability can be modeled using the actual values found in real single-fiber EMG recordings, provides simulated jitter values that are highly correlated with those observed in reality.

5.3. Modeling motor unit activation and firing strategies

5.3.1. Models for recruitment

Given a set of motor units of known sizes in the pool, the 'size principle' straightforwardly defines the order in which these motor units will be recruited with increasing excitation and decruited with decreasing excitation. The model, explained in (Fuglevand, 1993) and applied in other simulation studies (Yao, 2000; Farina, 2002; Zhou 2004; Gabriel 2009), aims to configure the recruitment threshold excitation (RTE) so that many MUs are assigned low thresholds, while relatively few MUs are assigned high thresholds. An exponential law similar to equation (XX) for the distribution of MUFN in the pool (see Section 5.2.1), was proposed for the RTE values. A motoneuron will remain inactive as long as the excitation target force (Fuglevand, 1993) or torque (Farina, 2002) level in the pool is lower than the motoneuron's threshold, and will start firing when the excitation level reaches that threshold.

A new perspective for recruitment modelling was offered by Wakeling (2009), who introduced two input functions, one excitatory and one inhibitory, for governing recruitment. When the excitation (demanded force) is increased from zero to a maximum level, this mechanism produces the recruitment of motor units of increasingly higher thresholds and the decruitment of motor units with low thresholds.

5.3.2. Models for rate coding

Rate coding models are characterized by three different elements concerning the pool of MUs: the minimum firing rate, the excitation-firing rate curves and the inter-spike interval (ISI) variability (Fuglevand, 1993).

Minimum. firing rate

Although there is a tendency for lower threshold MUs to have lower initial firing rates than higher threshold MUs (Erim, 1996), minimum firing rates are similar for all MUs in the pool (Monster, 1977; Fuglevand, 1993). In (Fuglevand, 1993; Yao 2000; Farina 2002; Zhou 2004) the minimum firing rate was given a constant value of 8 Hz for the whole pool of MUs.

Excitation-firing. rate curves

After the experimental work of Milner Brown (1973), the relationship between the firing rate of the MUs of the pool and the excitation has been modelled by means of a linear function (Fuglevand, 1993; Yao 2000; Farina 2002; Zhou 2004). Different behaviours in relation to the peak firing rates (PFR) of MUs, in combination with the slope of the excitation-firing rate curves (SEFRC), has led to different models for these curves:

a. SEFRC is the same for all MUs, and PFRs are in inverse proportion to the recruitment threshold (Fuglevand, 1993; Zhou, 2004) (Fig 8.A). This model is based on observations made in cats, monkeys and humans (Fuglevand, 1993) and is consistent with the 'onion skin' phenomenon (Erim, 1996).
b. SEFRC is the same for all MUs and the PFR is the same for all the MNs in the pool (Fuglevand, 1993; Farina 2002) (Fig 8.B). Several experimental works support this strategy (Fuglevand, 1993).
c. SEFRC is the same for all MUs and PFRs are proportional to MU recruitment thresholds (Fuglevand, 1993; Zhou, 2004) (Fig 8.C). In this case, peak firing rates are related to the mechanical outputs of the MUs in the sense that large force, fast contracting MUs are assigned higher PFRs than small force, slow contracting MUs. This model is also based on experimental observations (Fuglevand, 1993).
d. SEFRC increases with the recruitment threshold, so that all MUs finally reach the same PFR at maximum excitation (Zhou, 2004) (Fig 8.D).

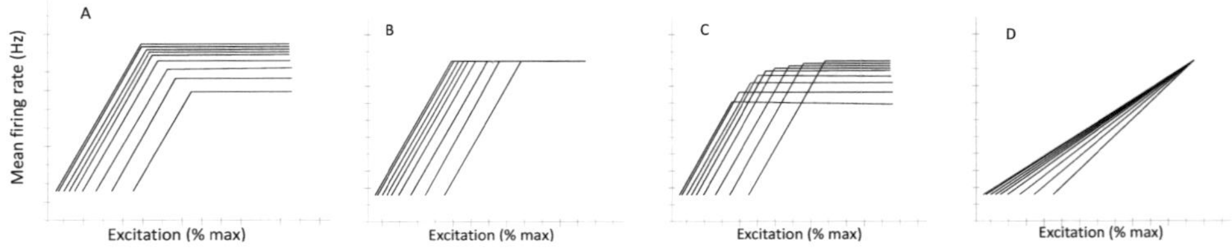

Figure 8. Linear excitation-firing rate curves.

ISI. variability

In most cases a Gaussian distribution has been confirmed to best fit the experimental data (Merletti, 2004; Fugglevand, 1993). But, a Poisson distribution and a gamma distribution have also been proposed (Merletti, 2004).

Physiological. models for the MU firing rate

A different model for firing rates of MUs was proposed by Matthews (1996). He considered that the repolarization phase of the membrane potential could be modelled by an exponential curve. When this curve crosses a certain threshold, a new action potential is fired. This leads to the repetitive firing of action potentials with a constant firing rate, which depends on the exponential decaying factor and on the threshold. Higher thresholds would lead to higher firing frequencies and *vice versa*. White Gaussian noise of zero mean was superimposed on the membrane exponential curves, thus introducing variability into the interspike intervals, which was directly related to the power of the noise.

Jiang et al. (2006) proposed a model for the generation of action potential trains in a small set of neurons, which included excitation neurons, motoneurons and synapses. In the particular example developed, one excitation neuron provided common input signals to two different MUs through corresponding synapses, which also received feedback information from the MN outputs (Fig 9). To compare the outputs of the model to data from real experiments, SEMG recordings were obtained from *biceps brachii* and *abductor pollicis brevis* muscles during slight isometric contractions. Real and simulated signals showed similar results regarding MN synchronization and common drive (see below).

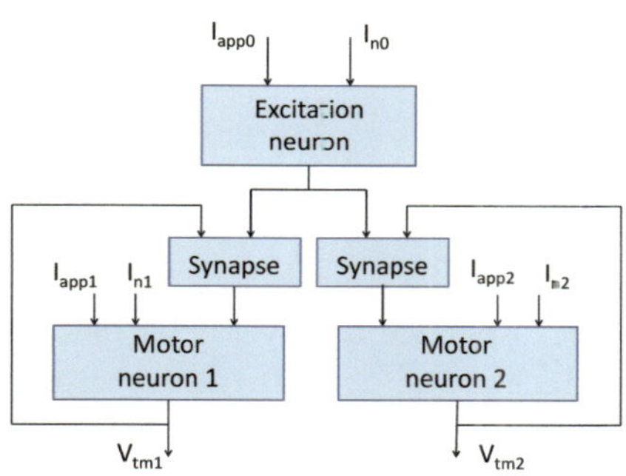

Figure 9. Jiang's model for the generation of action potential trains. I_{app}: applied currents, responsible of the neuron excitability, I_n: noise currents, V_{tm}: output potentials.

5.3.3. *Models for synchronization*

Yao et. al. proposed a model for MU synchronization which basically adjusts the firing instants of MUs in the pool so that they attain a certain degree of time proximity among them (synchronization) (Yao, 2000). This model is used to study the influence of synchronization on SEMG and output force as the neural excitations varies. Simulation results show that both the SEMG level and the variability of output force increase with synchronization, but the level of output force itself is not significantly influenced by it. The same conclusions were reported in the simulation study carried out by Zhou et. al. (2004)using Yao's model. This model was also used by Gabriel and Kamen (2009) in their inverse modelling study conducted to find out the physiological strategies responsible for elevating the force level in isometric voluntary contractions in *biceps brachii*. They concluded that either rate coding or synchronization could provide output data fit to the real data and that either of these two strategies, or a combination of the two, could be involved in the motor process.

A different model was proposed by Kleine et al. (2001), who slightly modified Matthews' firing rate model to introduce synchronization in a controlled way. In essence, the noisy input component is divided into two parts, one which is common to other MUs in the pool and one that is unique and independent of the other MUs. Simulation of SEMG signals correctly predicted the findings observed experimentally in isometric contractions of the trapezius muscle.

5.3.4. Modeling the common drive

Jiangs' physiological model for modeling the generation of MN firing trains also enables the simulation of common drive (Jiang, 2006). In the example explored (Fig. 9), there are independent MN inputs that determine their excitabilities (I_{app1} and I_{app2}). When these inputs are given a common oscillating signal, emulating interneural or afferent signals reaching the two MNs, their firing rates exhibit a clear correlation (common drive), although synchronization is not appreciably affected.

5.4. Models for the potentials recorded at the skin surface

Models for the potentials recorded at the skin surface usually follow the convolutional approach, that is, they try to find a 'weighting function' that provides the potential recorded at any point on the surface of the skin above the active fiber and caused by an elementary current source at the fiber. First of all, a geometric model of the muscle has to be defined, which might accommodate the existence of several tissue layers with different electrical properties (conductivities and capacitances). Together with the 'weighting function', a source function of the distribution of current sources in the fiber, such as one of those proposed for the single fiber case (Rodríguez et al, 2012), has to be used. Apart from the infinite homogeneous volume conductors, one of the first approximations for modeling the geometry of the muscle was the semi-infinite structure, which divides the complete (infinite) space into two parts separated by the skin plane: one with finite conductivity representing the muscle tissue, and one with zero conductivity, representing the other side of the skin plane (Merletti et al, 1999).

Muscle tissue presents higher conductivity in the direction longitudinal to the fibers than in the perpendicular direction. To include this behaviour into EMG models a new coefficient was included in the formulation of the 'weighting function': the anisotropy ratio (ratio between conductivities in the longitudinal and perpendicular directions) (Merletti et al, 1999). The effects of fat and skin layers, that have different electrical properties (conductivity and capacity), have also been incorporated into some models (Farina, 2001), (Block, 2002; Lowery 2002). The fat layer is normally considered isotropic, with conductivity appreciably lower than the muscle. Skin has a laminar structure with a highly resistant stratum corneoum and a deeper granular tissue with higher conductivity. However, it is normally modelled as a simple layer with homogeneous conductivity, although there is not general agreement about the values of skin conductivity), (Block, 2002; Lowery 2002). The effects of these layers have been studied through simulation; relative to models which only include one or two layers, multi-layer models generate potentials with peak amplitudes closer to those found in real recordings.

An important step forward in the construction of more elaborated EMG models is the inclusion of finite limb geometries. Cylindrical muscle models have been developed by several authors (Gootzen, 1989; Roeleveld, 1997; Farina, 2004) in which the fibers run parallel to the cylinder axis. But, fibers may also run radially within a cylindrical geometry, for example, in the anal sphincter (Farina, 2004) or have different fiber-pinnation angles (Mesin, 2004). More complicated geometries, which include bones and vessels, have also been included in the models (Mesin, 2008). As the geometrical structure and composition of layers of the EMG model is made more complicated, defining and solving the electrical equations of the problem becomes more difficult. Iterative computational approaches such as the finite-element method (FEM) or boundary element method (BEM) are called for. In (Lowery, 2002) a FEM model with cylindrical geometry was devised for a muscle. This included the muscle tissue, fat and skin layers and a bone, all of them with specific conductivities. Similarly, a FEM model with a realistic geometry taken from magnetic resonance images of a particular subject's muscle was also modelled (Lowery, 2004). Simulated signals from both models were compared to real EMG data from electrical stimulation of the upper arm. Both models presented similar features with regard to peak amplitude and power spectrum mean frequency as functions of the recording position. However, the more realistic model (Lowery, 2004) provided action potential shapes closer to those actually recorded (Lowery, 2002).

Finally, the effects of the surface EMG electrodes potentials should also be included in the model. In general, placing an electrode on the skin surface does not alter the potential field. This is due to the relatively high impedance "seen" by the conductor tissue, which is, in turn, due to the electrochemical double layer formed between the metal of the electrode and the tissue. The potential recorded by the electrode is then the average potential in the surface covered by the electrode (McGill, 2004). Analytical or numerical procedures may be used to calculate this average either in the spatial domain (Dimitrov, 1998; Merletti, 1999) or in the spatial frequency domain (Farina, 2004).

5.5. Conclusions and open research lines

A general perspective of EMG modeling has been displayed together with a description of the anatomical and functional physiological aspects, in which the described models are grounded. This panoramic view comprises models for the space and size distribution and architectural organization of MUs in the muscle; a view of the hierarchical organization of the motor control; models for the principal MU activation and firing strategies for muscle force production: MU recruitment, 'rate coding', MN synchronization and the 'common drive'; and models for the generation of potentials at electrodes placed on the skin surface.

Experimental research works sustaining evidences for the theories and concepts described in the chapter have also been included.

The research effort in modeling and simulating EMG signals in the last three decades has been paramount including both analytical as well as numerical orientations. The degree of complexity and detail has also run parallel to these developments with the aim of recreating the physiological EMG generation system on one hand and the temporal and spectral features of real EMG signals on the other hand. However, there is still room for improvement in several aspects:

- Most experimental observations related to force modulation mechanisms are referred to isometric contractions. The extent of the validity of existing models of such mechanisms in dynamic contractions is not solidly established yet, deserving more research attention.
- SMEG generation models with increasingly complex muscle geometry and fibers disposition have been developed (Messin 2004; Messin 2008; Lowery 2002). On the other hand, sophisticated models for the MU geometrical distribution and MUF innervations have been put forward (Navallas 2010). However, these two different and complementary modeling pieces have not been put together yet, as a unified approach of muscle architecture. Their combination could represent even better the complex physiological arrangement of fibers and MU in the muscle, permitting more refined simulation studies.
- The phenomena of MU substitution (Westgaard, 1999) and replacement (Bawa, 2009), which appears in prolonged contractions, can be considered as a fifth strategy for MU firing rate control. EMG models that include these phenomena are still missing.
- Fatigue, aging and neuromuscular disease are specific circumstances that degrade muscle performance. EMG models for these situations are scarce (Dimitrov, 2008; Nandedkar, 1989; Stalberg 2001; Enoka, 2003) but may be indeed very useful for better understanding the underlying mechanisms. More research attention should therefore be given to this important area of EMG modeling.

Author details

Javier Rodriguez-Falces, Javier Navallas and Armando Malanda
Department of Electrical and Electronic Engineering, Public University of Navarra, Pamplona, Spain

6. References

Albers, BA., Rutten, WLC., Wallinga, W., & Boom, HBK. (1988). Frequency domain modelling of volume conduction of single muscle fiber action potentials. *IEEE Trans Biomed Eng*, Vol. 35, pp. 328-333.

Andreassen, S., & Rosenfalck, A. (1981). Relationship of intracellular and extracellular action potentials of skeletal muscle fibers. *CRC Crit Rev Bioeng*, Vol. 7, pp. 267–306.

Aquilonius, SM., Askmark, H., Gillberg, PG., Nandedkar, S., Olsson, Y. & Stålberg, E. (1984) Topographical localization of end-plates in cryosections of whole human muscles. *Muscle Nerve,* Vol. 7, pp. 293–297.

Arai, T. & Kragic, D. (1999). Variability of Wind and Wind Power, In: *Wind Power,* S.M. Muyeen, (Ed.), 289-321, Scyio, ISBN 978-953-7619-81-7, Vukovar, Croatia

Basmajian, JV. & De Luca JC. (1985). Muscles alive. Their function revealed by Electromyography. Baltimore, USA: Williams and Wilkinson.

Bawa, P., Murnagham, C. (2009). Motor unit rotation in a variety of human muscles. J Neurophysiology 102, pp. 2265-2272.

Block, J.H., Stegeman, D.F. & Van Oosterom, A. (2002) Three-layer volume conductor model and software package for applications in surface Electromyography. *Annals Biomed Eng.* Vol. 30. pp. 566-577.

Bodine, SC., Garfinkel, A., Roy, RR. & Edgerton, VR. (1988) Spatial distribution of motor unit fibers in the cat soleus and tibialis anterior muscles: local interactions. *J Neurosci,* Vol. 8, pp. 2142-2152.

Bodine, SC., Roy, RR., Eldred, E. & Edgerton, VR. (1987) Maximal force as a function of anatomical features of motor units in the cat tibialis anterior. *J Neurophysiol,* Vol. 57, pp. 1730-1745.

Boyd, DC., Lawrence, PD., & Bratty, PJA. (1978). On modeling the single motor unit action potential. *IEEE Trans Biomed Eng,* Vol. 25, pp. 236–43.

Burke, RE. & Tsairis, P. (1973) Anatomy and innervation ratios in motor units of cat gastrocnemius. *J Physiol,* Vol. 234, pp. 749-765.

Burke, RE. (1981). Motor units: anatomy, physiology and functional organization. In: *Handbook of Physiology. The Nervous System. Motor Control,* pp. 345–422, Bethesda, MD: American Physiological Society.

Burke, RE., Levine, DN. & Zajac, FE. (1971) Mammalian motor units: physiological-histochemical correlation in three types in cat gastrocnemius. *Science,* Vol. 174, pp. 709-712.

Clark, J., & Plonsey, R. (1966). A Mathematical Evaluation of the Core ConductorModel. *Biophys J,* Vol. 6, No 1, pp. 95–112.

Clark, J., & Plonsey, R. (1968). The Extracellular Potential Field of the Single Active Nerve Fiber in a Volume Conductor. *Biophys J,* Vol. 8, No. 7, pp. 842–864.

Cohen, MH., Lester, JM., Bradley, WG., Brenner, JF., Hirsch, RP., Silber, DI. & Ziegelmiller, D. (1987) A computer model of denervation-reinnervation in skeletal muscle. *Muscle Nerve,* Vol. 10, pp. 826-836.

Datta, AK., Stephens, JA. (1990). Synchornization of motor unit activity during voluntary contractions in man. *J. Physiol. Lond.* Vol. 442, pp 397-419.

De Luca JC. (1993). Precision decomposition of EMG signals. *Meth Clin Nueurophysiol.* Vol 4. pp. 1-28.

De Luca, JC. & Erim, Z. (2002). Common drive in motor units of a synergistic muscle pair. *J. Neurophysiol.* Vol. 87, pp 2200-2204.

De Luca, JC. & Mambrito, B. (1987). Voluntary control of motor units in human antagonist muscles: coactivation and reciprocal activation. . *J. Neurophysiol.* Vol. 58, pp 525-542.

De Luca, JC., LeFever, RS., McCue, MP & Xenakis, P. (1982). Controls scheme governing concurrently active hunan motor units during voluntary contractions. *J. Physiol.* Vol. 329, pp 129-142.

Dimitrov, GV., & Dimitrova, NA. (1998). Precise and fast calculation of the motor unit potentials detected by a point and rectangular plate electrode. *Med Eng Phys*, Vol. 20, pp. 374–381.

Dimitrov, GV., Arabadzhiev, TY., Hogrel, JY. & Dimitrova NA. (2008). Simulation analysis of interference EMG during fatiguing voluntary contractions. part I: What do the intramuscular spike amplitude-frequency histograms reflect? *J Electromyogr Kinesiol*, Vol. 18, pp. 35-43.

Dimitrova, NA., & Dimitrov, GV. (2006). Electromyography (EMG) modeling. In: *Wiley encyclopedia of biomedical engineering*. Metin A, Hoboken, NJ: John Wiley & Sons.

Dimitrova, NA., Dimitrov, AG., & Dimitrov, GV. (1999). Calculation of extracellular potentials produced by inclined muscle fibers at a rectangular plate electrode. *Med Eng Phys*, Vol. 21, pp. 582–587.

Dimitrova, NA., Dimitrov, GV., & Dimitrov, AG. (2001). Calculation of spatially filtered signals produced by a motor unit comprising motor unit with a non-uniform propagation. *Med Biol Eng Compt*. Vol. 39, pp. 202–207.

Duchêne, J. & Hogrel JY. (2000) A model of EMG generation. *IEEE Trans Biomed Eng*, Vol. 47, pp.192-201.

Ekstedt, J. (1964). Human single fibre action potentals. *Acta Physiol Scand*, Vol. 61, No. 226, pp. 1-96.

Enoka RM, Christou EA, Hunter SK, Kornatz KW, Semmler JG, Taylor AM, Tracy BL. (2003) Mechanisms that contribute to differences in motor performance between young and old adults. J Electromyogr Kinesiol. Feb;13(1):1-12.

Erim, Z., De Luca CJ., Mineo, K. & Aoki, T. (1996). Rank-ordered regulation of motor units. *Muscle & Nerve*. Vol. 19. pp. 563-573.

Farina, D., Cescon, C. & Merletti, R. (2002) Influence of anatomical, physical, and detection-system parameters on surface EMG. *Biol Cybern*, Vol. 86, pp. 445-456.

Farina, D., Fosci, M. & Merletti, R. (2002). Motor unit recruitment strategies investigated by surface EMG variables. *J. Appl Physiol.* Vol. 92, pp 235-247.

Farina, D., Mertetti, R. (2002). A novel approach for precise simulation of the EMG signal detected by surface electrodes. *IEEE Trans Biomed Eng*, Vol. 48, pp. 637-646.

Farina, D., Messin, L., Martina, S., Mertetti, R. (2004). A surface EMG generation model with multilayer cylindrical description of the volume conductor. *IEEE Trans Biomed Eng*, Vol. 51, pp. 415-426.

Fuglevand, AJ., Winter, DA. & Patla, AE. (1993) Models of recruitment and rate coding organization in motor-unit pools. *J Neurophysiol*, Vol. 70, pp. 2470-2488.

Fuglevand, AJ., Winter, DA., Patla, AE., & Stashuk, D. (1992). Detection of motor unit action potentials with surface electrodes: influence of electrode size and spacing. *Biol Cybern*, Vol. 67, pp. 143–53.

Gabriel, DA., Kamen, G. (2009). Experimental and modelling investigation of spectral compression of biceps brachii SEMG activity with increasing force levels. *J Electromyogr Kinesiol.* Vol. 19. pp. 437-448.

Gath I. & Stålberg E. (1982) On the measurement of fibre density in human muscles. *Electroencephalogr Clin Neurophysiol*, Vol. 54, pp. 699-706.

George, RE. (1970). The summation of muscle fiber action potentials. *Med Biol Eng*, Vol. 8, pp. 357–65.

Gootzen, T., Stegeman, D., & Van Oosterom, A. (1991). Finit limb dimensions and finite muscle length in a model for the generation of electromyographic signals. *Electroenceph Clin Neurophysiol*, Vol. 81, pp. 152-162.

Gootzen, TH., Stegeman, DF. & Heringa A. (1989). On numerical problems of analytical calculation of extracellular fields in bounded cylindrical volume conductors. *J. Appl Physiol.* Vol. 66, pp. 4504-4508.

Griep, PAM., Boon, KL. & Stegeman, DF. (1978) A study of the motor unit action potential by means of computer simulation. *Biol Cybern*, Vol. 30, pp. 221-230.

Guyton AC. (1994). Anatomía y fisiología del sistema nervioso (2ª edición). Madrid, España. Editorial Médica Panamericana.

Hamilton-Wright, A. & Stashuk, DW. (2005) Physiologically based simulation of clinical EMG signals. *IEEE Trans Biomed Eng*, Vol. 52, pp. 171-183.

Helmholtz, H. (1853). Messungen über einige Gesetze der Vertheilung elektrischer Ströme in Körperlichen Leitern mit Anwendung auf die thierischelektrischen Versuche Ann Physik u Chem, Vol. 89, pp. 211–353.

Henneman, E., G. Somjem & D. O. Carpenter. (1965). Functional significance in cell size in spinal motoneuros. *J. Neurophysiol.* Vol. 28, pp 560-580.

Hilton-Brown, P., Nandedkar SD. & Stålberg EV. (1985) Simulation of fibre density in single-fibre electromyography and its relationship to macro-EMG. *Med Biol Eng Comput*, Vol. 23, pp. 541-546.

Hodgkin, AL., & Huxley, AF. (1952). A quantitative description of membrane current and its application to conduction and excitation in nerve. *J Physiol*, Vol. 117, pp. 500-544.

http://sciyo.com/articles/show/title/wind-power-integrating-wind-turbine-generators-wtg-s-with-energy-storage

Jiang, N., Parker, PA., Englehart, KB. Modeling of muscle motor unit innervation process correlation and common drive. *IEEE Trans Biomed Eng*, Vol. 53, pp. 1605-1614.

Kanda, K. & Hashizume, K. (1992) Factors causing differences in force output among motor units in the cat medialis gastrocnemius muscle. *J Physiol*, Vol. 448, pp. 677-695.

Kandel, ER., Schwartz, JH. & Jessel, TM. (1995). Essentials of neural science and behaviour. New York, USA: McGraw-Hill.

Keenan, KG. & Valero-Cuevas, FJ. (2007) Experimentally valid predictions of muscle force and EMG in models of motor-unit function are most sensitive to neural properties. *J Neurophysiol*, Vol. 98, pp. 1581-1590.

Keenan, KG., Farina, D., Merletti, R. & Enoka, RM. (2006) Influence of motor unit properties on the size of the simulated evoked surface EMG potential. *Exp Brain Res*, Vol. 169, pp. 37-49.

Kernell, D., Eerbeek, O. & Verhey, BA. (1983) Motor unit categorization on basis of contractile properties: an experimental analysis of the composition of the cat's muscle peroneus longus. *Exp Brain Res,* Vol. 50, pp. 211-219.

Kim , MS., Masakado, Y., Tomita, Y., Chino, N., Pae, YS., Lee, KE. (2001). Synchornization of single motor units during voluntary contractions in the upper and lower extremities. *Clin Neurophisiol.* Vol. 112. pp. 1243-1249.

Kleine, BU, Stegemean, DF., Mund, D. & Anders, C. (2001). Influence of motorneuron firing synchronization on SEMG characteristics in dependence to electrode position. *J. Appl Physiol.* Vol. 91, pp 1588-1599.

Kossev, A., Chistova, P. (1998). Discharge pattern of human motor units during dynamic concentric and eccentric contractions. *Electroenceph Clin Neurophysiol,* Vol. 109, pp. 345-255.

Li, B.; Xu, Y. & Choi, J. (1996). Applying Machine Learning Techniques, *Proceedings of ASME 2010 4th International Conference on Energy Sustainability,* pp. 14-17, ISBN 842-6508-23-3, Phoenix, Arizona, USA, May 17-22, 2010

Lieber, RL. (2010). Skeletal muscle structure, function, and plasticity, Baltimore, MD: Lippincott Williams & Wilkins.

Lima, P.; Bonarini, A. & Mataric, M. (2004). *Application of Machine Learning,* InTech, ISBN 978-953-7619-34-3, Vienna, Austria

Lorente de No, R. (1947). Analysis of the distribution of action currents of nerve in volume conductors. Studies from the *Rockefeller Inst. Med. Res.*, Vol. 132, pp. 384-485.

Lowery, M., Stoykov, NS., Dewald, JPA. & Kuiken, TA. (2004). Volume conduction in an anatomically based surface EMG model. *IEEE Trans Biomed Eng,* Vol. 51, pp. 2138-2147.

Lowery, M., Stoykov, NS., Taflove, A. & Kuiken, TA. A multiple-layer finite-element model of the surface EMG signal. *IEEE Trans Biomed Eng,* Vol. 49, pp. 446-454.

Ludin, H. (1973). Action potentials of normal and dystrophic human muscle fibers. In: *New development in electromyography and clinical neurophysiology,* pp. 400–406, Desmedt JE, Basel: Karger.

Matthews, PB. (1996). Relationship of firing intervals of human motor units to the trajectory of post-spike afterhypolarization and synaptic noise. *J. Physiol.*Vol. 492, pp 597-628.

McGill, KC., (2004). Surface electromyographic signal modelling. *Med Biol Eng Compt.* Vol. 42, pp. 446–454.

McGill, KC., Lateva, ZC., & Xiao, S. (2001). A model of the muscle action potential for describing the leading edge, terminal wave, and slow afterwave. *IEEE Trans Biomed Eng,* Vol. 48, pp. 1357–1365.

McIntosh, BR., Gardiner, PF. & McComas, AJ. (2006) *Skeletal muscle: form and function.* Human Kinetics, 2nd edition.

Merletti, R. & Parker, PA. (2004). Electromyography: physiology, engineering and noninvasive applications. New Jersey, USA: IEEE Press-John Wiley and Sons.

Merletti, R., Lo Conte, L., Avignone & Gugielminotti, P. (1999). Modeling of surface myoelectric signals-Part I: model implementation. *IEEE Trans Biomed Eng,* Vol. 46, pp. 810-820.

Mesin, L. (2008) Simulation of surface EMG signals for a multilayer volume conductor with a superficial bone or blood vessel. *IEEE Trans Biomed Eng*, Vol. 55, pp. 1647-1657.

Mesin, L., Farina, D. (2004). Simulation of surface EMG signals generated by muscle tissues with inhomogeneity due to fiber pinnation. *IEEE Trans Biomed Eng*, Vol. 51, pp. 1521-1529.

Miller-Larsson, A. (1980) A model of spatial distribution of muscle fibers of a motor unit in normal human limb muscles. *Electroencephalogr Clin Neurophysiol*, Vol. 20, pp. 281-298.

Milner-Brown, HS., Stein RB., & Yemm, R., (1973). Changes in firing rate of human motor units during linearly changing voluntary contractions. *J. Physiol. Lond.* Vol. 230, pp 371-390.

Monster, AW., Chan, H (1977). Isometric force production by motor units of extensor digitorum communis muscle in man. *J. Neurophysiol.* Vol. 40, pp 1432-1443.

Nandedkar, S. & Stålberg, E (1983) Simulation of single muscle fiber action potentials. *Med Biol Eng Comput*, Vol. 21, pp. 158-165.

Nandedkar, S., & Stalberg, E. (1983). Simulation of Macro EMG motor unit action potentials. *EEG Clin Neurophysiol*, Vol. 56, pp. 52–62.

Nandedkar, SD., Sanders, DB, Stålberg, EV. & Andreassen, S. (1988) Simulation of concentric needle EMG motor unit action potentials. *Muscle Nerve*, Vol. 11, pp. 151-159.

Nandedkar S.D., Sanders D.B., (1989). Simulation of myopathic motor unit action potentials. Muscle and Nerve 12, pp. 197-202.

Navallas & Stålberg (2009) Studying motor end-plate topography by means of scanning-electromyography. *Clin Neurphysiol*, Vol. 120, pp. 1335-1341.

Navallas, J., Malanda, A., Gila, L., Rodríguez, J. & Rodríguez, I. (2009a) Mathematical analysis of a muscle architecture model. *Math Biosci*, Vol. 217, pp. 64-76.

Navallas, J., Malanda, A., Gila, L., Rodríguez, J. & Rodríguez, I. (2009b) Comparative evaluation of motor unit architecture models. *Med Biol Eng Comput*, Vol. 47, pp. 1131-1142.

Navallas, J., Malanda, A., Gila, L., Rodríguez, J. & Rodríguez, I. (2010) A muscle architecture model offering control over motor unit fiber density distributions. *Med Biol Eng Comput*, Vol. 48, pp. 875-886.

Plonsey, R. (1974). The active fiber in a volume conductor. *IEEE Trans Biomed Eng*, Vol. 21, pp. 371–381.

Plonsey, R., &Barr RC. (2000). Bioelectricity. A quantitative approach, New York, USA: Kluwer Academic.

Rodríguez J, Navallas J, Gila L, Latasa I & Malanda A. (2012). Effects of changes in the shape of the intracellular action potential on the peak-to-peak ratio of single muscle fibre potentials. *J Electromyogr Kinesiol*. Vol. 22(1). pp. 88-97.

Rodriguez, J., Malanda, A., Gila, L., Rodríguez, I., & Navallas, J. (2011). Estimating the duration of intracellular action potentials in muscle fibres from single-fibre extracellular potentials. *J Neurosci Meth*, Vol. 197, pp. 221:230.

Roeleveld, K., Block, J.H., Stegeman, D.F. & Van Oosterom, A. (1997). Volume conductor models for surface EMG; confrontation with measurements. *J Electromyogr Kinesiol*. Vol. 7. pp. 221-232.

Schnetzer, MA., Ruegg, DG., Baltensperger, R. & Gabriel, JP. (2001) Three-dimensional model of a muscle and simulation of its surface EMG. *Proceedings of the 23rd Annual International Conference of the IEEE EMBS*, Vol. 2, pp. 1038-1043.

Sears, TA., & Stagg, D. (1976). Short term synchronization of intercostal motoneurone activity. *J. Physiol.* Vol. 263, pp 357-381.

Semmler, J.G., Nordstrom, MA., Wallace CJ. (1997). Relationship between motor unit short-term synchornization and common drive in human first dorsal interosseous muscle. *Brain Research*. Vol. 767. pp. 314-320.

Shenhav, R. & Gath, I. (1986) Simulation of the spatial distribution of muscle fibers in human muscle. *Comput Methods Programs Biomed*, Vol. 23, pp.3-9.

Siegwart, R. (2001). Indirect Manipulation of a Sphere on a Flat Disk Using Force Information. *International Journal of Advanced Robotic Systems,* Vol.6, No.4, (December 2009), pp. 12-16, ISSN 1729-8806

Stålberg, E. & Antoni, L. (1980) Electrophysiological cross section of the motor unit. *J Neurol Neurosurg Psychiatr*, Vol. 43, pp. 464-474.

Stålberg, E. & Karlsson, L. (2001) Simulation of the normal concentric needle electromyogram by using a muscle model. *Clin Neurophysiol*, Vol. 112, pp. 464-471.

Stalberg E., Karlsson, L. (2001). Simulation of EMG in pathological situations. Clinical Neurophysiology 112 pp. 869-878.

Stålberg, E. (1966) Propagation velocity in human muscle fibres in situ. *Acta Physiol Scand*, Vol. 70, suppl. 287, pp. 1-112.

Stålberg, E., & Trontelj J. (1979). Single fibre electromyography. Old Woking, UK: Raven Press.

Stålberg, E., & Trontelj J. (1992). Clinical neurophysiology: the motor unit in myopathy. In: *Handbook of clinical neurology*, pp. 49 – 84, Rowland LP. New York: Elsevier.

Stashuk, DW. (1993) Simulation of electromyographic signals. *J Electromyogr Kinesiol*, Vol. 3, pp. 157-173.

Van der Linden, S. (June 2010). Integrating Wind Turbine Generators (WTG's) with Energy Storage, In: Wind Power, 17.06.2010, Available from

Wakeling, JM. (2009). Patterns of motor recruitment can be determined by using surface EMG. J Electromyogr Kinesiol. Vol. 19. pp. 199-207.

Westgaard R.H., De Luca J.C., (1999). Motor unit substitution in long duration contractions of the human trapezius muscle. J Neurophysiol 82, pp. 501-504.

Wilson, F., MacLeod, A., & Barker, P. (1933). The distribution of the action currents produced by heart muscle and other excitable tissues immersed in extensive conducting media. *J Gen Physical*, Vol. 16, pp. 423–456.

Yao, W., Fugglevand, AJ., Enoka, RM. (2000). Motor unit synchronization increases EMG amplitude and decreases force steadiness of simulated contractions. *J. Neurophysiol.* Vol. 83, pp 441-452.

Zhou, P. & Rymer, WZ. (2004). Factors governing the form of relationship between muscle force and the EMG: a simulation study. *J. Neurophysiol.* Vol. 92, pp 2878-2886.

Chapter 2

Modelling of Transcranial Magnetic Stimulation in One-Year Follow-Up Study of Patients with Minor Ischaemic Stroke

Penka A. Atanassova, Nedka T. Chalakova and Borislav D. Dimitrov

Additional information is available at the end of the chapter

http://dx.doi.org/10.5772/50136

1. Introduction

Since its commercial advent in 1985, transcranial magnetic stimulation (TMS), a technique for stimulating neurons in the cerebral cortex through the scalp, safely and with minimal discomfort, has captured the imaginations of scientists, clinicians and lay observers [Wassermann et al, 2012]. Initially a laboratory tool for neurophysiologists studying the human motor system, TMS now has a growing list of applications in clinical and basic neuroscience. At cortical level, the abnormal amplitudes of the motor evoked potentials (MEP) may be due to the damage of the motoneurons themselves; as well as to their reduced capacity for repetitive excitation; deficit of the intracortical synaptic transmission (transfer); activation of motoneuron inhibitors, etc. At subcortical level the causes may be demyelinization, remyelinization, activation of the long-latent corticofugal fibres, axonal damage, etc. [Komori et al, 1993].

The human brain possesses a remarkable ability to adapt in response to changing anatomical (e.g., aging) or environmental modifications. This form of neuroplasticity is important at all stages of life but is critical in neurological disorders such as amblyopia and stroke [Sharma, 2012]. When MEP are obtained in the acute phase of stroke, the functional recovery of the motor deficit, as a rule, is to occur [Nowak et al, 2010; Dimyan, 2010]. The initially registered normal MEP amplitudes have a predictive value in the view of the long-term functional outcome [Stinear, 2010; Dimyan et al, 2010;].

The TMS approach was also used in the investigation of patients with lacunar strokes. The central motor conduction time (CMCT) and the threshold intensities for eliciting MEPs in the relaxed muscles were significantly increased on the affected side. MEP amplitude abnormalities were related to pyramidal signs (though they could be observed also in a patient without any motor impairment) and occurred independently of a specific clinical picture or a radiologically confirmed lacunar lesion [Abbruzzese et al, 1991; Hufnagel et al, 1990]. Earlier studies have shown that during the acute phase of the minor ischaemic stroke (MIS), MEP amplitudes can be registered in all investigated patients [Hadjipetrova et al, 1993]. To note, the increases in the latency of the M-response and CMCT have prognostic significance for early assessment of the outcome of ischaemic stroke [Stulin et al, 2003]. Earlier studies by Ferbert and collaborators [1992] have indicated that the MEP amplitudes are a more sensitive marker for the sublclinical damage of the pyramidal tract than CMCT. A significant correlation has also been reported among the recovery of muscle strength and the amplitude of MEP [Palliyath, 2000].

The aim of this study was to perform a *post-hoc* analysis of one-year follow-up data from 40 patients with MIS and to: (i) investigate the central motor conduction time (CMCT) and the amplitude of the motor evoked potential (MEP) during the acute phase of MIS; (ii) provide evidence for a subclinical damage of the pyramidal tract; and (iii) model and predict the outcome measures at month 12 after MIS as based on earlier changes in the acute phase.

2. Methods

2.1. Patient selection, diagnosis, data collection, and main characteristics

The Plovdiv project included hospital-based incident cases of patients with minor ischaemic stroke (MIS) that were followed for 12 months to determine the estimates of central motor conduction time (CMCT) and amplitudes of motor evoked potential (MEP) and their changes and correlations over time.

This is a *post-hoc* analysis and modelling study. The patient population has been described in more detail earlier [Atanassova, 1998; Atanasova & Vukov, 1998; Atanassova, Voukov & Tchalakova, 2002; Atanassova, Chalakova & Dimitrov, 2008a]. In particular, patients with cerebrovascular disease had been hospitalized in the Clinic of Cerebrovascular Diseases (Plovdiv Healthcare Region) and 56 consecutive patients with MIS were subjected to screening. All screened, eligible patients with MIS as an initial index event who provided a written, informed consent in accordance with the Declaration of Helsinki guidelines at discharge were immediately enrolled. During the lag interval from the index event until discharge (i.e., during the hospital stay), no vascular events were observed among the 56 screened eligible patients. Of these eligible patients, 54 patients (96.4%) provided written, informed consent and were included in the current follow-up study. The other 2 eligible patients did not provide informed consent at discharge and were not enrolled (**Figure 1**). Further, till month 12, a total of 14 patients were excluded or lost to follow-up and could not provide data on the outcome, therefore, 40 patients were subjected to statistical analyses and modelling in this study. The inclusion criteria were: patients with first MIS, age > 40 years and residence in Plovdiv for at least three months before identification and enrolment [Atanassova, Chalakova & Dimitrov, 2008a]. All evaluations were performed at Medical University Hospital of Plovdiv, Bulgaria. The University Ethical Committee approved the study protocol.

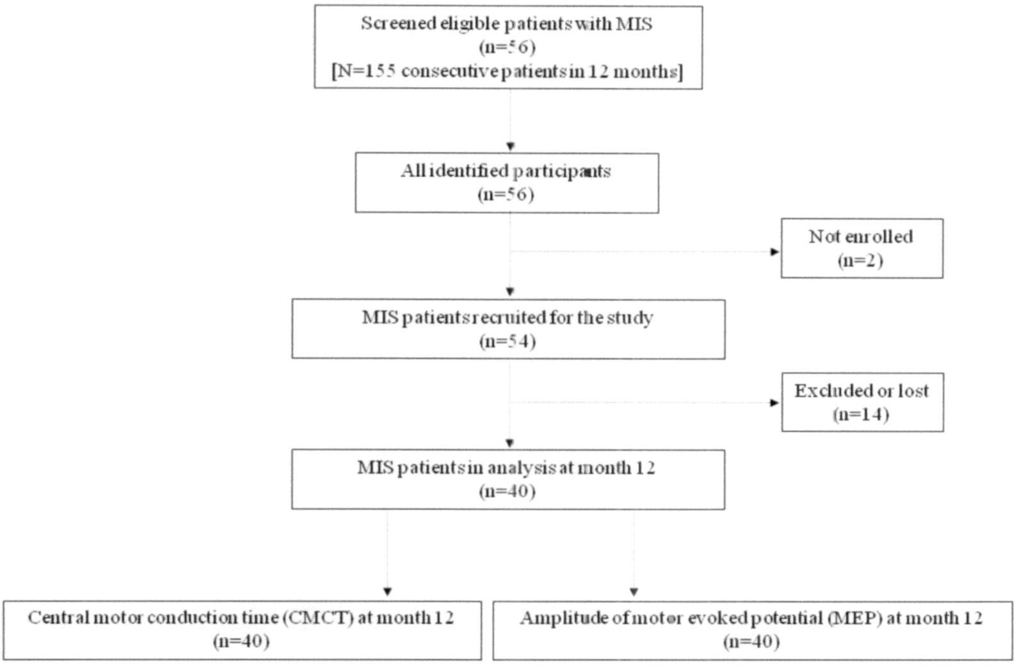

Figure 1. CONSORT flow-chart of study screening, enrolment and analysis.

Data were collected by instructed physicians and clinical (physical and neurological) examinations were conducted by study neurologists [Atanassova, Chalakova & Dimitrov, 2008a]. The assessments covered: hypertension, diabetes, dyslipidaemia, peripheral vascular disease, cardiac conditions, cigarette smoking, educational background, etc.

Initial stroke severity was assessed using the modified Rankin Scale [Bamford et al, 1990]. MIS diagnostic evaluations included CT or MRI of the brain and ultrasound evaluation and/or trans-thoracic or trans-oesophageal echocardiogram, as appropriate. A panel of stroke neurologists assessed every CV events subtype using standard diagnostic criteria and all available information for each patient. For this study, *MIS* was defined as a minor stroke if the score on the modified Rankin Scale was 1 at the first evaluation, or if the score was 0 or 1 at one-month follow-up (i.e., no symptoms, or minor symptoms that did not interfere with normal lifestyle) [Atanassova, 1998; Atanasova & Vukov, 1998; Atanassova, Voukov & Tchalakova, 2002]. In particular, acute onset was observed in 11 patients (20.4%). Extra-cranial ultrasound findings were recorded in 11 patients (20.4%). The main characteristics of the initial study cohort were as follows: 37 men (68.5%) and 17 women (31.5%), with male predominance in CV events (n=8 men) but with similar ages of 61.1±12.6 years in patients with CVE versus 62.2±9.2 years in patients without CVE ($p>0.05$). The mean follow-up time was 11.1±2.4 months with mean time to CV events of 5.8±2.7 months. For the purpose of this study, all MIS patients with subsequent stroke (n=8) as defined above, were excluded from the analysis.

2.1.1. Assessment of outcomes

The main outcome was defined as estimates of central motor conduction time (CMCT) and amplitudes of motor evoked potential (MEP) at month 12. We performed transcranial magnetic stimulation by MAGSTIM 200 after MIS (day 7 in month 1, month 3, and month 12) on the motor cerebral cortex bilaterally and on C7 with consecutive conduction of MEPs by surface electrodes from isometrically slightly contracted muscle *abductor policis brevis*. All measurements were taken as related to the symptomatic and asymptomatic hemispheres and differences between them were also analysed (Table 1). Normal values from 30 healthy subjects were also obtained for reference purposes.

Outcome parameters in MIS patients (n=40 patients)	Symptomatic hemisphere (n=40 cases*)	Asymptomatic hemisphere (n=40 cases*)	p-value
Central motor conduction time (CMCT) *[ms]*			
at Month 1 (day 7)	9.147 ± 1.862	7.550 ± 1.465	<0.05
at Month 3	8.038 ± 1.392	7.135 ± 1.052	<0.05
at Month 12	10.720 ± 1.831	8.550 ± 1.497	<0.05
Amplitude of motor evoked potential (MEP) *[mV]*			
at Month 1 (day 7)	6.083 ± 1.882	8.963 ± 1.925	<0.05
at Month 3	7.293 ± 1.876	10.350 ± 2.160	<0.05
at Month 12	7.290 ± 1.757	9.880 ± 1.986	<0.05

Notes: *Number of cases (measurements) in the MIS patients with TMS values; Data are mean ± standard deviation; °Difference at p<0.05 is considered statistically significant. Abbreviations: MIS, minor ischaemic stroke.

Table 1. Main outcomes of TMS in 40 MIS patients, followed prospectively for 12 months, as measured according to the existing symptomatics (symptomatic or asymptomatic hemisphere)

As secondary outcomes, the changes from month 1 onwards, as well as the correlations between the estimates, were also analysed. The role of the symptomatics (i.e., measures for symptomatic or asymptomatic hemisphere) as a predictor of the main outcome estimates at month 12, was also investigated. The presence/absence of non-fatal or fatal CV event after MIS was considered for the diagnosis of the MIS patients with a subsequent stroke, who were to be excluded from the analyses. Thus, two2 sub-categories for each secondary outcome were established as events classification: (i) non-fatal CVE; (ii) fatal CVE. Strict evaluations were conducted in 4 visits (at baseline, at month 1, month 3 and month 12), with telephone interview every other month, till month 12. Every evaluation was carried-out by contact with the patient, family member, or caregiver. Information was collected by somatic examination, inter-current symptoms, illness or hospitalization. The in-person visits were conducted at our clinic and included measuring vital signs, physical and neurological examination. A registry reporting system was used to identify study participants who experienced nonfatal or fatal vascular events, related hospitalization or death (vascular or nonvascular death). All records were reviewed for all outcome events, including death, and have been maintained. All outcome events were reviewed by a neurology specialist. Non-fatal strokes were validated by a study neurologist, and all deaths were to be validated, as well. Deaths were to be classified using death certificates and medical records.

Death as an eventual fatal outcome was defined as to be considered as due to stroke if there was clear documentation of a stroke from the death certificate or hospital records; deaths that would have occurred more than 30 days after the initial accident (i.e., secondary CV event) had to be considered related to the event on the grounds of a clinical judgment that relied on a clearly documented relationship to the stroke or its complications to the point of death in the medical records. Following the ascertainment procedures, all above mentioned death notifications, certificates, and autopsy protocols for all cases of death had to be collected and reviewed individually, especially for patients who died outside the hospital. In cases in which it was difficult to determine whether death was due to stroke, consensus was reached after discussion using the best available information.

2.2. Sample size, data elaboration and statistical analyses

2.2.1. Sample size estimation

The sample size of the initial follow-up cohort of 56 patients to be screened was calculated on the basis of the expected number of CV events, as described previously in more detail [Atanassova, Chalakova & Dimitrov, 2008a]. Having assumed a theoretical distribution from 0 to 50% for the non-events and based on the 3-year cumulative incidence of 24.5% for cerebrovascular events in MIS patients [Atanassova, Chalakova & Dimitrov, 2008b], 8.16% of CV events were to be expected in 12 months. Thus, it had been estimated that to give the study >95% power to detect such minimum event rate as statistically significant at $p<0.05$, 51 patients had to be included and analysed. A preliminary estimate of the prevalence of MIS patients that would satisfy the inclusion/exclusion criteria from all those referred to the Clinic of Cerebrovascular Diseases yearly had indicated that 56 patients with MIS had to be identified throughout a screening period of about 12 months (estimated maximum 10% drop-out). Given the pilot nature of the probabilistic modelling of the estimates and derivation of predictions at month 12 for both studied parameters (CMCT and MEP), no further sample size calculations were performed.

2.2.2. Data elaboration and statistical analyses

The main endpoint for both the central motor conduction time and amplitudes of motor evoked potentials was considered as an estimated mean (± standard deviation, S.D.) at month 12 (**Table 1**). Two other interim measures of the outcomes were also taken (at month 1 and month 3). A test for normality of distributions (Shapiro-Wilk test) was applied. The differences were analysed by two-tailed paired parametric (t-test, etc.) or non-parametric (Wilcoxon signed-rank) tests at $p<0.05$, as appropriate, as well as repeated-measures

ANOVA (general linear models) in the view of the symptomatic and asymptomatic hemispheres (**Figure 2 & Figure 3**). As appropriate, parametric and non-parametric correlations between CMCT and MEP at various times were also performed.

Parametric regression modelling was used to analyse the data and develop models to predict the outcomes at month 12 (**Table 2**). The significant relationships were later explored and confirmed by probabilistic artificial neural network (ANN) modelling, irrespectively of usual statistical constraints (**Figures 4 & Figure 5**). The stopping rule of learning was assumed when a state of maximum overall correctness of prediction with minimum average learning error was reached [Sarle, 1997]. The p-values less than 0.05 were considered statistically significant. The specialised software packages for statistical (SPSS ver.18) and probabilistic modelling (EasyNN ver.6.0i) were used.

3. Results

3.1. Descriptive statistics and basic comparisons

The recruited patient cohort consisted of 54 patients (37 males and 17 females), mean age of 62 years (SD 9.6). The neurological deficit by the Rankin's scale was assess at mRs=1 (37 patients), mRs=2 (16 patients) and mRs=3 (1 patient). Most frequent minor ischaemic strokes occurred in the left carotid system (53.7%), right carotid system (31.4%), both systems (9.3%) as well as in the vertebrobasilar system (5.6%). Most frequently observed are the syndromes of the middle cerebral artery (hemiparesis and involvement of VII and XII cranial nerves), aphasias after a damage of the dominant hemisphere, upper monoparesis and motor aphasia, etc. In particular, during the mean follow-up of 11.1±2.4 months, 8 secondary CV events (14.8%) were observed only in males within a mean period of 5.8±2.7 months. No difference in the age of patients with CV event (61.1±12.6 years) vs. those without (62.1±9.6 years) was found ($p>0.05$). The one-year risk for CVE was ≈15% (95%CI 7.1÷27.7%). The other main demographic and clinical parameters of the initial cohort of 54 patients were reported in a more detail earlier [Atanassova, Chalakova & Dimitrov, 2008a].

The main results are summarized in Table 1. Although the distributions of CMCT at month 12 in the asymptomatic hemisphere and MEP at month 1 in the symptomatic one were slightly skewed, two tendencies could be clearly observed. While there is clearly a difference in the TMS measures according to the existing symptomatics (i.e., symptomatic or asymptomatic hemisphere), the first one is an increase of CMCT over time with higher values in the symptomatic hemisphere, while the second one is again an increase of MEP over time, but the higher values this time are observed in the asymptomatic hemisphere ($p<0.05$).

An interesting pattern is, however, that while CMCT first decreased from month 1 to month 3 and then increased (Figure 2), the MEP amplitude, in parallel but opposite, increased in month 3 and then decreased slightly in month 12 (Figure 3). In particular, there was a significant change over time ($p<0.001$) in CMCT and a multivariate, combined effect of symptomatics and time (grand mean 8.523 ms, 95%CI 8.240-8.805, p=0.01). Notably, there was a statistically significant difference (adjusted for the baseline values at month 1) between the estimated marginal means of CMCT in the symptomatic (10.717 ms, 95%CI 10.191-11.244) and asymptomatic (8.023 ms, 95%CI 8.023-9.077) hemispheres (Figure 2).

There was a significant increase over time (p<0.001) in MEP amplitude, however, the multivariate, combined effect of symptomatics and time was not significant (grand mean 8.310 mV, 95%CI 7.922-8.697, p=0.309). Certainly, there was a statistically significant difference between the estimated marginal means of MEP amplitude in the symptomatic (6.888 mV, 95%CI 6.340-7.437) and asymptomatic (9.731 mV, 95%CI 9.182-10.279) hemispheres, but this was observed since month 1 and continued as such till month 12 (Figure 3).

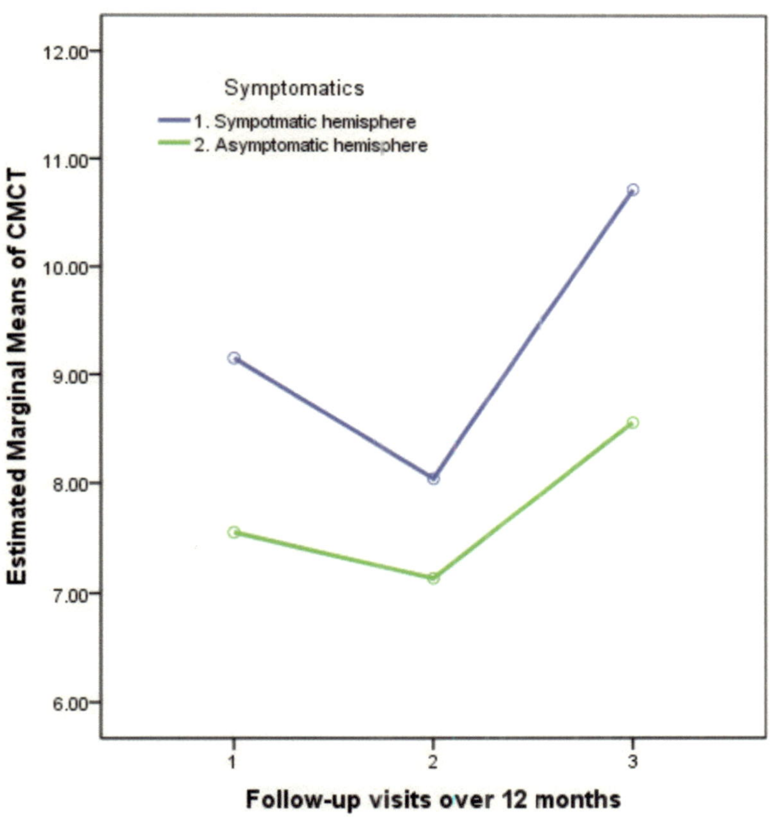

Figure 2. General linear modelling (repeated ANOVA) of CMCT changes from month 1 till month 12

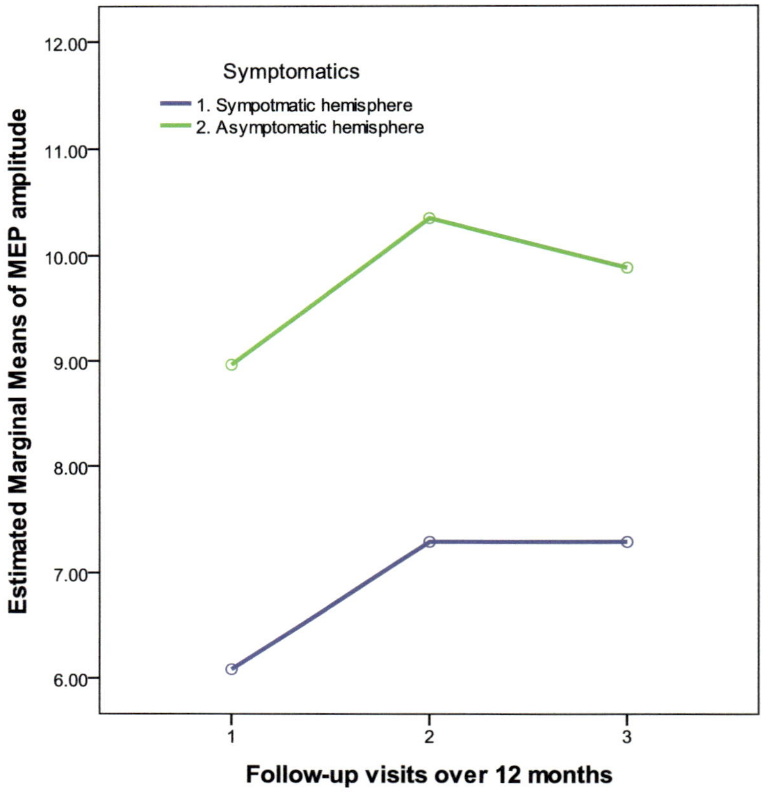

Figure 3. General linear modelling (repeated ANOVA) of MEP amplitude changes from month 1 till month 12

Since these changes appeared to be parallel, we tested also the correlations between the measurements of TMS parameters at different months. In particular, there was a weak inverse, but significant correlations between CMCT and MEP (Spearman's Rho=-0.45-0.46, p<0.05). Notably, the highest positive correlations were observed between CMCT at month 1 and the following months (0.60-0.81, p<0.05) as well as between MEP at month 1 and the following months (0.78-0.87, p<0.05). The latter relationships provided the opportunity to model and predict the outcome at month 12 in the two TMS parameters.

3.2. Statistical and probabilistic modelling of the outcome at 12 months

The parametric regression modelling indicated that the CMCT outcome at month 12 can be predicted by the initial values at month 1 and whether or not these have been observed in the symptomatic or asymptomatic hemisphere (Fmodel=33.323, p<0.001, Table 2). The same is valid for the MEP amplitude outcome at month 12 (Fmodel=55.0.09, p<0.001, Table 2), although the role of the symptomatic as a predictor is with a marginal statistical significance (p=0.051).

Outcome parameters in 40 MIS patients	Independent variables	Standardized coefficient β*	p-value
Central motor conduction time at month 12	CMCT at month 1	0.448	<0.001
	Symptomatics	-0.354	<0.001
Amplitude of motor evoked potential at month 12	Amplitude of MEP at month 1	0.642	<0.001
	Symptomatics	0.183	0.051

Notes: *The predictor "symptomatics" is a categorical variable referring to the particular hemisphere, with two categories: symptomatic and asymptomatic. The constants, unstandardized coefficients β and their standards errors are available from the authors upon request. Abbreviations: TMS, transcranial magnetic stimulation; CMCT, central motor conduction time; MEP, motor evoked potential.

Table 2. Parametric regression modelling to predict the TMS outcomes in 40 patients at month 12

The above relationships were further investigated by a probabilistic modelling, employing artificial neural network (ANN) methodology, which has not the usual constrains of a parametric regression analyses (Figure 4 & Figure 5). The ANN for modelling and predicting CMCT at month 12 contained 9 nodes with 2 hidden layers, with two potential predictors: CMCT at month 1 and symptomatics (symptomatic or asymptomatic hemisphere) (Fig. 4). The structure for predicting the resulting outcome node was obtained when the average error decreased below the target value of 0.049.

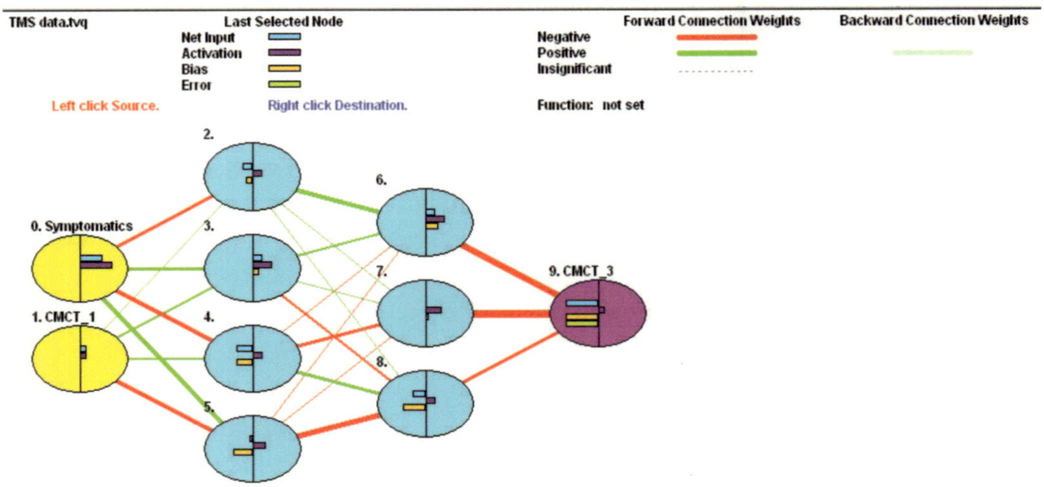

Legend: Yellow circles (No.0–1) on the left indicate 2 input variables. The magenta circle (No.9) on the right is the output variable (outcome). The nodes of two hidden layers are grouped vertically and coloured in cyan: hidden layer 1 (nodes No.2–5); hidden layer 2 (nodes No.6–8). ANN nodes description: Each node contains small bar charts indicating the basic functional parameters – net input (cyan bar), activation (magenta bar), bias (orange bar) and error (yellow bar). The hidden nodes are connected by lines, showing the type and strength of weights: the red and green lines indicate negative and positive weights, respectively. The thicker the line is, the heavier the weight.

Figure 4. Artificial neural network trained with 40 patients to predict the CMCT outcome at month 12

The modelling confirmed the finding from the parametric regression analysis (β=0.448, Table 2) for a slightly higher relative (predictive) importance of the CMCT at month 1 (0.301) than symptomatics (β=-0.354, relative importance = 0.290, not shown).

The ANN for modelling and predicting MEP at month 12 contained 16 nodes with 2 hidden layers, with two potential predictors: MEP at month 1 and symptomatics (symptomatic or asymptomatic hemisphere) (Fig. 5). The structure for predicting the resulting outcome node was obtained when the average error decrease below the target value of 0.049. The modelling confirmed the finding from the parametric regression analysis (β=0.642, Table 2) for a quite higher relative (predictive) importance of the MEP at month 1 (relative importance = 230.19) than symptomatics (β=0.183, relative importance = 62.06, not shown).

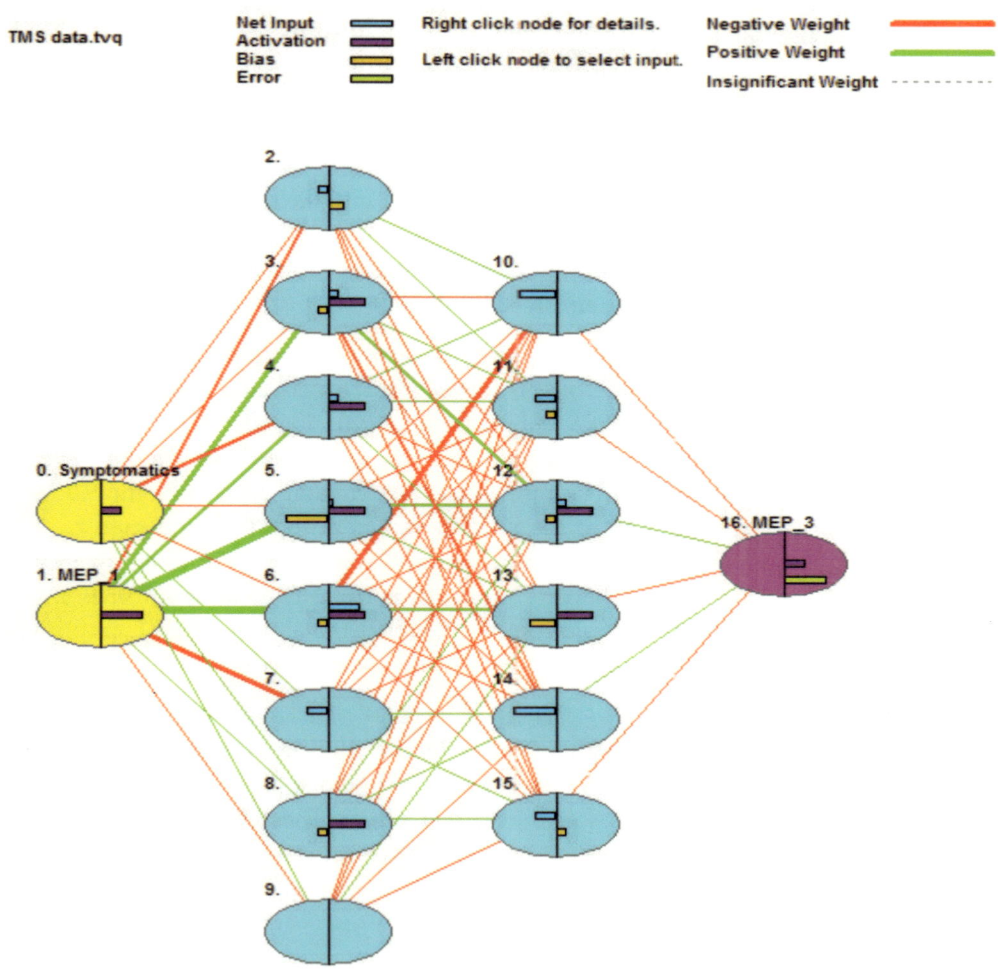

Legend: Yellow circles (No.0–1) on the left indicate 2 input variables. The magenta circle (No.16) on the right is the output variable (outcome). The nodes of two hidden layers are grouped vertically and coloured in cyan: hidden layer 1 (nodes No.2–9); hidden layer 2 (nodes No.10–15). ANN nodes description: Each node contains small bar charts indicating the basic functional parameters – net input (cyan bar), activation (magenta bar), bias (orange bar) and error (yellow bar). The hidden nodes are connected by lines, showing the type and strength of weights: the red and green lines indicate negative and positive weights, respectively. The thicker the line is, the heavier the weight.

Figure 5. Artificial neural network trained with 40 patients to predict the MEP amplitude outcome at month 12

4. Discussion

The one-year follow-up established a statistically significant dynamics in the MEP and CMCT outcomes. During the acute phase of the ischaemic stroke in the symptomatic hemisphere we found prolonged CMCT and reduced MEP amplitudes, similar to the findings by other authors [Segura et al, 1990]. When abnormal MEP amplitude is found, it is most likely the case of mainly functional disturbances of the pyramidal tract conduction, with a pathogenesis due to the acute disorder of cerebral circulation [Braune et al, 1996]. This may probably explain the prolonged latencies of MEP and reduced MEP amplitudes in the asymptomatic hemisphere. The decrease of the CMCT and the significant increase of the MEP amplitude (without reaching the normal values) at month 3, an according to Hadjipetrova et al [1993] – even at the 20-th day after the index event – could be explained with temporary functional compensation after MIS.

According to some authors, the MEP amplitudes are a more sensitive marker than CMCT in the view of assessing the damage of the corticospinal tracts as a result of the brain ischaemia. After the acute phase, there might be a facillitation at cortical level, which could allow an increase in the MEP amplitude and may eventually explain the increases in the MEP amplitude at month 3 in our patients. In particular, the MEP amplitudes in the asymptomatic hemisphere achieve the normal values at month 3 and month 12. In the same time, it is known that the minor ischaemic strokes are most likely of lacunar type (i.e., "deep", "subcortical"). The proportion of cortical clinical syndromes in our patients is relatively small and we could hypothesize that the abnormal MEP amplitudes might be present also in distant ischaemic lesion as it was shown earlier [Laloux et al, 1991].

At month 12, even in patients without neurological deficit and without recurrent cerebrovascular accidents, the CMCT is increased in both hemispheres. MEP amplitudes at month 12 are also reduced in the view of the normal values. These later changes are most likely due to the appearance of new asymptomatic structural changes of the corticospinal tracts during the progression of cerebrovascular disease.

Last but not least, following the revealed correlations, we were also able to create predictive models for the outcomes at month 12. For both the CMCT and MEP amplitude, the regression models were based on the initial measures at month 1 and symptomatics (i.e., pertaining to symptomatic or asymptomatic hemisphere). We confirmed our results further by using such probabilistic approach as artificial neural networks modelling. ANN proved to be very useful in the current analysis as it allowed us to assess the role of potential predictors of CMCT and MEP at month 12 as continuous outcomes, without the possible constraints of parametric models (e.g., normal distribution of the outcome, etc.). To note, ANN had been successfully used in other medical fields [Mecocci, 2002; Grossi, 2011; Azarkhish et al, 2012; etc.] and, in neurology, in particular [Mecocci, 2002; Shanthi et al, 2009; for a recent overview see Atanassova & Dimitrov, 2011].

5. Conclusions

This *post-hoc* analysis of one-year follow-up clinical trial data, obtained in 40 patients with minor ischaemic stroke, but without neurological deficit or recurrent cerebrovascular incidents, established a statistically significant dynamics in the MEP and CMCT outcomes after transcranial magnetic stimulation. During the acute phase of the ischaemic stroke (at day 7 in month 1) we performed an initial measurement on the motor cerebral cortex bilaterally and on C7 with consecutive conduction of MEPs by surface electrodes from isometrically slightly contracted muscle *abductor policis brevis* and found prolonged CMCT and reduced MEP amplitudes in the symptomatic hemisphere. By following consecutive measurements at the end of month 3 and month 12, we revealed that the CMCT was increased in both hemispheres and MEP amplitudes were reduced, thus both remaining with abnormal values. At the interim measurement, CMCT were shorter but still abnormal in both hemispheres while the MEP amplitudes were lower, mostly in the symptomatic hemisphere. The changes at the end of the follow-up are most likely due to the appearance of new asymptomatic structural changes of the corticospinal tracts during the progression of the cerebrovascular disease.

We observed a parallel dynamics and found correlations between CMCT and MEP at various times, preserving a significant asymmetry among the two hemisepheres. There was a statistically significant correlation between the initial values of CMCT and MEP and the outcome measurements at month 12. The parametric regression modelling indicated that CMCT outcomes at month 12 can be predicted by the initial values at month 1 and whether or not these have been observed in the symptomatic or asymptomatic hemisphere. The same is valid for the MEP amplitude outcomes at month 12, although the role of the symptomatics as a predictor is with a marginal statistical significance. The probabilistic ANN modelling confirmed the role of early CMCT (month 1) and hemisphere symptomatics in predicting the outcome at month 12. Given the dynamics of CMCT and MEP changes, we could postulate that cerebrovascular disease progression post-MIS may have most likely determined the subclinical damage of the pyramidal tract and its underlying mechanisms.

6. Future directions

Early MEP recordings in acute stroke patients provide valid prognostic information; they may become more useful for specific treatment decisions than presently available MRI surrogate parameters (Wohrle, 2004). The presence of MEP and disruption of the corticospinal tract on diffusion tensor tractography at the early stage of corona radiata infarct are indicative of a high probability of good and poor motor outcome at the chronic stage, respectively. We would suggest that further studies involving more parameters for TMS are warranted (Kwon, 2011).

Author details

Penka A. Atanassova and Nedka T. Chalakova
Department of Neurology; Medical University, Plovdiv, Bulgaria

Borislav D. Dimitrov
Department of General Practice, Division of Population Health Sciences, Royal College of Surgeons in Ireland, Dublin, Republic of Ireland

Academic Unit of Primary Care and Population Sciences, University of Southampton, Southampton, United Kingdom

7. References

Abbruzzese G, Morena M, Dall'Agata D et al (1991). Motor evoked potentials (MEP) in lacunar syndromes. *Electroencephalography & Clinical Neurophysiology*, 81, 202-208.

Azarkhish I, Raoufy MR, Gharibzadeh S (2012). Artificial intelligence models for predicting iron deficiency anaemia and iron serum level based on accessible laboratory data. *Journal of Medical Systems*, 36(3), 2057-2061.

Atanasova P, Vukov M (1998). Probability for arising of a repeated vascular incident after the primary brain infarction, with a complete clinical repair. *Social Medicine*, 1, 19-20 (In Bulgarian with English Abstr)

Atanassova P (1998). *Clinical and ElectrophysiologicalvStudy of Patients with Minor Stroke*, D.M. Thesis, MU-Plovdiv, Bulgaria.

Atanassova PA, Dimitrov BD (2011). Recent advances and challenges in the application of artificial neural networks (ANN) in the neurological sciences: an overview. In: Kwon SJ, editor. *Artificial Neural Networks*. Hauppauge, NY, USA, Nova Publishers, pp.61-69.

Atanassova P, Voukov M, Tchalakova N (2002). Prediction models for probable subsequent cerebral events in patients with reversible ischaemic neurological deficit. *Cerebrovasc Dis*, 2, 10-15 (In Bulgarian with English Abstr)

Atanassova PA, Chalakova NT, Dimitrov BD (2008a). Diastolic blood pressure cut-off predicts major cerebrovascular events after minor ischaemic stroke: a post-hoc modelling study. *Central European Journal of Medicine*, 3, 430-437.

Atanassova PA, Chalakova NT, Dimitrov BD (2008b). Major vascular events after transient ischaemic attack and minor ischaemic stroke: post-hoc modelling of incidence dynamics. *Cerebrovascular Diseases*, 25, 225-233.

Bamford J, Sandercock P, Dennis M, Burn J, Warlow C (1990). A prospective study of acute cerebrovascular disease in the community: The Oxfordshire Community Stroke Project 1981-1986. Incidence, case fatality rates and overall outcome at one year of cerebral infarction, primary intracerebral and subarachnoid haemorrhage. *J Neurol Neurosurg Psychiatry*, 53, 16-22.

Braune HJ, Fritz C (1996). Assymetry of silent period evoked by transcranial magnetic stimulation in stroke patients. *Acta Neurologica Scandinavica*, 93, 168-174.

Dimyan MA, Cohen LG (2010). Contribution of transcranial magnetic stimulation to the understanding of functional recovery mechanisms after stroke. *Neurorehabil Neural Repair*, 24(2), 125-135.

Ferbert A, Vielhaber S, Meincke U et al (1992). Transcranial magnetic stimulation in pontine infarction:correlation to degree of paresis. *J Neurol Neurosurg & Psychiatry*, 55, 294-299.

Grossi E (2011). Artificial neural networks and predictive medicine: a revolutionary paradigm shift. In: *Artificial Neural Networks - Methodological Advances and Biomedical Applications*. (K Suzuki, ed), Rijeka, Croatia, InTech, pp.139-150.

Hadjipetrova E, Chalakova-Atanassova N, Vassileva T et al (1993). Pathogenetic aspects of clinicoelectrophysiological differentiation of transient cerebral circulation disorders terminating with a complete clinical recovery, *Folia Medica*, XXXV, 122, 37-44

Hufnagel, A, Jaeger M, Elger C (1990). Transcranial magnetic stimulation : specific facilitation of magnetic motor evoked potentials. *J Neurology*, 237, 416-419.

Komori, T, Brown W (1993). Central Electromyography. In: *Clinical Electromyography* (WF Brown, CF Bolton, eds.), Chapter 1, Butterworth-Hainemann, Ltd, Boston, USA.

Kwon YH, Son SM, Lee J, et al. (2011). Combined study of transcranial magnetic stimulation and diffusion tensor tractography for prediction of motor outcome in patients with corona radiata infarct. J Rehabil Med 2011; 43: 430–434

Laloux P, Brucher JM (1991). Lacunar infarcts due to cholesterol emboli. *Stroke*, 22, 1440-1444.

Mecocci P, Grossi E, Buscema M, Intraligi M, Savarè R, Rinaldi P, Cherubini A, Senin U (2002). Use of artificial networks in clinical trials: a pilot study to predict responsiveness to donepezil in Alzheimer's disease. *J Am Geriatr Soc*, 50(11), 1857-1860.

Nowak DA, Bösl K, Podubeckà J, Carey JR (2010). Noninvasive brain stimulation and motor recovery after stroke. *Restor Neurol Neurosci*, 28(4), 531-544.

Palliyath S (2000). Role of central conduction time and motor evoked response amplitude in predicting stroke outcome. *Electromyogr Clin Neurophysiol*, 40(5), 315-320.

Sarle WS, ed (1997). Neural Network FAQ, part 1 of 7. Introduction, periodic posting to the Usenet newsgroup comp.ai.neural-nets URL: ftp://ftp.sas.com/pub/neural/FAQ.html (last accessed on 29 Apr 2012).

Segura MJ, Gandolfo CN, Sica RE (1990). Central motor conduction in ischaemic and haemorrhagic cerebral lesions. *Electromyography & Clinical Neurophysiology*, 30, Suppl, 1, 41-45.

Shanthi D, Sahoo D, Saravanan N (2009). Designing an artificial neural network model for the prediction of thromboembolic stroke. *International Journals of Biometric and Bioinformatics*, 3(1), 10-18.

Sharma N, Cohen LG. (2012). Recovery of motor function after stroke. *Dev Psychobiol*, 54(3), 254-262.

Stinear C (2010). Prediction of recovery of motor function after stroke. *Lancet Neurol*, 9(12), 1228-1232.

Stulin ID, Savchenko AY, Smyalovskii VE, Musin RS, Stryuk GV, Priz IL, Bagir' VN, Semenova EN (2003). Use of transcranial magnetic stimulation with measurement of motor evoked potentials in the acute period of hemispheric ischemic stroke. *Neurosci Behav Physiol*, 33(5), 425-429.

Wassermann EM, Zimmermann T (2012). Transcranial magnetic brain stimulation: therapeutic promises and scientific gaps. *Pharmacol Ther*, 133(1), 98-107

Wöhrle JC, Behrens S, Mielke O, Hennerici MG (2004). Early motor evoked potentials in acute stroke: adjunctive measure to MRI for assessment of prognosis in acute stroke within 6 hours. *Cerebrovasc Dis*, 18(2), 130-134.

Chapter 3

Relationships Between Surface Electromyography and Strength During Isometric Ramp Contractions

Runer Augusto Marson

Additional information is available at the end of the chapter

http://dx.doi.org/10.5772/48819

1. Introduction

From the many joints exposed to muscle-skeletal injuries, the knee joint is the one that more suffers consuming in the daily life, for both athletes and non-athletes [1], once for the maintenance of the corporal stability, it is necessary for the muscles of this joint to be the strongest as possible [2]. Such strengthening may be obtained through an isometric force training [3], which range from numbers of repetitions up to weekly frequencies [4,5].

The hamstrings muscle group is objeto de estudo devido seu papel como músculo bi-articular, bem como a sua função na insuficiência mecânica [6]. This group is composed of the *semitendinosus* (ST), *semimembranosus* (SM) and *biceps femoris caput longum* (BFCL) all of which are active during knee flexion. The activity of these muscles is often examined using surface electromyography (sEMG) [7,8,9].

The efficiency of muscle contraction depends on factors such as the fiber cross-section, the number of muscle fibers, the degree of fiber stretching, the traction angle and the type of contraction required [5,10].

Isometric exercise is one of several forms of exercise used to develop muscle force in humans. Isometric contraction occurs without any appreciable change in muscle length, such that although there is tension in the muscle there is little muscle movement for most of the time, hence the term static contraction [6,11].

A important fact that be associated with a force output is the neuromuscular fatigue. This can under certain conditions be reflected in a decreased performance and/or the failure point at wich the muscle is no longer able to sustain the requeried force or work output level [12,13,14].

Research by [15] Dimitrova & Dimitrov (2002) related that Muscle fatigue is recognized as a decline in force, or failure to maintain the required or expected force. It may occur at any point from the nervous centers and conducting pathways to the contractile mechanism of muscle fibers.

Study by [16] Moritani & Yoshitake (1998)Such changes have been shown to be related to hydrogen ion and metabolite accumulation and to sodium and potassium ion concentration shifts. These changes would in turn affect the muscle excitation traction coupling including the muscle membrane properties and muscle action potential propagation, leading to sEMG manifestations of muscle fatigue distinct from mechanical manifestations.

The increase in amplitude of the sEMG signal as an empirical measure of localized muscle fatigue or as an indicator of muscle fatigue [9,17]. The RMS-sEMG values tended increase with decreasing force as a function of the number of repetitions [6] phenomenon that determines the neuromuscular fatigue process.

The active motor units also discharge with increasing speed to compensate for the fall in the force of contraction of the fatigued fibers [13,18].

The surface electromyography behavior at different force levels is of particular importance. This can be either achieved by performing multiple isometric contractions at various force levels or using ramp contractions.

A ramp contraction is defined as a progressive linear increase in force over time and relationships sEMG-force is linear or quadratic [19], and then, sEMG parameters and phsyiologicasl events used ramp contraction in investigation, as well, motor unit recruitments, force produce and gender influence [20].

Study by [19] Bilodeau et al (2003), [20] Pérot et al (1996) and [21] Stulen and DeLuca (1981) related the relationship of curve in ramp contraction were this behavior can be confirmed between of recruitment of large, type II muscles fibers, with a higher muscle action potential conduction velocity, is associated with an increase in the median frequency or mean power frequency values of the power spectrum of sEMG [22].

In the decade 80 researches showed that the ramp contraction procedure might be replaced by procedure comprising a number of distinct and constant force contraction. Ramp contractions involve the registration of sEMG while the strength performance gradually increases his or her level of effort up to maximal or submaximal levels. Although the latter procedure seems to be easier to use in some investigation, the ramp procedure has gained a wider acceptance since then. They have been extensively applied to examine muscle activation strategies as well as in new protocols of electromyography analysis. [19,23]

The purpose of the present study was to investigate the relationships of sEMG and time during isometric strength ramp contraction in the hamstrings muscle group. Hamstrings muscle group is composed of the *semitendinosus* (ST), *semimembranosus* (SM) and *biceps femoris caput longum* (BFCL) all of which are active during knee flexion.

2. Material and methods

2.1. Subject

Twenty female healthy adults (age 19.5 ± 0.8 yrs, body mass 63.4 ± 1.5 kg, height: 1.65 ± 0.05 m), without muscle skeletal disorders and similar anthropometric measurement, subject in this study. Subjects were all right leg dominant. All subjects signed a written informed consent. The study was approved by the AESA Ethics Committee protocol 344/10.

2.2. Equipment and electrode placement

Surface electromyography activity was collected by an eight-channel unit (EMG System do Brazil Ltda®) consisting of a band pass filter of 20–500Hz, an amplifier gain of 1000, and a common rejection mode ratio >100dB. All data were acquired and processed using a 16-bit analog to digital converter (EMG System do Brazil Ltda®), with a sampling frequency 1024 Hz. A channel of the acquisition system was enabled for the utilization of the load cell (SF01 - EMG System do Brazil Ltda®) having an output between 0 and 20mV and a range up to 5kN.

The biosignals from the *semitendinosus* (ST), *semimembranosus* (SM) and *biceps femoris caput longum* (BFCL) muscles were recorded with pairs of bipolar silver–silver chloride surface electrodes (10 mm electrode diameter, fixed inter-electrode distance of 20 mm). Following skin abrasion with an alcohol soaked cotton pad, electrodes were placed with the recommendation of Marson [6].

2.3. Ramp contractions

This protocol was had increase of maximal voluntary contraction (MVC) (10, 20 30 e 40%). The knee was flexion to 90º and isometric contractions were done by pulling on a cable fixed to the ankle which was kept at 90º relative to the longitudinal axis of the leg. The cable length was adjusted to the size of the subject's leg.

The load cell traction was performed initial with 10% MVC during 20s, immediately increased to 20% MVC during 20s. This characteristic was used until 40% of MVC.

Initially the participant with the knee flexed 90°, is a traction against the cell load corresponding to 10% maintaining that drift for 20 seconds. Immediately the participant was asked to traction 20% and so on for 30 and 40% MVC (Figure 1).

Continuous samples were collected these traction. These collections take place without the participants to rest between them. The RMS-sEMG values there is a change in load has been discarded (Figure 2).

2.4. Signal processing

The sEMG signals were amplified with gain 1000. The analog channel band pass was set to 20-500 Hz and the sampling rate for analog-to-digital conversion was 1024 Hz.

For analyses time-domain the ramp contractions, sEMG-RMS value, were calculated from a 200 millisecond (ms) window at each the following force levels: 10%, 20%, 30% e 40% of MVC.

For signal processing of each isometric ramp contractions was used routine development by Matlab® and OriginLab©.

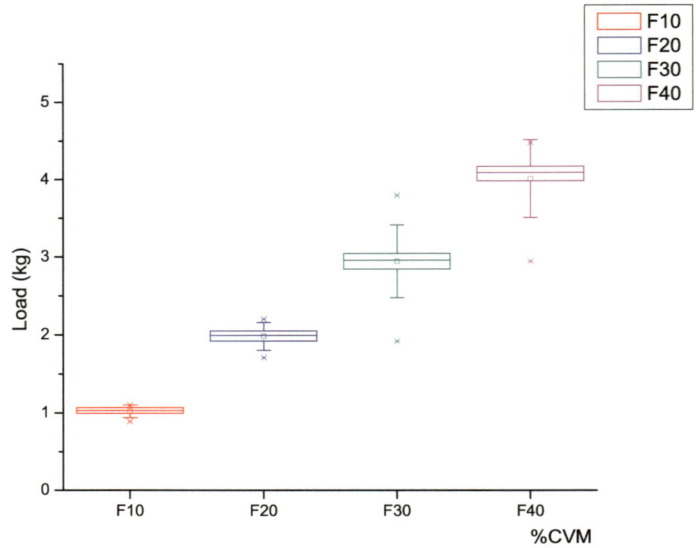

Figure 1. Box chart of mean,standard deviation and percentile (25,75) in 10% (F10), 20% (F20), 30%, (F30) and 40% (F40) of CVM

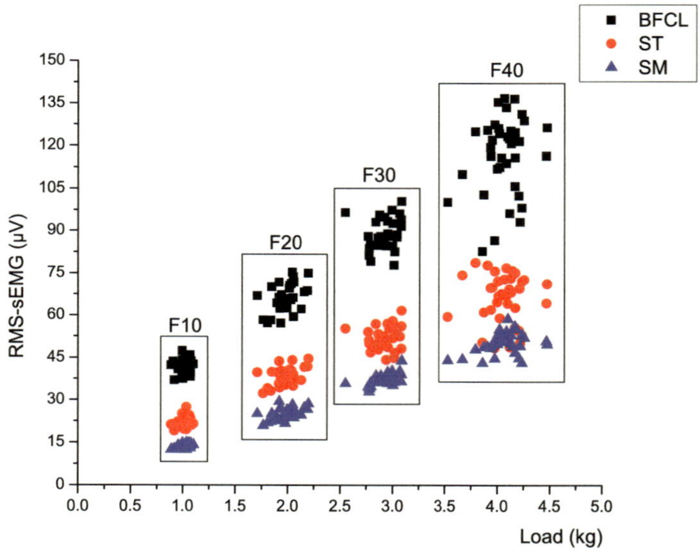

Figure 2. Relation of RMS-sEMG (μV) value versus CVM (kg). The rectangular box is the 10% (F10), 20% (F20), 30%, (F30) and 40% (F40) of CVM.

3. Results and discussion

Isometric exercises have shown a diversity of results regarding the strength gain and with it major changes have occurred regarding its inclusion within methods of strength training. This type of training is applied, mostly in clinics specializing in rehabilitation, physiotherapy and sports training centers aimed at improving muscle and joint injuries [8].

One of the most difficult physical qualities to be worked on is the strength, because a mistake in any application can lead to unpleasant consequences, such as stretching and muscle contractures. So the force is a physical quality that shows a vector quantity, it has magnitude and direction. The vectors are displayed graphically by a line of action, showing the direction and an attachment point of great importance for daily tasks as well as sports performance.

In the isometric there is a consensus response to an increase in sEMG as to alter some characteristic muscle joint as the increase in signal amplitude [13,24,25,26] changes the length and range of motion [27] and temperature [28,29,30].

Classic research shown that there is not always a tendency for this linearity. Research by [31] DeLuca & Lawrence (1983) studied the electromyographic behavior of the biceps brachii, deltoid and 1st dorsal interosseous fadigantes isometric contractions. They concluded that for the interosseous muscle was an almost linear relationship, but further analysis showed a characteristic polynomial 2nd order, the same is true for the biceps and deltoid muscles that showed a remarkable non-linearity of your data.

Studies [32] Clamann & Broecker (1979) who analyzed the triceps brachii, biceps, adductor pollicis and 1st interosseous, and [33] Woods & Bigland-Ritchie (1983) who analyzed the triceps brachii, biceps, adductor pollicis and soleus, showed that the electromyographic signal amplitude as a function of force applied to the interosseous muscle and adductor pollicis was always an almost linear relationship to the muscles and biceps, triceps and soleus this relationship was not linear, unless an exception of biceps brachii this relationship was almost linear [32].

Recent research report the nonlinear characteristic between amplitude of depolarization of motor units related to time and muscle strength [11,34]. This non-linear increase was also observed in this present study (Figure 3) in isometric ramp contraction test during time performance. The data presented in a slow onset, over time it has a rapid and finally back to grow slowly of sEMG amplitude.

According [35] Miyashita et al. (1981) and [11] Marson (2010) acting with incremental the amplitude of the electromyographic signal has an almost linear function of time to begin the individual fatigued. After the onset of muscular fatigue process the signal begins to have an increase predominantly curvilinear.

The electromyographic signal has quite often been used as a mean of assessment of muscle fatigue [17]. The increase in amplitude (Figure 3) of the EMG signal as an empirical measure of localized muscle fatigue or as an indicator of muscle fatigue [15].

Research by [15] Dimitrova & Dimitrov (2002) related that muscle fatigue is recognized as a decline in force, or failure to maintain the required or expected force. It may occur at any point from the nervous centers and conducting pathways to the contractile mechanism of muscle fibers.

Study by [16] Moritani & Yoshitake (1998) such changes have been shown to be related to hydrogen ion and metabolite accumulation and to sodium and potassium ion concentration shifts. These changes would in turn affect the muscle excitation traction coupling including the muscle membrane properties and muscle action potential propagation, leading to sEMG manifestations of muscle fatigue distinct from mechanical manifestations.

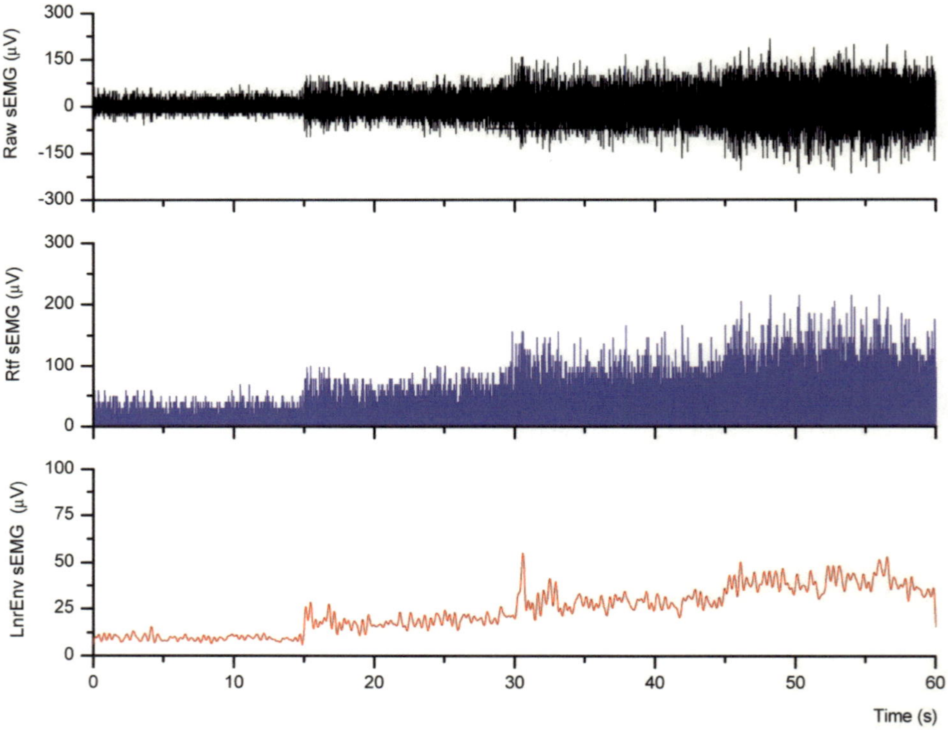

Figure 3. The raw sEMG (Raw sEMG), retificated (Rtf sEMG) and Linear envelope (LnrEnv sEMG) during ramp isometric contraction. Example figure.

The EMG amplitude increased progressively with increasing force in all muscles. The similar behavior was expressed as a percent of the RMS-sEMG value obtained during the brief pre-fatigue MVCs.

The data was fitting non linear by equation (1)

$$f(x) = \frac{A_1 - A_2}{1 + e^{(x_n - x_0)/d_x}} + A_2 \qquad (1)$$

The *f(x)* represents the data set in the RMS *x*-axis (time), A1 is the initial value of the RMS collected, the final value of *A2* RMS, *x0* is the point of inflection of the sigmoidal fit curve, i.e., the instant that there is a change from convex to concave curve which is found by the coordinate (*x0*,*y0*), where *y0* and found by equation (2). Since the coordinate *y0* is found the value of *x0* on the time axis.

$$y_0 = \frac{A1 + A2}{2} \tag{2}$$

The *dn* parameter is found using equation (3)

$$d_n = \frac{x_n - x_0}{\log(A_1 - A_2) - 1/y_n - A_2} \tag{3}$$

The *dn* parameter is the value obtained for each of the coordinate values *x* and *y*. After obtaining all the values of *dn* is done an average, and this is adopted with the value of the constant parameter *dx*.

Several studies report that the increase in the electrical function of time, fatiguing contractions, is characterized by the linearity between these data. Methods to assess muscle fatigue by surface electromyography are elaborated upon this predominance [11,34,36].

This nonlinear increase was also observed in this present study in ramp isometric contractions test. The data presented in the early slow growth over the same time is a rapid increase and eventually grow back slowly. With these data in hand a mathematical model was developed, based on the characteristic sigmoidal or logistic curve (Figure 4-6).

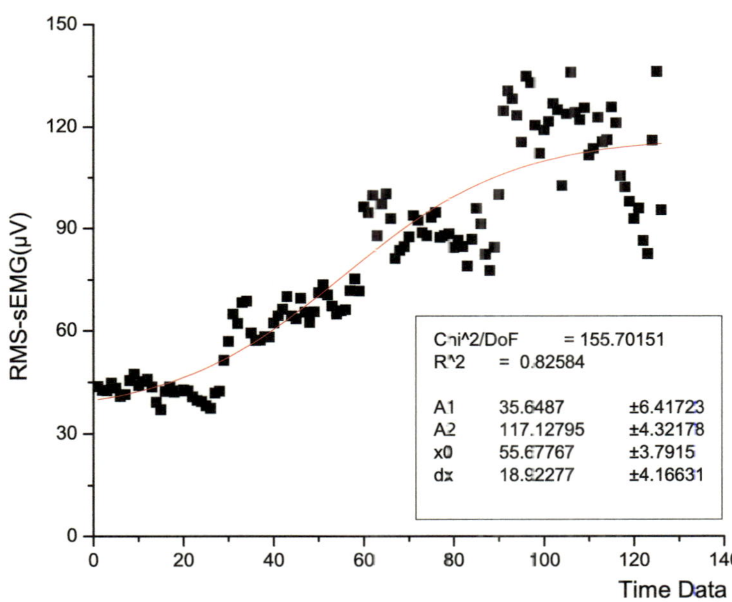

Figure 4. Relationship, adjust and parameter nonlinear of RMS-sEMG value. BFCL example.

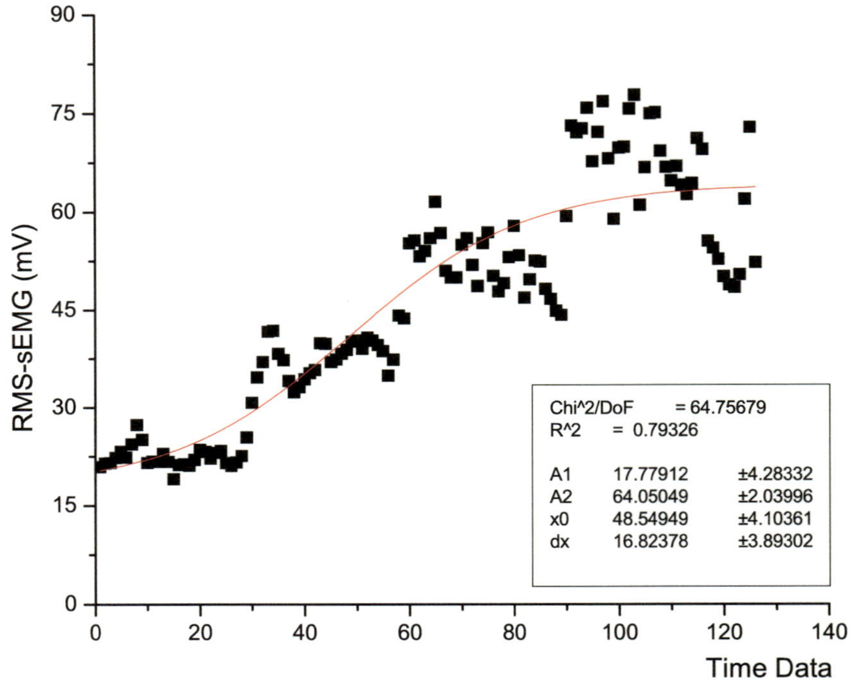

Figure 5. Relationship, adjust and parameter nonlinear of RMS-sEMG value. ST example.

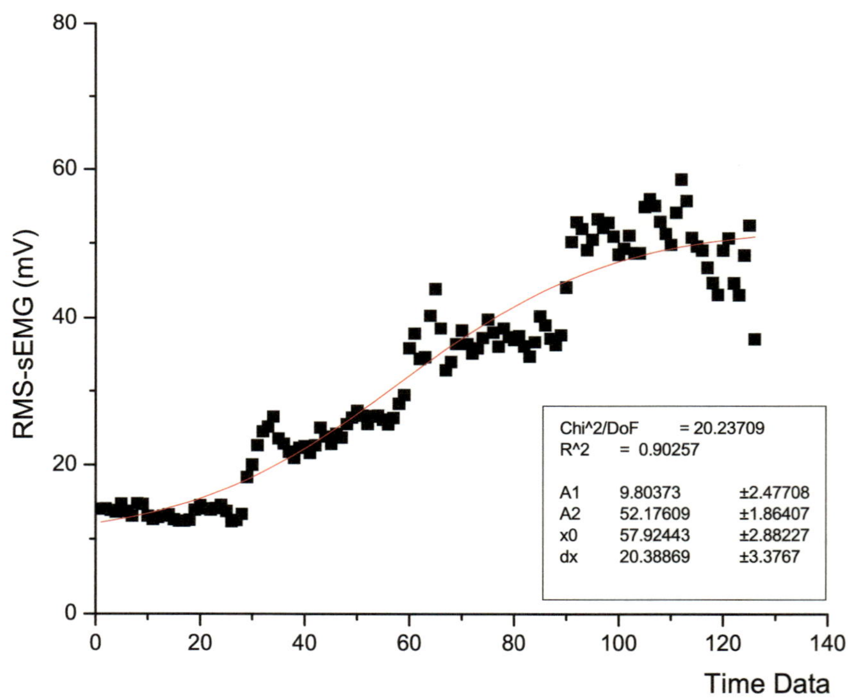

Figure 6. Relationship, adjust and parameter nonlinear of RMS-sEMG value. SM example.

The adjustment was made by equation 1. To verify that this setting was close to actual data (data collected) was analyzed the coefficient of determination (r^2) between the actual data and the adjusted data, where the r^2 values greater than 0.80.

According to [37] Enoka and Stuart (1992), [35] Miyashita et al. (1981) in incremental overhead fatiguing exercise with the amplitude of the electromyographic signal has an almost linear function of time until the individual begins to fatigue. After the onset of muscle fatigue process the signal begins to increase a predominantly curvilinear [38].

This characteristic presented in this mathematical adjustment points that are side left of the parameter *x0* which is the turning point of the concavity of the sigmoidal curve. This behavior provides a characterization of possible fatigue neuromuscular isometric ramp contractions.

4. Conclusion

Investigations have been concerned in the restricted use of the isometric contraction ramp during a single, non-fatiguing, and linearly increasing contraction force variation at short intervals, it is suggested that where the isometric ramp contractions can provide higher resolution in the entire spectrum force, less time required for data acquisition electromyography, and less susceptible to fatigue than contractions step. It is possible, however, that whereas the ramp and contraction power spectrum characteristic of the control strategies can incorporate various engine and comparing the dynamic and isometric contractions isokinetic step.

This present study revealed that the relationship between electromyography, force and time has characteristic sigmoidal. This demonstrates that the initial charges in a relationship are slowly increasing, but at intermediate loads this increase is more rapid and exponential. However, this behavior the load end presents a decrease in the rate of increase and maintenance of a depolarization of motor units at the end of execution of the isometric ramp contraction.

This sigmoidal relationship data is well described in the equation proposed for modeling (curve fitting) of hamstring muscle electromyographic signal analyzed, which is presented the start point (*A1*), the constant in equation (*dx*), the turning point the concavity of the curve (*x0*) and peak (*A2*) to be kept in mathematical adjustment of the curve in relation to actual curve acquired.

In summary, the results of this study indicate that RMS values of the hamstrings muscles tend to increase nonlinear whereas force with the number of isometric ramp contractions performed.

5. Future directions

Since these responses are characteristic of neuromuscular fatigue, the test described here may be useful for identifying muscle fatigue in ramp isometric contraction test. With this feature researches, in future studies, propose mathematical models to identify the turning point of the concavity of the sigmoid adjustment for the analysis and identification of the electromyographic fatigue. Therefore, in order to develop a new protocol for the identification of fatigue could be observed electromyographic initial characteristics of the sigmoid curve which is a slow increase over time data, which has an exponential characteristic. With these parameters can ascertain exponential models as the inflection point of the curve for possible identification of neuromuscular fatigue.

Understanding the importance of digital signal processing, in this case the surface electromyographic signal, the mathematical adjustment (mathematical modeling), presents itself as a tool to direct future research related to bioengineering, which may direct future investigations from the area of instrumentation to the development of new systems of man-machine synchronization.

Author details

Runer Augusto Marson

Laboratory of Biomechanics, Brazilian Army Physical Capacitation Research Institute, Rio de Janeiro, Brazil

Laboratory of Biomechanics and Kinesiology, Sport Center, Federal University of Ouro Preto, Minas Gerais, Brazil

6. References

[1] Zatsiorsky, V.M. 2000. *Biomechanics in Sport Performance: improvement and injury prevention.* 2000. Oxford: Blackwell Science LTD.

[2] Lippert, L. 2011. *Clinical kinesiology and anatomy,* 5th ed. Philadelphia: F. A. Davis Company.

[3] Kumar, S. 2004. *Muscle Strength.* Danver: CRC Press LLC.

[4] Verkhoshansky, Y. V. 2004. *Special Strength Training: a pratical manual for coaches.* Moscow: MOCKBA.

[5] Garfinkel S; Cafarelli E.1992. Relative changes in maximal force, EMG, and muscle cross-sectional area after isometric training. *Medice and Science in Sports and Exercise.* 24: 1220-27.

[6] Marson, R.A.; Gonçalves, M., 2003. Electromyographic behavior of the biceps femoris (caput longum) and semitendinosus muscles in the isometric contraction test. Brazilian *J. Morphol.* Sci.. 20:55-7.

[7] Solomonow M, Krogsgaard M. Sensorimotor control of knee stability: a review. *Scan J Med Sci Sports* 2001;11:64–80.

[8] Kellis,E; Katis, A. Reliability of EMG power-spectrum and amplitude of the semitendinosus and biceps femoris muscles during ramp isometric contractions. *J. Electromyograph Kinesiol* 18 (2008) 351–358.

[9] Marson Ra, Gonçalves M (2001) Comportamento eletromiográfico do músculo biceps femoris (caput longum) submetido a exercício isométrico. In: *Anais do IX Congresso Brasileiro de Biomecânica*. Gramado (RS), Brazil, 29 May-1 June. pp. 289-293.

[10] Garfinkel S; Cafarelli E.1992. Relative changes in maximal force, EMG, and muscle cross-sectional area after isometric training. *Med. Sci. Sports Exerc*. 24: 1220-27.

[11] Marson, R.A. Identificación de la fatiga electromiográfica en contracciones isométricas crecientes. *Lecturas Educación Física y Deportes*, 15:146 - Julio de 2010.

[12] Moritani T.; Nagata, A.; Devries, H.A.; Muro, M., 1981. Critical power as a measure of physical work capacity and anaerobic threshold. *Ergonomics*.24:339-50.

[13] BASMAJIAN JV; Deluca CJ. 1985. *Muscle Alive:* Their Function Revealed by Electromyography. Baltimore:Willians & Wilkins. p.201-222.

[14] Dimitrova Na; Dimitrov, GV. 2003. Interpretation of EMG changes with fatigue: facts, pitfalls, and fallacies. *J. Electromyograph Kinesiol*, 13:13-36.

[15] Dimitrova, Na; Dimitrov, GV. 2002. Amplitude-related characteristics of motor unit and M-wave potentials during fatigue. A simulation study using literature data on intracellular potential changes found in vitro. *J. Electromyograph Kinesiol*, 12:339-349.

[16] Moritani, T; Yoshitake, Y. 1998 ISEK Congress Keynote Lecture:The use of electromyography in applied physiology. *J Electromyograph Kinesiol*, 8:363-81.1998.

[17] Moritani, T.; Muro, M.; Nagata, A., 1986. Intramuscular and surface electromyogram changes during muscle fatigue. *J. Applied Physiol*. 60:1179-85.

[18] Petrofsky Js, Lind AR (1980) The influence of temperature on the amplitude and frequency components of the EMG during brief and sustained isometric contractions. Eur. *J. Appl. Physiol*. 44, 189-200.

[19] Bilodeau M, Schindler-Ivens S, Williams DM, Chandran R, Sharma SS. EMG frequency changes with increasing force and during fatigue in the quadriceps femoris muscle of men and women. *J Electromyogr Kinesiol* 2003;13:83–92.

[20] Pérot, C.; André, L.; Dupont, L.; Vanhouttle, C. Relative contributions of the long and shorts head of the biceps brachii during simple or dual isometrics tasks. *J. Electromyograph. Kinesiol.*, 6:3-11, 1996.

[21] Stulen, F.; Deluca, C.J. Frequency parameters of the myoeletric signal as a measure of muscle conduction value. IEEE Trans. *Biomed. Eng*. BME, 28:515-23, 1981.

[22] Dupont, L.; Gamet, D.; Pérot, C. Motor unit recruitment and EMG power spectra during ramp contraction of a bifunctional muscle. *J. Electromyograph. Kinesiol*, 10:217-24, 2000.

[23] Sanchez Jh, Solomonow M, Baratta Rv, D'ambrosia R. Control strategies of the elbow antagonist muscle pair during two types of increasing isometric contractions. *J Electromyograph Kinesiol* 1993;3:33–40.

[24] FarinA, D.; Holobar, A. Gazzoni, M.; Zazula, D.; Merletti, R.; Enoka, R.M. Adjustments differ among low-threshold motor units during intermittent isometric contraction. *J. Neurophysiol*, 101:350-359, 2009.

[25] Hug, F.; Nordez, A.; Guèvel, A. Can the electromyographic fatigue threshold be determined from superficial elbow flexors musclesduring an isometric sigle-joint task? *Eur. J. Appl. Physiol*, 101:193-201, 2009.

[26] James, C.R.; Scheuermann, B.W.; Smith, M.P. Effect of two neuromuscular fatigue protocols on landing performance. *J. Electromyograph Kinesiol.*, 20:667-675, 2010.

[27] Bandy, W.; Hanten, W.P. Changes in torque and electromyography activity of the quadriceps femoris muscles following isometric training. *Physical Therapic*, Danver, n.73, p.455-65, 1993

[28] Petrofsky, J.S.; Lind, A. R. The influece of temperature on the amplitude and frequecy components of the EMG during brief and sustained isometric contractions. *Eur J Applied Physiol*, Berlin, n. 44, p. 189-200, 1980.

[29] Kimura, T.; Hamada, T.; Ueno, L.M.; Moritani, T. Changes on contractile properties and neuromuscular propagation evaluated by simultaneous mechanomyogram and electromyogram during experimentally induce hypothermia. *J. Electromyograph Kinesiology*, 13: 433-440, 2003

[30] Farina, D.; Arendt-Nielsen, L.; Graven-Nielsen, T. Effect of temperature on spike-triggedere average torque and electrophysiological properties of low-threshold motor units. *J. Appl. Physiol.* 99:197-203, 2005.

[31] Deluca, C.J,; LAWRENCE, J.H. Effect of muscle on the EMG signal-force relationship. *J Applied Physiol*, Bethesda, v.13, p.77, 1983.

[32] Clamann, H.P.; Broecker, K.T. Relation beteween force and fatigability pad and pate skeletal muscles in man. *Am J Phys Medicine,* Baltimore, v.58, p.70-85, 1979.

[33] Woods J.J; Bigland-RitchiE, B. Linear and non-linear surface EMG/force relationships in human muscles. *Am. J Phys Medicine,* Baltimore, v.62, p.287, 1983.

[34] Marson, R.A. Study of muscular fatigue by EMG analysis during isometric exercise. In: ISSNIP *Biosignal and Biorobotics*,Conference, 2011.

[35] Miyashita, M.; Kanehisa, H.; Nemoto, I. EMG related to anaerobic threshold. *J Sports Med Physical Fitness*, London, v.21, p.209-17, 1981.

[36] DeVries HA (1968) Method for evaluation of muscle fatigue and endurance from electromyography fatigue curves. *Am. J. Physiol. Med.* 47, 125-135.

[37] Enoka, R.M.; Stuart, D.G. Neurobiology of muscle fatigue. *J. Applied Physiol.* 72:1631-48, 1992.

[38] Yao, W.; Figlevand, A.J.; Enoka, R.M. Motor-units synchronization increases EMG amplitude and decreases force steadiness of simulated contractions. *J. Neurophysiol.* 83:441-52, 2000.

Chapter 4

Comparison by EMG of Running Barefoot and Running Shod

Begoña Gavilanes-Miranda, Juan J. Goiriena De Gandarias and Gonzalo A. Garcia

Additional information is available at the end of the chapter

http://dx.doi.org/10.5772/47807

1. Introduction

Footwear is the "interface" between the locomotive system and the athlete's physical environment through which all the forces that act and react between the legs and the ground are transmitted.

According to Nigg (1986), the choice of footwear is based on the price, durability, comfort, colour, safety, weight, and performance; but, how footwear affects the human-ground interaction?

During jogging, running shoes have to reduce foot shock impact with the ground, to hold the foot, to control the pronation-supination, to direct the force at the time of propulsion for takeoff (Luethi & Stacoff 1987), and to increase efficiency.

Nowadays, more and more people practice sport, being jogging an activity common to many sports, besides being a sport specialty itself. Jogging is a complex activity requiring an exact timing of muscle activation and a precise control of movement. Many injuries occurred during jogging affect the musculoskeletal system: (1) tendonitis of: tibialis anterior, peroneus brevis, tibialis posterior, quadriceps, and Achilles tendon; (2) calcaneal apophysitis; (3) chronic syndromes: anterior and posterior compartments; (4) stress fractures; (5) plantar fasciitis; and (6) rupture of the hamstrings (Reber et al. 1993). Certain types of contractions may predispose the runner to a particular injury (Vaughan 1984).

The displacement speed is determined by the frequency and length of the stride. These variables are the result of the successful integration of many mechanical and neuromuscular processes.

The human body is a biological system that has many possibilities of action and reaction to external environmental influences. During the movement, the neuromuscular system is involved not only in the production of force to move the segments, but through different mechanisms sensory feedback is capable of reacting to small changes. Facilitation or reduction of these feedback mechanisms enable the human motor system for a wide variety of functions, such as: (1) control of the position and stiffness of joints, (2) shock absorption, (3) dynamic stability during the support, and (4) propulsion, facilitating that the involved muscles perform with suitable elastic and contractile characteristics (Gollhofer and Komi 1987).

During one cycle of jogging, lower extremities undergoes a phase of unipodal support (in which only of the feet is in contact with the ground), one of swinging, and two phases of flight (in which none of the feet are in contact with the ground): the first takes place before the swing phase and the second, after it. Support phase lasts less than 50% of the stride. Slocum & James (1968) divided the jogging stride in the following phases:

1. Support (or stand) phase: begins when one foot contacts the ground and ends when the first finger of the same foot is no longer in contact with the ground. This phase can be subdivided into three: (1.a) impact phase; (1.b) phase of medium support or of absorption: time when the whole foot is resting on the ground; and (1.c) propulsion or push phase, which begins when the foot is lifted off the ground and ends when the toes leave the ground.
2. Phase of no support or of recovery, which comprising three phases: (2.a) initial flight phase: begins when the first toe of the support foot is no longer in contact with the ground and ends when the heel of the contralateral foot (opposite one) touches the ground; (2.b) half swing phase: begins when the heel of the contralateral foot contacts the ground and ends when its first finger is no longer in contact with the ground; and (2.c) final flight phase: begins when the first finger of the opposite foot is no longer in contact with the ground and ends when the heel of the ipsilateral foot rests again on the floor.

Another way of dividing the non-phase support is as follows: period of follow-through (after leg takeoff, the hip stretches); forward period (the ipsilateral leg moves forward while the hip is flexed); and period of descend of the foot.

1.1. Movement of the joints

The displacement of the centre of gravity is due to the angular movement of the joints caused by the resultant of different forces: muscular force (caused by the neuromuscular system), ground reaction force, weight of the segments, misalignment of body weight, and the inertia of the moving segments. During jogging, the path of body's centre of gravity is sinusoidal, moving twice in the vertical direction, so there are two peaks for each stride. At the same time, when the centre of gravity loses height, it loses also horizontal speed, and the kinetic and potential energies are in phase, so large changes occur in the resultant of both forms of energy at each step. However, a significant amount of mechanical energy is conserved stored as potential elastic energy in the tissues. Another mechanism to save energy is its transferring between segments by two-joint muscles.

In jogging, the movements of the joints are larger in the sagittal (or anteroposterior) plane, even though the movements in the coronal and transverse planes facilitate the stability and progress in the sagittal plane, respectively. The movements are as follows:

1. Sagittal plane: the axis of rotation is medial-lateral and the movements are of flexion-extension.
   1.a. In the ankle: *support phase* –dorsiflexion (10°), plantar flexion (45°); phase of non support –dorsiflexion (45°).
   1.b. In the knee: *support phase* –flexion (20°), extension (18°); *phase of non support* – flexion (90°), extension (90°).
   1.c. In the hip: *support phase* –extension (35°): *phase of non support* – flexion (40°), extension (10°) (Milliron & Cavanagh, 1990; Mann et al. 1986).
   1.d. The pelvis has a rocking motion, respect to the anterior-superior iliac spine: forward or down and back or up. In the stance phase there are up and down movements; and in the no-support phase, down, up, and down.
2. Transverse plane: the lower limb segments rotate around a vertical axis, the direction of rotation is outward or inward and its development is the same in the components of the lower extremity: pelvis, thigh, and leg, but their magnitudes vary. The swing phase is characterized by the internal rotation of each segment; the more distal segments rotate faster and in a greater degree than the proximal ones. The average rotation of the pelvis is 5° and that of the tibia and femur 9°, summing up a total of 23°. In support phase the external rotation continues and then, halfway, its direction changes.
3. Coronal or frontal plane: the axis of rotation is anterior-posterior and the movements are of ab-adduction. The displacements of the pelvis and lower extremity in the frontal plane are not large but are very important to maintain balance. In the knee and ankle the movements are ab-adduction and are limited by the characteristics of the joints and the presence of lateral ligaments. During jogging, the hip is adduced during the support phase until half of it. In the swing phase occurs continuous abduction of the supporting leg and at half of the way, it changes its direction to adduction.
4. The movements of the ankle with the tibiofibular and subtalar joints produce the movement of supination-pronation.

1.2. Anatomy of the joints

From a biomechanical perspective, the factors that dictate the movement are our inherent structure and alignment, the joint range of motion, and the muscle strength available. The joint range is partly defined by the anatomical structure. In the following, the peculiarities of the joints of the legs and their angular displacements during locomotion are described (Testut 1971, Inman 1981, Perry 1992, Behnke 2001).

Each of the lower extremities is a system of articulated segments, with its own mechanical characteristics. The different joints involved are: (1) lumbosacral, (2) the two hips, (3) the two knees, (4) the two ankles, (5) the subtalar joints, and (6) the midtarsal joints. In studies on locomotion the foot is considered as a rigid segment (although it is formed by 26 bones) serving for the transmission of force between the body and the ground. During the movement, the body segments serve as levers (Perry 1992).

According to Arsenault et al. (1987) it seems clear that the kinematics of locomotion does not show high variability. From the data found in the literature, we describe the angular movements of different segments: pelvis, thigh, leg, and foot of the lower extremity in three planes: sagittal, coronal, and transverse during the different phases of the cycle locomotion.

In the sagittal plane, the movements are wider. In the other two planes the movements are small but are involved in the magnitude of the displacement of the center of gravity in the sagittal plane and also provide stability.

1.2.1. Ankle

The ankle is the only anatomical area where the vertical forces are transmitted to the horizontal support system, in this case the foot. The ankle includes the tibiofibular and the subtalar joints. The tibiofibular joint allows the movements of dorsiflexion and plantar flexion or extension in the sagittal plane. The lateral movement of the foot (or eversion) around the anterior-posterior and the medial movement (or inversion) are made in the subtalar joint in the frontal plane. Adduction and abduction movements occur around the vertical axis and the transverse plane. The combination of the movements of the tarsus with those of the ankle allows complex movements, such as: (1) supination, or inversion of the ankle with adduction of the foot and plantar flexion, and (2) pronation, or ankle eversion with abduction of the foot and dorsiflexion.

1.2.2. Knee

The knee is the binding site of two long bones, femur and tibia, which are the major body segments. Small range of motion produces significant changes in the foot or in the body.

The knee joint is very complex, bicondylar, characterized by a very wide range of motion in the sagittal plane and small arcs of motion in the coronal and transverse planes. During the movement of the knee in the sagittal plane, the tibia slides around the distal end of the femur so that the mediolateral axis of rotation displaces with movement.

The patella is the largest sesamoid bone in the human body. It modifies the thrust angle of the quadriceps femoris, affecting the production of muscle force components, so that the rotational component is greater (Nordin & Frankel, 2004).

During support, the knee is essential for the stability of the leg. During swinging, the flexibility of the knee is the main factor that determines the progress of the leg. The number of bicondylar muscles involved in controlling the knee indicates a great functional coordination with the hip and ankle.

The movement in the sagittal plane is used for progression through the support and during swing. During the phase of non support, the knee makes use of a range of movement widest than that of the any other joint. The rotation in the transverse plane accommodates changes in alignment when the body oscillates back and forth of the supporting leg. In walking, when the knee extends, the leg rotates externally; when the knee is flexed, the leg rotates internally. In jogging, the knee is flexed at the beginning of the stance phase while the leg is externally rotated (Novacheck 1998).

The movement in the coronal plane facilitates vertical balance on the leg, particularly during leg stance. In each cycle the knee moves into abduction and adduction. In support phase, the movement is of abduction. During oscillation, the knee returns to a more neutral position in adduction. In the transverse plane of a position of maximum external rotation at the end of the stance phase, the lower limb starts an internal rotation in the take-off of the leg and continues during the oscillation and the load response (initial part of the support phase).

1.2.3. Hip

The hip function differs from the other two joints in the following respects: (1) represents the junction between the passenger and the motor system, (2) allows movements in three planes of space with a specific control in each plane, although in the coronal plane movement is limited, but the mechanical demands are substantial.

In the sagittal plane hip extends in the phase of support and flexes in the non-support one. The hip has small arcs of motion in adduction and in abduction. At the initial contact of the heel with the ground, the hip is in adduced position. At the beginning of the swing phase, the hip is in a relative abduction of 5°. In the transverse plane, the internal rotation peak occurs at the end of the loading phase and maximum external rotation occurs at the end of the pre-swing phase.

1.2.4. Pelvis

During the stride, the pelvis moves in three directions asynchronously. The point of support is the hip of the leg that is in support. All its ranges of motion are small: in the sagittal plane it is a rocking motion of 4°; in the frontal plane, 7°; and in the transverse plane, 10°.

1.3. Differences in locomotion due to shoes

De Wit et al. (2000) describe different angular displacements of the knee and ankle when subjects ran barefoot and when running shod. During running, the body reacts to the external environment which produces the ground reaction force (GRF) that occurs in response to the force action transmitted by the leg in contact with the ground. The GRF reflects the net effect of the muscle action and the accelerations of the segments while the foot is in contact with the ground (Martin & Morgan 1992). All segments contribute to the total acceleration of the body in proportion to the acceleration of its centre of gravity and its relative mass.

The three components of the GRF (vertical, anterior-posterior, and medial-lateral) change their size when using footwear (Nigg 1983). The GRF reflects the acceleration and deceleration of the centre of gravity. The gravity eases the contact of the foot with the ground.

1.3.1. Vertical component (GRFv)

During movement, the GRFv varies above and below the body weight due to the positive and negative accelerations undergone by the body. The difference between the vertical component and the body weight is due to acceleration of the body. The direction of displacement of centre of gravity and acceleration influences also the magnitude of the vertical component.

The vertical component is biphasic and has a first peak of early impact (at 20ms after the impact), representing between 140% and 160% (and up to 200%) of body weight (BW), in the runners who touch the ground first with the heel, and a second peak in the stance phase, which appears at 80 ms and can almost triple the body weight. The two peaks have different slopes, the first very fast and the second more gradual. Contact time is about 0.25 s. The first peak is associated with heel strike and indicates pronation. It is surprising that this peak is smaller in magnitude than the second peak that is associated with the propulsion.

1.3.2. Antero-posterior component (GRF a-p)

When the foot contacts the ground, it is pushed forward and suffers a reaction force that slows it down. At the time the body passes over the foot that is resting on the ground, the horizontal component is zero. When the body moves over the foot which is resting, the foot is pushed against the ground and the antero-posterior component becomes positive, facilitating the forward propulsion. Its magnitude represents 50% of the BW during jogging.

1.3.3. Medial-lateral component (GRF m-l)

The medial-lateral component is the smallest of all components. It has two polarities, the first in reaction to the force transmitted by the foot on the medial direction, and the second in reaction to the force transmitted by the foot in the lateral direction. The polarity of this component of one leg is opposite to the polarity of this component in the contralateral leg. Thus the sign of the lateral component of the right foot would be first positive and then negative, and for the left foot would be reversed. The variation in magnitude of the vertical, antero-posterior, and medial-lateral components means that during the displacement, the speed is not constant, as the body moves faster in one point and slower in another.

The parameters related to the vertical component are the peak impact and the rate of increase of force (obtained with a force plate), and were used to examine the load under which the locomotor system is during locomotion (Nigg 1983). One of the main functions of the footwear is to cushion the strength of the action the subject exerts on the ground and to absorb the reaction force in order to protect the musculoskeletal system. In jogging, running shoes nullifies the impact peak and is involved in delaying the onset of the support vertical force by changing the gradient loading (Nigg 1983, De Wit et al. 2000). The anteroposterior force, which has two phases (braking and propulsion), is influenced by the friction introduced by the shoe sole. The medial-lateral component that guides us on the prono-supination movement can be modified by the shoes as they change the distance between the point of application of the GRF and the subtalar or calcaneo-talar joint.

Wakeling et al. (2001) speculated that the muscle activation levels in the lower extremities are adjusted depending on the loading speed of impact forces. Nigg & Wakeling (2001) suggested that the repetitive impact forces during physical activities are not responsible for possible injury but are the cause of changes in myoelectric activity (activation time and amplitude), and these changes are responsible for the injury. Gollhofer & Komi (1987) found differences in the electrical activity of muscles when subjects ran barefoot first, then shod; Gavilanes & Goiriena-de-Gandarias (2004) found changes in myoelectric activity throughout the gait cycle when the subjects walked barefoot or with two different types of footwear, with no differences due to types of footwear used. Wakeling et al. (2002) found that the muscle activity concomitant to the impact can be altered by changing the hardness of the shoe. Frederick (1986) concluded that footwear induces adjustments in the movement of the legs, which in turn have secondary effects on the kinetics.

As found in the literature, footwear induces adaptations in the motion of the joints of the lower extremities, changes in the reaction force, and modifications in the myoelectric activity. When designing and making shoes, different types of considerations are taken into account: (1) reduce excessive burden, by absorbing the impact, (2) improve the dynamic stability, (3) increase the performance, and (4) feel comfortable (Ramiro et al. 1988, Segesser & Nigg 1993). The impact absorption is carried out through the midsole of sport shoes that acts as a filter by changing the impact forces (Luethi & Stacoff 1987). The increase in performance with the use of the shoe has been an argument used by athletes and shoe manufacturers. The midsole of athletic shoes is a layer of resilient, deformable material that is interposed between the upper shoe and the outside. The main function is to provide a protective layer between the foot and the ground and soften the shock of impact. During the first stage of the stride of jogging, the midsole is compressed by the pressure of the foot and the forces acting on it do some work on the viscoelastic material of the sole. Part of this work becomes stored as deformation energy in the material (elastically deformed). When the load on the midsole is reduced, the material undergoes an elastic recovery to its original shape (Shorteen 1993).

The literature review reveals as well that the ability of sport shoes to mitigate the impact forces between the ground and the body has been examined by different researchers (Denoth et al. 1981, Bates et al. 1983, Nigg et al. 1986, Gollhofer & Komi 1987, Dufek JS et al. 1991, Forner et al. 1995, De Wit et al. 2000). Less studied are the effects of footwear on kinematics (Frederick 1986, Nigg et al. 1986), or muscle activity (Gollhofer & Komi 1987, Wakeling et al. 2001, Nigg & Wakeling 2001, Wakeling et al. 2002, Gavilanes & Goiriena de Gandarias 2004).

The design of sport shoes and the elasticity of the materials used in their sole influence, respectively, the location of the application point of the GRF and its magnitude. These parameters influence the ability to produce an angular movement of the joints. The elasticity of the materials can be characterized based on the concepts of elasticity, rigidity, deformability, hysteresis, resilience, and viscosity. Elasticity: ability of a body to recover its original shape once the force that has deformed it has disappeared. Stiffness: a body resistance to deformation. Deformability: the inverse of the stiffness, requiring little force per unit area to produce large deformation. Hysteresis: represents the energy dissipated between the deformation and recovery of the original shape. Resilience: the amount of energy returned by the deformed material during the discharge phase. Viscosity of a liquid or semiliquid substance is the resistance of a body to deformation in response to a load.

The duration of each phase of the jogging stride (support, flight, and swing) depends on the control of the muscles of each leg executed by the Nervous System: suprasegmental centres, spinal networks, and afferent information from the different senses and from the osteoarticular system. If the information from the feet changes due to modifications on the interface between the foot and the floor, it is expected that the muscular activity will be also modified.

The recording of electrical activity obtained during muscle contraction or electromyogram (EMG) reflects the muscle involvement in the movement of the joints and therefore in the kinetic response of the ground or reaction force. The EMG amplitudes are related both to the nervous system and to muscle tension, although the response of the mechanical system is not directly related to the nervous system signal (Bouisset 1973), as the mechanical response depends on more variables than the muscle activity (such as the length of the muscle, the rate of change of length, time of contraction, and the lever arm magnitude). The relationship between muscle activity and force is not straightforward; however, EMG amplitude, duration, and coordination among different muscles can provide information about the neural and mechanical systems. Therefore, the electromyography is a powerful tool in the study of the neuromusuclar control of movement. The EMG signal is not easily recorded, as it is very susceptible to interferences and cable movement, and it is quite small, varying its amplitude between microvolts and millivolts (Kleissen et al. 1998) being its maximum amplitude (peak-to-peak) only 5 mV when using surface electrodes (Winter 1979).

During locomotion, the muscles of the legs are used to meet the following mechanical demands: progression, dynamic stability, and improving the impact and energy conservation (Inman et al. 1981); if any of these tasks is altered, the record of the muscles electrical activity will provide information about its contribution.

The aim of our present study was to evaluate the influence of footwear on the electrical activity of muscles of both legs when running barefoot and running with two different types of sports footwear, in order to assess the effects on: the extent of muscle electrical signal, the profile of muscular electrical activity, the order of muscle involvement, and the coactivation of antagonist muscles.

2. Material and methods

2.1. Subjects

Ten (six male and four female) healthy subjects, 19 and 20 years old, with an average height of 1.73±0.10 m, with no history of neurological or musculoskeletal dysfunction, voluntarily participated in the study. All of them gave their written informed consent before participating in this research.

2.2. Experimental conditions

We have classified the hardness of the sole of each footwear type during jogging on the basis of their subjective hardness: barefoot condition was interpreted as the maximum hardness, as the outer protection and reduction of the shock at the beginning of the stance phase was minimal. The own athletic shoes of each subject (typically used to run) was the condition interpreted as the softest. The standard shoes were harder than the athletic shoes, and therefore feature less cushioning of the impact.

2.3. Proceeding

Prior to obtaining EMG recordings, subjects got used to carrying the electrodes and contact sensors (foot switches –FS) by walking freely in the laboratory until obtaining a normal gait.

For each individual there have been five successive records barefoot at spontaneous speed (no specific speed requested), five with a standard sports shoes and five with his/her own shoes. Subjects ran at ground level at their preferred speed in both the first registration and in the remaining four. When subjects were shod, they were given also some time to get habituated to the shoes, and moved at a freely chosen speed.

Each record registered the EMG corresponding to the cycles required to cross a distance of 10 m. From the cycles registered, clearly identified by the FS signal, only the central 2 were further analyzed; thus avoiding the effect of acceleration and deceleration on muscle activity. In order to calculate the average speed (in ms^{-1}), the time taken to cross the 10 m has been timed. Between each of the five records made for each condition, a pause of one minute was given.

The eight FSs (B & L, U.S.A.) facilitated the identification of the phases of the stride for each of the lower extremities. These sensors are flexible disks of two sizes: 18mm and 30mm. They were placed under the heel (30mm FS) and on the heads of the first and fifth metatarsal and toe tip (18mm FS). When subjects were shod, the FSs were placed on the bottom of the shoes at the sites corresponding to the outer edge of the heel, first and fifth metatarsal, and toe tip. A FS is activated when a pressure greater than 150 g is applied on it.

2.4. EMG

Visual monitoring of the signal from the FS eased the removal of stride records with deficiencies. The simultaneous recording of signals originating in the FS and the EMG has also allowed identifying the cycle phases (support, swing, or flight) in which the muscles were active. Prior to the start of the records, we checked the signals obtained through the electrodes and the FSs.

The electrode characteristics are presented in **Table 1**. The surface electrodes used were active, equipped with pre-amplifiers providing a gain of x320. EMG signal thus obtained is better than that achieved with passive electrodes respect to the level of noise. They are composed of three stainless steel electrodes, acting two as active electrodes and one as a common ground.

The leads used were bipolar, recording the difference signal between the two active electrodes ends. A general reference electrode was located on the right forearm of each subject.

Body size	50mm x 18mm x 7mm
Inter-electrode distance	Three 1/2" (1.27 cm) disks on 11/16" (0.16 cm) centres
Weight	30 grams (including connector)
Connector	LEMO, 5 pin male style
Cable Length	60 inches (1.5 metres)
Input Impedance	Greater than 100 MΩ
CMRR	>100dB at 60Hz
Bandwidth	10 Hz to 30KHz (-3dB)
Gain at 1kHz	320
Power Requirements	±4V to ±14V at 200μA

Table 1. Technical specifications of the active, surface electrodes used in this study.

The electrodes chosen for the study were of surface type, because they have the following advantages over intramuscular ones: do not cause pain or bleeding, are easier to apply, and as shown by Kadaba et al. (1985), they provide a more reproducible signal than that obtained with intramuscular electrodes.

The subject carried on his back a box with 14 channels (12 for EMG signal input from the 12 target muscles) and 2 for the signal from the FSs. Each channel had an additional gain range of 1 to 8. The 14 signals were transmitted through a optic fibre cable from the junction box to the electromyograph, a Motion Lab MA200 system equipped with a Pentium PC 64 MB of RAM, a CODAS acquisition card PGH DI 400, with 16 channel and 12 bit resolution. Through the Motion Lab software 900, reports of the actual electrical activity have been obtained and the linear envelop (LE) has been calculated. Afterwards, each LE has been expressed with respect to the normalized gait cycle. The display of the EMG signal in real time while being recorded has allowed us to assess the quality of the recording during movement, ensuring a good contact between the electrode and the skin and the absence of artefacts. The acquisition system (200 Motion Lab) has the following characteristics: level of signal output ± 5 V, bandwidth of 20 Hz to 1000 Hz, CMMR of 40 dB, and input impedance of 100 Ω.

The 12 muscles whose activity has been recorded have been forcibly superficial, as we were using surface electrodes. Four muscles were proximal: rectus femoris (RF), vastus medialis (VM), biceps femoris (BF) long portion, semitendinosus (ST); and two distal: tibialis anterior (TA) and lateral gastrocnemius (GN, or calf). These muscles were selected for their synergistic action and agonist-antagonist relationships. Biarticular muscles: rectus femoris, long head of biceps femoris, semitendinosus, and gastrocnemius; monoarticular: vastus medialis; through one of the joints examined: tibialis anterior. Architectural features of the muscles under study are shown in **Table 2**, and their function and innervation are shown in **Table 3**.

Muscle	Mass (g)	Muscular Length (ML) [mm]	Fibre Length (FL) [mm]	Pennation Angle [º]	Cross section area [cm2]	FL/ML
Rectus Femoris	84,3±14	316±5.7	66.0±1.5	5.0±0.0	12.7±1.9	0.209±0.002
Vastus Medialis	175±41	335±15	70.3±3.3	5.0±0.0	21.1±4.3	0.210±0.005
Tibialis Ant.	65,7±10	298±12	77.3±7.8	5.0±0.1	9.9±1.5	0.258±0.015
Biceps Femoris	128±28	342±14	85.3±5	0.0±0.0	12.8±2.8	0.251±0.022
Semitendinosus	76.9±7.7	317±4	158±2	5.0±0.0	5.4±1.0	0.498±0.0
Gastrocnemius	150±14	248±9.9	35.3±2	16.7±4.4	32.4±3.1	0.143±0.010

Table 2. Architectural characteristics of the studied muscles (from Wickiewiz et al. 1983).

The location of the electrodes was done by orienting the surfaces of the electrodes with respect to the direction of muscle fibres (Testut 1971, Wickiewiz et al. 1983, Lieber 1992), in order to obtain a signal of greater amplitude and frequency (De Luca 1997). The electrodes were placed following the recommendations of SENIAM (1999). Electrodes location was verified by performing specific muscular contractions before carrying out the records.

Muscles	Joint	Function (at each Plane)			Innervation
		Sagittal	Coronal	Transversal	
Rectus Femoris	hip	flexor	abductor		Crural Nerve L2-L4
	knee	extensor			Crural Nerve L2-L4
Vastus Medialis	knee	extensor			
Biceps Femoris	hip	extensor	adductor	external rotator	Sciatic Nerve L4-S2
	knee	flexor		external rotator	
Semitendinosus	hip	extensor	adductor	internal rotator	Sciatic Nerve L4-S2
	knee	flexor		internal rotator	
Tibialis Anterior	tibiofibular-talar	flexor			Tibial Nerve L4-S1
	subtalar		inverter	adductor	
Gastrocnemius	knee	flexor			Tibial Nerve L4-S3
	ankle	extensor			

Table 3. Muscles targeted in this study: function and innervation (Kendall 2000).

The optimum recording of action potentials require excellent preparation of the skin before placing on it the electrodes; i.e., waxing the area, removing debris with alcohol, and letting it to air dry. Each electrode was attached to the skin via hypoallergenic tape and bandage.

2.5. Signals analysis

The EMG signals and those from the pressure sensors were recorded digitally at a frequency of 3000 samples per second using an analog-to-digital card CODAS (DataQ Instruments, OH, USA). The records were afterwards selected for further processing based on the signal obtained with the pressure sensors.

In order to determine the intensity of the signal, peak amplitude (peak activity), and time of its appearance, it is necessary to use quantitative methods on the EMG signal such as the LE. The steps to obtain it are: (1) complete (full-wave) rectification of the raw EMG, and (2) obtaining the linear envelop window (LE window) by calculating the average amplitude values contained in a moving window of 50 points.

Further processing was carried out with the signals of six subjects (the records of four subjects were excluded because their signals were not fully valid). From each record, the activity corresponding to 2 (out of 5) cycles were used (5x2 = 10), for 6 subjects (10 x 6 = 60), so 60 cycles were used in each condition. Since there are 3 different conditions, we analyzed a total of 180 (60 x 3) cycles. Therefore, the database consisted of 180 files; each file containing the 51 values of the LE corresponding to each of the 12 muscles and the time length of the phases of the cycle for both feet.

Each file has been then processes in a spreadsheet to obtain time-space parameters and the 51 values of each of the 12 muscles' EMG signals expressed in mV and corresponding to each 2% of the normalized length of jogging cycle.

For each subject, the LE corresponding to the 2% for each consecutive cycle locomotion were averaged across the 10 selected strides resulting in a pattern "ensemble average" of EMG (EAV), which represents an average pattern of the intra-subject LE. Using the EAV of all subjects, the Great Ensemble Average (GEAV) was obtained.

Muscle activity, represented by its LE, was expressed between the 0% and the 100% of the duration of the cycle. The maximum amplitude and time of peak onset were obtained from the GEAV.

2.6. Statistical analysis

The influence of footwear on speed, the phases of locomotion, right-left legs symmetry, general effort, and on the maximum amplitude of the EMG activity of the 12 target muscles was evaluated by analysis of variance (ANOVA) for one factor with the statistical package of Matlab (The MathWorks, Massachusetts, USA), using the following factorial model: footwear, with three levels (barefoot, shod with standard shoes, and shod with athletic shoes). The statistic F has been analyzed and the significance level considered was $p < 0.05$.

3. Results

The aim of our study was to evaluate the influence of footwear on the electrical activity of muscles of both legs when jogging barefoot and jogging with two types of footwear featuring different geometry and damping characteristics. The barefoot condition was interpreted as the one in which the external protection and shock reduction at the beginning of the stance phase were minimal. The standard shoe was harder than the athletic one, cushioning less the impact.

For the realization of this goal we propose more specific objectives: to determine the profile of the muscle electrical activity and the order of muscle participation, to detect changes in the amplitude of the electrical signal muscles, and to measure the level of coactivation of antagonistic muscles. The different phases of the gait cycle were measured based on the records obtained by the pressure sensors (see **Figure 1**) located under the foot or shoe sole.

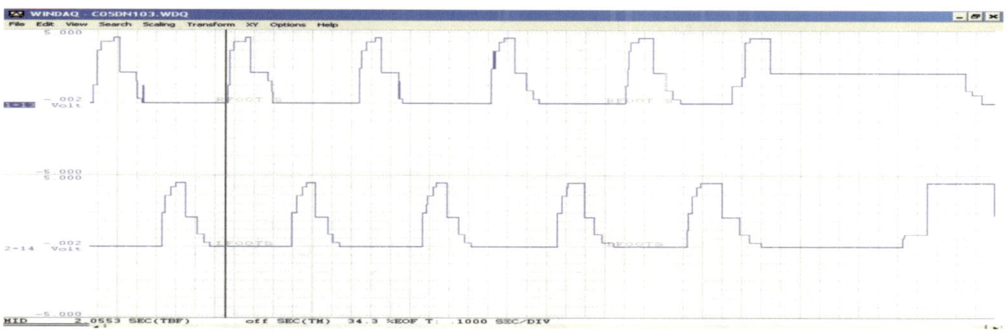

Figure 1. Bilateral support and non-support patterns from each foot obtained with pressure sensors.

The speed was higher when jogging with the own athletic shoes, and of a similar magnitude when jogging barefoot than when using standard sneakers. **Figure 2** shows the mean values of the speed and, for both legs, the mean values of the phases of: support, non support, and double flight. When running shod, the duration of the phases of the stride was different with respect the barefoot condition. The stance phase was shorter and the non-support phase, longer. The time length of the double flight increased. Between the two types of footwear used (standard and athletic) there were differences in speed but not in phases.

3.1. Muscular activity: EMG

Figure 3 shows the EMG signal, processed and expressed as GEAV for the three conditions. To assess the influence of footwear, we have divided the stride into two phases: (1) support phase and (2) non-support phase, each of which exhibited its own characteristics in muscle activity.

In order to check whether there are differences in the muscular effort depending on the locomotion condition, we calculated the area under each muscle's GEAV for each condition and used it as an estimation of that effort. The ANOVA found that there is no statistically significant difference between the three conditions with respect to the general effort required for the locomotion.

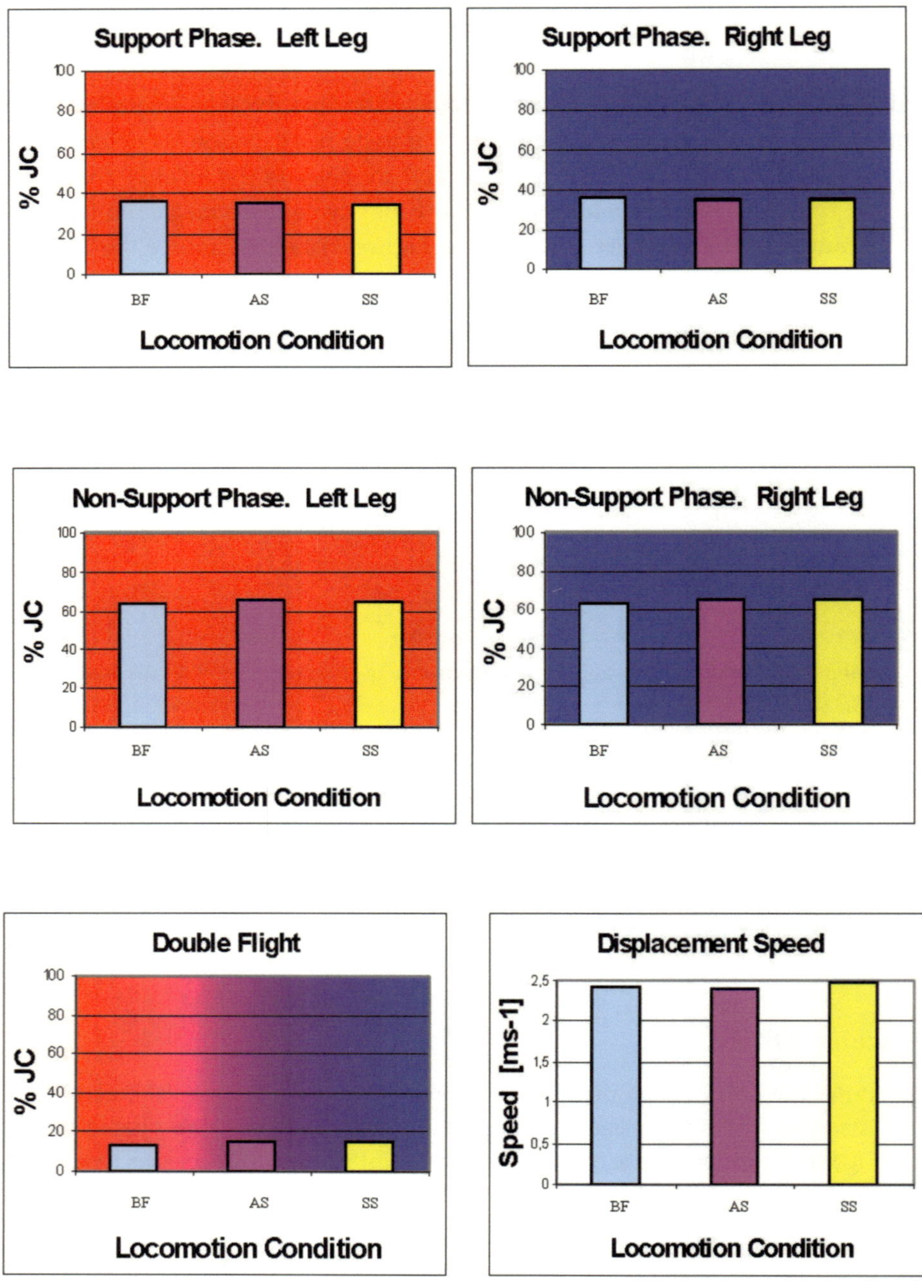

Figure 2. Space-temporal parameters expressed respect to the percentage of the jogging cycle (JC). Locomotion Conditions: BF –barefoot, AS –wearing athletic shoes, SS –wearing standard shoes.

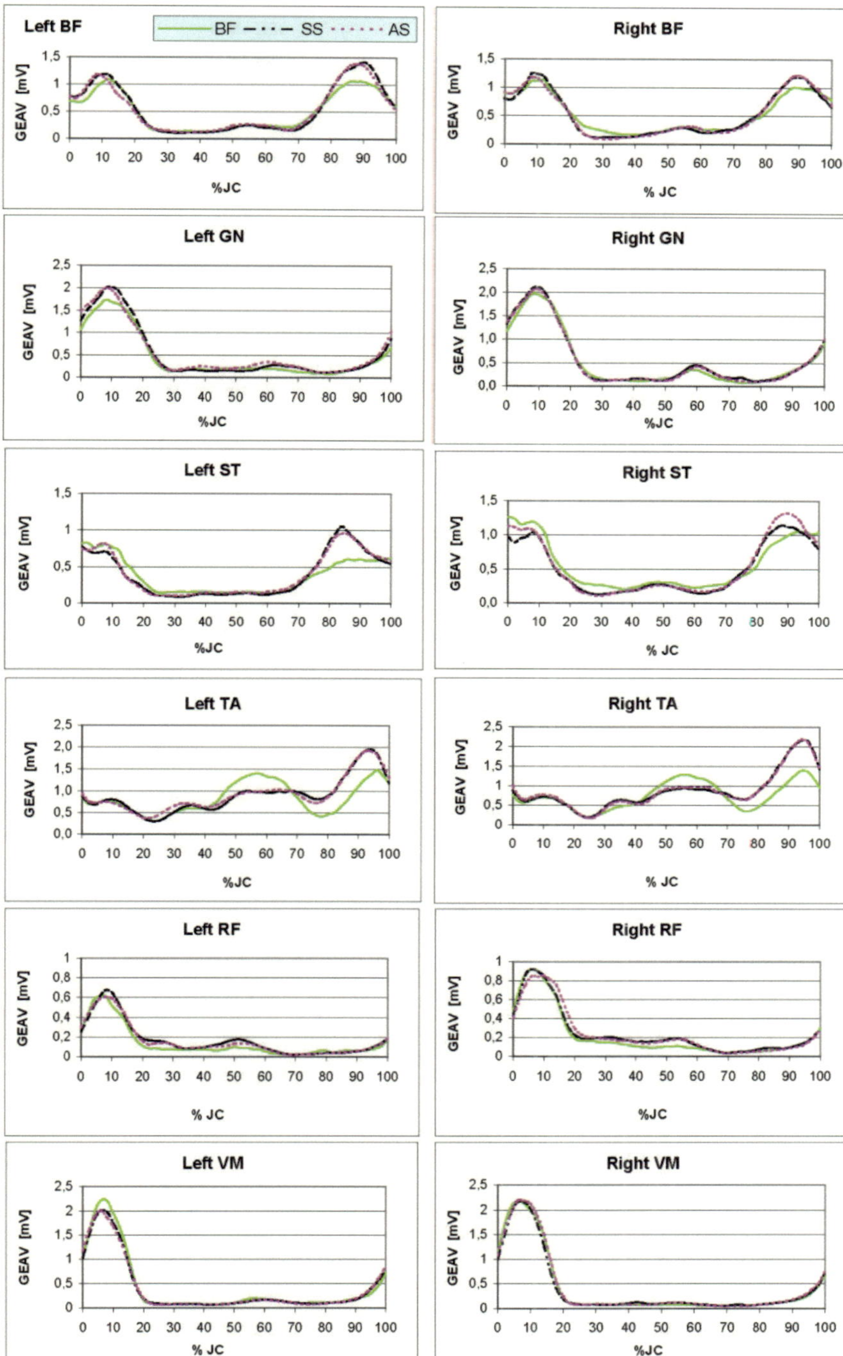

Figure 3. Profile of the GEAV for each muscle and for each locomotion condition (BF: barefoot, SS: standard shoes, and AS: athletic shoes).

3.2. Order of muscle participation

From the GEAV signal, the order of participation of each muscle can be seen. This order remained constant in all three conditions: tibialis anterior, hamstrings, gastrocnemius, and quadriceps. The AT muscle was the first one to be activated during the stride; it was activated before the flight of the ipsilateral foot, in the last part of unipodal support. The BF and ST were activated after the TA, but in the swing phase, i.e., when the contralateral leg was resting on the floor. The GN was activated in the final flight. Vastus medialis and RF were also activated in the final flight, but after the GN.

3.3. Profile of muscular electrical activity

The profile of the electrical activity is characterized by the length of time of muscle activity, the peak (maximum amplitude), and the time of its appearance. Changes in muscle activity can occur in any of the variables: amplitude, time, and frequency. In all three conditions muscle electrical activity was present for short periods of time.

The functions of the muscles varied through the cycle of jogging. There is no statistically significant difference between the three conditions with respect to the activity profile of the jogging cycle.

Rectus femoris, VM, and GN had a peak at the beginning of the stance phase. Tibialis anterior showed two peaks: one in the swing phase and another in the final flight. Biceps femoris and ST showed two peaks, one at the end of the non-support phase, and one in the initial support.

3.3.1. Time of onset of maximum intensity

Table 4 gives the exact percentages of jogging cycle at which the maximum amplitude occurred. For five muscles there were no differences in the time of peak onset in their GEAV, maintaining their patterns of activity in the three conditions. As shown in Figure 3, the peak of the RF, VM, and GN appeared in the support phase; the peak of the BF, ST, TA, in the non-support phase.

In both legs, the peak appears in very similar times. Depending on the footwear, the time of occurrence of the peak is slightly modified. In general, muscles that have their peak after the impact when shod may appear a little later; and muscles that have their peak before impact when shod can occur earlier.

The peak of the RF, VM, and GN appeared between 6% and 10% in the three conditions and in both legs. The TA peaks between 94-96% in the final flight; the highest peak of the BF appeared between 88% and 90%. Semitendinosus peak appeared about 84%-90% in the shod condition, ahead respect to the barefoot condition, which appeared between 94-98%.

3.4. Maximum amplitude

The changes of amplitude or intensity of muscle activity can be evaluated considering: (1) the entire cycle, (2) the stance phase after impact, and (3) the non-support, before impact. We will describe the changes in that order.

Locomotion condition	Left leg muscles					
	RF	VM	GN	TA	BF	ST
Barefoot	8	6	8	96	90	98
Standard shoes	8	6	10	94	90	84
Athletic shoes	8	6	8	94	88	84
Locomotion condition	**Right leg muscles**					
	RF	VM	GN	TA	BF	ST
Barefoot	6	6	8	94	88	94
Standard shoes	6	8	10	94	90	88
Athletic shoes	10	6	10	94	90	90

Table 4. Time of occurrence (in % of the jogging cycle) of the GEAV peak in each of the three different locomotion conditions.

3.4.1. Maximum amplitude along the entire cycle

Figure 4 shows the maximum activity displayed during the entire cycle by each of the twelve muscles. In all three conditions the muscles that had the highest amplitude were the VM, GN and TA. The muscles that showed less activity were the BF, ST and RF.

The maximum amplitude of homologous muscles was of the same order of magnitude for both legs, as shown in **Figure 5**.

There is no statistically significant difference between the three conditions with respect to the value of the amplitude peak.

3.4.2. Maximum amplitude during the support phase after impact

Figure 6a shows the maximum activity during the support phase produced after the impact of the heel. The TA, GN, and BF muscles in both legs increased their activity with both types of shoes. The behaviour of RF, VM, and ST varied positively and negatively.

The evolution of electrical activity in buffer muscles (RF and VM) during the loading phase was not the same in both legs, neither with both types of shoes.

Figure 7 shows the increase (not normalized, in mV) of EMG activity with respect to the barefoot condition. When subjects wore standard shoes with hard soles, the RF of the left leg increased its maximum amplitude after impact, and the left VM decreased their activity.

When subjects wore their own shoes, the RF of the left leg decreased its peak amplitude after impact. The left VM decreased its activity; and the one of the right, increased.

When the shoe was harder, the left RF increased its activity and the VM of both legs decreased. When the shoe was softer, the RF of both legs and the VM of the left leg decreased its activity, and the right VM slightly increased its activity.

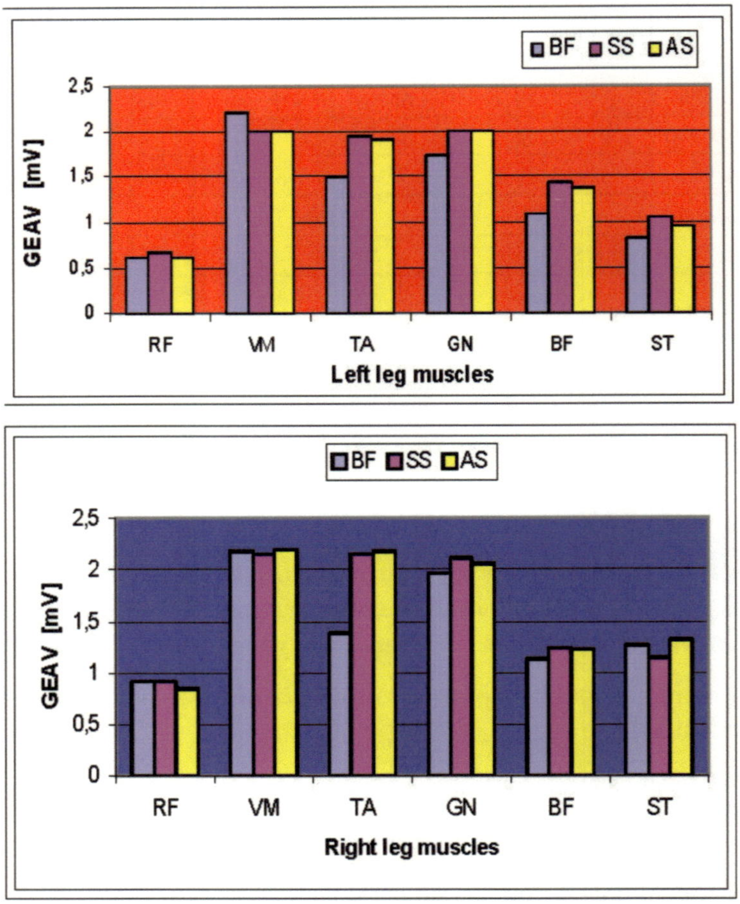

Figure 4. Peak of EMG during the whole cycle, for the left (upper graph) and right (bottom) legs muscles for each Locomotion Condition (BF: barefoot, SS: standard shoes, and AS: athletic shoes).

The TA of both legs increased their activity. The right TA increased more than the left one. In both legs, the TA increases more its maximum amplitude in the condition of own jogging shoes; perhaps because this type of shoe offers more cushioning. The GM activity in the condition of standard jogging shoe increased more than in the own shoe condition. When the hardness of the sole was higher, the translational velocity was lower and higher GM activity. Perhaps this trend has to do with balance, because when the speed is less, dynamic stability decreases.

The BF of both legs and both conditions increased their activity. In the standard shoe condition, it increased more. The ST in both conditions decreased its activity.

The response of the agonist muscles from the same muscle group is not the same when the shoe condition changes. Thus, with the standard shoe RF activity increased and decreased the one of VM, the BF increased, and ST decreased.

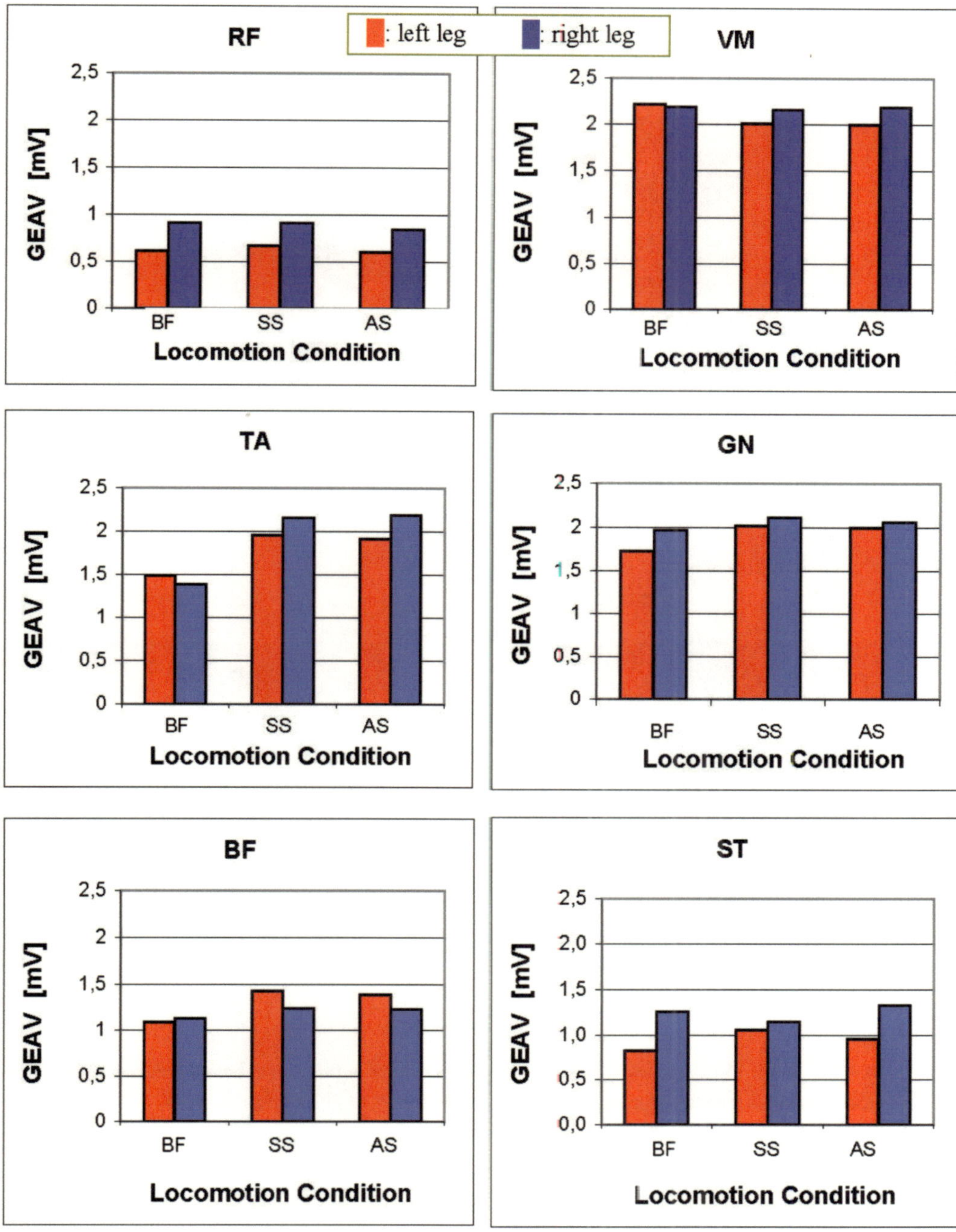

Figure 5. Maximum amplitude of the EMG from homologous leg muscles (red: left, blue: right; RF: rectus femoris, VM: vastus medialis, TA: tibialis anterior, GN: lateral gastrocnemius, BF: biceps femoris, ST: semitendinosus) for each locomotion condition (BF: barefoot, SS: standard shoes, and AS: athletic shoes).

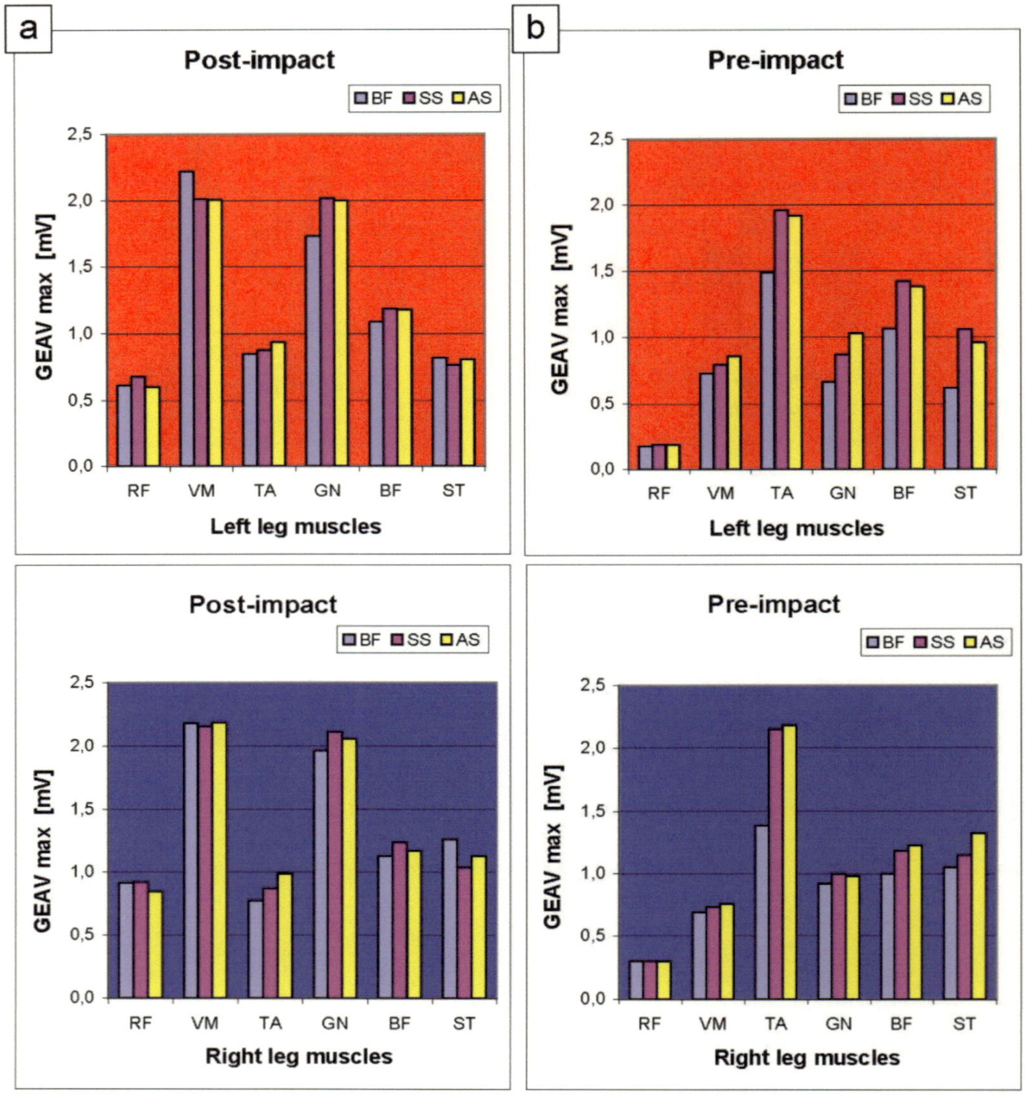

Figure 6. Maximum amplitude of the GEAV post - and pre-impact (after and before initial contact) for the 12 studied muscles for each locomotion condition (BF: barefoot, SS: standard shoes, and AS: athletic shoes).

3.4.3. Maximum amplitude before impact

As shown in **Figure 6b**, for both legs, five out of the six muscles (TA, GN, BF, ST, and VM) increased their activity in the non-support phase in shod condition. The RF maintained its level of activity; unlike what happened in the stance phase, in which the RF, VM, and ST decreased their activity.

Figure 7 shows that the EMG signal before contact of the heel exhibited greater increase than in the signal after contact. The intensity of the myoelectric activity showed differences between both types of shoes. In both shod conditions the TA muscle activity increased more in absolute terms. The ST, BF and GN increased their activity more than the VM, the activity of which increased very little.

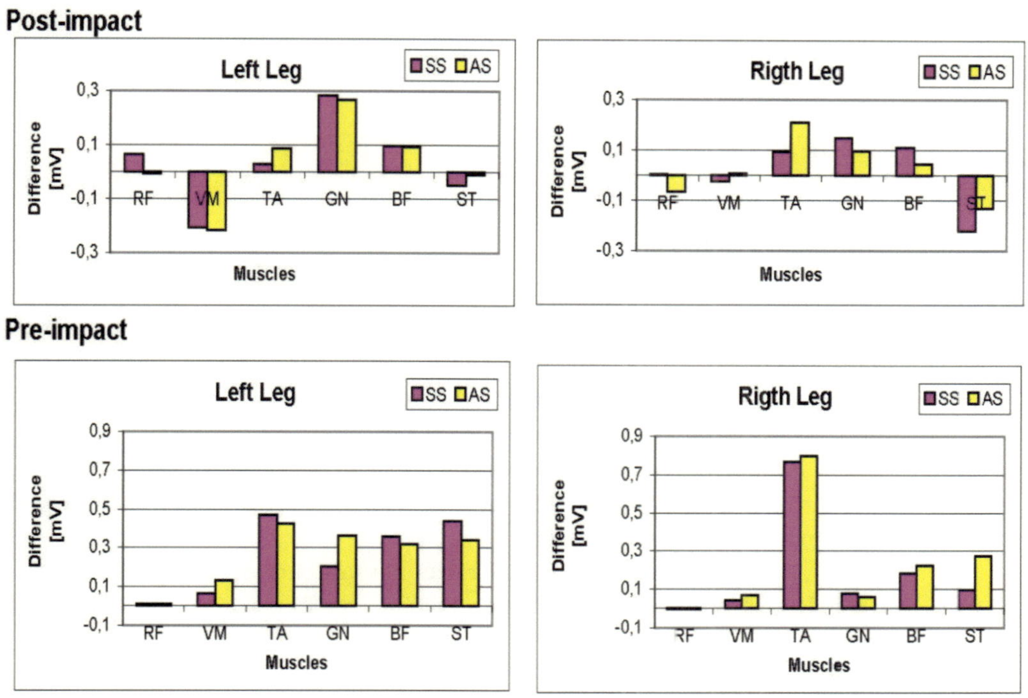

Figure 7. Absolute GEAV peaks amplitude increments respect to barefoot condition for the other two locomotion conditions (SS: standard shoes and AS: athletic shoes) for both legs muscles after impact (upper graph) and before impact (bottom graph).

In the left leg, the TA, BF, and ST were more active in the standard shoe condition. The increased activity of the semitendinosus was more important than that of the biceps femoris. In the right leg, the TA, BF, ST, and VM activity increased more in the athletic shoe condition than in the standard shoe condition. The electrical activity of the muscles of both legs showed different evolution depending on the type of shoe.

3.5. Activity of antagonist muscles

In order to evaluate the coactivity of agonist-antagonist muscles, we have established an index obtained as the ratio between the peak of the agonist muscle activity and the activity of the oppose muscle or muscles (antagonists). That index can be higher (agonist's peak is bigger than that of the antagonist) or below (opposite case) one (see **Figure 8**). To establish the role of a muscle as agonist or antagonist, we rely on the movement of joints:

- In the support phase, between 6% and 10% of the jogging cycle, the peaks of the following muscles occur: GN, RF, and VM; there is also a second peak of lesser magnitude in the activity of the BF and ST muscles. Concomitant to the important activity of these muscles, ankle dorsiflexion, knee flexion, and hip extension occur.
- In the phase of non support, the peak of the TA, BF, and ST are concomitant with an ankle dorsiflexion, knee extension, and hip extension.

There is no statistically significant difference between the three conditions with respect to the level of coactivation.

3.5.1. Coactivation during support phase

3.5.1.1. Barefoot

- Coactivation of tibialis anterior (agonist) / gastrocnemius (antagonist): the peak activity of GN occurs between 8% and 10% of the jogging cycle. The TA shows no peak in the stance phase. The index is below unity. The LG shows greater activity during dorsiflexion.
- Coactivation of hamstring (agonist) / rectus femoris (antagonist): index above unity. The BF (hip extensor) shows increased activity.
- Coactivation of hamstring (agonist) BF / vastus medialis (antagonist): the index is less than unity and therefore smaller than that showed by the antagonist muscles BF and RF because the activity of VM is much higher.
- Coactivation of semitendinosus (agonist) / rectus femoris (antagonist): index greater than one, but less than that found between the BF and RF because the ST has less activity than the BF.
- Coactivation of semitendinosus (agonist) / vastus medialis (antagonist): the index is less than unity and therefore is less than that presented by the antagonist muscles BF and RF because the ST activity was smaller than that of the BF, and the activity of the VM is much higher.

The peaks of RF and VM were not taken into account because they occur while acting as antagonists.

3.5.1.2. Shod

- Coactivation of tibialis anterior (agonist) / gastrocnemius (antagonist): both muscles increase their activity, so the index remained similar.
- Coactivation of semitendinosus (agonist) / vastus medialis (antagonist): the index is maintained because the two muscles decrease their respective activity.
- Coactivation of hamstring (agonist) / vastus medialis (antagonist): the index increases slightly because the BF activity increases and that of the VM decreases.
- Coactivation of semitendinosus (agonist) / rectus femoris (antagonist): the index decreases because the ST activity decreases.
- Coactivation of biceps femoris (agonist) / rectus femoris (antagonist): the index decreases because the RF activity increases.

The antagonist muscles showed more activity than agonist ones in the ankle and knee joints, for all the three conditions. In the hip, agonist muscles were more active, mainly in shod condition.

3.5.1.3. Coactivation during non-support phase

In the ankle and knee joints, agonist muscles showed a slightly higher activity than the antagonists. In the hip and knee, agonist muscles activity was higher.

The peaks of TA, BF, and ST muscles occur in the non-support phase (see Figure 3), concomitant with the dorsiflexion, the extension of the knee, and the hip extension. In all three conditions, the agonist muscles show greater activity than the antagonist muscles, as shown by the coactivity index being higher than one (see Figure 8). The results about the muscular coactivity during jogging barefoot and shod are just preliminary, but indicate that it is worth a study in greater depth on the subject.

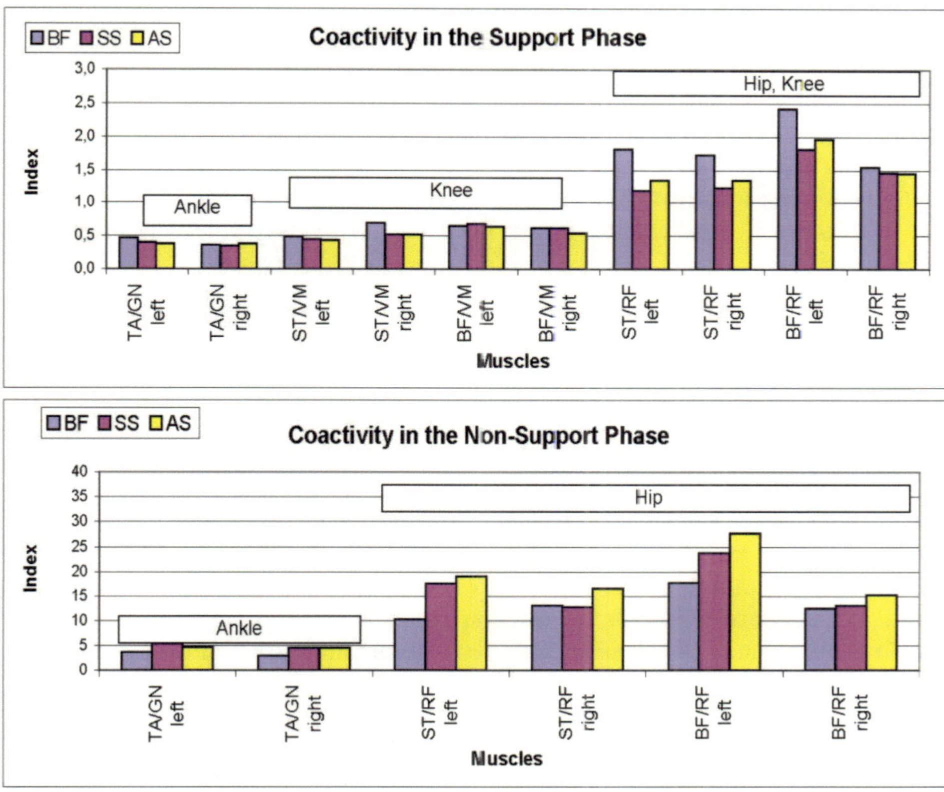

Figure 8. Coactivity of ago- and antagonist muscles during support (upper graph) and non-support (bottom graph) phases.

4. Discussion

The aim of our study was to evaluate the influence of footwear on the electrical activity of muscles of both legs when jogging barefoot and shod with two types of shoes, with different geometry and damping features. Our findings show that shoes increase the intensity of muscle activity, especially in the non-support phase. These results are consistent with those of Nigg et al. (2003) that showed specific changes in the intensity of muscle activation before heel strike.

The speed increase is concomitant with decreased activity of the VM and ST in the stance phase. The increase in the intensity of TA in the stance phase is less than in the non-support phase, a result consistent with Komi et al. (1987).

The speed of jogging at which the EMG activity was recorded in the three conditions was freely chosen by the subjects because previous research (e.g., Kadaba et al. 1985) have shown that EMG activity is more reproducible when the speed is chosen freely than when it is imposed.

We note that the footwear influences the speed of locomotion, increasing it in the athletic shoe condition. This result suggests that the speed has to be one more parameter to consider when assessing the influence of footwear on the interaction between man-shoe-surface. The speed in similar condition of hardness (barefoot and standard shoe) was similar, but muscle activity was different in both conditions, being more similar that of the standard shoe and athletic shoe conditions.

In the different conditions under study, the pattern of muscle activity kept its profile. The starting and ending times of the activity were constant, but the amplitude of the EMG signal changed when using footwear. Also, the duration of the phases in the shod condition was reversed with respect to the bare condition, decreasing the stance phase and increasing the non-support one.

A limitation of this work was that has considered only 6 muscles out of the 57 having each of the lower extremities. The advantage over previous studies is that it has analyzed those six muscles from both legs simultaneously. The fact that the homologous muscles of both legs have similar amplitude allows us to use their absolute values.

The timing of muscle activity was assessed using visual inspection of the actual records, which is the detection method used to interpret the real surface EMG signal. Usually, visual inspection provides a high level of accuracy because all the details of the signal can be measured. Detecting the beginning and end of the activity by using different types of algorithms is based on establishing a threshold, usually based on intuitive criteria. In the end, both visual interpretation and detection using algorithms are based on subjective criteria. The advantage of the subjectivity of the experimenter is based on the acquisition of the ability to interpret the EMG signal and experience that allows the evaluator to use the capabilities of the human brain to perform a more sophisticated interpretation of highly variable data (Staude & Wolf 1999).

The order of participation of the muscles studied did not vary with the type of shoes. First, the TA muscles activated, afterwards the muscles of the posterior part of the thigh (BF and ST), followed by the activation of the GN of the back of the leg, and finally the activation of the RF and VM of the anterior part of the thigh.

The length of time of muscle activity in the three conditions did not vary with respect to the normalized jogging cycle. In all conditions, muscle activity was present in the first half of the stance phase, disappearing in the second, when the body weight fell on the forefoot. In absolute values, the time of activity would be different because the stance phase was shorter in the condition of athletic shoes and the phase of non support was longer. Thus, the time of muscle activity would be greater in the stance phase and lower in the non-support phase.

It is interesting to find that during the jogging, as happens in walking, there are phases in which no muscle activity is taking place, although there are movements that would make one expect some muscular activity. This result is consistent with other studies that have shown that the main goal of locomotion is to transport the body from one position to another using lower limb locomotor coordination and effective mechanisms. The nervous system integrates the movement of different body segments and controls the activity of the muscles to decrease energy expenditure (Inman 1968).

This lack of muscle activity is not surprising. In jogging, the decrease of kinetic and potential energies in the first part of the support is concomitant with the accumulation of elastic energy in the tendons of the muscles; this energy is later released during the remainder of the stance phase to facilitate the progression and stability dynamics. Margaria and Cavagna (1965) found that during jogging, elasticity accounts for 50% of the work. During the unipodal support, the contralateral leg swing provides a second pushing force generated by the acceleration of the leg. Once the centre of gravity has shifted over the foot on the ground, the weight of the body becomes a driving force. When the contralateral leg is slowed by the hamstring muscles, the ipsilateral leg acquires kinetic energy, which is used to start the double flight. Inman (1968) argues that the slowdown of the swing leg during walking can contribute more to the forward movement of the body that the thrust of the ipsilateral leg. Once the leg is in motion, as the first law of Newton states, a force is needed to stop it, and that is the role of the hamstrings when they become active at the end of the swing phase. While the hamstrings are active, the RF and VM become activated to improve the accuracy of the landing of the foot.

The amplitude of the myoelectric activity, expressed in absolute values, varied when using the two different types of footwear; these results are consistent with those found by Gollhofer & Komi (1987), who found differences in the electrical activity of muscles when subjects were at first barefoot and then shod. The effects of athletic shoes on the amplitude of muscle activity were significant. Changes in hardness and shape of the shoe did not affect the muscle activity.

Different considerations have led us to not normalize the EMG signal amplitude: (1) to assess absolute muscle activity when a sole is interposed between the foot and the ground, and (2) to maintain the electrodes in place when the geometry of the footwear and the elasticity of the sole varied.

The subjects ran faster in the athletic shoe condition and muscle activity was similar in the two footwear conditions: higher in the non-support phase. There is no statistically significant difference between the three conditions with respect to the speed of locomotion.

There was similar muscle activity in both shod conditions, which was different from the barefoot condition. In this paper we have classified the hardness of footwear subjectively. Although the interaction subject-shoe-ground occurs only during the stance phase, the intensity of the EMG activity was modified both during the stance phase and during the phase of non support. At first, one might think that the presence of the sole alters the physical characteristics of the force of action and reaction and influences the feedback mechanisms of muscle activity. The results show that although the interaction subject-shoe-ground occurs only during the stance phase, the amplitude of the EMG activity was modified both in the stance and in the swing phases, the major changes occurring in the non-support phase.

Before the foot contacts the ground, there is no information available from the ground; therefore, no feedback mechanism is in use and muscle activity would be controlled by forward mechanisms. The changes in the amplitude of muscle activity in the two footwear conditions were more homogeneous in both legs during the post-impact than during the pre-impact. This finding is in agreement with those of Nigg (2003), who suggests that the EMG activity before and after impact corresponds to two different events. Before the foot contact with the ground, there is no information available from the ground, then no feedback mechanism is in use. It is speculated that this would be some pre-programmed muscle activity based on the expected impact and would be related to the "muscle tuning" and controlled by a forward mechanism. Thus, the configuration of the leg when the heel hits the floor is prepared beforehand during the non-support phase, following the strategy adopted (De Wit et al. 2000). In the other hand, the activity that appears after heel contact is due to a reflex effect. In this context, one can understand the variability of electrical activity in the pre-impact and its consistency in the post-impact.

The changes in the impact force described under the influence of footwear may be a consequence of changes in muscle activity in the non-support phase to reduce soft tissue vibrations during locomotion. Wakeling et al. (2002) explains how the frequencies of the impact force and the soft tissues may overlap during walking and running. It can be expected that the impact forces will cause vibrations within the range of vibration of the soft tissues. However, observations show that such vibrations are minimal. Wakeling et al. (2002) proposed that muscle activity is adjusted before impact in order to reduce possible vibrations resulting from the impact.

The reflex effect has to be understood in the context that the heel contact with the ground is a stimulus that triggers feedback mechanisms. This stimulus does not trigger the onset of muscle activity, which had already begun in all muscles during the swing phase or during the final flight phase (or even during the initial flight phase), but could just change it. The reflex time is around 110 ms in the normal population (Kroll & Clarson 1978), and is divided into a latency time of 20 ms and a motor time of 90 ms. A peak muscle activity for most of the muscles studied appears on the 8% of 700ms-long jogging cycle, i.e. at 56 ms, which correspond well with the reflex motor time.

The maximum activity peak appears in the three conditions in the same phase. The increase in mean activity increased recruitment of motor units and increased force production. The decrease means the opposite. The observation of decreased activity of the VM in the post-impact is consistent with previous findings (De Wit et al. 2000) about the influence of shoes on the ground reaction force. In the shod condition, impact peak appears later perhaps due to decreased activity of the damper (shock absorber) muscles. The loading speed is influenced by muscle activity, which affects the acceleration of the segments.

When wearing footwear, the right and left BF increased their activity at the end of the swing phase, in the final flight, and in the onset of the stance phase. At the end of the swing phase, those muscles act as antagonists of the extension of the knee and of the hip flexion in the swing phase; from the final flight phase, they act as agonists of the extension of the hip.

The increased activity of BF in the shod condition at the end of the swing phase could be justified by the higher speed and greater participation of these muscles to slow down the flexion of the thigh. In principle, its action would facilitate the advancement of the leg by inertia, and then its action would stop the leg being extended to facilitate the support of the foot on the floor. Perhaps, the increased activity in the phase of non-support has an effect on increasing the speed of the contralateral leg, as suggested by the studies of Inman (1968). At the beginning of the stance phase, the BF and ST intervene as agonists of the extension of the hip and knee flexion, cooperating synergistically with the torque that has the lower extremity and maintained as a result of inertia when the foot has been slowed by friction with the ground. When the sole absorbs more impact, shock muscles (RF and VM) decreased its activity. When the shoe was harder, the left RF increased its activity and that of the VM of both legs decreased.

The fact that the muscles of both legs do not modify its maximum amplitude in the same percentage is understood in the context that the activity of a leg is adapted to the activity of the other. However, in the left leg there are significant differences in the activity of some of its muscles when wearing different types of footwear (see for example O'Connor 2005).

The lower activity of the RF and of the VM observed at the beginning of the stance phase may facilitate hip extension and knee flexion caused by increased activity of the hamstrings. This finding is consistent with the results of De Wit et al. (2000) who found that the knee is more flexed in the medium supporting phase in the shod condition. Also in that condition, the TA increased its activity in the final flight and at the beginning of the stance phase, being its activity lower during part of the swing. The role of the TA in the final flight and at the beginning of the stance phase is to promote dorsiflexion. The increased activity in the final flight can be explained based on segmental geometry: the hip extends and the foot flexes dorsally to avoid bumping into the ground until the proper stride length has been obtained. When jogging without shoes, De Wit et al. (2000) reported increased plantar flexion at the beginning of the support phase. Our results are consistent with their findings: the lower activity of the TA muscle in this condition would favour plantar flexion, apparently intended to reduce the pressure, which is higher in the barefoot condition because the impact force is increased and occurs in a shorter time.

One explanation for the decreased activity of ST in the stance phase in the shod condition could be the following: this muscle is extensor and adductor of the hip, and also flexor and rotator of the knee. Shod, the movement from supine-pronation can be affected by the change in the distance between the point of application of the GRF and the subtalar or calcaneus-talus joint. The shoes would favour a faster decrease of the inversion with a faster rotation of the knee in a lower limb that is externally rotated, favouring a twist in the knee. If the ST does not decrease its activity, it would increase that twisting torque affecting the knee. A more active GN in the stance phase could influence the stability of the ankle. In the shod condition, there is more damping of the impact force. Cushioning and stability are conflicting (Perry 1992): more cushioning brings less stability.

Nigg et al. (2003) speculated that the body reacts to changes in input signal to adapt the muscle activity to reduce the vibrations of the soft tissues. In principle, the proximal muscles would be less required than the distal ones. These authors found that the TA activity increased more than that of the proximal ones (BF and ST). Our results are consistent with those findings respect to the TA and the ST; but not for the BF.

According to Mundermann et al. (2003), changes in the intensity of leg muscles activity predict better the differences in comfort than changes in the impact force. As the muscle activity decreased in the stance phase, the kinematic differences between the conditions disappeared (De Wit et al. 2000). This result is consistent with the absence of muscle activity. The signal amplitude indicates the level of activation of the muscle: there is a relationship between activity and strength, implying that increased activity is the source of increased muscle strength. The change in muscle electrical activity may be due to the role of the muscles to adapt to the characteristics of elasticity and friction of the shoes used.

According to Arsenault et al. (1987), it seems clear that the kinematics of locomotion is not very variable. From the scientific literature one can obtain the parameters describing the movement and explain muscle activity during jogging in different conditions. When the peak of the RF, VM, GN, BF, and ST muscles appears, the hip stretches, the knee flexes, and the ankle flexes dorsally. Rectus femoris and VM undergo an eccentric contraction, BF and ST concentric, and GN concentric in the knee and eccentric in the ankle. Biceps femoris and GN promote the flexing of the knee and the GN transfers energy from the ankle to the knee.

The activation of the muscles acting as antagonists (i.e., contracting eccentrically) promote the absorption of energy recovered in the immediate concentric contraction. In the condition barefoot, the BF presented electrical activity at the end of the swing phase, in the final flight, and at the onset of stance phase, acting first as antagonist and then as agonist. With shoes, the activity increased in both phases, increasing the energy absorbed in the non-support phase. During the concentric contraction at the beginning of the stance phase, the increased activity means more power generation. The increase of the absorbed energy and the energy produced could be interpreted as an effort at the beginning of the stance phase in order to do hip extension, perhaps to counterbalance the increased frictional force that opposes the advance in the shod condition. At the beginning of the support phase, the GN, RF, and VM are active in eccentric contraction. The reduction of the duration of the support phase in the shod condition may improve the efficacy of the stretching-shortening cycle.

The potential problem of crosstalk was reduced using a double differential technique, which is based on a single amplifier fed with three electrodes (De Luca & Merletti, 1988; Winter, 1990; Winter et al., 1994). It is already widely accepted that double-differential technique reduces the level of cross-talk (see, *e.g.*, De Luca & Merletti, 1988; and Meinecke et al., 2004). In any case, cross-talk cannot ever be fully cancelled.

As the human body is a biological system that has many possibilities of action and reaction, it would be advisable to evaluate the electrical activity of other additional muscles when changing the subject-shoe-ground interface. According to Ferris et al. (1999), persons adjust the degree of stiffness of the legs when they run on different surfaces. The stiffness is given by the coactivation of the ago-antagonists muscles that cross the joints. In the support phase, the coactivation in the shod condition was greater than in the barefoot condition. At the stage of non support, the coactivation in the shod condition was not homogeneous, neither for both legs nor for all muscles, as it may decrease or increase respect to the barefoot condition.

A major function of footwear is to cushion both the strength of action the subject performs on the ground and absorb its reaction force, in order to protect the musculoskeletal system. Athletic shoes diminish –or even nullify- the impact peak of the vertical component and are involved in delaying the onset of the vertical support force, by changing the load gradient (Nigg 1983, De Wit et al. 2000).

The impact force acts as an input signal in the body and influences the vibration of the soft tissues (Nigg et al. 2000). The vertical component is biphasic and has two peaks: the impact peak appears after 20 ms of the impact, representing 140-160% -200% of BW, in those runners that support the heel first in the ground. A second peak, in the stance phase, appears at 80 ms and can almost triple the BW. Previous works (De Wit et al. 2000, Nigg 1983) have shown that in jogging, the magnitude of the passive and active peaks of the vertical component of the GRF does not vary with the shoes. The load gradient was lower in the shod condition due to the later occurrence of the impact force (33 ms against 11 ms).

In our study, peak muscle activity appeared in the following cycle time: 2-6% for the ST, 6-8% for the VM and RF, 8-10% for GN. In absolute values, the 2% amounts to 14 ms, 6% to 42 ms, and 10% to 70 ms. The activity peak of four muscles occur between the peaks of the vertical component of the reaction force. Despite finding a second peak of greater magnitude in the shod condition, muscle activity was higher in only three of the six muscles studied. In two of the other muscles (VM and ST) in the shod condition the activity was lower. In the RF, the activity response was not constant.

The increased activity of the TA in the shod condition could lead to the appearance of the anterior compartment syndrome of the lower leg. The results here presented about the increased EMG signal amplitude suggest further studies to corroborate or refute the argument used by athletes and shoe manufacturers on increased performance with the use of athletic footwear.

Author details

Begoña Gavilanes-Miranda
Faculty of Physical Activity and Sport Science, University of Basque Country, Vitoria, Spain

Juan J. Goiriena De Gandarias
Faculty of Medicine, University of Basque Country, Bilbao, Spain

Gonzalo A. Garcia*
Biorobotics Department, TECNALIA, Bilbao, Spain

* Corresponding Author

Acknowledgement

Authors thank the volunteers who participated in the experiments carried out for the present work. Thanks also to J. de la Cruz (Department of Applied Economy, University of Basque Country, Spain), F. Ainz (Department of Physiology, University of Basque Country, Spain), and to J. Bilbao (Department of Statistics, University of Basque Country, Spain) for their participation in the analysis of the data; and to S. Rainieri (Food Research Division, AZTI-Tecnalia, Spain) for helpful comments on the original manuscript.

This study was supported by the Foundation *Jesús de Gangoiti Barrera*. G.A.G. was supported by a European Marie Curie Post-doctoral Fellowship (ADCOMP project; Contract MEIF-CT-2006-025056). The CONSOLIDER INGENIO 2010 must be acknowledged for supporting partially this work through grant CSD2009-00067.

5. References

Arsenault AB, Winter DA, Marteniuk RG (1987). Is there a 'normal ' profile of EMG activity in gait?. Medical & Biological Engineering & Computing 337-343.

Bates BT, Osterninig JA, Sawhill JA (1983). An assessment of subject variability, subject inter-action, and the evaluation of running shoes using ground reaction force data. J Biomec 16: 181-191.

Behnke R (2001). Kinetic Anatomy. Human Kinetics, Champaign,IL.

Bouisset S (1973). EMG and force in normal motor activities. In: Desmedt JE ed. New developments in electromyography and clinical neurology. Base: Karger: 547-583.

De Luca CJ (1997). The use of surface electromyography in biomechanics. Journal of Applied Biomechanics 13: 135-167.

De Luca CJ & Merletti R. (1988). Surface myoelectric signal cross-talk among muscles of the leg. Electromyography and Clinical Neurophysiology; 1988, 69:568-75.

De Wit B, De Clercq D, Aerts P (2000). Biomechanical analysis of the stance phase during barefoot and shod running. J Biomech Mar;33(3):269-78.

Dufek JS, Bates BT, Davis HP, Malone LA (1991). Dynamic performance assessment of selected sport shoes on impact forces. Medicine and Science in Sports and Exercise 23 (9): 1062-1067.

Denoth J and Nigg B (1981). The influence of various sport floors on the load on the lower extremities. In : Biomechanics VII-B,A. Morecki, K Fidelus ,K Kedzior and A Wit (eds). Baltimore: University Park Press, 100-106.

Ferris DP, Liang K, Farley CT (1999). Runners adjust leg stiffness for their first step on a new running surface. J Biomech. 32: 787-794.

Forner A, Garcia AC, Alcantara E, Ramiro J, Hoyos JV, Vera P (1995). Properties of shoe insert materials related to shock wave transmission during gait. Foot Ankle Int Dec;16(12):778-86

Frederick EC (1986). Kinematically mediated effects of sport shoe design: a review. J Sports Sci 4 (3): 169-184.

Gavilanes MB, Goiriena de Gandarias JJ (2004). Muscle activity in shod and barefoot healthy young subjects during walking. In : International proceedings of XVth Congress of the International Society of Electrophysiology & Kinesiology. Boston U.S.A. 2004:105

Gollhofer A, Komi PV (1987). Measurement of Man-Shoe-Surface interaction during locomotion. Medicine Sport Sci, 26: 187-199.

Inman VT (1968). Conservation of energy in ambulation. In: Bull Procc Res BPR 1968; 10:(9):26-35.

Inman VT, Ralston HJ, Todd F (1981). Human walking. Baltimore, MD, Williams and Wilkins Company.

Kadaba MP, Wootten ME, Gainey J, Cochran GV (1985). Repeatability of phasic muscle activity: performance of surface and intramuscular wire electrodes in gait analysis. J Orthop Res. 1985;3(3):350-9.

Kendall FP, Mccreary EK, Provance PG (2000). Músculos: pruebas funcionales, postura y dolor. Willinams & Wilkins. Baltimore.

Kleissen RFM, Buurke JH, Harlaar J, Hof AL, Zilvold G. C (1998). Electromyography in the biomechanical analysis of human movement and its clinical application. Gait & Posture 8 : 143-158.

Komi PV, Gollhofer A, Schmidtbleicher D, Frick U. (1987) Interaction between man and shoe in running: considerations for a more comprehensive measurement approach. Int J Sports Med. 1987 Jun;8(3):196-202

Kroll W & Clarson PM (1978). Fractionated reflex time, resisted and unresisted fractionated reaction time under normal and fatigued conditions. In DM Landrers & RW. Christina (Eds), Psychology of Motor Behaviour and Sport 1977 (pp 106-129) Champaign ,IL: Human Kinetics.

Lieber RL (1992). Skeletal muscle response to injury. In: Skeletal muscle structure and function. John P Butler, Ed. Baltimore/Williams § Wilkins, 1992: 260-292

Luethi S, Stacoff A (1987).The influence of shoes on foot mechanics in running. Med. Sport Sci., 25:72-85.

Mann RA, Moran GT, Dogherty SE (1986). Comparative electromyography of the lower extremity in jogging, running and sprinting. The American Journal of sports Medicine 14 (6): 501-510.

Margaria R, Cavagna GA (1965). The mechanics of walking. J Physiol (Paris). Sep-Oct;57(5):655-6.

Martín PE, Morgan DW (1992). Biomechanical considerations for economical walking and running. Med. Sci. Sports Exerc. 24 (4):467-474.

Meinecke L., Disselhorst-Klug C., & Rau G. (2004): Crosstalk and Coactivation in Bipolar Surface EMG Data: A New Methodology for Detection, Discrimination and Quantification; in the 25th Congress of the International Society of Electrophysiological Kinesiology (ISEK), Boston, Massachusetts, June 2004, p. 87.

Milliron M, Cavanagh PR (1990). Sagittal plane kinematics of the lower extremity during distance running. In Biomechanics of distance running. Human Kinetics Books, Champaign Illinois.

Mundermann A, NiggBM, Humblew RN, Stefanyshyn DJ (2003). Foot orthotics affect lower extremity kinematics and kinetics during running. Cl Biom18: 254-262.

Nigg BM (1983). External force measurements with sport shoes and playing surfaces; in Nigg Kerr, Biomechanical aspects of sport shoes and playing surfaces 11-23 (University Printing, Calgary).

Nigg BM, Bahlsen HA, Denoth J, Luethi SM, Stacoff A (1986). Factors influencing kinetic and kinematic variables in tuning. In: Biomechanics of running shoes. BM Nigg (ed.). Pp 139-159. Champaign, IL: Human Kinetics Publishers.

Nigg BM, Wakeling JM (2001). Impact forces and muscle tuning: a new paradigm. Exerc Sport Sci Rev 29(1):37-41.

Nigg BM, Mundeermann A, Stefanyshyn DJ, Cole G, Stergiou P, Miller J (2003).The effect of material characteristics of shoe soles on muscle activation and energy aspects during running.J Biom 36: 569-575.

Novacheck TF (1998). The biomechanics of running. Gait & Posture 7: 77-95.

Perry J (1992). Gait analysis sistems in gait analysis: normal and pathological function. Thorofare, NJ: Slack 353-411.

Nordin M and Frankel VH (2004). Biomecanica de la rodilla. In: Biomecanica basica del sistema musculoesqueletico. McGraw Hill/Inteamérİcana de Espana, S.A.U.

O'Connor KM, Hamill J (2005).The role of selected extrinsic foot muscles during running. Clin Biomech (2004) Jan;19(1):71-7.

Ramiro J, Ferranids R, Sánchez J, Alepuz R, Latorre P, Dejoz R, Candela F (1988). Evaluación de la técnica del calzado deportivo. Archivos Medicina del Deporte V (18): 161-168.

Reber L, Perry J, Pink M (1993). Muscular control of the ankle in running. Am J Sports Med 21 (6):805-810.

SENIAM (1999). European recommendations for surface electromyography.

Segesser B, Nigg BM (1993). Orthopedic and biomechanical concepts of sports shoe construction Sportverletz Sportschaden 7 (4) 150-162.

Shorteen MR (1993). The energetics of running and running shoes. J Biom 26 (1): 41-51.

Slocum DB, James SL (1968). Biomechanics of running. JAMA. 1968 Sep 9;205(11):721-8.

Staude G, Wolf W (1999). Objective motor response onset detection in surface myoelectric signals. Medical Engineering & Physics 21:449-467.

Testut L, Latarjet A (1971). Tratado de Anatomía Humana. Barcelona: Salvat editores.

Vaughan, CL (1984). Biomechanics of running. Crit Rev Biomed Eng 12:1-48

Wakeling JM, Von Tscharner V, Nigg BM, Stergiou P (2001). Muscle activity in the leg is tuned in response to ground reaction forces. J Appl Physiol Sep;91(3):1307-17.

Wakeling JM, Pascual S, Nigg B M (2002). Altering muscle activity in lower extremities by running with different shoes. Med. Sci. Sports Exerc. 34 (9): 1529-1532.

Winter DA (1979). Mechanical work, energy and power. In: Biomechanics of human movement. Pp 84-107. Toronto: John Wiley and Sons.

Winter DA (1990). Biomechanical and motor control of human movement, 2nd edn. New York:Wyley, 1990.

Winter DA, Fugelvand AJ, & Archer SE (1994). Crosstalk in surface electromyography: theoretical and practical estimates. Journal of Electromyography and Kynesiology 1994;4:15-26.

Wickiewiz TL, Roland R, Perry L, Powell BS, Edgerton R (1983). Muscle architecture of the human lower limb. Clinical Ortopaedics and Related Research 179: 275-283.

Chapter 5

Influence of Different Strategies of Treatment Muscle Contraction and Relaxation Phases on EMG Signal Processing and Analysis During Cyclic Exercise

Leandro Ricardo Altimari, José Luiz Dantas, Marcelo Bigliassi,
Thiago Ferreira Dias Kanthack, Antonio Carlos de Moraes and Taufik Abrão

Additional information is available at the end of the chapter

http://dx.doi.org/10.5772/50599

1. Introduction

For a long time we work with muscular activity, trying to answer questions related to fatigue, muscle activity and other issues related to neuromuscular system. In this way we started to use the electromyography (EMG) as a tool to achieve better results in our studies, since it appeared to us as a truthful method to access the muscle activity inside a lot of perspectives we had been working with.

In this chapter we will try to bring some research results that we found on the GEPESINE laboratory in the last couple of years about regarding the EMG analysis. Firstly there are relevant issues that arise during the use of EMG as a tool in others works. It is not hard to find studies that use EMG signal as a way to measure the muscle activity [1-3], muscle fatigue [4] and also in studies involving healthy issues [5]. Most of those studies try to access the activity or fatigue slope of the muscle during some motor task, mostly trying to access performance or just to categorize an activity according to the muscle(s) accessed. The real problem is that most of those studies use isometric movements or even isokinetic, leaving a remarkable problem for the researchers who decide to work with dynamic contractions, once the available protocols are most based on and suitable isometric studies.

We have decided to take a different look to the process on how to treat the EMG signal and how to analyze it. For instance, in order to have a more trustful signal, founds in literature recommend filtering, smoothing the raw and also rectifying the signal, which the last step does not affect the signal power. However, the filtered root mean square (RMS) signal could not be the best way to pre-process the EMG signal. Other current concern, in EMG signal pre-processing, is about the use of the total signal against evaluation only the burst-time segments of the signal. Those concerns are explained and analyzed along this chapter. In an epistemological language, we take a more critic look into the EMG signal processing. We hope the reader also to have the same look, not only into the results and conclusions, but also, into methods and thoughts, since the intention herein is not to bring an irrefutable true, but the real intention is to discuss and point out valuable arguments for the reader in order to he/she thinks about it by himself or herself, and apply it properly.

2. Theory

2.1. The importance of electromyography in cyclic exercises

Cyclic exercises correspond to modalities such as bicycle, running, walking and swimming. Inside those we can already imagine a lot of different sports with a great repercussion over the media, a few examples include: street bike, mountain bike and tour, like the famous Tour of France; marathon, 400 meters, race walking and putting in just one thing, the triathlon. You may notice that the swimming sports are not exemplified above, it's because it is still hard to access the muscle activity through electromyography in those sports due to the environment where they happens. This discussion was set aside for our future work

So, keeping in mind that some of the most important sports have a cyclic dynamic as characterization, for the evolution of them, new technologies need to be able to help the coaches and physical trainers. Nowadays individual time-trial sports are reaching world records that we would never imagine, and every new record is followed by a technology behind it helping in training or even during the task if is not prohibited. To be able to access the muscle activity with a good reliability in different moments of the exercise could give us the weak and the strong moments of one athlete during the task, and allow us to create the better strategy and also create new training cycles that can improve the weakness. It is worth noting the electromyography is useful to access not only muscle activity -- in order to enhance the performance in sports --, but also be deployed in exercises evaluation aiming healthy improvement.

2.2. Time and frequency domain

Talk about frequency domain is talk about: how many times a event occurs in a time space, in this way, to use this component we need transform the signal in different points presented in a frequency spectrum capable to show us the energy of cue obtained in the determined muscle. This energy in the most part of the time appears represented in some bands, where your intensity and duration has more amplitude. To find and use the spectrum, we must find a source that gives us the possibility to produce this figure, when sometimes the Fast Fourier Transform proves as algorithm in a simple calculus to find discrete signals. A series of recommendations are proposed to this technique, since the establishment of sample number, duration intervals, window apply and many aspects as signal stationary is a complicated thing to deal with, which leads us to use a wavelet transform, more appropriate to cyclic activities as cycling and running for example [6-9].

Independently of technique used we should get some variable from this analyses to compare, relate or make our considerations, in this case, the most common variable toke from frequency domain is the median frequency, representative of fatigue aspect in the muscular activity from decrease of conduct fibers velocity, is exactly the point that divided the spectrum in two equal parts and gives us a good representation of reduction in the force produced.

Time domain is used when the intention is to achieve the contractibility of the muscle, meaning that as stronger the signal the most number of motor units are been activated. The most common variable used inside this domain is the Root Mean Square (RMS) [9]. To get this variable some procedures are required, like the filtration, rectification and smoothing, those will be better explained later. Just like the frequency domain, a correct time window is necessary and follows the frequency domain also when talking about the use of wavelet transform.

2.3. Treating the EMG signal

Now you already know about how the domains work and how to use them for different analysis depending on the applications necessity. During the subchapter "Analysis of the EMG signal" we hope it became clear that we have some procedures until the real signal is accessed, especially without noises. The raw signal can already give us some information, like the muscle innervations or even the change in the signal size. Depending of the intention, these qualitative variables can be very useful. An easy and good way to simple control some noises when there is no intention of further computer treatment to remove it, is to be sure to have a good baseline, meaning that the line that should appear at the EMG signal must be as close as it can to zero when the muscle with the electrode connected is not in contraction. That doesn't mean that when the muscle starts to contract the signal that will appear will only be from the muscle activity, especially in dynamic contractions. There are three main differences in noises on static contractions and dynamic ones, they are: the non-stationarity of the signal for the constant contraction and relaxing of the muscle, the change of the electrode distance relative to the origin of the action potential and the changes in the conductivity of the tissues properties [10].

A better way to understand what a noise is, is looking at it, the figure 1 under is an EMG signal with a closer look in the burst moment. Notice that the areas surrounded with black circles have a peculiar difference, it has a horizontal straight shaped line, which means that those parts don't have a corresponding negative part, and so, it is considered a noise. Of course in this same image you can find some more of those, not only the surrounded ones, but the intention here is only to show how a noise appears inside an EMG signal.

When the signal appears to us in the computer screen those details are impossible to see without a zoom look. So, lets talk now about how the treatments can influence in the signal value.

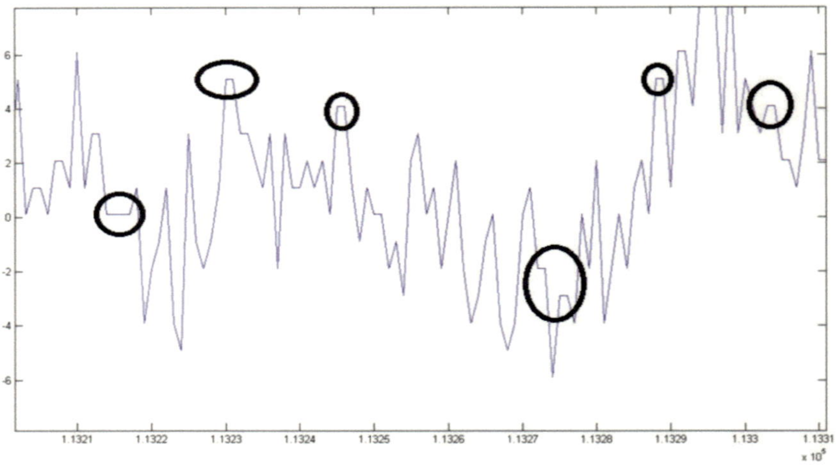

Figure 1. Noises in the EMG signal

Note the figure 2 under, pay even more attention to the baseline in the raw signal, it is close to zero because it almost creates a straight line, considering that the muscle in this case is the vastus lateralis in a bike-like exercise, we can imagine that in the beginning of the exercise he is not much triggered, probably because the recto femuralis is doing almost all the job, but as time goes and also the exercise, its starts to have stronger signal, so we can imagine that the other muscles, like the recto femuralis is entering in fatigue process, so the vasto lateralis as a co-worker has to get part of this charge in order to maintain the exercise, that is the kind of qualitative analyze that was told before, without even knowing the values numbers, we can visually access an ideia about the use of vasto lateralis in a cicliergometer exercise.

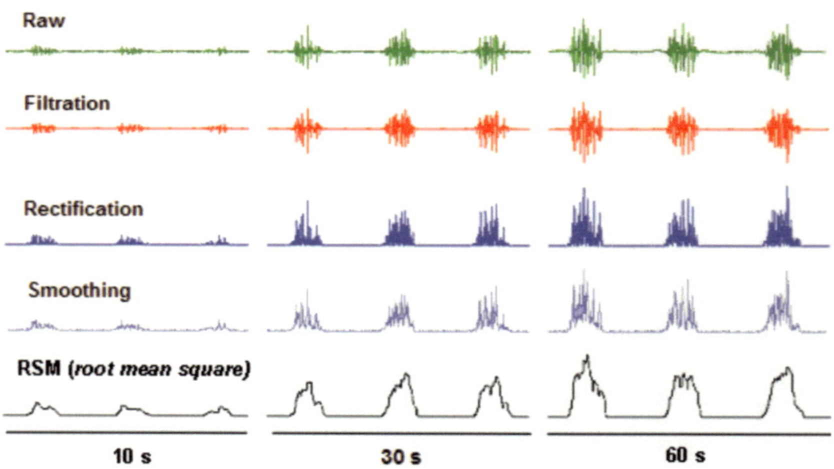

Figure 2. EMG signal process recommended. Green: The raw signal, no treatment was applied until this moment; Red: Filtrated signal, a limit was created for the signal, excluding everything out of it; Blue: Rectified signal, all negative values were transformed in positive ones and added; Purple: the smoothed signal, a linear enveloped was created and the extreme parts of the signal was excluded; Black: The RMS values after all the treatments.

With the intention of clearing the EMG signal, and make it more reliable and truthful, some computer processes are used before analyzes, they are: Filtration, Rectification and Smoothing. The image below shows the same signal from raw until the smoothed in order to obtain the RMS values for the vastus lateralis muscle in an exercise in 100% of the maximal watts in a cicloergometer during 60 seconds. Those process, expecially the Filtration and the Smoothing has the purpose of giving us the possibility to evaluate only the signal coming from the muscular contraction, without mechanical or electromagnetic interferences [2,11].

2.3.1. Signal filtering

In a first moment the filtration occurs when the signal is been collected. With the objective to avoid interferences the EMG signal passes through a 50 to 60 Hz filter (notch filter), if it's necessary. This filter already starts rejecting the frequency band of 60 Hz once that in this band is where the ambient interferences like pressure appear, arrangement or closer apparatus. In a second moment, the EMG signal must pass through a pass-band; this pass-band frequency must be decided by the analyzer, once it can depend on the intentions of the study. Normally, this frequency is fixed between 20 and 450 Hz, because normally 80% of the muscular energy is concentrated [12-13]. But, as said before, it is a free choice for the user, once that this frequency can differ from muscle to muscle, so, it's important for the user to know exactly the band of the muscle that is been assessed to make sure that the pass-band will cut off only the signal that doesn`t belong to that muscle, and at the same time guarantee as precisely as it can that it won't let noises get inside the signal. Basically, it limits the signal inside a previous decided range to maintain it inside the muscle activation site.

The visual difference between the raw and the filtrated signal can be really hard to notice especially when the collected process is well cared, however, if we take a rigorous look to both of them, the difference will appear to our eyes, but remembering that the main reason of using those treatments is to obtain the quantitative values of the signal.

2.3.2. Signal rectification

This procedure has the purpose to turn all the signal values integrative, submitting them to the cut of all negative values, that means, to delete the values that are under the baseline, or to turn all this negative values to positive adding the values, making them integrative. The second option is more recommended if the intention is to achieve the total muscle signal, if you cut off the negative part, half of the signal will be lost, so turning all of them positive is a more used and more interesting when it comes to final results. This procedure doesn't affect the signal noises like the filtration and the smoothing, which will be explained in sequence. However it is still recommended and made part of the studies involving this chapter, so it's important for the reader to know how we used and what it means.

This procedure is simple, and it can be easily understood by the figure above. Note that until the filtration moment the signal had both positive and negative side in the burst moments, taking the baseline as a zero mark, and once that the signal was rectified it became not only positive, but also increased the positive side size, that mean that we didn't exclude the negative part, we added it to the positive side. If the reader wants to know how the same signal without the adding of the negative values would be, you just have to take the filtrated signal and cut the down part, always considering the baseline as a zero mark. Look at the figure 3 under and try to make a qualitative analyze of the two methods.

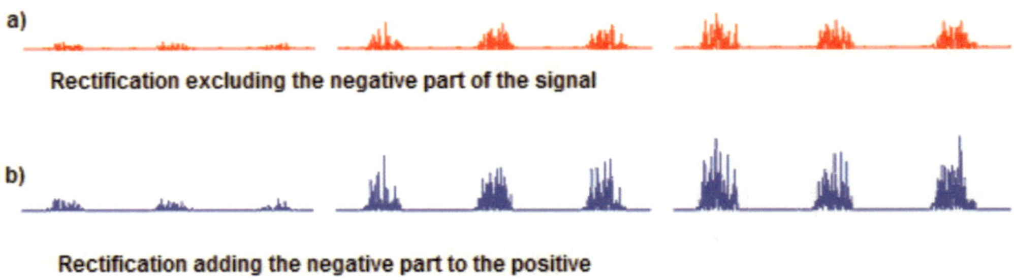

Figure 3. a) Half-wave rectification: rectification excluding the negative part of signal amplitude; **b**) Full-wave rectification: aggregating the negative part (reducing the ripple) of EMG signal.

Notice that for a visual analysis excluding the negative parte can bring an error, it's hard to say that the three last bursts of the red signal are different from the three before it, but in the blue signal is much easier to assume that. Thus in the first one I could say that the muscle had reached his maximal power, while in the second I could not make the same affirmation.

2.3.3. Signal smoothing

The Smoothing and the filtration have some similar parameters, mostly because both have the intention of taking out the extremes, the parts that are considering noises. Smoothing creates a linear envelope in the signal, leaving only a center part of the signal. The mainly difference between the smoothing and the filtration, is that filtration take in account the muscle activation range, and the smoothing the signal obtained itself. If the filter is strong enough or considered really good, it can even make the smoothing unnecessary. However, it's recommended to use both, especially in cyclic dynamic contractions, that as we already saw, have a bigger chance to have noises interferences. Looking at the Figure again, the smoothed signal is also really easy to realize, it creates visually a much cleaner signal, creating almost a line, which means, it excludes the extremes, leaving only the signal that is considered the muscle activation signal.

2.4. Burst and silence

During the obtainment of the EMG signal we can separate two parts of it, the Silence and the Burst, as showed in the figure 4.

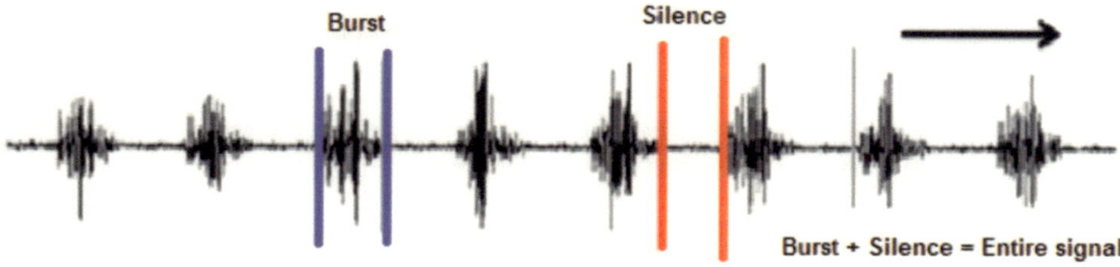

Figure 4. Burst and silence moments in an electromyography signal during a Wingate test in a cicloergometer. The break between the blue lines show a burst moment and the break between the red lines is the silence moment. Unification of Burst and Silence generates the full signal.

The Burst moment is the muscle contraction moment, easily noticed by the sudden break in the baseline, and so, the Silence moment is when no contraction is occurring, so the signal stays at zero, or at least should stay, as said before in the treatment discussions. That's another important reason to maintain a baseline close to zero; it is easier to separate the onset and the end of the Burst from the Silence moment. When a signal is collected it's normal to treat it as an Entire signal, which means that it takes to account both Burst and Silence moments of the signal. The figure showed above is from the recto femoral muscle in a cyclic exercise in a cicloergometer during a Wingate test. As expected in this kind of exercise, it is found a lot of Burst and Silence moments, differing from isometric exercises for example, that would appear only a Burst moment, which would lose strength as time goes by for the fatigue process.

The problem is the use of the entire signal, or only the Burst moments, taking into account that if the intention is to read only the muscle activity it can be assumed that should be used only the Burst moment once that a cyclic exercise will have a lot of Silence moments, and this could make the final results to become smaller, to decrease the meaning. Thus, to know if the Silence moment affects the final results in time and frequency domains variables is of great importance for the researchers that works especially with cyclic exercises. That is one of the problems that will be further discussed on this chapter.

2.5. Time windows

The term "time windows" is used to determine the size of the cuts that will be made in the EMG signal for further analyzes. The most normal is to use the 1 second window, and in case of short tasks it can easily be done once that the signal is short and it is easy to separate the total task time in 1 second parts. However, for longer tasks it can be really difficult for the researcher to separate a signal of 10 minutes in 600 windows of 1 second each for example. Thus, a study from [14] brought that to use a 5 second window and a 1 second in a cyclic exercise can provide the same result of muscle activity for further analyzes, providing for the EMG researchers an excitement about using the method in long tasks. To bring a better example, the figure 5 under shows us a signal and how it would be analyzed if it was cut in one second windows.

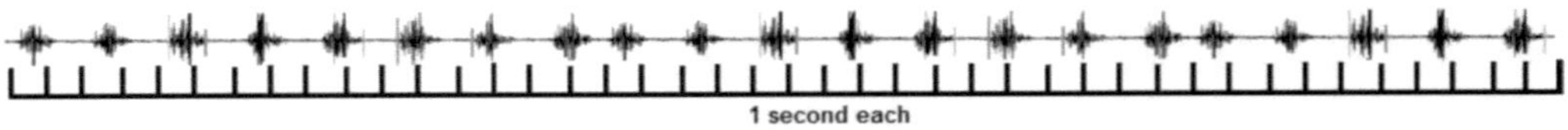

Figure 5. An EMG signal divided in 1 second time windows.

In the same signal, the next image has the cuts made in five seconds windows (Figure 6). The biggest importance about using a bigger window is not just because it would be hard for the researcher to divide the signal, but also because some routines that treat the signal don`t accept too much windows to process.

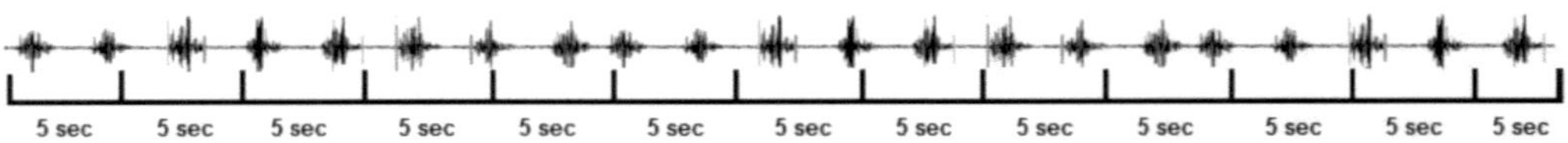

Figure 6. The same EMG signal of Figure 5, now divided in 5 seconds windows.

3. Methodology

3.1. Influence of the treatments (First study)

The Signal processing in EMG is a complex matter to adopt in determined studies, in several times the signal process used is based on the mainly recommendations and the needs of researcher, but sometimes the instructions are not so clear and are not based in studies that contemplate the new tendencies in contemporary researches. However, the main objective of this chapter is to show the great possibility of using the different treatments to find the same outcome of an EMG signal, using many combinations of process (filtration, rectification and smoothing) in a variable of time domain (RMS) and discover if bursts are capable to interfere in the final result of a dynamic exercise in high intensity that is more capable to induce great noises. In that way, we keep our efforts in test these intriguing questions about the signal processing in EMG with a considerable method to involve the main exercise capable of producing the high amount of noises in the signal and test in this sequence the differences in use several proceedings in dynamic exercise (cycling). To introduce this perspective we assessed in a first period 20 men (27,5 ± 4,1 years old; 83,1 ± 8,2 kg; 184,5 ± 4,5 cm), healthy and active physically.

Briefly the subjects passed for a session of familiarization in the protocols and the instruments of the test, basically to know the cycle simulator and find/keep adjusts in bench and foot pedals. In the next step the men did a maximal incremental test (MIT) until exhaustion to determine the maximal work load (MWL). The information obtained in MIT was used to find the intensity of effort in constant load tests (CLT) in three different intensities in severe domain: 80% MWL, 100% MWL and 110% MWL, see figure 7 for better understanding. The different intensities in severe domain were chosen with the intention to allow us to make affirmations including all domains. Each subject was tested in the same hour of day to minimize the effects of the circadian variations.

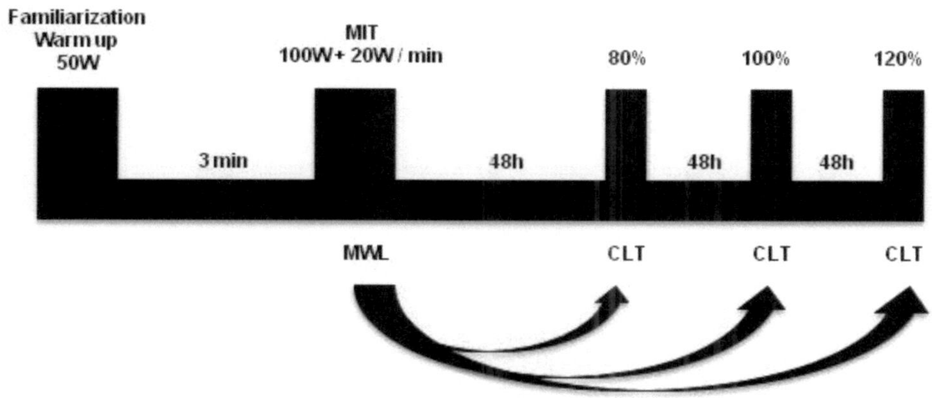

Figure 7. Illustrative representation of the first study, involving signal treatments for RMS obtainment.

Initially it was realized the MWL with initial load in 100W and 20W of increments each minute until voluntary exhaustion, remain a cadence of 70 revolutions per minute (rpm). The MWL was preceded of a warm-up with a load of 50W, with a period of three minutes, follow by three minutes in rest. The MWL was defined as a higher work load maintained for 30 seconds at least, this was assumed so we could make sure to achieve the MWL and not the peak load.

From the information obtained in the MWL, the subjects were oriented to realize three constant load tests (CLT) in different intensities, these being: submaximal (80%MWL), maximal (100%) and supramaximal (110%). Every test was realized in a cyclesimulator (Computrainer™, Racer Mate®, USA). The tests occur with at least 48 hours between then. The CLT was preceded of three minutes of warm-up with 50W, followed by three minutes of rest. After that the tests occur until exhaustion. The subjects were instructed to keep their cadence in 90 rpm, could not pedal less than that, and the test was interrupted when the subjects reported voluntary exhaustion or showed inability to keep the cadence stipulated on the test. The verbal encouragement was used.

The EMG signal was obtained during all period of realization in CLT using an electromyography with 16 channels, model MP150™ (Biopac System®, USA) with a sampling rate of 2000 samples/second, in agreement with ISEK [15]. Before the beginning of each CLT, the subjects were submitted to asepsis and curettage. The electrodes used were active and bipolar, model TSD 150™ (BIOPAC Systems®, USA), with distance among electrodes fixed in two centimeters, putted above superficial muscles of quadriceps femoral of right leg: vastus lateralis (VL), vastus medialis (VM) and rectus femoris (RF), following the standard of SENIAM [12], as showed by the white circles on the figure 8.

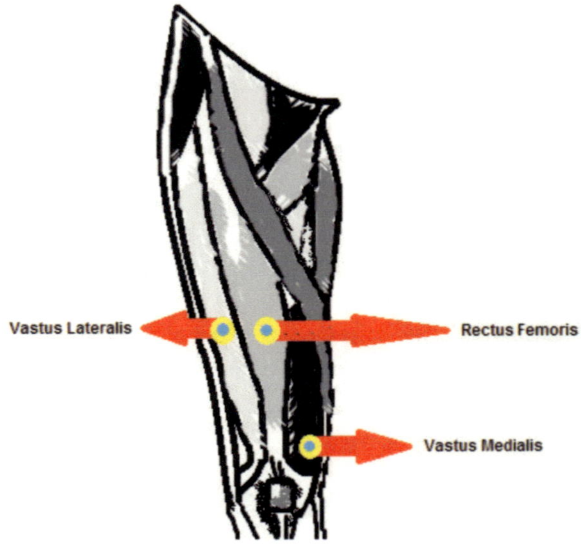

Figure 8. Electrode position used; SENIAM recommendations [12].

The relation of rejection common mode was >95dB and the limits of entrance of established signal in ± 5 mV. The reference electrode was positioned in the right elbow (lateral epicondyle). To capture and process the signal was used the software AcqKnowledge 3.8.1™ (BIOPAC Systems®, USA) and the software MatLab 7.0 (Mathworks®, South Natick, MA, USA).

The EMG signal was treated to obtain the RMS (root mean square) values in time windows with five seconds in the first minute of the test in different intensities. The first twenty seconds of each signal were discarded with the intention to avoid possible inertial influences. After that, it was used proceedings recommended to exclude artifacts and noises from EMG signal, divided in conditions: raw (R), Filtration (F), Filtration + smoothing (FS), filtration + smoothing + rectification (FSR). The filtration was done using a pass-band digital filter Butterworth with frequencies of 20 and 500 Hz. The smoothing process was done through a mobile mean with three points. The process of rectification was done considering all signals, without discards of negative part. The table 1 present the mean values of the load used in the constant load test in 80, 100 and 110% of MWL and the respective times to exhaustion.

Condition	**Load (W)**	**Time (s)**
CLT 80%	212.6 ± 23.5^{a}	1070.0 ± 250.5^{a}
CLT 100%	268.5 ± 33.6^{b}	282.3 ± 75.5^{b}
CLT 110%	301.5 ± 31.7^{c}	110.3 ± 22.3^{c}

Note: different letters show significant differences between loads and times to exhaustion, ($P<0.05$).

Table 1. Loads and times to exhaustion (mean and standard deviation) on constant load tests in 80, 100 and 110% of MWL.

3.2. Influence of the burst and silence in treatment of EMG signal (Second Study)

To test the possibility of bursts get in the way of an EMG signal and change the final outcome, we used a similar method, assessing 27 healthy students (14 men, age = 28,2 ± 2,7 years and 13 women, age = 23,2 ± 2,7 years). The test proposed was the Wingate supramaximal test (WST) used with a purpose to reach a higher intensity in exercise matched with a short duration. The index of performance was defined in a software (WINGATE TEST®, CEFISE, BRASIL) to determine the power by each second during the test, beyond the relative peak power (RPP) ($W.kg^{-1}$), relative mean power (RMP) ($W.kg^{-1}$), fatigue index (FI) (%) and the peak power instant (PPI). The figure 9 represents the second study protocol.

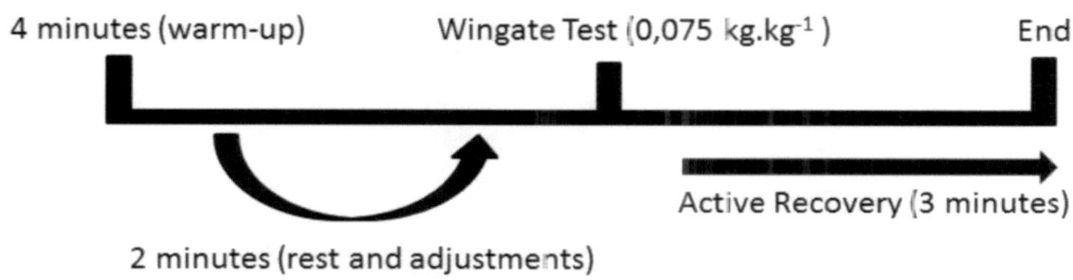

Figure 9. Illustrative representation of second study protocol, involving burst analyze.

The protocol consisted of 4 minutes warm-up in a mechanic cycle ergometer to lower limbs (MONARK 324E, SWEDEN) with 50 W load, with a pedal cadence in 70 rpm and the beginning of each minute the subjects realized a sprint during 6 seconds. After warm-up, the subjects rest for two minutes and they began the test, with a 0,075 $kg.kg^{-1}$ load until finish the test in 30 seconds. The same muscles were analyzed with the same EMG protocol and the same equipment's and procedures in the previous study. However, for this study in addition to the RMS also analyzed spectral parameters. To spectral analyses or frequency domain, was obtained the parameters from median frequency (MF), variance and slope, those values were determined using Wavelet Daubechies db4 (DWT) [6,8]. Was considered the analyses of EMG signal in the contraction phase (bursts) and during all signal (bursts + silence).

The table 2 present a descriptive analyze referent of subject performance.

Variables	Men n=14	Women n=13
RPP ($W.kg^{-1}$)	10.0 ± 0.9	7.7 ± 0,9
RMP ($W.kg^{-1}$)	7.3 ± 0.5	5.6 ± 0.6
FI (%)	52.9 ± 9,0	51.1 ± 11.9

Note: relative peak power (RPP), relative mean power (RMP), and fatigue index (FI).

Table 2. Mean values ± standard deviation of subject performance.

4. Results

4.1. Influence of the treatments (First study)

The figure 10 shows a comparative analyses of the RMS mean values from quadriceps integrated, obtained in submaximal intensity. We can see that no differences were found among different kinds of EMG treatment (p>0.05), although it shows a tendency to decrease the values encountered in the measure that the procedure of analyses are added to treatment.

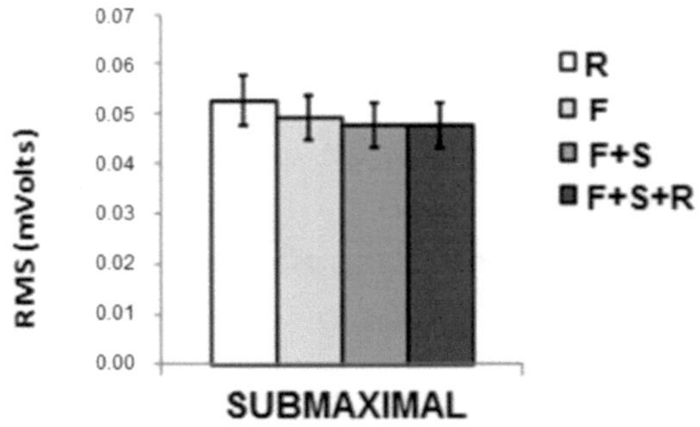

Figure 10. RMS values (mean and standard deviation) from quadriceps integrated muscles ([VL + VM+ RF] ÷ 3) in the different kinds of treatments to submaximal intensity exercise. R = Raw, F = Filtered, S = Smoothing. No differences were found (p>0.05).

The figure 11 shows a comparative analyses of the RMS mean values from quadriceps integrated, obtained in maximal intensity. We can see that no differences were found among different kinds of EMG treatment (p>0.05), although, like the submaximal intensity, it shows a tendency to decrease the values encountered in the measure that the procedure of analyses are added to treatment.

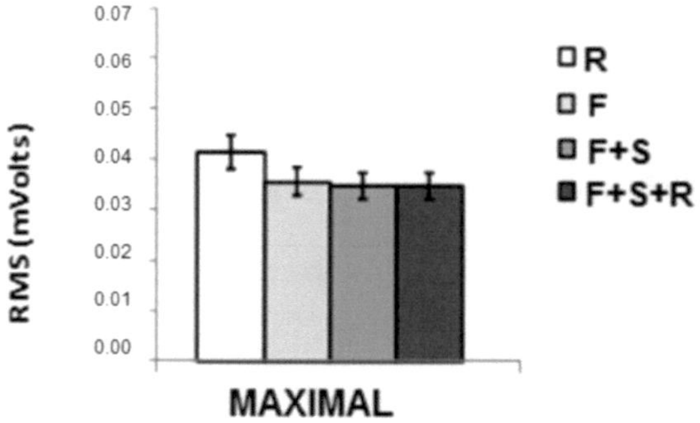

Figure 11. RMS values (mean and standard deviation) from quadriceps integrated muscles ([VL + VM+ RF] ÷ 3) in the different kinds of treatments to maximal intensity exercise. R = Raw, F = Filtered, S = Smoothing. No differences were found (p>0.05).

The figure 12 shows a comparative analyses of the RMS mean values from quadriceps integrated, obtained in supramaximal intensity. Once again we can see that no differences were found among different kinds of EMG treatment (p>0.05), although, like the other two intensities, it shows a tendency to decrease the values encountered in the measure that the procedure of analyses are added to treatment.

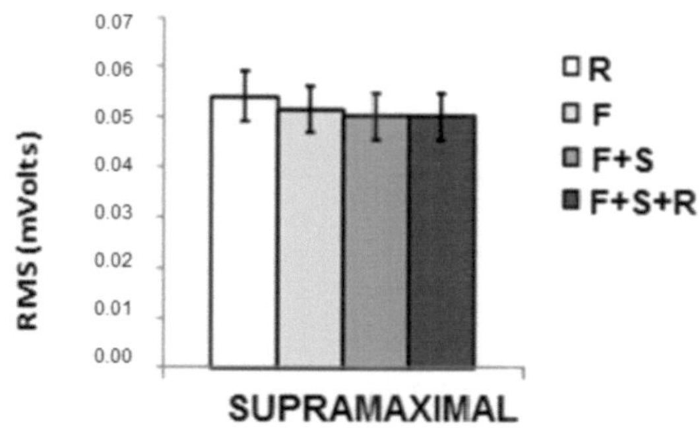

Figure 12. RMS values (mean and standard deviation) from quadriceps integrated muscles ([VL + VM+ RF] ÷ 3) in the different kinds of treatments to supramaximal intensity exercise. R = Raw, F = Filtered, S = Smoothing. No differences were found (p>0.05).

This last one is the one that most called our attention, once that an exercise in this intensity should cause a lot of noises, coming from the exercise (Cross-talk, muscular and skin movement, changes in the conductor tissues) and from the devices (electrode, wire movement, quickly distance change from the devices that capture and record the signal).

The Bland-Altman test shows good concordance between different methods of treatment in the neuromuscular activity to obtain the RMS in all muscles. In submaximal, maximal or supramaximal intensity differences among data weren`t found using as reference always the FSR method.

In trying to find possible influences of the EMG treatments procedures for the RMS value, the results allow us through the comparison and concordance tested to affirm a similar achievement in mVolts, for the muscles in any intensity. Those results shall bring us some perspective about the protocol imposed, where the principal recommendations are the filtering, rectification and smoothing [11]. The final results founded for the treatment of the muscular activity has a identification with a specific baseline achievement always close to zero [15]. Thus, the EMG is a very detailed and disturbed situation because of the sequence of noises, often caused by different reasons of difficulty control. It is worth to say the cross-talk influence, defined by the capitation of electric signal from synergic muscles. This interference normally doesn't surpass 15% of the total signal, but make it very clear the importance of a good location for the electrode. Also, a lot of different reasons can bring those noises, like the pressure, the environment and even the evaluator experience [16,18-20]. Thus, it's clear the necessities of procedures that can eliminate those noises, and give us a signal that really represents the muscular activity.

SUBMAXIMAL (n=20)			BLAND and ALTMAN TEST(μVolt)			
TREATMENTS			ICC	BIAS	LD	UD
RF FRS	and	RF R	0.927	-0.0030	-0.0120	0.0060
RF FRS	and	RF F	1.000	-0.0002	-0.0010	0.0006
RF FRS	and	RF FS	1.000	0.0000	0.0000	0.0000
TREATMENTS RF			0.980	--------	--------	--------
VM_FRS	and	VM_R	0.958	-0.0058	-0.0275	0.0154
VM FRS	and	VM F	1.000	-0.0008	-0.0023	0.0008
VM FRS	and	VM FS	1.000	0.0000	0.0000	0.0000
TREATMENTS VM			0.989	--------	--------	--------
VL FRS	and	VL R	0.830	-0.0050	-0.0247	0.0143
VL FRS	and	VL F	0.999	-0.0008	-0.0023	0.0008
VL FRS	and	VL FS	1.000	0.0000	0.0000	0.0000
TREATMENTS VL			0.959	--------	--------	--------
MAXIMAL (n=20)			BLAND and ALTMAN TEST (μVolt)			
TREATMENTS			ICC	BIAS	LD	UD
RF FRS	and	RF R	0.950	-0.0038	-0.0151	0.0074
RF FRS	and	RF F	1.000	-0.0006	-0.0018	0.0006
RF FRS	and	RF FS	1.000	0.0000	0.0000	0.0000
TREATMENTS RF			0.987	--------	--------	--------
VM FRS	and	VM R	0.994	-0.0039	-0.0075	-0.0004
VM FRS	and	VM F	0.998	-0.0022	-0.0047	0.0003
VM FRS	and	VM FS	1.000	0.0000	0.0000	0.0000
TREATMENTS VM			0,999	--------	--------	--------
VL FRS	and	VL R	0.969	-0.0070	-0.0209	0.0067
VL FRS	and	VL F	0.999	-0.0015	-0.0032	0.0003
VL FRS	and	VL FS	1.000	0.0000	0.0000	0.0000
TREATMENTS VL			0.992	--------	--------	--------
SUPRAMAXIMAL (n=20)			BLAND and ALTMAN TEST (μVolt)			
TREATMENTS			ICC	BIAS	LD	UD
RF FRS	and	RF R	0.970	-0.0022	-0.0063	0.0019
RF FRS	and	RF F	0.999	-0.0004	-0.0016	0.0008
RF FRS	and	RF FS	1.000	0.0000	0.0000	0.0000
TREATMENTS RF			0.993	--------	--------	--------
VM FRS	and	VM R	0.992	-0.0048	-0.0114	0.0016
VM FRS	and	VM F	0.999	-0.0020	-0.0042	0.0003
VM FRS	and	VM FS	1.000	0.0000	0.0000	0.0000
TREATMENTS VM			0.998	--------	--------	--------
VL FRS	and	VL R	0.992	-0.0039	-0.0087	0.0009
VL FRS	and	VL F	0.999	-0.0018	-0.0040	0.0004
VL FRS	and	VL FS	1.000	0.0000	0.0000	0.0000
TREATMENTS VL			0.998	--------	--------	--------

RF: Rectu Femoris; VM: Vastus Medialis; VL: Vastus Lateralis; FRS: Filtered, Rectified, Smooth; R: Raw; F: Filtered; FS: Filtered, Smooth.

Table 3. Intraclass Correlation Coefficient (ICC), Bias Level of treatment (BIAS) and Lower Dispersion (LD) Upper Dispersion (UD) from BIAS in submaximal, maximal and supramaximal exercise.

4.2. Influence of the burst and silence in treatment of EMG signal (Second Study)

The figure 13 present us the RMS comparison between different kinds of analyze (all signal phase and contraction phase) respectively, among muscles: RF, VM and VL in the Wingate Test, no differences were found between methods ($p>0.05$).

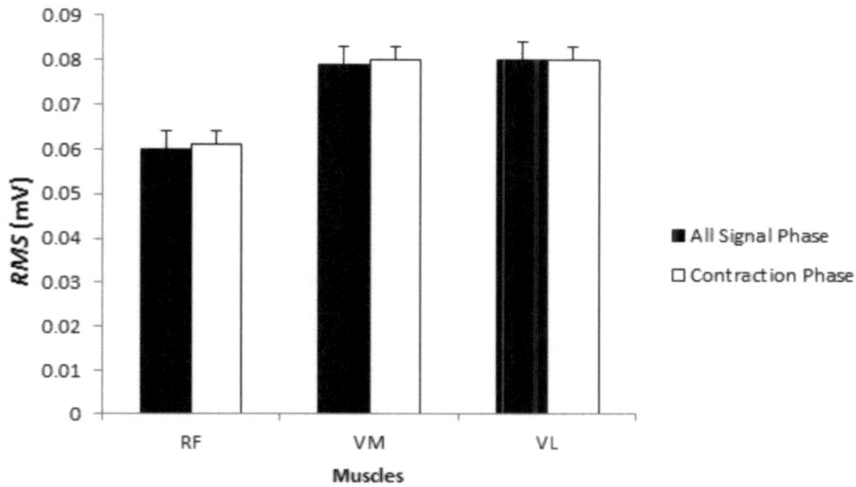

Figure 13. Comparison of root mean square (RMS) between three different muscles from quadriceps femoris (RF = rectus femoris, VM = vastus lateralis, VL = vastus lateralis) in a Wingate Test ($p>0.05$).

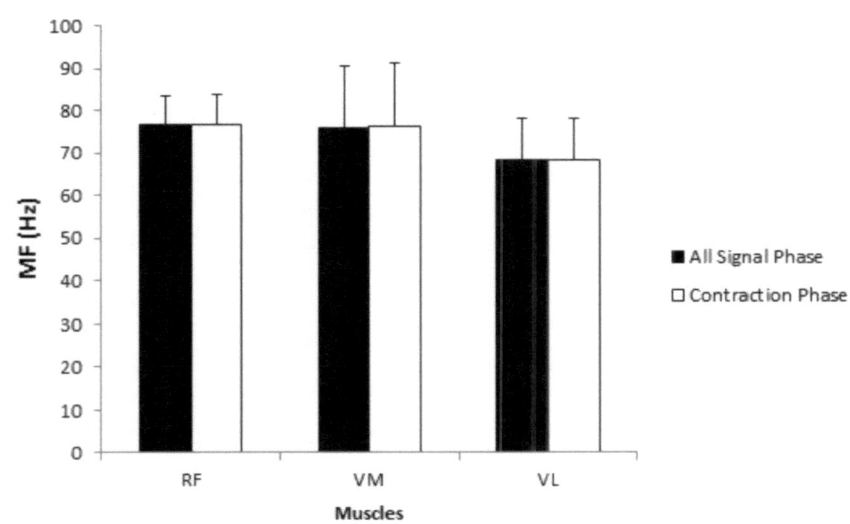

Figure 14. Comparison of Median Frequency (MF) between three different muscles from quadriceps femoris (RF = rectus femoris, VM = vastus lateralis, VL = vastus lateralis) in a Wingate Test ($p>0.05$).

The figure 14 present us the MF comparison between different kinds of analyze (all signal phase and contraction phase) respectively, among muscles: RF, VM and VL in the Wingate test, no differences were found between methods ($p>0.05$).

The results presented above show us that there were no significant difference between the two analyzes. Probably, these results were found because despite the silence moment has power gradient, the amount of lost energy is not enough to change the EMG signal parameters when the whole signal is analyzed. This result should not be transferred to others activity like the golf or to a martial art kick or punch for example due to the different characteristics, where in this sports the motor activity should be analyzed per complete, because during the whole time there is a contraction, so there is a signal amplitude [21-22].

5. Conclusions

We concluded that, although exist many orientations and recommendations to use and apply the electromyography method, sometimes these components can be a path too complex to understand and to respect with closed eyes. In a considerable perspective of study we were able to show with a model of exercise in high intensity, which was capable to produce a lot of noises and variations on the signal, that different methods of process to achieve the muscular activity do not change the final result if used the complete signal or just the burst parts, or still using all sequence of treatment with filtration, rectification and smoothing in many combinations of analyses. Moreover, should be noted that only filtration was sufficient to improve the quality of EMG signal, making us think in keeping the use at least the filtration in electromyography analyses, still this procedure is used to at least maintain the signal inside the muscle activity range, so, it should not be took out just because no significant differences were founded, we have to consider all the process, as said before, like the devices used and the investigator experience. These outcomes show us that we have remained with a critical knowledge to many things and test the main recommendations to use some techniques. In order to make those results clearer and give us more confidence when use the treatments in EMG analyzes. Some studies creating different noises in computer should be made. This way we can be more secure about the removing of noises, securing that the absence of difference is not because a good pre-acquisition was made, securing not enough noises to be cut.

These results and conclusion takes in consideration only cyclic exercise with the intensity used in the studies. Exercises such as isometric or acyclic have different signal waves and so, could have different results to the same treatments. Also, exercises with lower load could change mainly the results in the Burst + Silence (Second Study) results, once that a task such as 10 km in low intensity, would be realized with less intense movements, creating not only different power signals but also different silence and burst time duration.

Still, a more accuracy statistic method could be used, such as The Smallest Worthwhile Change [23], capable to find minimal and almost invisible differences between different methods, that can contribute with good perspective to sports domain when obscure changes exist among several techniques to data process in EMG analysis and if we use a classical statistic we may not identify with probabilities these modulations.

6. Future directions

Although, we should now take the conclusions and think in considerable applicability with our outcomes, we should remain our critical thinking about the theme, about our limitations and keep our considerations related just to our results in this study with these methods and these subjects. We expect that our findings encourage new experiences inside a positive vision in his complete trend to refute ours dogmas and explain in a better way how we should use and respect the recommendations and orientations to electromyography application in human studies, involving different kind of exercise in several intensities and oscillating between isometric and isotonic conditions, testing many aspects that stays around electromyography process and show to the scientific world a great amount of specificities to use this technique taking into account these variables capable to confuse and change the signal with noises, underestimating or overestimating the final value.

Such design, as showed on this chapter should be applied to others tasks with the same characteristics, like running or any other cyclic exercises that has different muscles involved with different activation ranges and other kinds of possible noises, and silence and burst times. Also, different data process should be tested for spectral analyses, like Wavelet families and Fast Fourier Transform (FFT) for different exercises modalities, until it comes to conclusion about the correct use of this technique involving the correct results achievement, signal process and interpretation.

7. Nomenclature

EMG – Electromyography
RMS – Root Mean Square
MIT – Maximal Incremental Test
MWL – Maximal Work Load
CLT – Constant Load Test
Rpm – Revolution per Minute
ISEK - International Society of Electrophysiology and Kinesiology
SENIAM – Surface Electromyography for Non-Invasive Assessment of Muscles
R- Raw signal
F – Filtrated Signal
FS – Filtrated and Smoothed signal
FSR – Signal Filtrated, Smoothed and Rectified
RF – Rectus Femoris
VM – Vastus Medialis
VL – Vastus Lateralis
ICC – Interclass Correlation Coefficient
BIAS – Bias Level of Treatment

LD – Lower Dispersion from BIAS
UD – Upper Dispersion from BIAS
FI – Fatigue Index
PPI – Peak Power Instant
MF – Median
RPP – Relative Peak Power
RMP – Relative Mean Power

Author details

Leandro Ricardo Altimari, José Luiz Dantas,
Marcelo Bigliassi and Thiago Ferreira Dias Kanthack
Group of Study and Research in Neuromuscular System and Exercise,
CEFE - State University of Londrina, Brazil

Antonio Carlos de Moraes
GPNeurom - Laboratory of Electromyography Studies, FEF - State University of Campinas, Brazil

Taufik Abrão
Department of Electrical Engineering, CTU - State University of Londrina, Brazil

Acknowledgement

We are thankful to everyone of the Laboratory of Telecomunications and DSP (Department of Electrical Engineering/CTU, State University of Londrina) and to Dra. Maria Angelica O. C. Brunetto (Department of Computing/CCE, State University of Londrina) that helped with the development of MatLab routine to process the electromyography data and give us the possibility to understand in different perspectives the same cue. The authors thank still the Fundação Araucária do Paraná, the Fundação de Amparo a Pesquisa do Estado de São Paulo (FAPESP), and Conselho Nacional de Desenvolvimento Cientifico e Tecnológico (CNPq) for post-graduate scholarships and supported financially. Finally we say thanks to everybody that meticulously contributed with this work, in your write or review process, and additionally keep in thankful to professor Dr. Ganesh Naik for given us the possibility to be part of this wonderful work, helping others to understand the electromyography in cyclic activities.

8. References

[1] Medved, V. & Cifrek, M. Kinesiological electromyography. Biomechanics in applications.4(7) 2010; 349-366.

[2] Massó, N., Rey, F., Romero, D., GuaL, G., Ccosta, L. & Germám, A. Surface electromyography applications in the sport. Apunts Medicina del I'Esport. 2010;45(165) 121-130.

[3] Camata, T. V., AltimarI, L. R., Bortolotti, H., Dantas, J. L. et al. Electromyographic Activity and Rate of Muscle Fatigue of the Quadriceps Femoris During Cycling Exercise

in the Severe Domain. Journal Strength and Conditioning Research.2011;25(9) 2537-2543.

[4] Andrade, M. M., nascimento, F. A. O. Análise tempo-frequência de sinais eletromiográficos de superfície para a avaliação de fadiga muscular em cicloergômetro. Tese de doutorado, UNB. Brasília. 2006.

[5] Ocarino, J. M., Silva, P. L. P., Vaz, D. V., Aquino, C. F., Brício, R. S., Fonseca, S. T. Eletromiografia: interpretação e aplicações nas ciências da reabilitação. Fisioterapia. Brasil. 2005;6(4) 305-310.

[6] Dantas, J. L., Camata, T. V., Brunetto, M. A. O. C., Moraes, A. C., Abrao, T., Altimari, L. R. Fourier (STFT) and Wavelet (db4) spectral analysis of EMG signals in isometric and dynamic maximal effort exercise. IEEE Engineering in Medicine and Biology Society. Conf. 2010:1(1) 5979-5982.

[7] Vitor-Costa, M., Pereira, L. A., Oliveria, R. S., Pedro, R. E., Camata, T. V., Abrao, T., Brunetto, M. A. O. C.,Altimari, L. R. Fourier (STFT) and Wavelet (db4) spectral analysis of EMG signals in maximal cosntant load dynamic exercise. IEEE Engineering in Medicine and Biology Society. Conf. 2010 : 1(1) 4622-4625.

[8] Camata, T. V., Dantas, J. L., Abrao, T., Brunetto, M. A. O. C., Moraes, A. C., Altimari, L. R. Fourier (STFT) and Wavelet (db4) spectral analysis of EMG signals in supramaximal constant load dymic exercise. IEEE Engineering in Medicine and Biology Society. Conf. 2010: 1(1) 1364 - 1367.

[9] Kamen, G. & Gabriell, D. A. Essentials of electromyography. Champaign, IL: Human Kinetics. 2010.

[10] Farina, D. Interpretation of the surface electromyogram in dynamic contractions. Exercise and Sports Science Review; 2006(34)3 121-7.

[11] Konrad, P. The ABC of EMG: A Practical Introduction to Kinesiological Electromyography. Version 1.0 April, Noraxon INC. USA. 2005

[12] Hermens, H, J., Freriks, B., Disselhorst-klug, C. & Rau, G. Development of recommendations for SEMG sensors and sensor placement procedures. Journal of Electromyography and Kinesiology. 2000;10(5) 361-374.

[13] Pezarat, C. P. & Santos, P. A Electromiografia no Estudo do Movimento Humana. Faculdade de Motricidade Humana. Lisboa. 2004.

[14] Camata, T. V., et al. Association between the electromyographic fatigue threshold and ventilatory threshold. Electromyography and Clinical Neurophysiology. 2009;49(6-7) 102-108.

[15] De luca, C. J., Gilmore, L. D., Kuznetsov, M. & Roy, S. R. Filtering the surface EMG signal: Movement artifact and baseline noise contamination. Journal of Biomechanics. 2010;43 (8) 1573-9

[16] Merletti, R., et al. Surface electromyography for noninvasive characterization of muscle. Exercise and Sports Sciences Reviews. 2001;29(1) 20-25.

[17] Finsterer, J. EMG-interference pattern analysis. Journal of Electromyography and Kinesiology.2011;11(4) 231-46.

[18] Clancy, E. A., Morin, E. L. & Merletti, R. Sampling, noise-reduction and amplitude estimation issues in surface electromyography. Journal of Electromyography and Kinesiology. 2002;1(12) 1-16.

[19] Mclean, L., Chislett, M., Murphy, M. & Walton, P. The effect of head position, electrode site, movement and smoothing window in the determination of a reliable maximum voluntary activation of the upper trapezius muscle. Journal of Electromyography and Kinesiology. 2003;2(13) 169–180.

[20] Disselhorst-klug, C., Schmitz-rode, T. & Rau, G. Surface electromyography and muscle force: Limits in sEMG–force relationship and new approaches for applications. Clinical Biomechanics. 2009;3(24) 225-235.

[21] Vencesbrito, A. M. et al. Kinematic and electromyographic analyses of a karate punch. Journal of Electromyography and Kinesiology. 2011; 21(6) 1023-1029.

[22] Farber, A. J. et al. Electromyographic analysis of forearm muscles in professional and amateur golfers. American Journal of Sports Medicine. 2009;37(2) 396-401.

[23] Hopkins, W. G., et al. Progressive statistics for studies in sports medicine and exercise science. Medicine and Science in Sports and Exercise. 2009; 41(1) 3-13.

Section 2

EMG Analysis and Applications

Chapter 6

Nonlinear Analysis of Surface EMG Signals

Min Lei and Guang Meng

Additional information is available at the end of the chapter

http://dx.doi.org/10.5772/49986

1. Introduction

The aim of this chapter is to answer the essence of SEMG and to explore the potential use of nonlinear analysis as a tool in the clinical and biomechanical applications. The technical tools include nonlinear time series test, time series analysis based on chaos theory, multifractal analysis.

In Section 2, we discuss the two methods of nonlinear time series test: surrogate data test method and Volterra-Wiener-Korenberg (VWK) model test method. Theoretically, the two methods can detect the nonlinearity of the data indirectly. The surrogate data method is used to analyze the SEMG. The result shows that the SEMG has deterministic nonlinear components. Meanwhile, we introduce the VWK model test method and compare it with the surrogate data method. The nonlinearity of SEMG during muscle fatigue can be detected by the VWK.

In Section 3, we describe the time series analysis based on chaos theory. The chaos definition and chaotic characteristics are discussed. The embedding theory of the attractor reconstruction is investigated for the dynamical system. From the view of the fractal structure of the chaotic attractor, the correlation dimension is used to test the chaotic characteristics of the SEMG during arm movements. The Largest Lyapunov exponent is also studied. Then, we investigate the influence of measure noise, internal noise and sampling interval on the principal components of chaotic time series. The symplectic principal component analysis is given. We illustrate the feasibility of this method and give the embedding dimension of the action surface EMG signal.

In Section 4, the self-affine fractal definition and nature are described. The power spectrum and frequency relationship is used to calculate the self-affine fractal dimension of the time series, such as SEMG. Then, the multifractal dimension is given for the SEMG.

The conclusion and future research are shown in Section 5. Here, it is necessary to note that this chapter is actually the result of many years work. The new methods presented here build on a broad and strong foundation of nonlinear time series analysis and chaotic dynamical theory.

2. Detecting nonlinearity of the surface EMG signals

In many areas of science and engineering, it is a critical issue to determine whether an observed time series is purely stochastic, or deterministic nonlinear, even chaotic. One may know about the intrinsic properties of the observed phenomenon by distinguishing between nonlinear deterministic dynamics and noisy dynamics from a time series. In this section, we review and discuss the surrogate data test method[1] and Volterra-Wiener-Korenberg (VWK) model test method[2] for identifying the nonlinearity of a time series. These methods have been successfully used to detect and characterize nonlinear dynamics from recordings in biology and medicine[2-5].

Surrogate analysis is currently an important empirical technique of testing nonlinearity for a time series. The aim is to test whether the dynamics are consistent with linearly filtered noise or a nonlinear dynamical system[1, 6]. The basic idea of the surrogate data method is to first specify some kind of linear stochastic process as a null hypothesis that mimics "linear properties" of the original data. According to the null hypothesis, surrogate data sets are generated. Then, a discriminating statistic is calculated for the original and for each of the surrogate data sets. If the statistic of the original data is significantly different from those of surrogate data sets, the null hypothesis can be rejected within a certain confidence level. It shows that the original data is from a nonlinear dynamical system. The method is demonstrated for numerical time series generated by known chaotic systems and applied to the analysis of SEMG.

VWK test method is a kind of nonlinear detection of time series based on linear and nonlinear Volterra-Wiener-Korenberg model [2, 5]. That is, it first produces the linear and nonlinear predicted data from the original time series and then compares their information criterions to detect the nonlinearity of the raw data. VWK test technique is capable of robust and highly sensitive statistical detection of deterministic dynamics, including chaotic dynamics, in experimental time series. This method is superior to other techniques when applied to short time series, either continuous or discrete, even when heavily contaminated with noise or in the presence of strong periodicity. Later, an extension of the Volterra algorithm (called the numerical titration algorithm) was given to detect and quantify chaos in noisy time series[7]. Here, the surrogate data method and VWK test approach are used to analyze the nonlinearity of surface EMG signals.

2.1. Surrogate data test method

Surrogate data method includes two parts: a null hypothesis and a test statistic. The null hypothesis is a specific process which may or may not adequately explain an origin of the data. The test statistic provides a quantitative description to demonstrate the data sources.

2.1.1. Null hypotheses and algorithms[1]

The null hypotheses usually specify some certain properties of the original data that reflect some structure characteristics of the dynamical system, such as mean and variance, and possibly also the Fourier power spectrum. Different null hypotheses describe different specific dynamical systems. In terms of the corresponding null hypothesis, the surrogate data can be generated so as to test the corresponding specific dynamical system class.

Null hypothesis 1 The observed data is produced by independent and identically distributed (IID) random variables.

For this hypothesis, the corresponding surrogate data can be generated by shuffling the time-order of the original time series so that it has the same mean, variance and amplitude distribution as the original data. But any temporal correlations of the original data are destroyed in the surrogate data. Schienkman and LeBaron[8] applied this hypothesis to analyze stock market returns. Breeden and Packard also used this hypothesis to demonstrate that a time series of quasar data which were sampled nonuniformly in time has some dynamics structure[9].

The algorithm of the null hypothesis is that one first create gaussian random numbers from 1 to N, where N is the length of the original data x. Then, the original data x is permuted by the random numbers to generate the surrogate data.

Null hypothesis 2 The observed data is produced by the Ornstein-Uhlenbeck process.

The surrogate data generated by the Ornstein-Uhlenbeck process is a sequence that has the simplest time correlation. The Ornstein-Uhlenbeck process can be given as follows.

$$x_t = a_0 + a_1 x_{t-1} + \sigma e_t \tag{1}$$

where e_t is a Gaussian random with zero mean and unit variance. The coefficients a_0, a_1, and σ work together to determine the mean, variance, and autocorrelation time of the time series x_t. In this case, its autocorrelation function is exponential form. Let $\lambda = -\log a_1$, $\langle \cdot \rangle$ denotes an average over time t. That is,

$$A(\tau) \equiv \frac{\langle x_t \cdot x_{t-\tau} \rangle - \langle x_t \rangle^2}{\langle x_t^2 \rangle - \langle x_t \rangle^2} = e^{-\lambda|\tau|} \tag{2}$$

In order to generate the surrogate data that is consistent with this hypothesis, the algorithm is that one first calculates the mean μ, variance γ and autocorrelation $A(1)$ (in Eq. (2)) from the original data x. Then, the coefficients in Eq. (1) can be estimated: $a_1 = A(1)$, $a_0 = \mu(1 - a_1)$, and $\sigma^2 = \gamma(1 - a_1^2)$. The Gaussian e_t can be generated by a pseudorandom number generator. Finally, the surrogate data can be produced by iterating Eq. (1).

Null hypothesis 3 The observed data is produced by the linear autocorrelated gaussian process with the mean and variance of the original time series.

The hypothesis has been usually used to test whether the original time series contains nonlinear components. It can be described by using a linear autoregressive (AR) model.

$$x_t = a_0 + \sum_{k=1}^{q} a_k x_{t-k} + \sigma e_t \tag{3}$$

There are the two algorithms to produce the surrogate data in accord with this hypothesis. One algorithm is to directly use Eq.3. That is, the coefficients are firstly identified by using the original data. Then, the surrogate data is generated by repeatedly iterating Eq.3. However, the performance of this algorithm is very unstable. If the values of the coefficients are mis-estimated slightly, this algorithm may lead to the iterative results which easily diverge to infinity. The alternative algorithm is that a surrogate data is generated by randomizing the phases of a Fourier transform. According to the Weiner-Khintchine theorem, the two algorithms are equivalent in essence[1, 10]. The surrogate data has the same Fourier spectrum as the original data. Meanwhile, the algorithm based on the Fourier transform is stabler in the numerical calculation than the first algorithm. The following is the steps of this algorithm.

Let an observed data as $x(n)$. The Fourier transform of $x(n)$ is computed as follows[3]:

$$X(k) = \sum_{n=0}^{N-1} x(n) e^{-2\pi ink/N} \tag{4}$$

The Fourier transform has a complex amplitude at each frequency. One can randomize the phases of the Fourier transform by multiplying $e^{i\varphi}$,

$$X'(k) = X(k) \cdot e^{i\varphi} \tag{5}$$

where φ is independently chosen for each frequency from the [0, 2π]. In order to the inverse Fourier transform to be real (no imaginary components), the phases must satisfy the antisymmetric condition $\varphi(k) = -\varphi(N-k)$. Meanwhile, $\varphi(0) = 0$, $\varphi(N/2) = 0$ (when N is even), so that

$$X'(k) = \overline{X'(N-k)} \tag{6}$$

This point can be easily proved[11].

Proof:

According to the nature of DFT of a real time series $x(n)$, if $x(n) \in R$, then

$$\phi(k) = -\phi(-k) \tag{7}$$

where $\phi(k)$ is the phase angle of $X(k)$. k = 0, 1, … N-1. N is the period of Fourier Transform. Then, for $k = 0$, $k = N/2$ (N is even), there are

$$\phi(0) = -\phi(0), \tag{8}$$

$$\phi(N/2) = -\phi(-N/2) = -\phi(N/2) \tag{9}$$

In order to ensure that the inverse Fourier transform results are real values, there must be

$$\phi(0)=0,\ \phi(N/2)=0.$$

In practical, if the data length N is odd, $\varphi(f_1)=0$, $\varphi(f_i)=-\varphi(f_k)$, $i=2\sim(N+1)/2$, $k=N\sim(N+1)/2+1$; If N is even, $\varphi(f_1)=0$, $\varphi(f_{N/2+1})=0$, $\varphi(f_i)=-\varphi(f_k)$, $i=2\sim N/2$, $k=N\sim N/2+2$. Thus, the surrogate data $x'(n)$ given by the inverse Fourier transform is a sequence of real numbers.

$$x'(n)=\frac{1}{N}\sum_{k=0}^{N-1}X'(k)\cdot e^{2\pi ink/N} \tag{10}$$

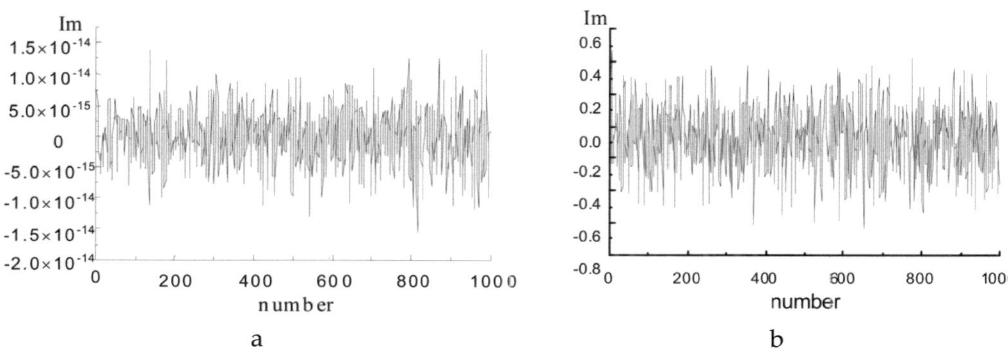

Figure 1. The imaginary components of surrogate data by our (a) and previous (b) FT algorithm

Thus, there are no imaginary components (see Fig. (1a)). The values of the imaginary parts are very little (magnitude 10^{-14}) so that they can be regarded as computing precision errors. The surrogate data has the same Fourier transform spectrum as the original data by using this algorithm. The reproduced "pure" frequencies are very well. Fig.(1b)shows that the previous FT algorithm[1] cannot make the imaginary components of Fourier inverse transform to be zero. So, if one only uses the real part of Fourier inverse transform as surrogate data and omit its imaginary components, the obtained surrogates would have the two limitations[1, 12].

Null hypothesis 4 The observed data is produced by the static nonlinear transform of linear gaussian process.

The static nonlinear transform is that the observation or measure function is nonlinear. The static means that the measure data x_t only depends on the state y_t of the dynamic process at the time t, not on derivatives or values in the past. Let h be a measure function, then

$$x_t = h(y_t) \tag{11}$$

The generated surrogate data not only contain the linear correlated characteristic, but also can reflect the static, monotonic nonlinearity of the original data. Strictly speaking, time series in this class are nonlinear. But this nonlinearity is not from the dynamics. This hypothesis can be used to indicate whether the nonlinearity is from the dynamical system or the amplitude distribution (i.e. the measure process).

For generating surrogate data corresponding to this null hypothesis, an algorithm is described. The aim is to shuffle the time-order of the data x_t and to preserve the linear correlations of the underlying time series $y_t = h^{-1}(x_t)$. The first step is to make a Gaussian time series y_t, where each element is generated independently from a Gaussian pseudorandom number generator. Next, we rescale y_t in accordance with the time-order of the original data x_t. The re-ordered y_t has a time series which "follows" the static, monotonic nonlinearity of the original data. Then, the data y_t' is created by using the above FT algorithm to deal with the re-ordered y_t. Finally, the raw data x_t is rescaled in terms of the time-order of the data y_t' to generate the surrogate data x_t'. The "underlying" time series (y_t and y_t') are Gaussian and have the same Fourier power spectrum. The produced x_t' matches the amplitude distribution of the raw data x_t.

2.1.2. Test statistics[6]

The test statistic is a value which estimates some certain aspects of the time series. To compare the raw data to its surrogate data sets, a suitable test statistic must be selected. A useful statistic should be pivotal and independent of the way that surrogate data sets are generated. In other words, for every data set z and every realization z_i of any $F_i \in F_\phi$, their test statistics should be different, i.e.

$$T(z) \neq T(z_i) \tag{12}$$

where F_ϕ represents the null hypothesis process. Meanwhile, the distribution of T under the null hypothesis does not depend on μ or σ. Here we give two discriminating statistics as follows:

$$T = \overline{(x-\overline{x})^4} \Big/ \overline{(x-\overline{x})^2}^{\,2} \tag{13}$$

$$T = \frac{1}{n-1}\sum_{i=1}^{n-1} \left|(x(i)-\overline{x}) \cdot (x(i+1)-\overline{x})\right| \Big/ \overline{(x-\overline{x})^2} \tag{14}$$

where "$\overline{}$" denotes the average of the data. The mean μ and variance σ have no effect on the T value in Eq. (13). Therefore, some linear structure characteristics can be determined except for the mean and variance. The T value in Eq.(14) can judge if the surrogate data are consist with the raw data in the view of the correlation with the mean and variance. The T value in Eq. (15) is a simple skewed difference statistic that is both rapidly computable and often quite powerful.

$$T = \left\langle (x_{t+m} - x_t)^3 \right\rangle \Big/ \left\langle (x_{t+m} - x_t)^2 \right\rangle \tag{15}$$

where $\langle\cdot\rangle$ is mean operator, m is time delay. This statistic T provides a more significant rejection of the hypothesis of the static nonlinear filter of an underlying linear process. Informally, this statistic indicates the asymmetry between rise and fall times in the time series.

2.1.3. *Performance of surrogate data method based on our FT algorithm[3, 13, 14]*

The surrogate data method is suitable to detect the nonlinearity of a short, noisy time series. Here, a Gaussian data and a Logistic chaotic time series are used to study the performance of surrogate data method. For a two-sided test, the probability of rejecting the null hypothesis is given by the confidence level p, the surrogate data sets B must be at least as large as $B_{\min} = 2/(1-p)-1$. For 95% confidence level, there should be 39 sets of surrogate data.

A Gaussian data x is a random time series with zero mean and unit variance produced by the pseudorandom generator. The data length is 1000 points. According to the null hypothesis 3, 39 sets of surrogate data are generated by using our above FT algorithm. The T value is calculated by Eq. (13) and Eq. (14), respectively. In the Figure (2a and b), there are no statistical discrepancy between the test statistic T of the raw data x and those of surrogate data.

The statistic T values of the raw data are on the range of the empirical distribution of T given by the surrogate data. The results show that the generated surrogate data has the same Fourier transform spectrum as the raw data besides the same mean and variance as the raw data because the T value in Eq. (14) is a measure of the time irreversibility of the data. The null hypothesis 3 is accepted at the confidence level 95%. The raw data is consistent with the stochastic process of the null hypothesis 3. The surrogate data produced by the above FT algorithm is equivalent to the raw data. The generated surrogate data reflects the null hypothesis 3.

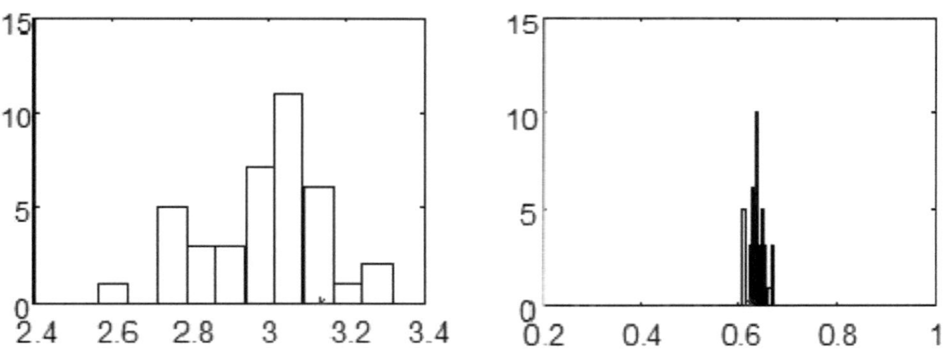

a. T calculated by Eq. (13) b. T calculated by Eq. (14)

Figure 2. The histogram is T distribution of surrogate data given by FT algorithm, * is T value of the original data, where abscissa is T, ordinate is the number of surrogate data sets

To further test that the surrogate data based on the above FT algorithm can be used to detect nonlinearity of a time series, we apply the Logistic chaotic system to produce a chaotic time series as follows.

$$x_{t+1} = \alpha x_t (1 - x_t) + e \tag{16}$$

where $\alpha = 3.9$, $x_0 \in [0,1]$, e is white noise with mean 0, variance 0.001^2. If e takes part in the evolution process of the above equation, it is called as interior noise (or dynamic noise); otherwise it is called as measure noise.

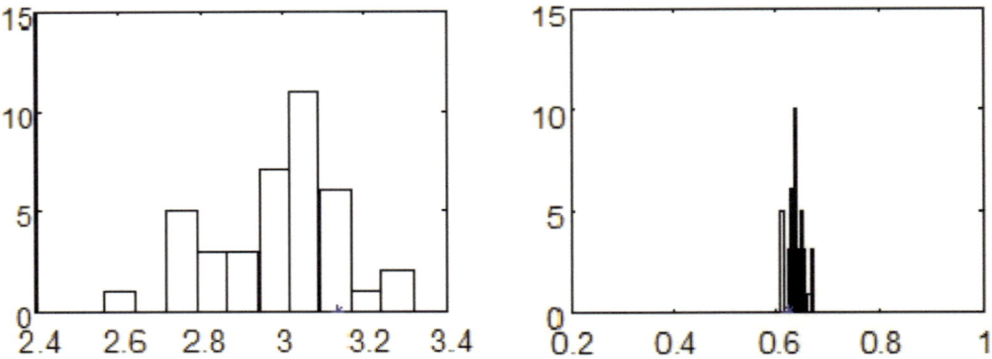

a. The length N=5000 of the raw time series b. The length N=500 of the raw time series

Figure 3. *T* calculated by Eq. (13), histogram is *T* distribution of surrogate data, * is *T* value of the original data, where abscissa is *T*, ordinate is the number of surrogate data sets

For the case without noise $e = 0$, we use Eq. (16) to compute the two Logistic chaotic time series with the length of 5000 points and 500 points. 39 surrogate data generated by the above FT algorithm contain the linear properties of the original data in terms of the null hypothesis 3. In Fig.3, we can see the obvious difference between the original data and its surrogate data, regardless of the length of 5000 points or 500 points. The null hypothesis can be rejected in 95% confidence level. The original data has nonlinear components. The results show that the data length has little effect on the surrogate data method based on the above FT algorithm. In Figure 4, we study the nonlinear test of Logistic chaotic time series with measure noise and interior noise, respectively. The data length is 1000 points. According to the null hypothesis, 39 sets of surrogate data are generated. The statistic *T* for the original data is significantly different from the values obtained for the surrogate data sets. The null hypothesis 3 can also be rejected in 95% significance. The nonlinearity of the original data can be detected. To sum up, the length and noise has no impact on the surrogate data method based on our FT algorithm.

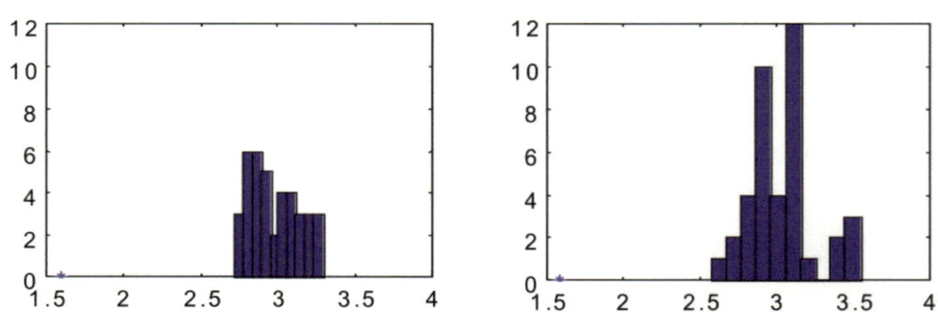

a. Chaos time series with measure noise b. Chaos time series with interior noise

Figure 4. *T* calculated by Eq.(13), histogram is *T* distribution of surrogate data, * is *T* value of the original data, where abscissa is *T*, ordinate is the number of surrogate data sets

2.1.4. Nonlinear test of surface EMG signal based on surrogate data[3, 13, 14]

The nature of SEMG plays an important role in neuromuscular disorder diagnosis, muscle fatigue monitoring, prosthesis control, etc. Here the analyzed data are collected from physiological instruments. Humid surface electrode and AD12-16LG collecting card of physiology signal are used in the whole experiment that was done at Hua Shan Hospital in Shanghai. The data are sampled at 1kHz for the action surface EMG (ASEMG) [3]and the fatigue surface EMG (FSEMG) when one hand carries a 1kg heavy thing [15](see Fig. 5). The length of data for ASEMG is 1000 points during the beginning of action because this time span contains the information of the forearm movement. In the case of carrying a 1kg heavy thing, the length of FSEMG data is also 1000 points when the arm has been fatigue.

For these surface EMG signals, 39 surrogate data are produced by the null hypothesis 2. The surrogate data analysis is given for the action surface EMG signal and the fatigue surface EMG signal, respectively(see Fig. 6). The results show that for action surface EMG signal and fatigue surface EMG signal, their T values are obviously different from those of surrogate data in terms of Eq.13. The null hypothesis 2 can be rejected in 95% degree of confidence. The action surface EMG signal and fatigue surface EMG signal is not stochastic signal produced by a linear stochastic process, but contains nonlinear components. However, this result could not ensure that this nonlinearity must be from the dynamic system.

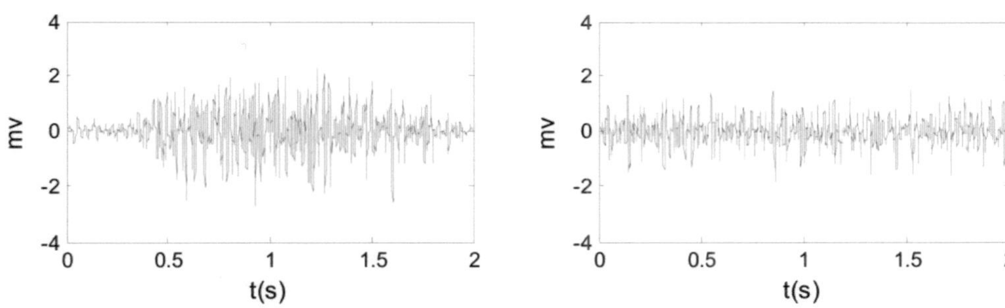

a. a typical action surface EMG wave

b. a typical fatigue surface EMG wave

Figure 5. The surface EMG signals

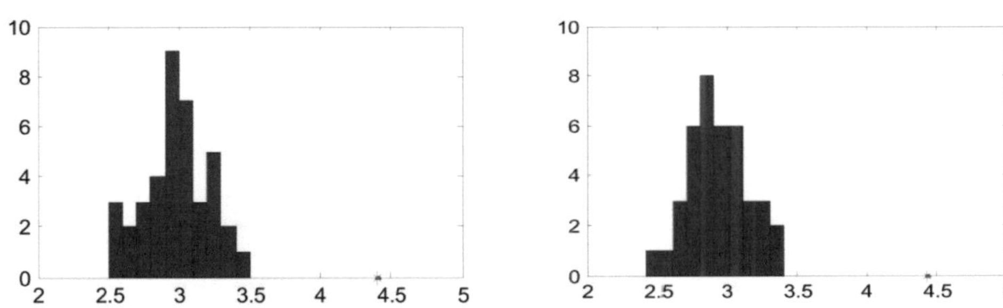

a. action surface EMG signal

b. fatigue surface EMG signal

Figure 6. Surrogate data analysis of surface EMG signal. * is T_{orig}, histogram is T_{surr} distribution of surrogate data

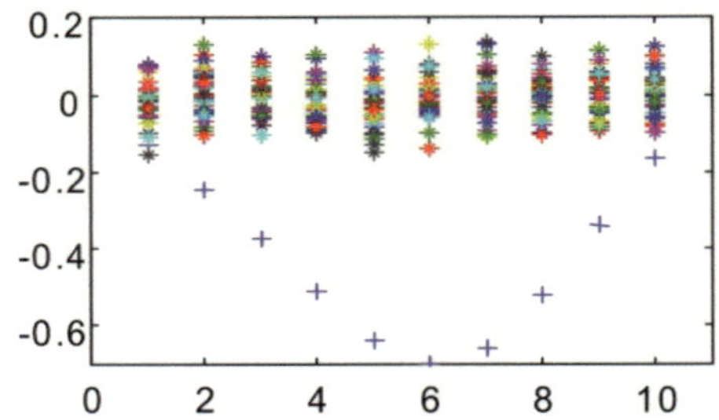

Figure 7. Surrogate data test of surface EMG signal during movement, where surrogate data sets are 39 sets; * is *T* value of surrogate data by the null hypothesis 4, +is *T* value of EMG signal, where *T* is calculated by Eq. 15

In order to test that the nonlinear components are intrinsic deterministic, we further assume that ASEMG is stochastic signal consistent with the null hypothesis 4. Fig.7 gives the *T* values of ASEMG and surrogate data calculated by Eq. 15. This statistic indicates the asymmetry between rise and fall times in the time series. From this figure, we can see that there is the difference between data and surrogates, and the null hypothesis 4 is rejected in 95% credibility. This result shows that the nonlinearity of ASEMG is intrinsic and deterministic.

2.2. Volterra-Wiener-Korenberg test method

2.2.1. Volterra-Wiener-Korenberg test model[2]

For a dynamic system, an observed time series $\{y_n\}_{n=1}^{N}$ can be treated as a closed loop Volterra series by utilizing the feedback of y_n. Suppose the time series is univariate. A discrete Volterra-Winner-Korenberg series can be calculated as follows:

$$\begin{aligned} y_n^{cala} &= a_0 + a_1 y_{n-1} + a_2 y_{n-2} + \cdots + a_k y_{n-k} + a_{k+1} y_{n-1}^2 + a_{k+2} y_{n-1} y_{n-2} + \cdots + a_{M-1} y_{n-k}^d \\ &= \sum_{m=0}^{M} a_m z_m(n) \end{aligned} \tag{17}$$

where the memory *k* and combination degree *d* correspond to the embedding dimension and the degree of nonlinearity of the model, respectively. The coefficients a_m are recursively estimated through a Gram-Schmidt procedure from linear and nonlinear autocorrelations of the data itself with a total dimension $M=(k+d)!/(d!k!)$.

There is the following information criterion in accordance with the parsimony principle:

$$C(r) = \log \varepsilon(r) + r/N \tag{18}$$

$$\varepsilon(k,d)^2 \equiv \frac{\sum_{n=1}^{N} (y_a^{calc}(k,d) - y_n)^2}{\sum_{n=1}^{N} (y_n - \bar{y})^2} \tag{19}$$

where $r \in [1, M]$ is the number of polynomial terms of the truncated Volterra expansions from the given pair $\{k, d\}$, $\varepsilon(k,d)^2$ is a normalized variance of the error residuals, $\bar{y} = \frac{1}{N}\sum_{n=1}^{N} y_n$. For d=1, VWK model is linear, whereas the model is nonlinear for d>1.

For each data series, there is the following numerical procedure to search for the optimal pair $\{k_{opt}, d_{opt}\}$:

1. when d=1, search for k_{opt} which minimizes $C(r)$.
2. with k=k_{opt}, increasing d>1, search for d_{opt} which minimizes $C(r)$.
3. calculate $C^{lin}(r)$ with d=1 and k=M-1, and $C^{nl}(r)$ with d=d_{opt} and k=k_{opt}.
4. Compare $C^{lin}(r)$ and $C^{nl}(r)$, if $C^{nl}(r)$ is obviously smaller than $C^{lin}(r)$, then the original system dynamics is nonlinear, the obtained time series is nonlinear, even chaos; otherwise, the original system dynamics is linear, the raw data is linear.

Note that when k_{opt} is rather large, M is quite large, too, then the computational time will rapidly go up. In this case, k and d should be adjusted synchronously to search for k_{opt} and d_{opt} so as to make $C^{nl}(r) < C^{lin}(r)$. Furthermore, one can obtain the corresponding linear and nonlinear models for surrogate data generated by the FT algorithm according to the null hypothesis 3 so that $C_{orig}^{lin}(r), C_{surr}^{lin}(r), C_{surr}^{nl}(r) > C_{orig}^{nl}(r)$ in the statistical sense.

2.2.2. *Analysis of SEMG based on VWK method[15, 16]*

Here, the VWK method is used to deal with the surface EMG signals in Fig.5. For the action surface EMG signal, $C^{lin}(r)$ is almost equal to $C^{nl}(r)$, i.e. $C^{lin}(r) \approx C^{nl}(r)$, this technique can hardly detect its nonlinearity (see Fig.8a). For the fatigue surface EMG signal, $C^{nl}(r)$ is distinctly smaller than $C^{lin}(r)$ so that its nonlinear component can be detected (see Fig.8b). So VWK technique can effectively detect the nonlinear dynamic speciality of fatigue surface EMG signal but fails to test the nonlinearity of the action surface EMG signal. In other words, VWK technique can not be used directly to deal with the action surface EMG signal.

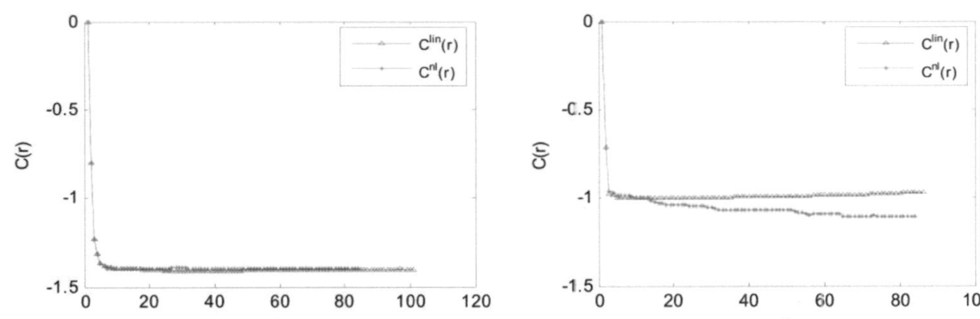

a. The action surface EMG signal   b. The fatigue surface EMG signal

Figure 8. VWK test analysis of surface EMG signal

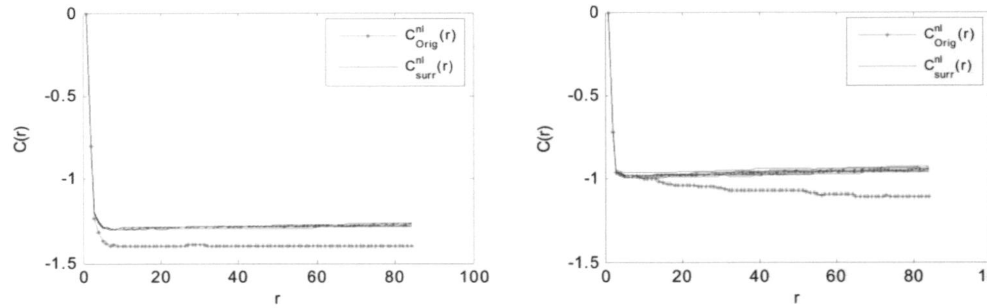

a. The action surface EMG signal   b. The fatigue surface EMG signal

Figure 9. VWK combined with surrogate analysis of surface EMG signal. solid is $C^{nl}_{surr}(r)$, * is $C^{nl}_{orig}(r)$

2.2.3. Analysis of SEMG based on VWK method with surrogate data[16]

In order to detect the nonlinearity of the action surface EMG signal, 39 FT-based surrogate data are used according to the null hypothesis 3. The generated surrogate data contain the linear properties of the raw data. Figure 9 is the analysis of surface EMG signal based on VWK with surrogate data. We can see that no matter whether it is the action or fatigue EMG signal, $C^{nl}_{orig}(r)$ is always smaller than $C^{nl}_{surr}(r)$. The null hypothesis 3 can be rejected in 95% significance. The results illuminate that the action and fatigue surface EMG signals contain nonlinear dynamic properties.

3. Analysis of the surface EMG signals based on chaos theory

The discovery of chaotic phenomena is the third major breakthrough in the 20th century physics scientific community following the creation of relativity and quantum mechanics. It organically combines the two major theoretical systems of determinism and probabilism that have long been debated to create a scientific model of a new paradigm, so that people can use some simple rules to explain seemingly stochastic information in the past[17-19]. The practical significance that finds chaotic phenomena is to recognize that a deterministic nonlinear system can have inherent uncertainty. Perhaps a system has only a few degrees of freedom, but it can produce complex, similar to the random output signal. In the past, one could only denote a random-looking data as a random process from the view of the traditional time series analysis. The statistical methods or random time series models were used to analyze the data. Since the chaotic phenomenon was discovered by Lorenz[17], people have begun to reunderstand and restudy these random-looking signals so as to reveal the inherent deterministic mechanisms of these signals. That is, it is to explore that the systems which generate these signals may contain essentially deterministic characteristics. Chaos phenomenon breaks the path that the regularity is found in a lot of completely different systems. This will lead to a revolution in the field of influence of various disciplines. It is chaos to lead people to explore the complexity in nature.

At present, the idea of Chaos has been introduced into the analysis of time series to create the field of chaotic time series analysis. Since the inception of chaotic time series analysis, it has quickly been penetrated into other disciplines and engineering fields. Thus it becomes the most active branch of the modern nonlinear dynamics. This section describes the chaos definition and the phase space reconstruction of chaotic time series, discusses some parameters that are used to analysis chaotic time series, such as the correlation dimension and Lyapunov exponent, study the principal component analysis methods based on SVD, and propose the symplectic principal component method based on symplectic geometry. Then we use these methods to investigate the surface EMG signals.

3.1. Chaos and its definition

Chaos is "order in disorder". The order means its deterministic nature. The disorder means that the final results can be unpredictable for a long time. As a scientific concept, chaos generally denotes that the long-term dynamical behavior of a deterministic nonlinear system manifests as a random-looking behavior. Mathematically speaking, "chaos" has not been a unified strict definition. For the definition of chaos, there are at least nine different definitions, where the three definitions given by Li-Yorke, Devaney, Marotto are more commonly used. Here describes the definition of chaos by Li-Yorke[18].

Li-Yorke Theorem: Let $f(x)$ as a continuous self-map in $[a,b]$. If $f(x)$ has a periodic point with period 3, then for any positive integer n=1, 2, 3, ..., there is a periodic point with period n.

This is the famous period 3 theorem. It becomes a milestone in the development history of chaos theory and promotes the creation and development of chaos theory. From this theorem, the first formal mathematical definition of the chaos is given.

Chaos definition: Let $f(x)$ as a continuous self-map in closed interval I, i.e.

$$f: I \to I \subset R^m, \quad y = f(x) \tag{20}$$

where $x, y \in I$. If $m=1$, f is one-dimensional mapping. If $m \neq 1$, f is multi-dimensional mapping. Denote the n times iteration of f as $f^n(x)$. If Eq.20 satisfies the following conditions, then it has chaotic motion:

1. The period of periodic point of f has no upper bound.
2. There is an uncountable set $S \subset I$, which satisfies the following conditions:

$$\lim_{n\to\infty} \sup \left| f^n(x) - f^n(y) \right| > 0, \qquad \forall x, y \in S, \quad x \neq y \tag{21}$$

$$\lim_{n\to\infty} \inf \left| f^n(x) - f^n(y) \right| = 0, \qquad \forall x, y \in S \tag{22}$$

$$\lim_{n\to\infty} \sup \left| f^n(x) - f^n(p) \right| > 0, \qquad \forall x \in S, \quad \forall p \in P(f) \tag{23}$$

where $P(f) \underline{\underline{\Delta}} \{x \mid x \text{ is a periodic point of } f\}$.

This definition explains "existence" of chaos in mathematics. According to the above theorem and the definition, the description of chaotic motion is different from the general periodic and quasi-periodic motion. Its motion is not a single periodic orbit but an envelope for a bunch of tracks, where the infinite number of countable stable periodic orbits and uncountable stable aperiodic orbits are embedded densely. Meanwhile, there is at least one unstable aperiodic orbit. Overall, the chaos not only contains some inherent regularity, but also shows that the system has ergodicity. That is, the system has a long-term unpredictability. In other words, the long-term behavior of the system can not be predicted if the system displays the so-called "sensitive dependence on initial conditions". The meaning of this definition is that the aperiodicity of chaotic system is exhibited accurately. For a dynamical system, the observable behaviour was called stochastic in the past. In fact, it can be random-looking, i.e. "stochastic behaviour occurring in a deterministic system". Therefore, it is challenging to quantitatively describe the nature of chaotic dynamics and distinguish between the so-called random and chaotic motions from a time series, especially from an experimental time series. At present, chaotic time series analysis methods have been widely attention in fields of mathematics, physics, biology, biomedicine, robotics, geology, engineering, economics, finance, and so on.

3.2. Phase space reconstruction theory

3.2.1. Phase space reconstruction

Phase space reconstruction is generally the first step of chaotic time series analysis from a time series data. The dynamic characteristic of the system can be explored through phase space reconstruction of the original time series so that the mechanism of the original system can be revealed from the original time series[20]. It has been proved by the so-called Takens' embedding theorem[21]. According to the theorem, the reconstructed phase space can maintain the invariance of geometry for the original dynamical system[22], such as the characteristic value of the fixed point, the fractal dimension of the attractor, the Lyapunov exponent in the phase space orbit, and so on.

Definition 1: Let (N,ρ) and (N_1,ρ_1) as two metric spaces. If the mapping $\varphi : N \rightarrow N_1$ satisfies ① φ is a surjection; ② $\rho(x,y) = \rho_1(\varphi x, \varphi y)$, then (N,ρ) and (N_1,ρ_1) are called as the isometric isomorphism.

Definition 2: If (N_1,ρ_1) is isometric isomorphism with a subspace (N_0,ρ_2) of another metric space (N_2,ρ_2), then (N_1,ρ_1) can be embedded into (N_2,ρ_2).

Theorem 1: Let M be a compact manifold of dimension m. For pairs (φ, x), $\varphi : M \rightarrow M$ a smooth diffeomorphism and $x : M \rightarrow R$ a smooth function, it is a generic property that the map $\phi_{(\varphi,x)} : M \rightarrow R^{2m+1}$ is an embedding, where $\phi_{(\varphi,x)}(y) = \{x(y), x(\varphi(y)), \cdots, x(\varphi^{2m}(y))\}$.

In terms of the above definitions and theorem, $\phi_{(\varphi,x)}(y) = \{x(y), x(\varphi(y)), \cdots, x(\varphi^{2m}(y))\}$ is a subspace of R^{2m+1}. $\phi_{(\varphi,x)}$ and the subspace are isometric isomorphic. Then the manifold M of dimension m can be embedded into R^{2m+1}. In other words, $\phi_{(\varphi,x)}$ is an embedding of

$M \to R^{2m+1}$. For a practical time series $\{x_t\}$, the state of the original system is equivalent to the m-dimensional manifold M. In fact, $\{x_t\}$ is a signal observed in the m-dimensional manifold M. If let $\varphi : y_t \to y_{t-\tau_d}$, φ is a smooth diffeomorphism. y_t denotes the state of the system M at time t. τ_d is the delay time. The signal observed in M at time t consist of $\{x_t, x_{t-\tau_d}, \cdots, x_{t-2m\tau_d}\}$, where $x_t = x(y_t)$, $x_{t-\tau} = x(y_{t-\tau_d}) = x(\varphi(y))$, ..., $x_{t-2m\tau_d} = x(\varphi^{2m}(y))$. $\phi_{(\varphi,x)} = (x_t, x_{t-\tau_d}, \cdots, x_{t-2m\tau_d})$ is an embedding of $M \to R^{2m+1}$. The manifold M is diffeomorphic with $\{x_t, x_{t-\tau_d}, \cdots, x_{t-2m\tau_d}\}$. If the embedding dimension is greater than 2 times the dimension m of the attractor of the original system, the phase space with the base of the practical signal delay time coordinates is equivalent to the state space of the original system. That is, Takens' embedding theorem states that if the time series is indeed composed of scalar measurements of the state from a dynamical system, then under certain genericity assumptions, a one-to-one image of the original set $\{x\}$ is given by the time-delay embedding, provided d is large enough. At present, the delay coordinate method has been widely used to give the phase space reconstruction from the original signal.

For a time series $x(t)$ observed by the measure function h, i.e.

$$x(t) = h(Y) \tag{24}$$

the vector $\overline{X}_t$ can be constructed as follows,

$$\overline{X}_t = (x(t), x(t-\tau_d), x(t-2\tau_d), \cdots, x(t-(d-1)\tau_d))^T \tag{25}$$

where τ_d is an integer multiple of the sampling interval τ, called as the lag time or delay time. d is and embedding dimension, $d \geq 2m+1$. m is an attractor dimension of the original system.

3.2.2. *Problems in phase space reconstruction*

Takens' embedding theorem offers in the absence of noise, the possibility of reconstructing n-dimensional dynamics from one-dimensional infinite data of one observable-measurable system. This means that in the case of any delay time, a time series can always be embedded into the state space of the system, and when the embedding dimension is sufficiently large, reconstructed space and embedded space is almost one-to-one correspondence. Therefore, one can reconstruct a phase space from an experimental time series so as to estimate dynamical invariants of the time series, such as dimensions, Lyapunov exponents, entropies[21, 23, 24] and so on. However, the embedding theorem does not directly answer how to choose embedding dimension d and delay time t. In practical application, the experimental data is always limited and noisy so that the estimation of the above parameters presents some difficulties[25, 26]. Accuracy of the phase space reconstruction is critically important to the estimation of invariant measures characterizing system behavior. The choice of delay time τ_d and embedding dimension d always has a great impact on the phase space reconstruction.

Some researchers have studied the choice of delay time τ_d [26-30]. If the delay time τ_d is too small, the reconstructed attractor will be crowded around the main diagonal, which is called as redundance. If τ_d is too large, the dynamic shape of the attractor will be broken, which is called as irrelevance, and the phase space reconstruction is no longer representative of the true dynamics in the real system[28]. In normal circumstances, in order to make the elements of $\overline{Y}_t$ independent, τ_d is the same for all the embedding dimension *d*[27-29]. The autocorrelation function method and mutual information technique[30] have been most commonly used to give the delay time τ_d although the issue of the delay time choice has still been completely resolved.

For the embedding dimension *d*, there are three methods that are usually used to choose the appropriate embedding dimension, including the correlation dimension, singular value decomposition(SVD), the false neighbors[21, 31, 32]. The correlation dimension method is to estimate appropriate dimension *d* in terms of the correlation theorem[8, 21, 33]. By increasing the embedding dimension, one notes an appropriate dimension d when the value of the correlation dimension stops changing. Broomhead and King[31] used the singular value decomposition (SVD) technique to determine an appropriate embedding dimension *d* directly from the raw time series. The false neighbor method is based on the fact that choosing a too low embedding dimension results in points, which are far apart in the original phase space, being moved closer together in the reconstruction space[32]. Besides, there are also some other methods and modified extensions developed based on the above methods. However, there are still problems on how to determine the appropriate embedding dimension from a scalar time series[34-38].

3.3. Correlation dimension

If a system is chaotic, the strange attractor in a region of the phase space constitutes an infinite hierarchy of self-similar structure, i.e. a fractal structure. One can use quantitative measures to define the fractal nature. The correlation dimension is a useful measurement. Grassberger and Proccacia give a kind of computation method, called GP algorithm[33, 39, 40].

3.3.1. GP algorithm of correlation dimension

Let $X_1, X_2, \ldots, X_n$ be a point of the attractor in phase space. $C_l(X_j)$ is denoted as a hypersurface sphere with the radius l at the reference point X_j. $\mu[C_l(X_i)]$ is the probability that X_i (i=1, ..., n) falls into $C_l(X_j)$, as follows.

$$\mu[C_l(X_j)] = \frac{1}{n}\sum_{i=1}^{n}\theta(l - \|X_i - X_j\|) \tag{26}$$

where $\|\bullet\|$ is Euclidean norm. $\theta(r)$ is Heaviside function whose value is 1 if $r \geq 0$, otherwise, zero.

Then a correlation integral function is defined as

$$C(l) = \frac{1}{n^2} \sum_{i=1}^{n} \sum_{j=1}^{n} \theta(l - \|X_i - X_j\|) \tag{27}$$

with $l \to 0$, there are a scaling relation $C(l) \propto l^{D_2}$ between the correlation integral $C(l)$ and l. A correlation dimension D_2 is defined.

$$D_2 = \lim_{l \to 0} \frac{\ln C(l)}{\ln(l)} \tag{28}$$

In practical computation, D_2 is the slope of log C vs log l curve over a selected straight line range.

3.3.2. Correlation dimension theorem[41]

Theorem 2: Let a map $G: R^n \to R^n$. A is an attractor of map G that has only a finite number of periodic points of period P. Under a natural probability measure μ, the correlation dimension of A is $D_2(\mu)$. For a measure function h of A, $h: R^n \to R$, define a delay coordinate map $F_h: R^n \to R^d$ as

$$F_h(X) = [h(X), h(G^{-1}(X)), \cdots, h(G^{-(d-1)}(X))] \tag{29}$$

where $d \geq P$. $F_h(\mu)$ is a natural probability measure in R^d of $F_h(A)$. If $d \geq D_2(\mu)$, then for almost every h, $D_2(F_h(\mu)) = D_2(\mu)$.

The theorem says that with the embedding dimension increasing, the slope of corresponding correlation integral curve will converge to the correlation dimension D_2 of the original system attractor. Therefore, the optimal embedding dimension can be estimated by using the correlation dimension D_2. That is, if the embedding dimension $d \geq D_2$, the slope of the correlation integral curve is equal to the correlation dimension. This also indicates that the dimension estimation actually does not have to meet the requirements of the embedding theorem on the embedding dimension $d \geq 2D_2 + 1$. When the embedding dimension $d \geq D_2$, the reconstructed attractor can contain the fractal structural feature of the original system attractor to reflect the chaotic characteristics of the original system. Correlation dimension has been widely used in the analysis of chaotic time series.

3.3.3. Chaotic test based on correlation dimension

Chaos has a fractal structure so that the corresponding correlation dimension D_2 is a fractional value. The estimation of correlation dimension D_2 from a time series can be used to determine whether the time series is chaotic. If D_2 is fractional, the original time series can have chaotic features, otherwise, it cannot be chaotic. According to the correlation dimension theorem, when the embedding dimension d of the reconstructed phase space is increased to a certain value, the correlation dimension D_2 will be saturated. Then, the optimal embedding dimension d will be given from a time series. The corresponding correlation dimension D_2 is called as the correlation dimension of this time series.

Lorenz chaotic time series is given by the state variable x of Lorenz system as follows.

$$\begin{cases} \dfrac{dx}{dt} = \sigma(y - x) \\ \dfrac{dy}{dt} = rx - y - xz \\ \dfrac{dz}{dt} = -bz + xy \end{cases} \tag{30}$$

where σ=10, b=8/3, γ=28, initial conditions: $x(0)$=5, $y(0)$=5, $z(0)$=15. The sampling interval τ=0.1. The sampling points N=1000. For delay time $\tau_d=\tau$, the corresponding correlation dimension values are given in Table 1 when the embedding dimension d is increased from 2 to 12. From this table, we can see that the correlation dimension of the time series is about 2.07. The result shows that the reconstructed attractor has a fractal structure to reflect the chaotic feature of the system. The time series can reconstruct the state space of the original system when the embedding dimension d=6.

Logistic chaotic time series $\{x_n\}_{n=1}^{N}$ is given by Logistic system in Eq.16 with α=3.9 and e =0. The length N is 1000 points. Here, τ_d=1 (i.e. discrete time series interval). With increasing the embedding dimension d, the corresponding correlation dimension is 0.97 (see Table 2). The optimal embedding dimension is 2.

For finite sampling number (e.g. N=1000), the reconstructed attractor will be broken when the embedding dimension d is increased continuously to a higher value. The estimation of correlation dimension will fail during computation. Therefore, embedding dimension d should not be unlimitedly increased.

d	2	3	4	5	6	7	8	9	10	11	12
D_2	1.8009	1.9284	1.9718	2.0389	2.0737	2.0966	2.086	2.0788	2.0705	2.0760	2.0753

Table 1. The analysis of correlation dimensions of Lorenz chaos time series

d	1	2	3	4	5	6	7	8	9	10	11
D_2	0.9598	0.9718	0.9689	0.9713	0.9718	0.9591	0.9774	0.9621	0.9827	0.9826	0.9839

Table 2. The analysis of correlation dimensions of Logistic chaos time series

3.3.4. The analysis of surface EMG signal based on correlation dimension

From the above analysis, we can see that the surface EMG signal has deterministic nonlinear component. Here, the correlation dimension is further used to study whether its nonlinear component are chaotic. Figure 10a shows a raw data for forearm pronation. Figure 10b gives the correlation integral curve of the data under the embedding dimension from 2 to 12. In the recontructed phase space, the delay time τ_d is chosen as the sampling interval. With the increase of embedding dimension, the straight line segments of the computed correlation integral curves will tend to be parallel and keep unchange in the range.

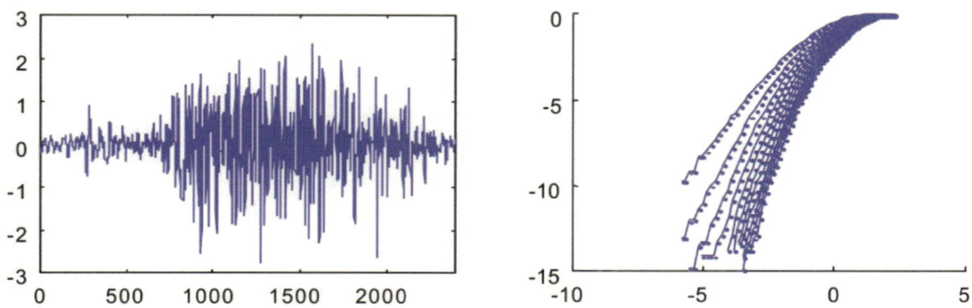

a. The original data

b. The correlation integral curves of data in Fig. a

Figure 10. The correlation dimension analysis of surface EMG signal

The corresponding slope value is the correlation dimension of the surface EMG signal, about 3.8050 ± 0.0560(see Table 3). The result indicates that the surface EMG signal during movement has fractal feature to reveal the implied chaotic motion behavior. Table 3 shows that the reconstructed attractor contains the nature of the raw system when the embedding dimension is over 6.

d	2	3	4	5	6	7	8	9	10	11	12
D_2	1.9315	2.7037	3.2808	3.4837	3.8047	3.7597	3.8511	3.8864	3.8129	3.7160	3.8039

Table 3. The analysis of correlation dimension of surface EMG signal during movement

3.3.5. Study of surrogate data test method based on correlation dimension

The correlation dimension is a quantitative index that describes the fractal structure of chaotic attractor. It measures the freedom degree and complexity of the system. For the raw data and all data of $F \in F_{\phi}$, in the case of the same embedding dimension, the corresponding test results will be obviously significant[42]. Here, the correlation dimension is used as a test statistic to analyze the surface EMG signal. According to the null hypothesis 3, 39 sets of surrogate data are produced in confidence level 95%. In order to quickly obtain the correlation dimension in a variety of circumstances, the linear parts of all correlation integral curves are taken as the same. Though these values are not accurate, this test algorithm is great effective to test the chaotic fractal feature of the experimental data.

When the sampling interval τ=1, Figure 11a and b show the results of the surrogate data test analysis for Lorenz chaotic time series based on correlation dimension. There are significant differences between the original data and its surrogate data in m = 5 (see Fig. 11a). This result explains that the null hypothesis can be rejected in confidence level 95%. The

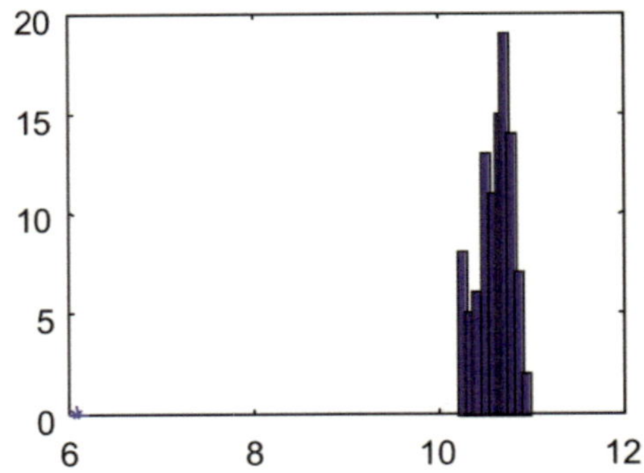

a. * is D_2 value of raw data in $m = 5$, $\tau = 1$ histogram is D_2 distribution of surrogate data, abscissa is D_2, ordinate is histogram

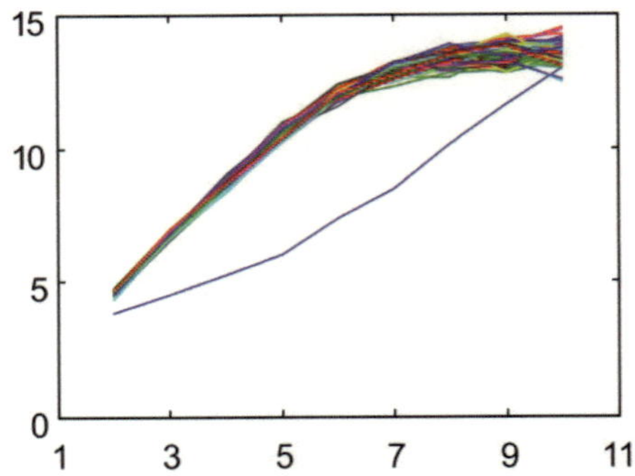

b. The D_2 curves of raw data and surrogate data with m, abscissa is m=2~10, ordinate is D_2

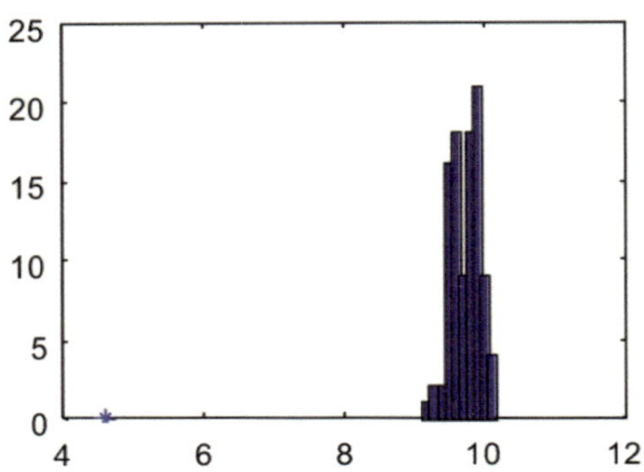

c. * is D_2 value of raw data in $m = 4$, τ=0.1 histogram is D_2 distribution of surrogate data, abscissa is D_2, ordinate is histogram

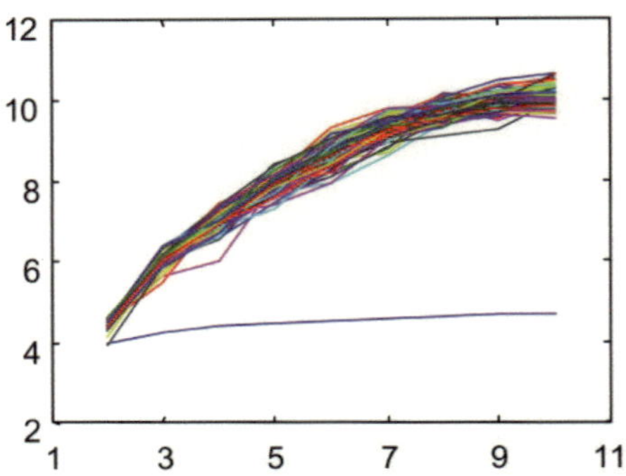

d. The D_2 curves of raw data and surrogate data with m, abscissa is m=2~10, ordinate is D_2

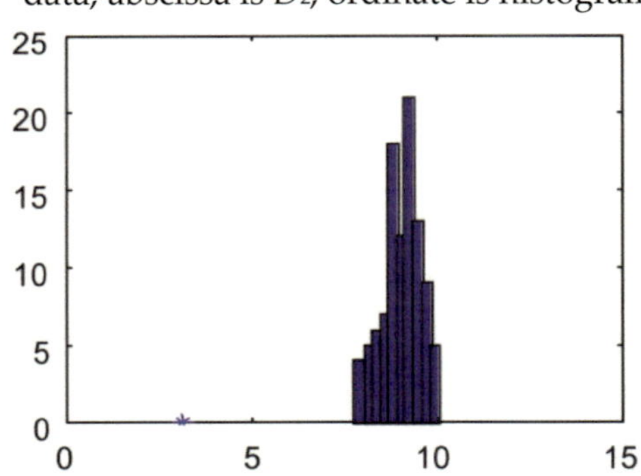

e. * is D_2 value of raw data in $m = 2$, τ=0.005 histogram is D_2 distribution of surrogate data, abscissa is D_2, ordinate is histogram

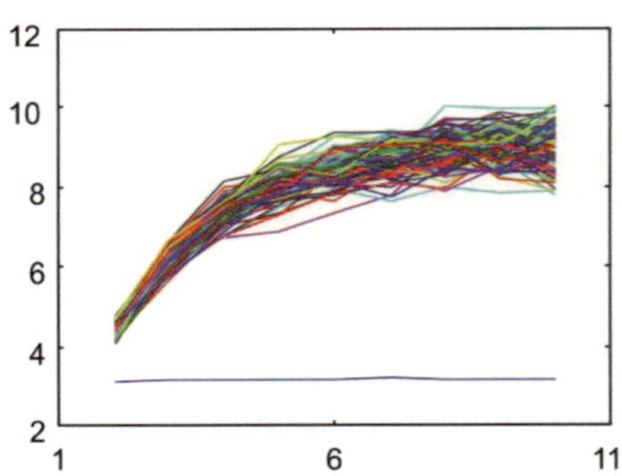

f. The D_2 curves of raw data and surrogate data with m, abscissa is m=2~10, ordinate is D_2

Figure 11. The surrogate data test analysis based on correlation dimension for Lorenz chaos time series by sampling intervals differences disappear between the raw data and its surrogate data in $m = 10$ (see Fig. 11b). This illustrates that the reconstructed attractor appears broken. The reconstructed phase space is similar to that of the surrogate data with linear stochastic noise characteristics.

Figure 11c and d show the results with τ=0.1. The differences between the raw data and its surrogate data can be seen in Fig. 11c ($m = 4$). When $m>2$, these differences become larger as m increases. Figure 11e and f show the results with τ=0.005. Figure 11e shows the surrogate data test histogram in $m = 2$. The correlation dimension curves of the raw data and its surrogate data are given in $m = 2 \sim 10$ (see Fig. 11f). Even in the case of oversampling, the correlation dimension as test statistic can also make the surrogate data method very effective.

3.3.6. *The surface EMG signal analysis based on the surrogate data and correlation dimension*

Figure 12 shows the surrogate data analysis for the surface EMG signal in Fig. 12a based on correlation dimension. When $m = 6$, the correlation dimension value of the raw data is different from those of its surrogate data generated by the null hypothesis 3. The correlation dimension curves of the raw data and its surrogate data are given when $m = 2 \sim 8$ in Fig. 12b. We can see the differences between the original data and its surrogate data. The null hypothesis 3 can be rejected in confidence level 95%. The result indicates that the surface EMG signal has deterministic nonlinear components, even chaotic.

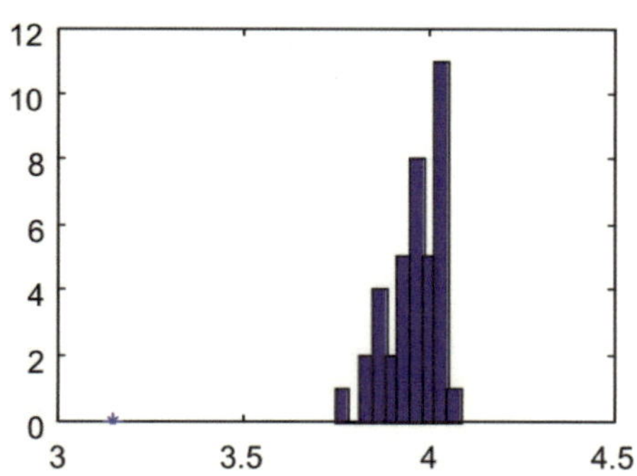

a. * is D_2 of surface EMG in $m = 6$, histogram is D_2 distribution of surrogate data, abscissa is D_2, ordinate is histogram

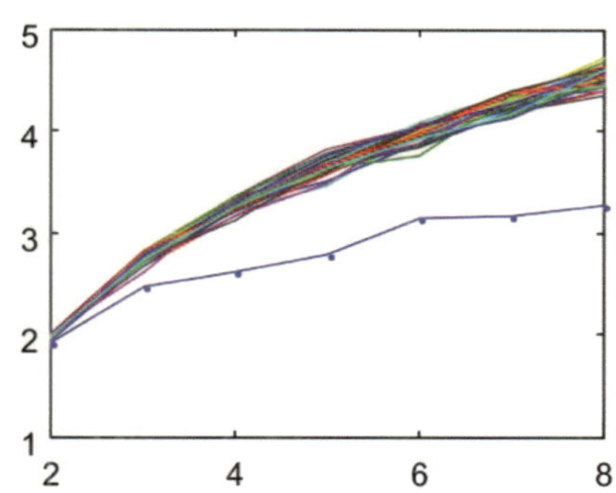

b. The curves of surface EMG and surrogate data with m, abscissa is m=2~8, ordinate is D_2

Figure 12. The surrogate data test analysis based on correlation dimension for surface EMG signal.

3.4. Largest Lyapunov exponent

The Lyapunov exponent method is to directly identify whether a system is chaotic. If the system is chaotic, the Lyapunov exponent is positive. Otherwise, the Lyapunov exponent is negative. For this, the Lyapunov exponent can be used to test the chaotic feature of a signal under study. The first algorithms developed computed the whole Lyapunov spectrum by

Wolf et al. [43] and Sano et al. [44]. Meanwhile, the largest Lyapunov exponent is sufficient for assessing the presence of chaos. At present, there are many algorithms to estimate the largest Lyapunov exponent from a time series, such as an algorithm given by Rosenstein et al.[45]. This algorithm is aimed specifically at estimating the largest Lyapunov exponent from short data.

3.4.1. Algorithm of largest Lyapunov exponent estimation[45]

For a short time series, Rosenstein et al. present a robust estimation algorithm of the largest Lyapunov exponent. First, the attractor is reconstructed, refer to Eq. 25. Next, the algorithm locates the closest neighbor of each point X_i on the trajectory, with respect to the Euclidian distance. Then, one defines the distance between two neighboring points at instant n=0 by:

$$d_i(0) = \min_{X_j} \left\| X_j - X_i \right\| \tag{31}$$

where $\left\| \bullet \right\|$ is the Euclidian norm. Here, the temporal separation of the nearest neighbors should be greater than the mean period of the time series.

$$\left| i - j \right| > mean \quad period \tag{32}$$

According to time, the average distance between two neighboring vectors can be simply

$$d_i(n) = \left\| X_{j+n} - X_{i+n} \right\| \tag{33}$$

Assume that the system is controlled by the largest Lyapunov exponent only. Then, the distance between two neighbor points obey the following relationship:

$$d(t) = Ce^{\lambda t} \tag{34}$$

For $t = n\Delta t$, there is:

$$d_i(n) \approx C_i e^{\lambda n \Delta t} \tag{35}$$

$$\lambda = \frac{1}{n \cdot \Delta t} \ln \frac{d_i(n)}{C_i} \tag{36}$$

$$n \cdot \lambda = \frac{1}{\Delta t} (\ln d_i(n) - \ln C_i) \tag{37}$$

$$\begin{aligned} n\langle \lambda \rangle &= \frac{1}{\Delta t} \langle \ln d_i(n) \rangle - \frac{1}{\Delta t} \langle \ln C_i \rangle \\ &= \frac{1}{\Delta t} \langle \ln d_i(n) \rangle - b \end{aligned} \tag{38}$$

where $b = \frac{1}{\Delta t} \langle \ln C_i \rangle$.

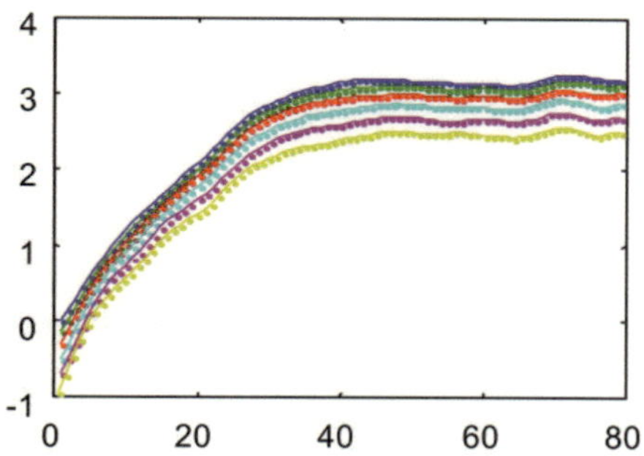

a. $y(n)$ curves of time series x of Lorenz chaos system sampled by τ=0.01, embedding dimension m=2~8

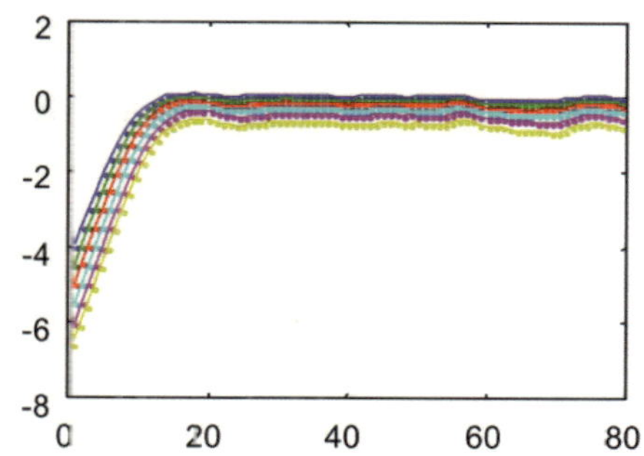

b. $y(n)$ curves of time series x of Logistic chaos system in α=3.9, embedding dimension m=2~8

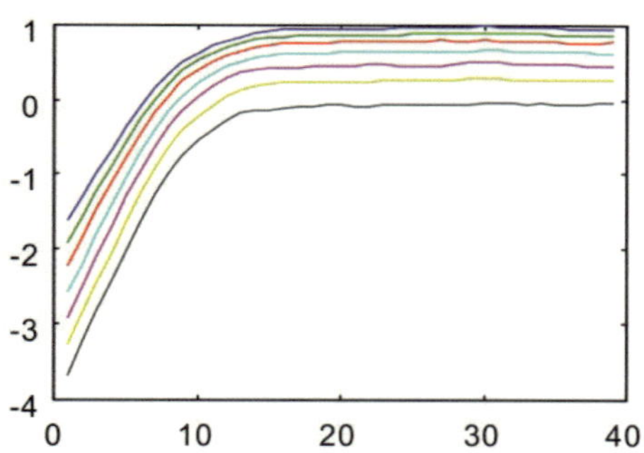

c. $y(n)$ curves of Henon chaos series embedding dimension m=2~8

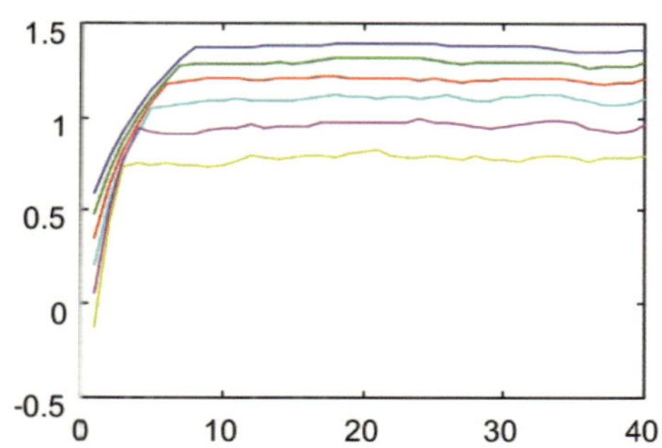

d. $y(n)$ curves of gaussian noise embedding dimension m=2~8

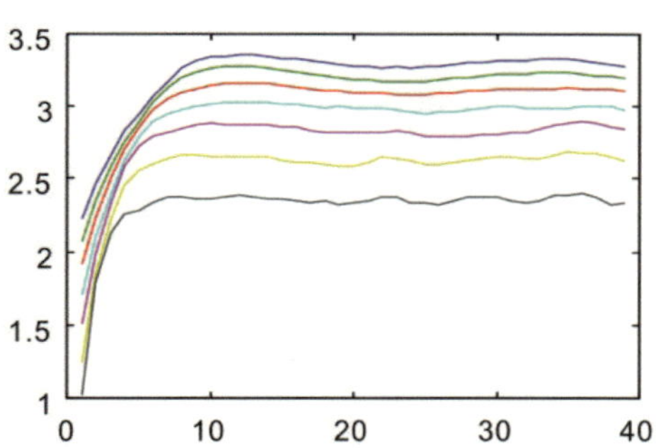

e. $y(n)$ curves of linear stochastic process embedding dimension m=2~8

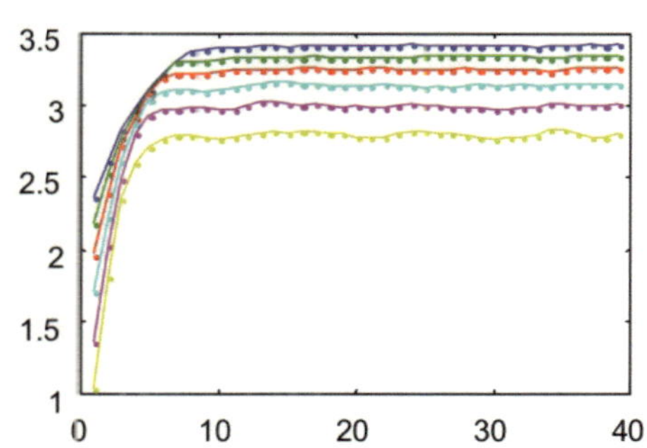

f. $y(n)$ curves of Lorenz chaos series in $\tau = 1$, embedding dimension m=3~8

Figure 13. $y(n)$ curves of signals, abscissa is n, ordinate is $y(n)$

Then, the Lyapunov exponent can be given by using a least-squares fit to the "average" line:

$$y(n) = \frac{1}{\Delta t}\langle \ln d_i(n) \rangle \tag{39}$$

where $y(n) = n\langle \lambda \rangle + b$. The largest Lyapunov exponent λ is the slope of $y(n)$ in the above equation.

This method is deduced directly from the largest Lyapunov exponent definition. The accurate evaluation of λ depends on the full use of the data. In practice, the curve $y(n)$ will tend to saturation. The largest Lyapunov exponent λ is given by computing the slope of the linear part in the curve $y(n)$.

3.4.2. Chaos test based on largest Lyapunov exponent

In general, if the signal is chaotic, the slope of the curve $y(n)$ will be independent of the embedding dimension. Otherwise, if the signal is not chaotic, the slope of the curve $y(n)$ will depend on the embedding dimension. When the embedding dimension m is chosen from 2 to 8, the Lyapunov exponent of the curve $y(n)$ of the signal is shown in Figure 13. For a chaotic signal, a good illustration is given (see Figure 13a, b and c). The $y(n)$ curves are different from those of a non-chaotic signal (compare with Figure 13d and e). However, even for chaotic signals, the $y(n)$ curves are not always parallel. For example, in the case of undersampling ($\tau = 1$), the $y(n)$ curves of Lorenz chaotic time series are similar to those of linear stochastic process(compare with Figure 13e and f). In the literature[23], the $y(n)$ curves of the Ikeda chaotic time series are also not parallel.

3.4.3. The analysis of surface EMG signal based on the largest Lyapunov exponent

Figure 14 gives the curves of Lyapunove exponent $y(n)$ for the surface EMG signal. The $y(n)$ curves are not very parallel for the surface EMG signal. It is difficult to distinguish the curves of $y(n)$ for the surface EMG signal from those of Figure 13d, f and g. The surface EMG signal can not be determined as chaotic, or as stochastic. But it can be a high-dimensional system.

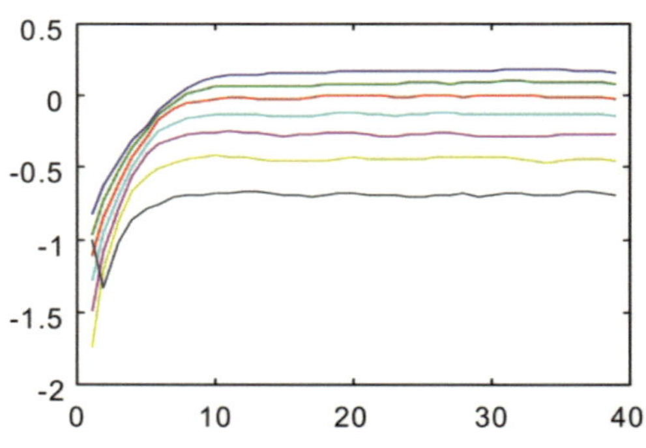

Figure 14. $y(n)$ curves of surface EMG signal, embedding dimension m=2~8, abscissa is n, ordinate is $y(n)$

3.5. Principal component analysis

Broomhead and King[31] proposed the idea of singular system analysis that determines an appropriate embedding dimension d directly from the raw time series. It provides its convenience for the further analysis of the given system. Numerical experience, however, led several authors to express some doubts about reliability of singular system analysis in the attractor reconstruction[46-48]. Palus and Dvorak[37] explain why singular-value decomposition(SVD), the heart of the singular system analysis and by nature a linear method, may become misleading technique when it is used in nonlinear dynamics studies that reconstruction parameters are time-delay, embedding dimension (or embedding windows). For this, we propose a novel nonlinear analysis method based symplectic geometry, called symplectic principal component analysis(SPCA)[49].

3.5.1. *Principle and algorithm of principal component analysis*

Let a time series $x_1, x_2, \ldots, x_n$ be the measured signal by sampling interval t_s, n is the number of samples. According to Takens' embedding theorem, a trajectory matrix X can be given by time delay coordinates method, refer to Eq. 25(τ_d=1):

$$X = \begin{bmatrix} X_1^T \\ X_2^T \\ \vdots \\ X_m^T \end{bmatrix} = \begin{bmatrix} x_1 & x_2 & \cdots & x_d \\ x_2 & x_3 & \cdots & x_{d+} \\ \vdots & \vdots & \cdots & \vdots \\ x_m & x_{m+1} & \cdots & x_n \end{bmatrix} \tag{40}$$

where d is embedding dimension. $m=n-d+1$ is the number of points in d-dimension reconstruction attractor, $X_i^T, i = 1, \cdots\cdots, m$, denotes a point in the attractor. For the matrix X, there are a $m \times d$ orthogonal matrix V and a $d \times d$ orthogonal matrix. The matrix X can be decomposed as follows.

$$X = VSU^T \tag{41}$$

where S is $d \times d$ diagonal matrix, whose elements are defined

$$S_{ij} = \delta_{ij}\sqrt{\sigma_i m}, \qquad i, j = 1,2,\cdots, d \tag{42}$$

Since the matrix V is orthogonal, then

$$(V^T \cdot V)_{ij} = \delta_{ij} \tag{43}$$

Meanwhile, for the matrix U, there are

$$(U^T \cdot U)_{ij} = (U \cdot U^T)_{ij} = \delta_{ij} \tag{44}$$

In order to facilitate the calculation, Broomhead et al. applies the covariance matrix C of the matrix X to replace the matrix X. The details are as follows:

$$C = \frac{1}{m} \cdot X^T \cdot X \tag{45}$$

$$C_{ij} = \frac{1}{m} \sum_{k=1}^{m} x_{i+k-1} x_{j+k-1}, \qquad i, j = 1, 2, \cdots, d \tag{46}$$

Its values reflect the degree of correlation between the time delay coordinate variable *i* and *j*.

$$C = \frac{1}{m} \cdot X^T \cdot X = \frac{1}{m} \cdot U \cdot S \cdot S \cdot U^T = \frac{1}{m} \cdot U \cdot S^2 \cdot U^T \tag{47}$$

$$U^T \cdot C \cdot U = \frac{1}{m} \cdot (XU)^T \cdot XU = \frac{1}{m} \cdot S^2 \tag{48}$$

Let $Y=XU$, then:

$$U^T \cdot C \cdot U = \frac{1}{m} \cdot Y^T \cdot Y = \frac{1}{m} \cdot S^2 \tag{49}$$

where U^TCU is the covariance matrix of the matrix *Y*. Its elements are zero, except that the diagonal elements are equal to σ_i. This means that the variables *i* and *j* of the matrix *Y* are independent. The coordinate system is orthogonal, which is constituted from the variables of the matrix *Y* after the above transformed. The σ_i is called the principal component or singular value in accordance with the order of the largest to the smallest. The orthogonal vector U_i corresponding to the principal component σ_i is called the principal axis. The principal component describes the distribution of the signal energy. That is, the value of the principal component reflects the projection of the signal energy in the corresponding principal axis. In the different principal axes, a distribution value is given as $\sigma_i / \sum_{i=1}^{d} \sigma_i$, where $\sum_{i=1}^{d} \sigma_i$ is the total energy of the signal. If $\sigma_{i+1} \approx \cdots \approx \sigma_d$, the distribution values are called a noise floor. The distribution can be used to estimate the dimension of the dynamical system that generates a time series or to filter out the noise. Let $\overline{U}_i$ be the principal axes corresponding to the principal components over the noise floor. Zero vector describes the principal axes corresponding to the noise floor. Thus, for $\sigma_i >$ noise floor, a new coordinate transform matrix is made up of:

$$\overline{U} = [\overline{U}_1, \overline{U}_2, \cdots, \overline{U}_i, 0, \cdots, 0] \tag{50}$$

In order to filter out noise, the trajectory matrix *X* is first projected into the coordinate system *U*.

$$Y = XU \tag{51}$$

The variables in the matrix *Y* are independent. Then, the original coordinate system is updated by using the matrix *Y*:

$$\overline{X} = Y\overline{U}^T = (XU) \cdot \overline{U}^T \tag{52}$$

That is, $\overline{X}$ is a new time delay coordinate system.

3.5.2. Influence of noise on the principal component spectrum of chaotic time series

Figure 15a shows the principal component spectrum of Logistic attractor from a Logistic chaotic time series without noise. The principal component spectrum has not a significant noise level. When the interior noise is Gaussian noise with zero mean and 0.001^2 variance, the principal component spectrum is given for Logistic attractor. Figure 15c and d give the principal component spectrum of Logistic attractor with the measurement noise $\sigma^2=0.001^2$ and $\sigma^2=0.8^2$, respectively. It can be seen that the Logistic attractor with the internal noise has the same principal component spectrum as the attractor without noise. The curves of the principal component spectrum are also slanting. The total energy is significantly distributed into each principal axes. The principal components are declining with the index *i* so that there is no noise floor. It is difficult to choose an appropriate embedding dimension *d*. For the larger measurement noise, the corresponding principal component spectrum of Logistic attractor slant into a floor area with increasing the embedding dimension. In the floor area, the principal components keep unchanged and do not decline with the index *i*, called noise floor. Broomhead and King[31] have suggested that this noise floor can be used to determine the embedding dimension and filter out noise from the data. The signal energy will be focused on the truncated principal components and the corresponding principal axes

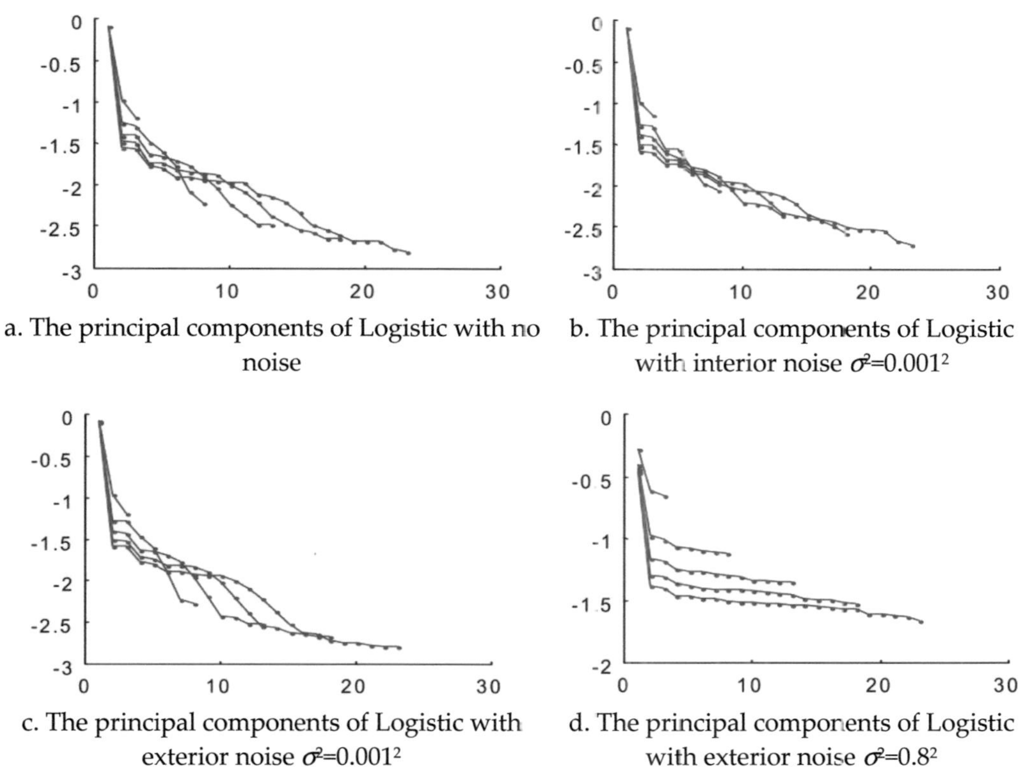

a. The principal components of Logistic with no noise

b. The principal components of Logistic with interior noise $\sigma^2=0.001^2$

c. The principal components of Logistic with exterior noise $\sigma^2=0.001^2$

d. The principal components of Logistic with exterior noise $\sigma^2=0.8^2$

Figure 15. The principal component analysis of Logistic chaos series with different noises based on SVD, d=3 : 2 : 23, abscissa is *d*, ordinate is $\log(\sigma_i / tr(\sigma_i))$

when the principal components above noise floor are only held. The number of the principal components above the noise floor is the optimal embedding dimension.

Besides, the new coordinate system corresponding to the principal axes can eliminate the noise floor to reduce the noise from the data. However, the truncated position of the principal components depends on the signal-noise-ratio, especially for the measurement noise. The principal components of the chaotic time series based on SVD spectrum more easily subject to the measurement noise so that the embedding dimension estimation is directly affected. For the smaller noise, there is the more number of principal components above the noise floor. For the larger noise, the number of the corresponding principal components will be reduced. Here, the above calculation accuracy is 2.2204e-016, which does not consider the numerical calculation error.

3.5.3. Influence of sampling interval on the principal component spectrum of chaotic time series[49]

The Lorenz chaotic system is considered to give the state variable x in order to study the influence of sampling interval on the principal component spectrum. The principal component spectrum slant and have no floor for the chaotic time series x with τ=0.005 (see Fig. 16a). When τ=0.1 (see Fig. 16b), the principal component spectrum are basically similar

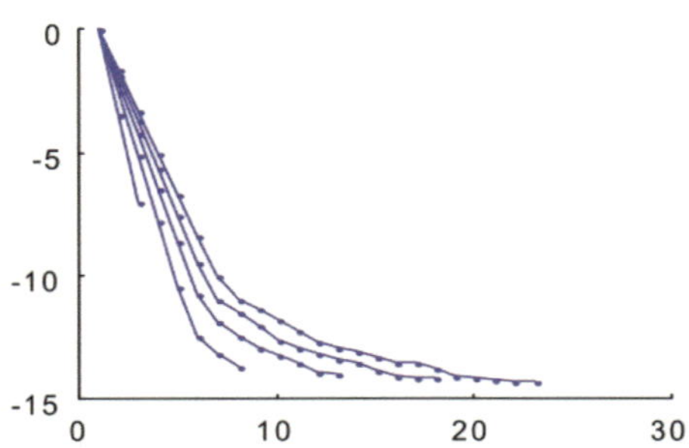

a. The principal components of Lorenz chaos time series, τ=0.005

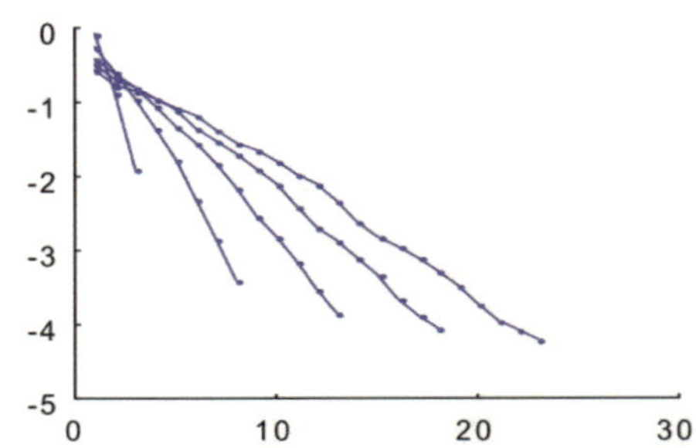

b. The principal components of Lorenz chaos time series, τ=0.1

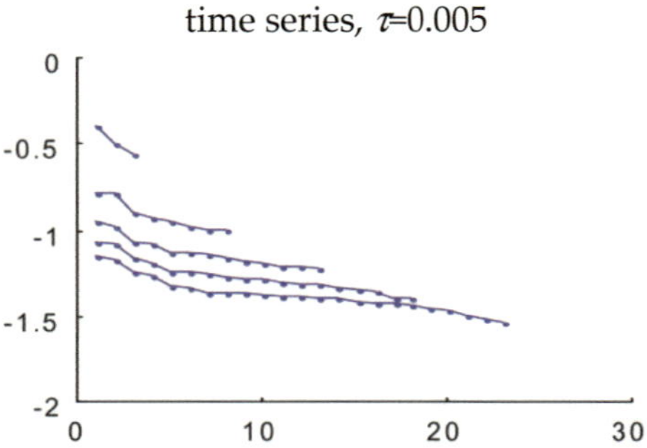

c. The principal components of Lorenz chaos time series, τ=1

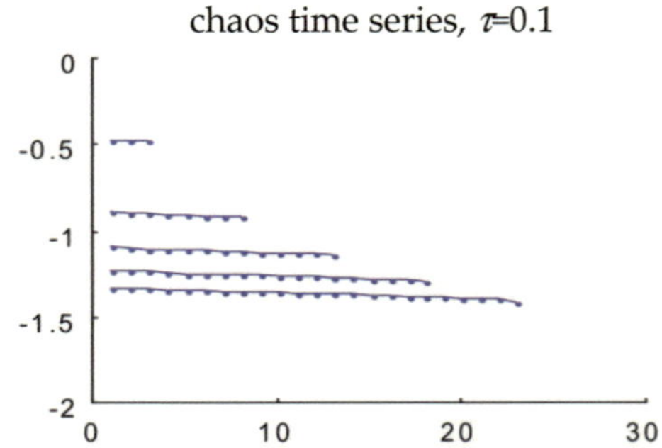

d. The principal components of noise, n=10000

Figure 16. The principal component analysis of gaussian noise and Lorenz chaos time series by different sampling intervals based on SVD, d=3 : 2 : 23, abscissa is d, ordinate is $\log(\sigma_i / tr(\sigma_i))$

to those in the Figure 16a. When τ=1, each line is separated from each other and tends to horizontal line in the case of different embedding dimensions(see Fig. 16c). It shows that the distribution of the total energy has little difference in each principal axis, like the Gaussian noise (see Fig. 16d). For the Gaussian noise, its principal component spectrum curves are horizontal lines, where N=10000. It shows that every principal component is equal to each other. The energy distributes into every principal axis averagely. Therefore, it can be seen that sampling interval affects the determination of embedding dimension. When the sampling interval is not undersampling, the determination of embedding dimension depends the amount of signal-noise-ratio. In the case of undersampling, the chaotic time series is similar to noise so that the embedding dimension seems to be estimated as 1.

3.6. Symplectic principal component analysis

The symplectic geometry is a kind of phase space geometry. Its nature is nonlinear. It can describe the system structure, especially nonlinear structure, very well. It has been used to study various nonlinear dynamical systems[50-52] since Feng Kang[53] has proposed a symplectic algorithm for solving symplectic differential. However, from the view of data analysis, few literatures have employed symplectic geometry theory to explore the dynamics of the system. Our previous works have proposed the estimation of the embedding dimension based on symplectic geometry from a time series[49, 54-56]. Subsequently, Niu et al. have used our method to evaluate sprinter's surface EMG signals[57]. Xie et al[58] have proposed a kind of symplectic geometry spectra based on our work. Subsequently, we show that SPCA can well represent chaotic time series and reduce noise in chaotic data[59, 60].

In SPCA, a fundamental step is to build the multidimensional structure (attractor) in symplectic geometry space. Here, in terms of Taken's embedding theorem, we first construct an attractor in phase space, i.e. the trajectory matrix X from a time series. That is, for a measured data (the observable of the system under study) x_1, x_2, ..., x_n recorded with sampling interval t_s, the corresponding d-dimension reconstruction attractor, $X_{m\times d}$ can be given (refer to Eq.40).Then we describe the symplectic principal component analysis (SPCA) based on symplectic geometry theory and give its corresponding algorithm.

3.7. Symplectic principal component method

SPCA is a kind of PCA approaches based on symplectic geometry. Its idea is to map the investigated complex system in symplectic space and elucidate the dominant features underlying the measured data. The first few larger components capture the main relationship between the variables in symplectic space. The remaining components are composed of the less important components or noise in the measured data. In symplectic space, the used geometry is called symplectic geometry. Different from Eulid geometry, symplectic geometry is the even dimensional geometry with a special symplectic structure. It is dependent on a bilinear antisymmetric nonsingular cross product——symplectic cross product:

$$[x, y] = \langle x, Jy \rangle \tag{53}$$

where, $$J = J_{2n} = \begin{bmatrix} 0 & +I_n \\ -I_n & 0 \end{bmatrix} \tag{54}$$

When $n = 1$, $x = [x_1, x_2]$, $y = [y_1, y_2]$,

$$J = \begin{bmatrix} 0 & 1 \\ -1 & 0 \end{bmatrix} \tag{55}$$

$$\begin{aligned} [x, y] &= [x_1 \ x_2] J \begin{bmatrix} y_1 \\ y_2 \end{bmatrix} \\ &= \begin{vmatrix} x_1 & y_1 \\ x_2 & y_2 \end{vmatrix} \end{aligned} \tag{56}$$

The measurement of symplectic space is area scale. In symplectic space, the length of arbitrary vectors always equals zero and without signification, and there is the concept of orthogonal cross-course. In symplectic geometry, the symplectic transform is the nonlinear transform in essence, which is also called canonical transform, since it has measure preserving characteristics and can keep the natural properties of the original data unchanged. It is fit for nonlinear dynamics systems.

The symplectic principal components are given by symplectic similar transform. It is similar to SVD-based PCA. The corresponding eigenvalues can be obtained by symplectic *QR* method. Here, we first construct the autocorrelation matrix $A_{d\times d}$ of the trajectory matrix $X_{m\times d}$. Then the matrix *A* can be transformed as a Hamilton matrix *M* in symplectic space.

Definition 1 Let *S* is a matrix, if $JSJ^{-1} = S^{-*}$, then *S* is a symplectic matrix.

Definition 2 Let *H* is a matrix, if $JHJ^{-1} = -H^*$, then *H* is a Hamilton matrix.

Theorem 1 Any *dxd* matrix can be made into a Hamilton matrix. Let a matrix as *A*, so $\begin{pmatrix} A & 0 \\ 0 & -A^T \end{pmatrix}$ is a Hamilton matrix. (Proof refers to appendix A)

Theorem 2 Hamilton matrix *M* keeps unchanged at symplectic similar transform. (Proof refers to appendix A)

Theorem 3 Let $M \in C^{2d\times 2d}$ as Hamilton matrix, so e^M is symplectic matrix.

Theorem 4 Let $S \in C^{2d\times 2d}$ as symplectic matrix, there is $S = QR$, where *Q* is symplectic unitary matrix, *R* is upper triangle matrix.

Theorem 5 The product of sympletcic matrixes is also a symplectic matrix. (Proof refers to appendix A)

Theorem 6 Suppose Household matrix *H* is：

$$H = H(k,\omega) = \begin{pmatrix} P & 0 \\ 0 & P \end{pmatrix} \tag{57}$$

where $P = I_n - \frac{2\varpi\varpi^*}{\varpi^*\varpi}$, $\varpi = (0,\cdots,0;\omega_k,\cdots,\omega_d)^T \neq 0$

so, H is symplectic unitary matrix. ϖ^* is ϖ conjugate transposition. (Proof refers to appendix A)

For Hamilton matrix M , its eigenvalues can be given by symplectic similar transform and the primary $2d$ dimension space can be transformed into d dimension space to resolve[17-19], as follows:

i. Let $N = M^2$

$$M^2 = \begin{bmatrix} A^T & G \\ F & -A \end{bmatrix}^2 \tag{58}$$

ii. Construct a symplectic matrix Q,

$$Q^T N Q = \begin{bmatrix} B & R \\ 0 & B^T \end{bmatrix} \tag{59}$$

where B is up Hessenberg matrix ($b_{ij}=0$, $i>j+1$). The matrix Q may be a symplectic Household matrix H. If the matrix M is a real symmetry matrix, M can be considered as N. Then one can get an upper Hessenberg matrix (referred to equ. 13), namely,

$$\begin{aligned} HMH' &= \begin{pmatrix} P & 0 \\ 0 & P \end{pmatrix} \begin{pmatrix} A & 0 \\ 0 & -A' \end{pmatrix} \begin{pmatrix} P & 0 \\ 0 & P \end{pmatrix}' \\ &= \begin{pmatrix} PAP' & 0 \\ 0 & -PA'P' \end{pmatrix} \\ &= \begin{pmatrix} B & 0 \\ 0 & -B' \end{pmatrix} \end{aligned} \tag{60}$$

where H is the symplectic Householder matrix.

iii. Calculate eigenvalues $\lambda(B) = \{\mu_1, \mu_2, \cdots, \mu_d\}$ by using symplectic QR decomposition method; if M is a real symmetry matrix, the eigenvalues of A is equal to those of B:

$$\mu = \lambda(B) = \lambda(A) \tag{61}$$

$$\lambda(A) = \lambda^2(X) \tag{62}$$

iv. These eigenvalues $\boldsymbol{\mu} = \{\mu_1, \mu_2, \cdots, \mu_d\}$ are sorted by descending order, that is

$$\mu_1 > \mu_2 > \cdots > \mu_k >> \mu_{k+1} \geq \cdots \geq \mu_d \tag{63}$$

Thus the calculation of $2d$ dimension space is transformed into that of that of d dimension space. The $\boldsymbol{\mu}$ is the symplectic principal component spectrums of A with relevant symplectic orthonormal bases. In the so-called noise floor, values of μ_i, $i = k+1,\cdots,d$, reflect the noise level in the data[49, 55]. The corresponding matrix Q denotes symplectic eigenvectors of A.

3.7.1. Proposed algorithm of symplectic principal component method

For a measured data $x_1, x_2, \ldots, x_n$, our proposed algorithm consists of the following steps:

1. Reconstruct the attractor $X_{m\times d}$ from the measured time series, where d is the embedding dimension of the matrix X, and $m = n-d+1$.
2. Remove the mean values X_{mean} of each row of the matrix X.
3. Build the real $d\times d$ symmetry matrix A, that is,

$$A = (X - X_{mean})'(X - X_{mean}) \tag{64}$$

Here, d should be larger than the dimension of the system in terms of Taken's embedding theorem.

4. Calculate the symplectic principal components of the matrix A by QR decomposition, and choose the Householder matrix H instead of the transform matrix Q. It is easy to prove that H is a symplectic unitary matrix (Proof refers to appendix A) and H can be constructed from real matrix (refer to appendix B).
5. Construct the corresponding principal eigenvalue matrix W according to the number k of the chosen symplectic principal components of the matrix A, where $W \subseteq Q$. That is, when $k=d$, $W=Q$, otherwise $W \subset Q$. In use, k can be chosen according to Eq.63.
6. Get the transformed coefficients $S = \{S_1, S_2, \ldots, S_m\}$, where

$$S_i = W'X_i, \quad i = 1,\cdots,m \tag{65}$$

7. Reestimate the X_s from S,

$$X_{si} = WS_i \tag{66}$$

Then the reestimation data $x_{s1}, x_{s2}, \cdots, x_{sm}$ can be given.

8. For the noisy time series, the first estimation of data is usually not good. Here, one can go back to the step (6) and let $X_i = X_s$ in Eq.(65) to do step (6) and (7) again. Generally, the second estimated data will be better than the first estimated data.

Besides, it is necessary to note that for the clean time series, the step (8) is unnecessary to handle.

3.7.2. Performance evaluation

SPCA, like PCA, can not only represent the original data by capturing the relationship between the variables, but also reduce the contribution of errors in the original data. Here, the performance analysis of SPCA is studied from the two views, i.e. representation of chaotic signals and noise reduction in chaotic signals.

Representation of chaotic signals

We first show that for the clean chaotic time series, SPCA can perfectly reconstruct the original data in a high-dimensional space. We first embed the original time series to a phase space. Considering the dimension of the Lorenz system(see Eq. 30) is 3, d of the matrix A is chosen as 8 in our SPCA analysis. To quantify the difference between the original data and the SPCA-filtered data, we employ the root-mean-square error (RMSE) as a measure:

$$RMSE = \sqrt{\frac{1}{N}\sum_{i=1}^{N}[x(i) - \hat{x}(i)]^2} \tag{67}$$

where $x(i)$ and $\hat{x}(i)$ are the original data and estimated data, respectively.

When $k = d$, the RMSE values are lower than 10^{-14} (see Figure 17). In Figure 17, the original data are generated by Eq. 30. The estimated data is obtained by SPCA with k=d. The results show that the SPCA method is better than the PCA. Since the real systems are usually unknown, it is necessary to study the effect of sampling time, data length, and noise to the SPCA approach. From the Figure 17 and 18, we can see that the sampling time and data length have less effect on SPCA method in the case of free-noise.

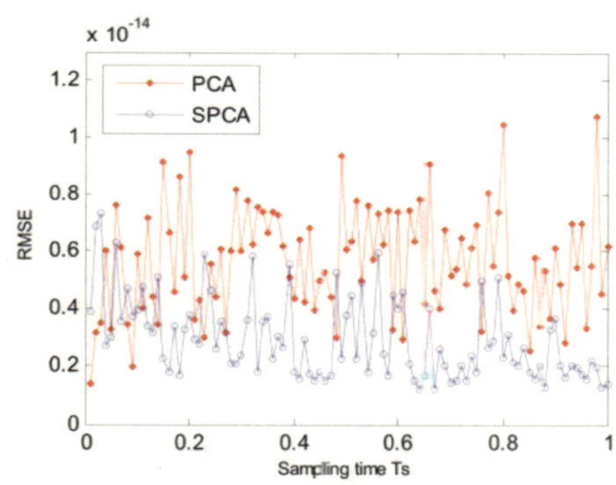

Figure 17. (Color online) RMSE vs. Sampling time curves for the SPCA and PCA.

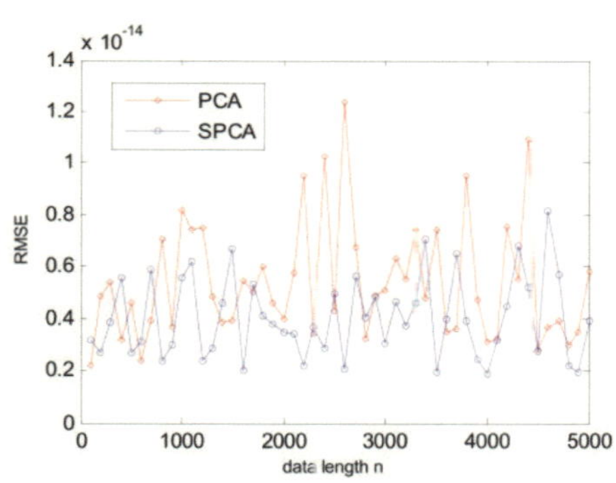

Figure 18. (Color online) RMSE vs. data length curves for the SPCA and PCA.

For analyzing noisy data, we use the percentage of principal components (PCs) to study the occupancy rate of each PC in order to reduce noise. The percentage of PCs is defined by

$$P_i = \frac{\mu_i}{\sum_{i=1}^{d} \mu_i} \times 100\% \tag{68}$$

where d is the embedding dimension, μ_i is the i-th principal component value. From the Figure 19, we find that the first largest symplectic principal component (SPC) of the SPCA is a little larger than that of the PCA. It is almost possessed of all the proportion of the symplectic principal components. This shows that it is feasible for the SPCA to study the principal component analysis of time series.

Next, we study the reduced space spanned by a few largest symplectic principal components (SPCs) to estimate the chaotic Lorenz time series (see Fig. 20). In Figure 20, the data x is given with a sampling time of 0.01 from chaotic Lorenz system. The estimated data is calculated by the first three largest SPCs. The average error and standard deviation between the original data and the estimated data is -6.55e-16 and 1.03e-2, respectively. The

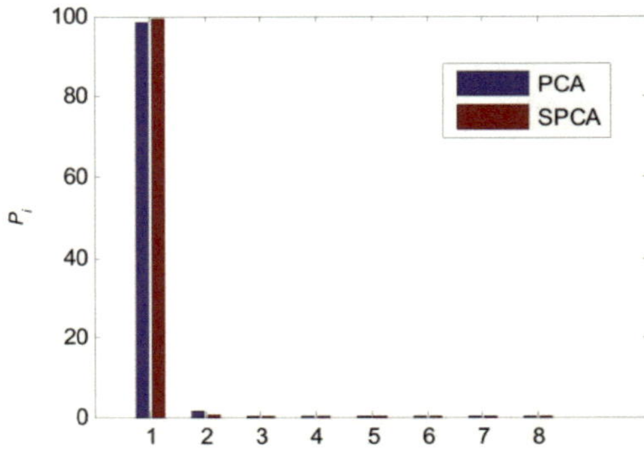

Figure 19. (Color online) The percentage of principal components for the SPCA and PCA.

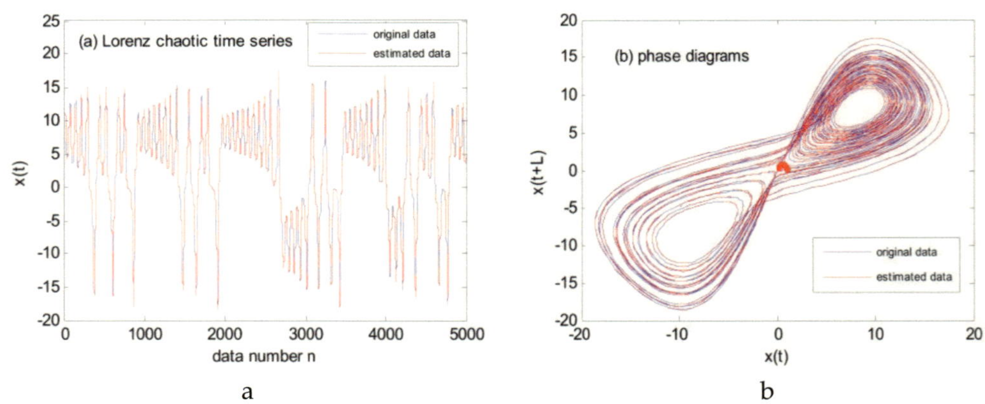

Figure 20. (Colour online) Chaotic signal reconstructed by the proposed SPCA algorithm with k=3, where (a) the time series of the original Lorenz data x without noise and the estimated data; (b) phase diagrams with L =11 for the original Lorenz data x without noise and the estimated data. The sampling time $t_s = 0.01$.

estimated data is very close to the original data not only in time domain (see Figure 20a) but also in phase space (see Figure 20b). We further explore the effect of sampling time in different number of PCs. When the PCs number k =1 and k =7, respectively, the SPCA and PCA give the change of RMSE values with the sampling time in Figure 21. We can see that the RMSE values of the SPCA are smaller than those of the PCA. The sampling time has less impact on the SPCA than the PCA. In the case of k = 7, the data length has also less effect on the SPCA than the PCA(see Fig. 22).

Comparing with PCA, the results of SPCA are better in the above Figures. We can see that the SPCA method keep the essential dynamical character of the primary time series generated by chaotic continuous systems. These indicate that the SPCA can reflect intrinsic nonlinear characteristics of the original time series. Moreover, the SPCA can elucidate the dominant features underlying the observed data. This will help to retrieve dominant patterns from the noisy data. For this, we study the feasibility of the proposed algorithm to reduce noise by using the noisy chaotic Lorenz data.

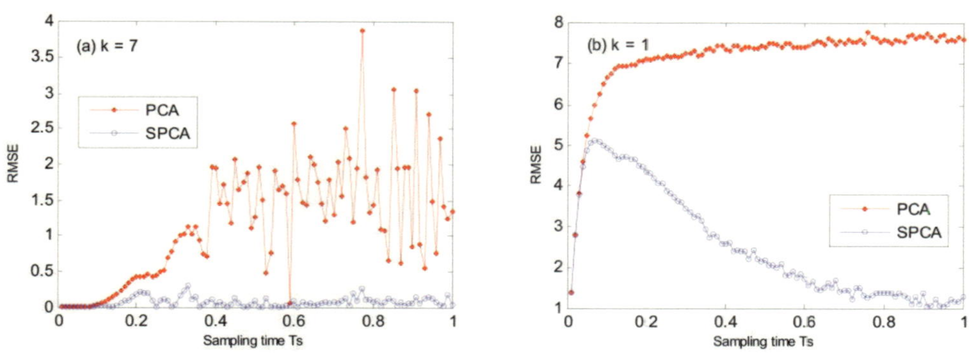

Figure 21. The RMSE values vs. the sampling time for the SPCA and PCA, where (a) the PCs number k =7; (b) k =1.

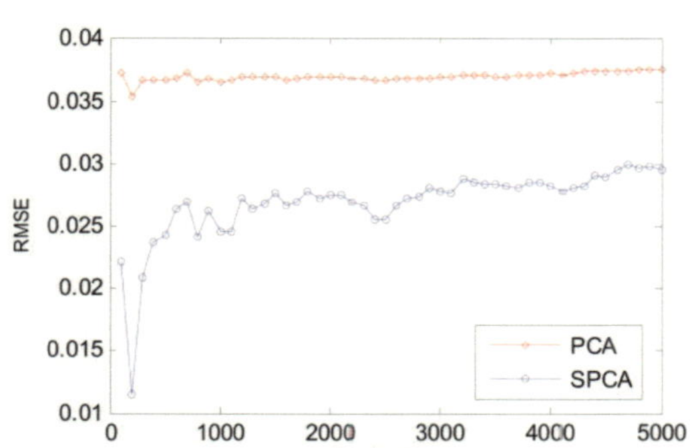

Figure 22. The RMSE vs. the data length for the SPCA and PCA, where k =7. The sampling time is 0.1.

Noise reduction in chaotic signals

For the noisy Lorenz data x, the phase diagrams of the noisy and clean data are given in Figure 23a and 23b. The clean data is the chaotic Lorenz data x with noise-free (see Eq. 30).

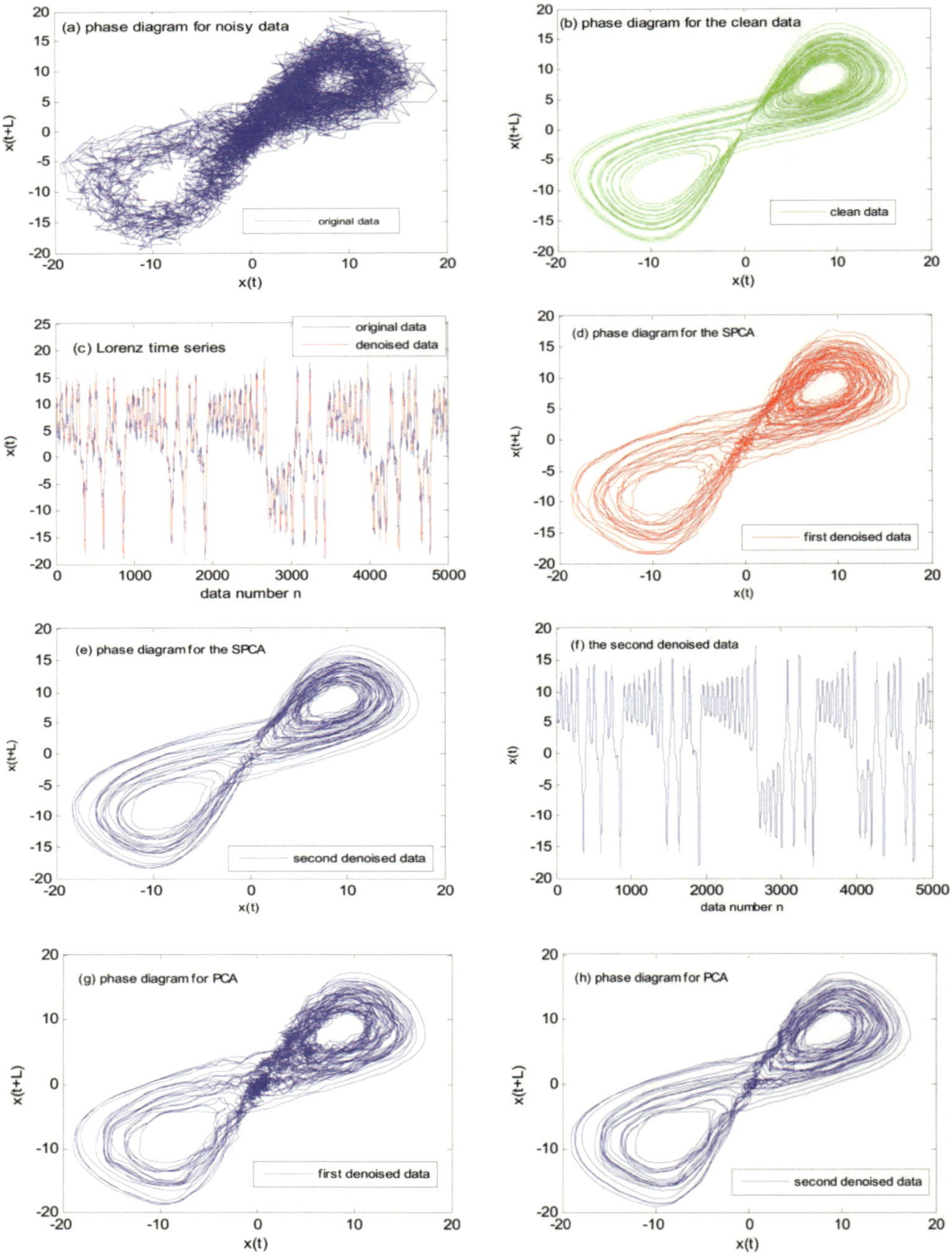

Figure 23. The noise reduction analysis of the proposed SPCA algorithm and PCA for the noisy Lorenz time series, where L=11.

The noisy data is the chaotic Lorenz data x with Gaussian white noise of zero mean and one variance (see Eq. 30). The sampling time is 0.01. The time delay L is 11 in Figure 23. It is obvious that noise is very strong. The first denoised data is obtained in terms of the proposed SPCA algorithm (see Figure 23c- f). Here, we first build an attractor X with the embedding dimension of 8. Then the transform matrix W is constructed when k=1. The first denoised data is generated by Eq.(65) and (66). In Figure 23c, the first denoised data is compared with the noisy Lorenz data x from the view of time field. Figure 23d shows the corresponding phase diagram of the first denoised data. Compared with Fig. 23a, the first denoised data can basically give the structure of the original system. In order to obtain better results, this denoised data is reduced noise again by the step (8). We can see that after the second noise reduction, the results are greatly improved in Fig. 23e and 23f, respectively. The curves of the second denoised data are better than those of the first denoised data whether in time domain or in phase space by contrast with Fig. 23c and 23d. Figure 23g shows that the PCA technique gives the first denoised result. We refer to our algorithm to deal with the first denoised data again by the PCA (see Figure 23h). Some of noise has been further reduced but the curve of PCA is not better than that of SPCA in Figure 23e. The reason is that the PCA is a linear method indeed. When nonlinear structures have to be considered, it can be misleading, especially in the case of a large sampling time (see Figure 24). The used program code of the PCA comes from the TISEAN tools (http://www.mpipks–dresden.mpg.de/ ~tisean).

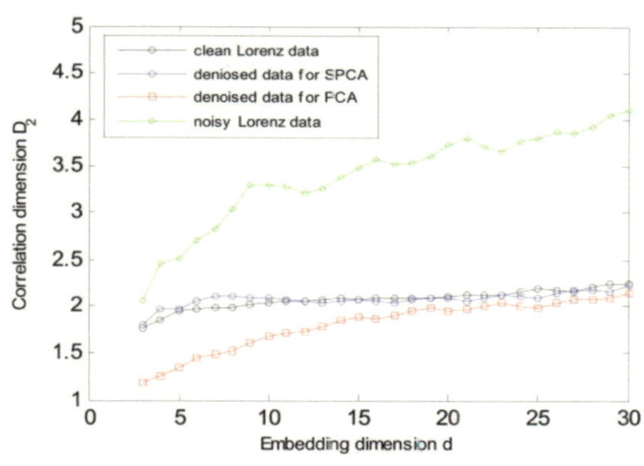

Figure 24. (Color online) D_2 vs. embedding dimension d

Figure 24 shows the variation of correlation dimension D_2 with embedding dimension d in the sampling time of 0.1 for the clean, noisy, and denoised Lorenz data. We can observe that for the clean and SPCA denoised data, the trend of the curves tends to smooth in the vicinity of 2. For the noisy data, the trend of the curve is constantly increasing and has no platform. For the PCA denoised data, the trend of the curve is also increasing and trends to a platform with 2. However, this platform is smaller than that of SPCA. It is less effective than the SPCA algorithm. This indicates that it is difficult for the PCA to describe the nonlinear structure of a system, because the correlation dimension D_2 manifests nonlinear properties of chaotic systems. Here, the correlation dimension D_2 is estimated by the Grassberger-Procaccia's algorithm[33, 40].

3.7.3. Estimation of embedding dimension based on symplectic geometry

In terms of Eq. 63, the values of μ_i, i=k+1, ..., d, are far smaller than μ_k. These values form a noise floor. Therefore, the embedding dimension of the reconstruction system can be determined by the noise floor. Here, the noise and nonlinear time series are used to investigate the feasibility of the embedding dimension estimation based on symplectic geometry.

For noise (which is generally regarded as Gauss white noise with mean value 0 and variance 1 in practical systems), symplectic geometry spectrums of this noise give the even distribution of its total energy (see Fig. 25a). From this figure, we can see that the symplectic geometry spectrums of noise can reflect the characteristic of noise very well when N=1000. This shows SG method can reflect noise level in the condition of short data length. For the time series of state variable x in Logistic chaos system without noise interference, the symplectic geometry spectrums (see Fig. 25b) are slant in the beginning then turn into plane area with the increase of index i. In other words, the distribution of total energy on the different axes is obviously different and with increasing the embedding dimension, the slants of symplectic geometry spectrums transit into noise floor. So one can determine embedding dimension from the number of symplectic geometry spectrums over noise floor, in which its determining criterion is similar to that in [37]. From Fig. 25b, the embedding dimension of Logistic chaotic time series can be estimated at 4 because the symplectic geometry spectrums begin to turn into noise floor at index 5. In a similar way, for Lorenz chaos time series without noise, when sampling interval τ=0.005, the embedding dimension can be estimated at 6 (see Fig. 25c).

Comparison of the results of our method (see Fig. 25b and 25c) and the results of SVD method (see Fig. 25d and 25e) shows that in SG method, the position of the noise floor is determined by the intrinsic dynamical structure of the nonlinear dynamic system rather than the numerical accuracy of the input data and the computation precision, but in SVD method, the noise floor was determined reversely[8, 37, 61].

In a word, the numerical experiments discuss that for the nonlinear dynamic systems, SG method can give the appropriate embedding dimension from their time series but SVD method cannot. So SG method is fit to deal with nonlinear systems.

3.7.4. Robustness of the embedding dimension estimation based on symplectic geometry

It is well known that the recent methods about embedding dimension are almost more or less subjective, or are affected by changes of the data length, noise, time lag, or sampling time, etc. Here, it is necessary that the robustness of the SG method is studied.

The effect of data length

In order to avoid the effect of the characteristics of the nonlinear system, this paper only considers and uses the noise to analyze the effect of data length. For Gauss white noise with mean value 0 and variance 1, when N=1000, the SG method can give better results than the SVD method (see Fig. 26a) because the total energy is distributed equably (see Fig. 25a).

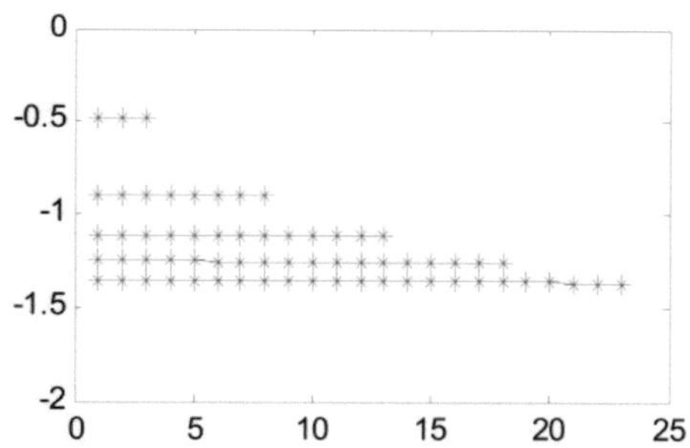

a. The symplectic geometry spectrums of Gauss white noise with mean value 0 and variance 1

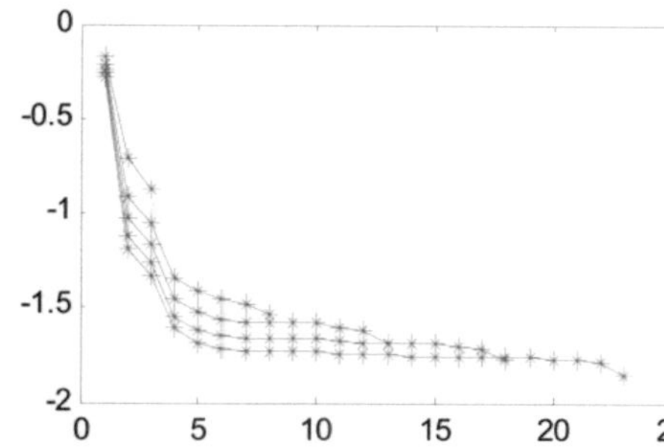

b. The symplectic geometry spectrums of Logistic chaotic series with no noise

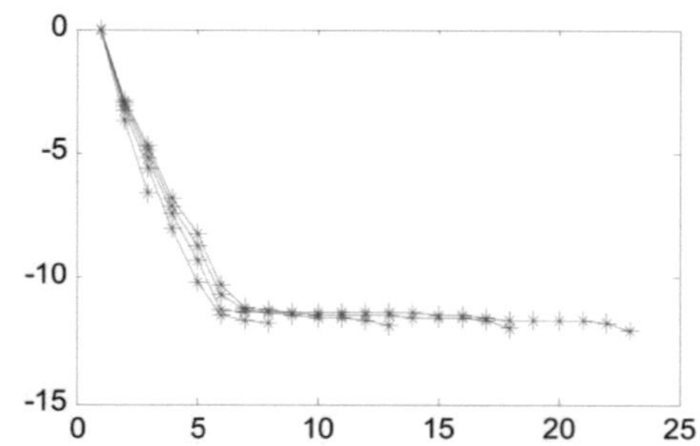

c. The symplectic geometry spectrums of Lorenz chaotic series with no noise, τ=0.005

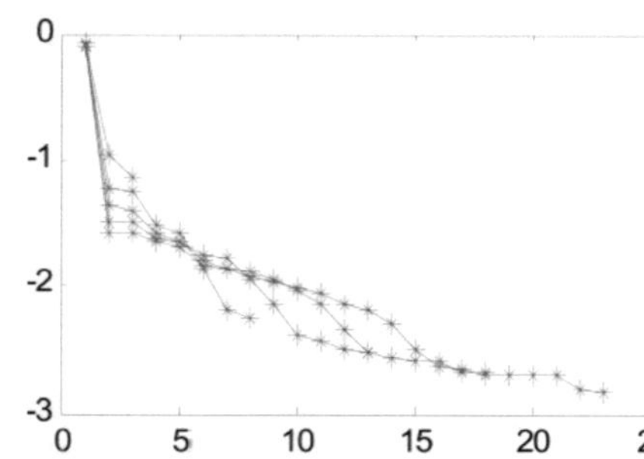

d. The SVD principal components of Logistic chaotic series with no noise

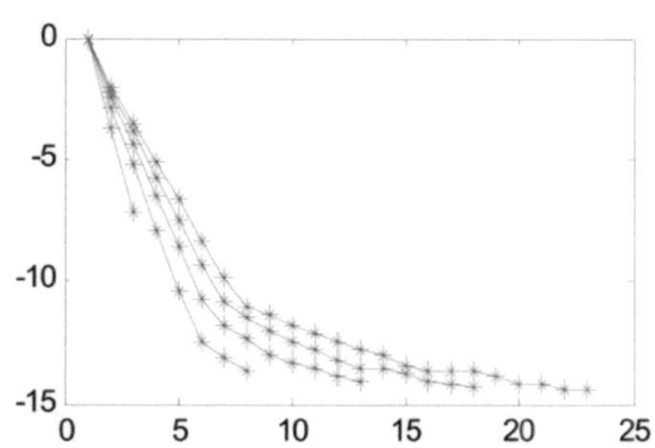

e. The SVD principal components of Lorenz chaotic series with no niose, τ=0.005

Figure 25. The study of embedding dimension based on symplectic geometry algorithm, *N*=1000, *d*=3, 8, 13, 18, 23, abscissa is *d*, ordinate is $\log(\mu_i / tr(\mu_i))$

And yet when *N* is rather large, e.g. *N*=10000, the SVD method can just have the similar results (see Fig. 26b) with Fig. 25a. These show that the SG method is more robust to changes of the data length than the SVD method. Then the SG method is fitter to the analysis of short time series.

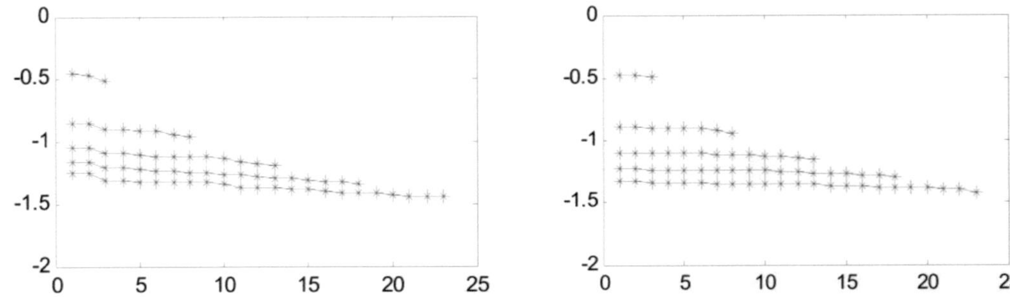

Figure 26. The analysis of SVD principal components of noise with different data length, *d*=3, 8, 13, 18, 23, abscissa is *d*, ordinate is $\log(\mu_i / tr(\mu_i))$

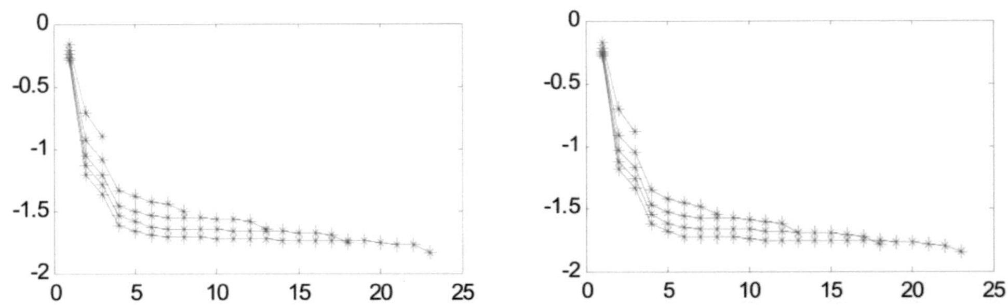

a. The symplectic geometry spectrums of Logistic chaos series with interior noise, $\sigma^2 = 0.001^2$

b. The symplectic geometry spectrums of Logistic chaos series with exterior noise, $\sigma^2 = 0.001^2$

$\sigma^2 = 0.001^2$ $\sigma^2 = 0.001^2$

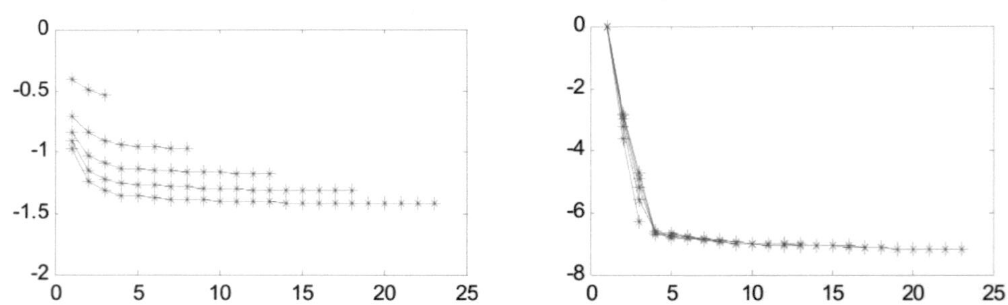

c. The symplectic geometry spectrums of Logistic chaos series with exterior noise, $\sigma^2 = 0.8^2$

d. The symplectic geometry spectrums of Lorenz chaos series with exterior noise, $\sigma^2 = 0.01^2$

Figure 27. The study of symplectic geometry spectrum analysis in different noises, *N*=1000, *d*=3, 8, 13, 18, 23, abscissa is *d*, ordinate is $\log(\mu_i / tr(\mu_i))$

The effect of noise

At present, there are many estimators of appropriate embedding dimension, but it has gradually been realized that such estimators are useful only for low-dimensional noise-free systems; such systems, however, seem hardly to occur in the real life. Therefore, this paper studies the robustness of the SG method under noise. For the signal obtained from the real system, it is always contaminated by noise (inner noise or/and outer noise). Although contaminated by inner or/and outer noise, the embedding dimension of Logistic system can always be noted at 4 by using the SG method because the noise floor begins at the embedding dimension 5 (see Fig. 27a and 27b). These show either inner noise or outer noise has little impact on the symplectic geometry spectrums. On the further increase of noise, the position of noise floor is obviously raised from the Figure 27c, but the appropriate embedding dimension 2 can still be obtained. In the similar way, for Lorenz chaos time series without and with noise, when sampling interval τ=0.005, the embedding dimension is 6 without noise and 3 with noise, respectively (see Fig. 25c and Fig. 27d). These results show that the SG method is useful for Lorenz system with noise, too. Meanwhile, we find that the SG method can obtain the results similar to nonlinear high singular spectrum algorithm[62]. Thus, it further shows that the SG method can reflect intrinsic nonlinear characteristics of the raw data.

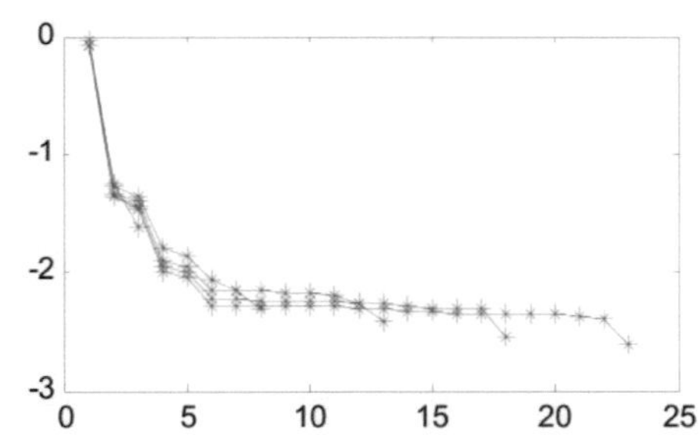

a. The symplectic geometry spectrums, τ=0.1

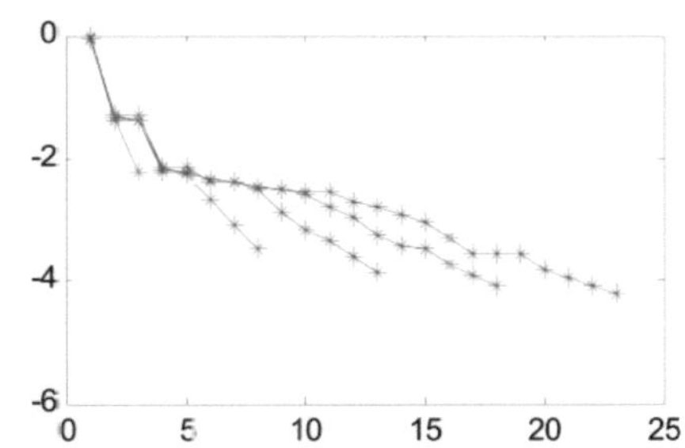

b. The principal components based on SVD, τ=0.1

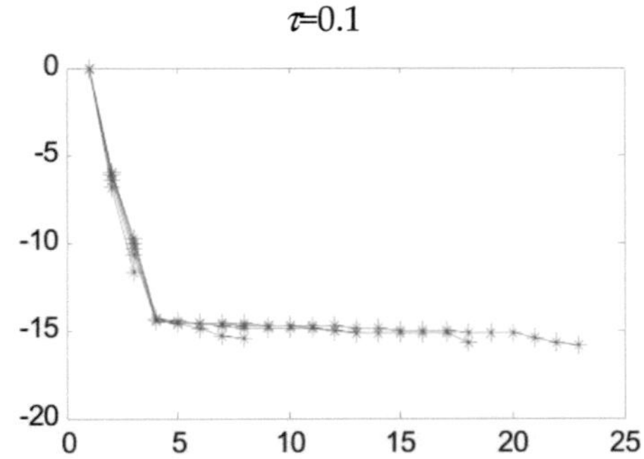

c. The symplectic geometry spectrums, τ=0.005

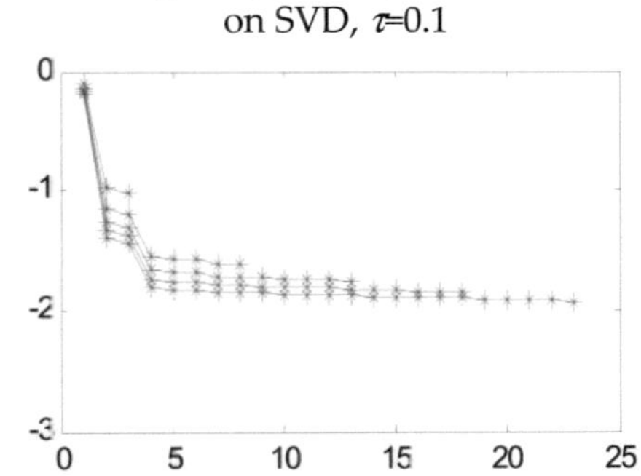

d. The symplectic geometry spectrums, τ=1

Figure 28. The symplectic geometry spectrum analysis of Lorenz chaos series by different sampling intervals, *N*=1000, *d*=3, 8, 13, 18, 23, abscissa is *d*, ordinate is $\log(\mu_i / tr(\mu_i))$

The effect of sampling interval

For the changes of the sampling interval from τ=0.005 to τ=0.1, this paper finds that the embedding dimension can be estimated at 6 from the corresponding symplectic geometry spectrums of Lorenz chaos time series (see Fig. 25c and Fig. 28a), although the position of noise floor is constantly driven up. However, in the same condition, SVD method cannot give the appropriate embedding dimension (see Fig. 25e and 28b), the results of which are similar to the results of the literature[61]. Besides, no matter the sampling interval is over sampling or under sampling, SG method can always give the appropriate embedding dimension d of Lorenz chaos time series (see Fig. 28c and 28d) because the correlation dimension m of Lorenz system is 2.07, in general, if $d>m$, d is viable.

3.7.5. Analysis of the surface EMG signal based on symplectic geometry

For the action surface EMG signal (ASEMG) collected from a normal person, SVD method cannot give its appropriate embedding dimension (see Fig. 29a). The method based on correlation theory can do it but costs much time for computation. Here, SG method can fast obtain its embedding dimension. Figure 29b is the symplectic geometry spectrums of action surface EMG signal. The embedding dimension can be chosen as 6, which is the same as that of correlation dimension analysis[3]. This further shows that the SG method has stronger practicability for the small sets of experiment data.

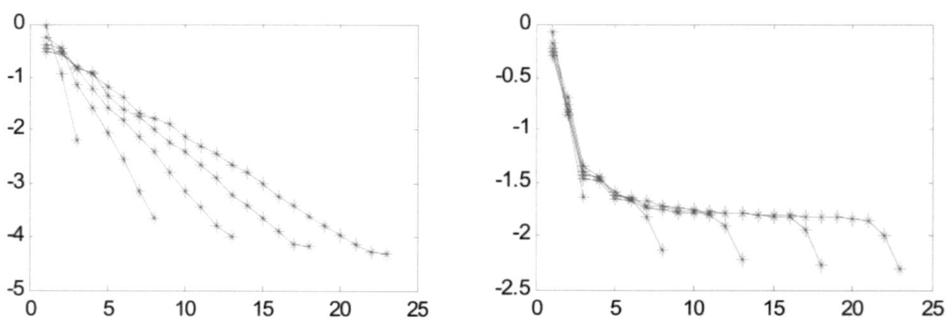

a. The SVD principal component spectrums b. The symplectic geometry spectrums

Figure 29. The analysis of action surface EMG signal, d=3, 8, 13, 18, 23, abscissa is d, ordinate is $\log(\mu_i / tr(\mu_i))$

4. Study of nonlinear dynamical systems based on multifractal theory

Fractal is a kind of geometry structures that have similarity in structure, form or function between the local and the whole. In nature, almost every object is very complex and performs a self-organization phenomenon that is a spatiotemporal structure or state phenomenon by forming spontaneously. From the view of geometry structure, this object has its own self-similarity properties in many parts, called a multifractal system. This structure can often be characterized by a set of coefficients, such as multifractal dimension, wavelet multifractal energy dimension. The multifractal theory reflects the complexity and richness of the nature in essence.

4.1. Self-affine fractal[63-65]

Definition 1 Let the mapping $S: R^n \to R^n$. S is defined by

$$S(x) = T(x) + b \tag{69}$$

where T is a linear transformation on R^n. b is a vector in R^n. Thus, S is a combination of a translation, rotation, dilation and, perhaps, a reflection, called an affine mapping. Unlike similarities, affine mappings contract with differing ratios in different directions.

Theorem 1 Consider the iterated function system given by the contractions{ $S_1, \cdots, S_m$ }on $D \subset R^n$, so that

$$|S_i(x) - S_i(y)| \le C_i |x - y|,\ \forall x, y \in D \tag{70}$$

with $\exists C_i < 1$ for each i. Then there is a unique attractor F, i.e. a non-empty compact set such that

$$F = \bigcup_{i=1}^{m} S_i(F) \tag{71}$$

Moreover, if we define a transformation S on the class ϕ of non-empty compact sets by

$$S(E) = \bigcup_{i=1}^{m} S_i(E) \tag{72}$$

For $E \in \phi$, and write S^k for the kth iterate of S (so $S^0(E) = E$ and $S^k(E) = S(S^{k-1}(E))$ for $k \ge 1$), then

$$F = \bigcap_{k=1}^{\infty} S^k(E) \tag{73}$$

for every set $E \in \phi$ such that $S_i(E) \subset E$ for all i.

If an IFS consists of affine contractions $\{S_1, \cdots, S_m\}$ on R^n, the attractor F guaranteed by Theorem 1 is termed a self-affine set.

Since self-affine time series have a power-law dependence of the power-spectral density function on frequency, .self-affine time series exhibit long-range persistence. For a practical data, one can use the relationship of power spectrum and frequency to determine if the data has the self-affine fractal characteristic.

4.2. Spectrum analysis[65, 66]

Let a time series be $x(t)$, $t \in [0, T]$. Its spectrum is given by

$$X(f,T) = \int_0^T x(t) e^{2\pi i f t} dt \tag{74}$$

where f is frequency. The power spectrum of f is defined by

$$S(f) = \frac{1}{T} |X(f,T)|^2 \tag{75}$$

If the power spectrum obeys a power law

$$S(f) = K \cdot f^{-\beta} \tag{76}$$

for large f, the time series $x(t)$ has the self-affine fractal characteristic. The self-affine fractal dimension D is given

$$D = (5 - \beta)/2 \tag{77}$$

$S(f)$ is plotted as a function of f with log-log scaling. β is the negative of the slope of the best-fit straight line in the range of large f. Note that the value of β is a measure of the strength of persistence in a time series. $\beta>1$ reflects strong persistence and nonstationary. $1>\beta>0$ describes weak persistence and stationary. $\beta=0$ shows uncorrelated stationary. $\beta<0$ indicates antipersistence and stationary. In all cases, however, a self-affine time series with a non-zero β has long-range (as well as short-range) persistence and anti-persistence. For small β, the correlations with large lag are small but are non-zero. This can be contrasted with time series that are not self-affine; these may have only short-range persistence (either strong or weak).

Although the self-affine mapping are varied in a continuous way, the dimension of the self-affine set need not change continuously. Unfortunately, the self-affine fractal situation is much more complicated. It is quite difficult to obtain a general formula for the dimension of self-affine sets. It is not enough that only one fractal dimension is used to describe the self-affine fractal time series. The multifractal dimensions have been proposed to describe this kind of the time series[67-72].

4.3. Multifractal dimension

For a measured time series of a multifractal system, its trajectory in phase space is often attracted to a bounded fractal object called strange attractor for which a whole set of dimension D_q has been introduced which generalize the concept of the Hausdorff dimension. Let X_1, ..., X_n be a point of the attractor in the phase space. The probability that the trajectory point is found within a ball of radius l around one of the inhomogeneously distributed points of the trajectory is denoted by

$$\mu(C_i) = \frac{1}{n}\sum_{i=1}^{n}\theta(l - \|X_i - X_j\|) \tag{78}$$

where $\theta(X)$ is the Heaviside step function. If $X \geq 0$, $\theta(X) = 1$; otherwise, $\theta(X) = 0$.

The q-order correlation integral is defined by

$$C_q(l) = (\frac{1}{n}\sum_{j=1}^{n}(\mu(C_i))^q)^{1/(q-1)} \tag{79}$$

The multifractal dimension D_q can be computed by the following equation:

$$D_q = \lim_{l\to 0}\frac{\ln(C_q(l))}{\ln(l)} = \begin{cases} \dfrac{1}{q-1}\lim\limits_{l\to 0}\dfrac{\ln\sum\limits_{i=1}^{N(l)}[\mu(C_i)]^q}{\ln(l)} & q \neq 1 \\ \lim\limits_{l\to 0}\dfrac{\sum\limits_{i=1}^{N(l)}\mu(C_i)\ln\mu(C_i)}{\ln(l)} & q = 1 \end{cases} \tag{80}$$

The above D_q is the multifractal dimension method based on Grassberger and Procaccia. The generalized correlation integral $C^q(l)$ which can be obtained from an experimental time series yields in a plot $\ln C^q(l)$ vs $\ln l$ straight lines with slopes D_q. For q=0, the D_0 is called the topological dimension, fractal dimension or capacity dimension. For q=1, the D_1 is called the information dimension. For q=2, the D_2 is called correlation dimension. The function D_q is monotonically decreasing with q and gives information about the inhomogeneity of the attractor. For simple fractals, called monofractals, such as a homogeneous attractor, the multifractal dimension D_q is constant. In the general case of multifractal objects, the values of D_q monotonically decrease as q increase[67]. The shape of the D_q can be considered a criterion confirming that the object is a nonuniform fractal. Furthermore, it can be determined if the object is a nonlinear, complex structure by using the multifractal dimension of the signal.

4.4. Analysis of surface EMG signal based on multifractal dimension

The surface EMG signal is a complicated physiological signal. Its distribution is clearly uneven (see Figure 30). When the surface EMG signal is studied by using the fractal method, one should first determine if the surface EMG signal is fractal. Then, its corresponding fractal dimension D can be estimated by Eq.(77) under a certain resolution. Figure 30 shows the self-affine fractal analysis of the surface EMG signals from Channel 1 during finger flexion, finger tension, forearm pronation and forearm supination (the results of Channel 2 are similar to those of Channel 1). It can be seen that the surface EMG signals have self-affine fractal characteristics. The results explain the physiological mechanism of the surface EMG signals.

In view of self-affine fractal characteristics, only one single fractal dimension is not easy to characterize the dynamics of surface EMG signals for different actions (see Table 4). There is little difference for the self-affine fractal dimensions of the four actions, where each type of action signals was chosen 100 sets of the data. The data length is 1000 points. In other words, it is difficult to identify the surface EMG signals of the different actions by using a single fractal dimension. The multifractal dimension values should be used to describe the action surface EMG signals during the arm movements.

	Finger flexion	Finger tension	Forearm pronation	Forearm supination
Channel 1	-0.2402±0.0725	-0.2571±0.0947	-0.0280±0.3250	0.0692±0.1418
Channel 2	0.0738±0.5734	-0.3199±0.2842	-0.0901±0.2591	-0.2343±0.2134

Table 4. The self-affine D of surface EMG signals during movements

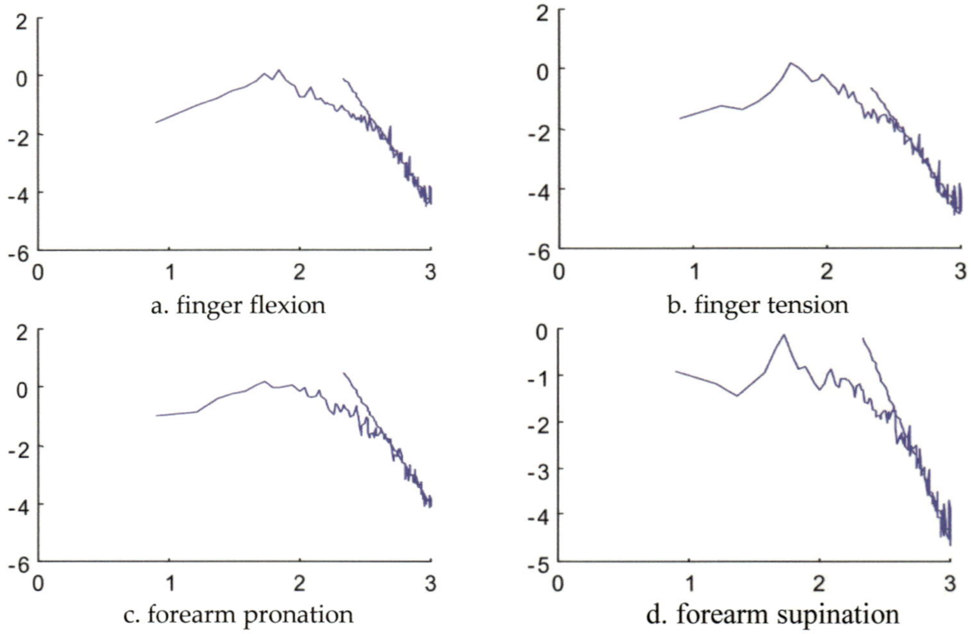

Figure 30. The analysis study of self-affine of surface EMG signal: Curve is power spectrum of surface EMG signal, line is straight line fit related part of curve; Abscissa is lg(*f*), ordinate is lg(Psd)

Here, we use the above multifractal dimension theory to analyze the action surface EMG signals. For the surface EMG signals of the four actions in channel 1, the multifractal analysis results are shown in Figure 31. The results of channel 2 are omitted since they are similar to those of channel 1. In the figure, the D_q-q curves are calculated under q =8, 7, 6, 5, 4, 3, 2, 1, 0, -1, -2, -3, -4, -5, -6, -7, -8. It can be seen that the D_q-q curves have a certain range. The results indicate that the surface EMG signals are non-uniform fractal structure signals. These are consistent with the results of the above self-affine fractal analysis. The parameter values with q can be used to classify the data. In theory, it will be more reasonable that multifractal dimensions are used to describe the surface EMG signals. However, the actual calculation process of the multifractal dimensions is very time-consuming. For the surface EMG signals, it is extremely difficult to meet the requirements of real-time classification.

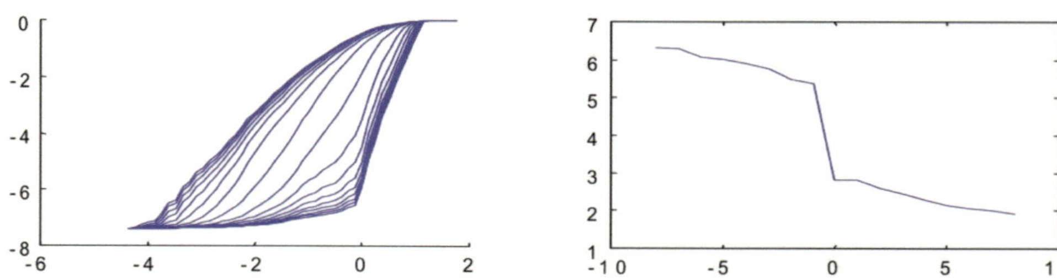

a. The multi-fractal curves of EMG signal during finger flexion; abscissa is ln(l), ordinate is ln($C_q(l)$)

b. The multi-fractal dimensions of curves in Fig. a; abscissa is q, ordinate is D_q

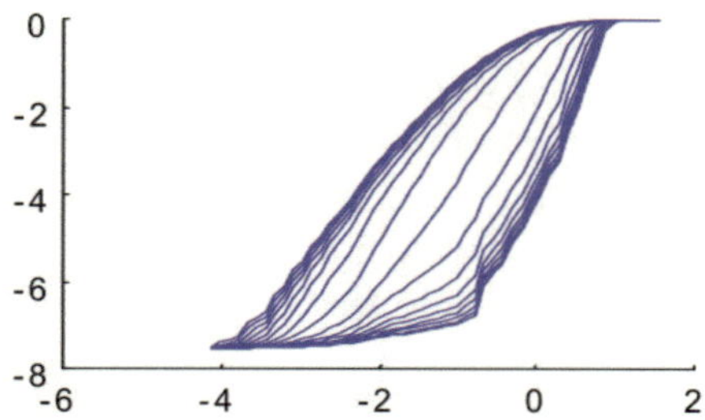

c. The multi-fractal curves of EMG signal during finger tension; abscissa is $\ln(l)$, ordinate is $\ln(C_q(l))$

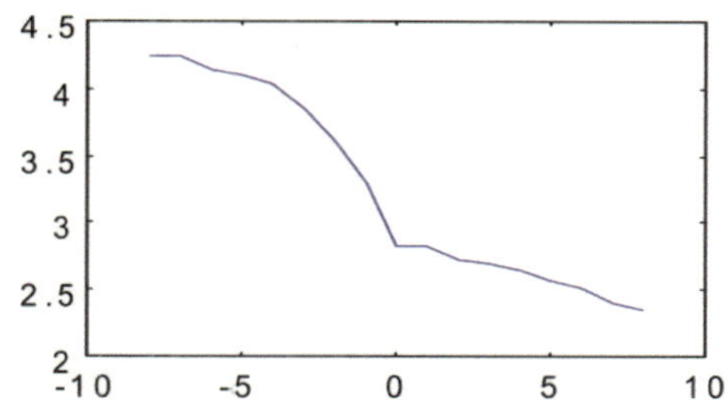

d. The multi-fractal dimensions of curves in Fig. c; abscissa is q, ordinate is D_q

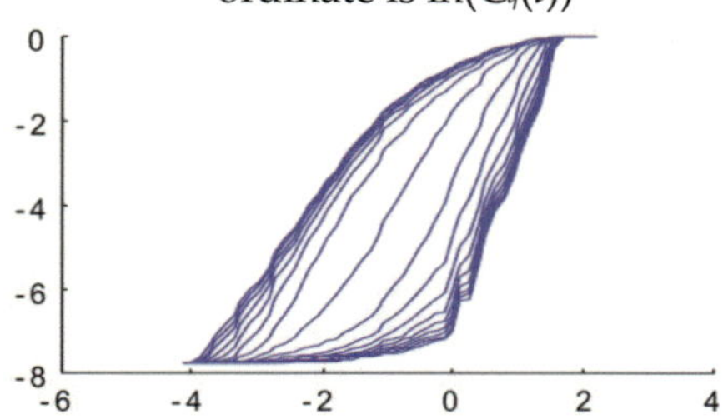

e. The multi-fractal curves of EMG signal during forearm pronation; abscissa is $\ln(l)$, ordinate is $\ln(C_q(l))$

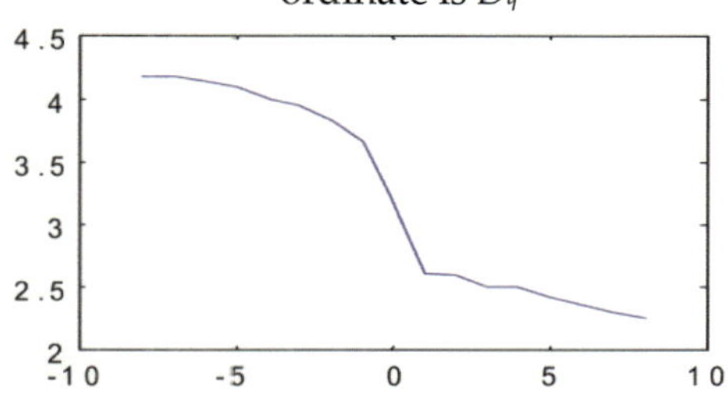

f. The multi-fractal dimensions of curves in Fig. e; abscissa is q, ordinate is D_q

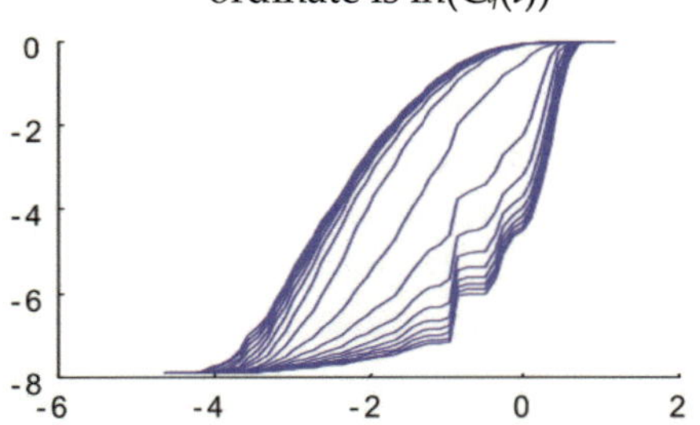

g. The multi-fractal curves of EMG signal during forearm pronation; abscissa is $\ln(l)$, ordinate is $\ln(C_q(l))$

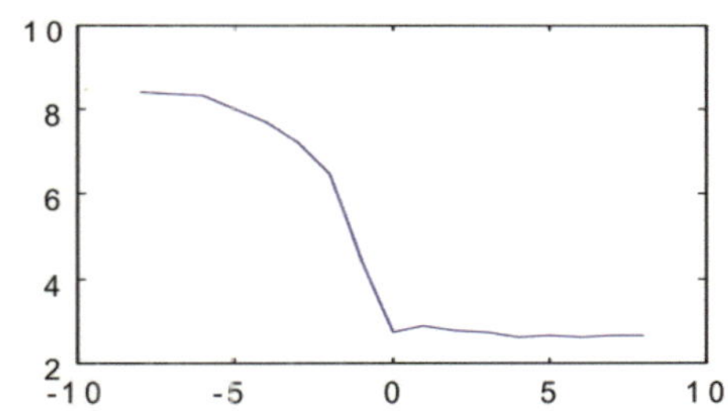

h. The multi-fractal dimensions of curves in Fig. e; abscissa is q, ordinate is D_q

Figure 31. The multi-fractal analysis of surface EMG signals during movements

5. Conclusion and future research

In order to investigate whether the essence of the surface EMG signal is stochastic or deterministic nonlinear (even chaotic), some emerging nonlinear time series analysis approaches are discussed in this chapter. These techniques are based on detecting and describing determinisitic structure in the signal, such as surrogate data method, VWK model method, chaotic analysis method, symplectic geometry method, fractal analysis method, and so on.

The surrogate data method and VWK model mehtod are used to detect the surface EMG signal for arm movement and muscle fatigue. The results show that the surface EMG signal has deterministic nonlinear components. Moreover, our algorithm of surrogate data based on the null hypothesis 3 is proved that can completely satisfy the requirment of the null hypothesis 3. The VWK method with surrogate data can illuminate that not only the action but also fatigue surface EMG signals contain nonlinear dynamic properties.

Chaotic analysis techniques are reviewed and applied to investigate the surface EMG signals. The results show that the surface EMG signals have high-dimension chaotic dynamics by using correlation dimension and largest Lyapunov expoent techniques. For the estimation of embedding dimension, symplectic principal component analysis method is introduced and discussed. In comparison with correlation dimension algorithm and SVD analysis, symplectic geometry analysis is both very simple and reliable. The results show that symplectic geometry method is useful for determining of the system attractor from the experiment data.

The fractal theory is applied to study the fractal feature of the action surface EMG signal collected from forearm of normal person. The results show that he action surface EMG signal possesses the self-affine fractal characteristic. So, it is difficult to describe the surface EMG signals by using a single fractal dimension. The multifractal dimensions are used to analyze the action surface EMG signals during the arm movements. The results indicate that the surface EMG signals are non-uniform fractal structure signals. The multifractal dimension values can be used to identify the surface EMG signals for different movements.

For the nonlinear characteristics of the surface EMG signals, chaos and fractal theories will play the leading role in the nonlinear study of the surface EMG signals. The related methods need to be further researched and developed although these techniques have been applied to analyze the surface EMG signals. It provides a new way for the study of the quantitative analysis of physiology and pathology, sports medicine, clinical medical diagnostics and bionics of robot limb motion.

Apendix A

Theorem 1 proof:

$$\begin{aligned}
\because \quad & J\begin{pmatrix} A & 0 \\ 0 & -A^* \end{pmatrix} J^{-1} \\
&= \begin{pmatrix} 0 & I_n \\ -I_n & 0 \end{pmatrix}\begin{pmatrix} A & 0 \\ 0 & -A^* \end{pmatrix}\begin{pmatrix} 0 & I_n \\ -I_n & 0 \end{pmatrix}^{-1} \\
&= \begin{pmatrix} -A^* & 0 \\ 0 & A \end{pmatrix} \\
&= -\begin{pmatrix} A & 0 \\ 0 & -A^* \end{pmatrix}^*
\end{aligned} \tag{81}$$

$\therefore$ According Definition 2, $\begin{pmatrix} A & 0 \\ 0 & -A^* \end{pmatrix}$ is a Hamilton matrix. □

Theorem 2 proof:

Let S as a symplectic transform matrix, M as a Hamilton matrix. Then S^{-1} is also symplectic matrix. According Definition 1 and 2, there is

$$\begin{aligned} & J\left(SMS^{-1}\right)J^{-1} \\ & = JSJ^{-1}JMJ^{-1}JS^{-1}J^{-1} \\ & = S^{-*}\left(-M^*\right)S^* \\ & = -\left(SMS^{-1}\right)^* \end{aligned} \tag{82}$$

$\therefore SMS^{-1}$ is also a Hamilton matrix.

$$\therefore SMS^{-1} \sim M \tag{83}$$

So Hamilton matrix M keeps unchanged at symplectic similar transform. □

Theorem 5 proof:

Let $S_1, S_2, \ldots, S_n$ as symplectic matrix, respectively. According Definition 1, there are

$$\begin{aligned} & JS_1J^{-1} = S_1^{-*} \\ & JS_2J^{-1} = S_2^{-*} \\ & \cdots \\ & JS_nJ^{-1} = S_n^{-*} \end{aligned} \tag{84}$$

$$\begin{aligned} & J(S_1S_2\cdots S_n)J^{-1} \\ & = JS_1J^{-1}JS_2J^{-1}J\cdots J^{-1}JS_nJ^{-1} \\ & = S_1^{-*}S_2^{-*}\cdots S_n^{-*} \\ & = \left(S_1S_2\cdots S_n\right)^{-*} \end{aligned} \tag{85}$$

So the product of sympletcic matrixes is also a symplectic matrix.

Theorem 6 proof:

In order to prove that H matrix is symplectic matrix, we only need to prove $H^*JH = J$.

$$\begin{aligned} H^*JH & = \begin{pmatrix} P & 0 \\ 0 & P \end{pmatrix}^* J \begin{pmatrix} P & 0 \\ 0 & P \end{pmatrix} \\ & = \begin{pmatrix} 0 & P^*P \\ -P^*P & 0 \end{pmatrix} \end{aligned} \tag{86}$$

$$\because P = I_n - \frac{2\varpi\varpi^*}{\varpi^*\varpi}$$

$$\therefore \quad P^* = P$$

$$\begin{aligned} P^*P &= P^2 \\ &= \left(I_n - \frac{2\varpi\varpi^*}{\varpi^*\varpi}\right)\left(I_n - \frac{2\varpi\varpi^*}{\varpi^*\varpi}\right) \\ &= I_n - \frac{4\varpi\varpi^*}{\varpi^*\varpi} + \frac{4\varpi(\varpi^*\varpi)\varpi^*}{(\varpi^*\varpi)(\varpi^*\varpi)} \\ &= I_n \end{aligned} \tag{87}$$

where $\varpi = (0,\cdots,0;\omega_k,\cdots,\omega_n)^T \neq 0$.

Plugging Eq.(87) into Eq.(86), we have:

$$H^*JH = J \tag{88}$$

$\therefore$ H is symplectic matrix.

$$\begin{aligned} H^*H &= \begin{pmatrix} P & 0 \\ 0 & P \end{pmatrix}^* \begin{pmatrix} P & 0 \\ 0 & P \end{pmatrix} \\ &= \begin{pmatrix} P^*P & 0 \\ 0 & P^*P \end{pmatrix} \\ &= I_{2n} \end{aligned} \tag{89}$$

$\therefore$ H is also unitary matrix.

$\therefore$ H is symplectic unitary matrix. □

Apendix B

Theorem 7 suppose x and y are two unequal n dimension vectors, and $\|x\|_2 = \|y\|_2$, so there is elementary reflective array $H = 1 - 2\omega\omega^T$, which make $Hx = y$, where $\omega = \frac{x-y}{\|x-y\|_2}$.

It can be easily deduced from theorem 5, for non zero n dimension vector $x = (x_1, x_2, \cdots, x_n)^T$, notes $\alpha = \|x\|_2$, there is

$$Hx = \alpha e_1 \tag{90}$$

$$H = 1 - 2\varpi\varpi^T \tag{91}$$

$$e_1 = (1,0,\cdots,0)^T \tag{92}$$

$$\varpi = \frac{1}{\rho}(x - \alpha e_1) \tag{93}$$

$$\rho = \|x - \alpha e_1\|_2 \tag{94}$$

Then $\|\omega\|_2 = 1$, and H is elementary reflective array.

It's easy to testify, elementary reflective array H is symmetry matrix $(H^T = H)$, orthogonal matrix $(H^T H = 1)$ and involution matrix $(H^2 = 1)$.

For real symmetrical matrix A, Householder matrix H can be constructed as follows[73]. Notes A:

$$A = \begin{pmatrix} a_{11} & a_{12} & \cdots & a_{1n} \\ a_{21} & a_{22} & \cdots & a_{2n} \\ \vdots & \vdots & \cdots & \vdots \\ a_{n1} & a_{n2} & \cdots & a_{nn} \end{pmatrix} = \begin{pmatrix} a_{11} & A_{12}^{(1)} \\ \alpha_{21}^{(1)} & A_{22}^{(1)} \end{pmatrix} \tag{95}$$

First, suppose $\alpha_{21}^{(1)} \neq 0$, otherwise this column will be skipped and the next column will be considered until the ith column of $\alpha_{2i}^{(1)} \neq 0$. Set first column vector of A:

$$S^{(1)} = \left(a_{11}^{(1)}, a_{21}^{(1)}, \cdots, a_{n1}^{(1)}\right)^T = \left(a_{11}, a_{21}, \cdots, a_{n1}\right) \tag{96}$$

select elementary reflective array $H^{(1)}$:

$$H^{(1)} = I - 2\varpi^{(1)}(\varpi^{(1)})^T \tag{97}$$

where

$$\begin{cases} \alpha_1 = \left\|S^{(1)}\right\|_2 \\ E^{(1)} = (1, 0, \cdots, 0)^T \qquad n\times 1 \\ \rho_1 = \left\|S^{(1)} - \alpha_1 E^{(1)}\right\| \\ \varpi^{(1)} = \dfrac{1}{\rho_1}\left(S^{(1)} - \alpha_1 E^{(1)}\right) \end{cases} \tag{98}$$

so, after $H^{(1)}$ transform, A is changed to a matrix with the first column is all zero except the first element is α_1, namely:

$$H^{(1)}A = \begin{pmatrix} \sigma_1 & a_{12}^{(2)} & \cdots & a_{1n}^{(2)} \\ 0 & a_{22}^{(2)} & \cdots & a_{2n}^{(2)} \\ \vdots & \vdots & \ddots & \vdots \\ 0 & a_{n2}^{(2)} & \cdots & a_{nn}^{(2)} \end{pmatrix} = A^{(2)} \tag{99}$$

Second, the same method is adopted to the second column vector of $A^{(2)}$, let

$$S^{(2)} = \left(0, a_{22}^{(2)}, \cdots, a_{n2}^{(2)}\right)^T \tag{100}$$

construct $H^{(2)}$ matrix：

$$H^{(2)} = I - 2\omega^{(2)}(\varpi^{(2)})^T \tag{101}$$

where,

$$\begin{cases} \alpha_2 = \left\| S^{(2)} \right\|_2 \\ E^{(2)} = (0, 1, 0, \cdots, 0)^T \qquad n\times 1 \\ \rho_2 = \left\| S^{(2)} - \alpha_2 E^{(2)} \right\| \\ \varpi^{(2)} = \dfrac{1}{\rho_2}\left(S^{(2)} - \alpha_2 E^{(2)} \right) \end{cases} \tag{102}$$

Using $H^{(2)}$, the second column of $A^{(2)}$ can be changed to all zero vector except the first and second elements, namely:

$$H^{(2)} A^{(2)} = A^{(3)} \tag{103}$$

Householder matrix H can be obtained by repeating above mentioned method until $A^{(n)}$ becomes an upper triangle matrix:

$$H = H^{(n)} H^{(n-1)} \cdots H^{(1)} \tag{104}$$

Author details

Min Lei and Guang Meng
Institute of Vibration, Shock and Noise, State Key Laboratory of Mechanical System and Vibration, Shanghai Jiao Tong University, Shanghai, P R China

Acknowledgement

This work was supported by the National Natural Science Foundation of China (No. 10872125 and No.69675002), Science Fund for Creative Research Groups of the National Natural Science Foundation of China(no. 50821003), State Key Lab of Mechanical System and Vibration，Project supported by the Research Fund of State Key Lab of MSV, China (Grant no. MSV-MS-2010-08) , Key Laboratory of Hand Reconstruction, Ministry of Health, Shanghai, People's Republic of China, Shanghai Key Laboratory of Peripheral Nerve and Microsurgery, Shanghai, People's Republic of China, Science and Technology Commission of Shanghai Municipality (no.06ZR14042). We also thank Chinese Academy of Engineering GU Yudong and Professor Zhang Kaili very much for providing related data and valuable discussions.

6. References

[1] J Theiler, S Eubank, A Longtin, et al., Testing for nonlinearity in time series: the method of surrogate data. Physica D, 1992. 58: 77-94.
[2] M Barahona and C-S Poon, Detection of nonlinear dynamics in short, noisy time series. Nature, 1996. 381: 215-217.
[3] M Lei, Z Z Wang, and Z J Feng, Detecting nonlinearity of action surface EMG signal. Phys. Lett. A, 2001. 290(5-6): 297-303.

[4] M Palus and D Hoyer, Detecting nonlinearity and phase synchronization with surrogate data. IEEE Engineering in Medical and Biology, 1998. 17(6): 40-45.

[5] C-S Poon and K M Christopher, Decrease of cardiac chaos in congestive heart failure. Nature, 1997. 389: 492-495.

[6] J Theiler and D Prichard, Constrained-realization Monte-Carlo method for hypothesis testing. Physica D, 1996. 94: 221-235.

[7] C S Poon and M Barahona, Titration of chaos with added noise. Proceedings of The National Academy of Sciences of The United States of America, 2001. 98(13): 7107-7112.

[8] J A Scheinkman and B LeBaron., Nonlinear dynamics and stock returns. Journal of Business, 1989. 62(3): 311-337.

[9] J L Breeden and N H Packard, Nonlinear analysis of data sampled nonuniformly in time. Physica D, 1992. 58(1-4): 273-283.

[10] A R Osborne and A Provenzale, Finite correlation dimension for stochastic systems with power-law spectra. Physica D, 1989. 35(3): 357-381.

[11] M Lei, Nonlinear Time Series Analysis and Its Applied Study in Surface EMG Signal. 2000, Shanghai Jiao Tong University (in chinese).

[12] T Schreiber and A Schmitz, Improved surrogate data for nonlinearity tests. Phys. Rev. Lett., 1996. 77(4): 635-638.

[13] M Lei and Z Z Wang, Application of surrogate data method in electromyograph analysis. Journal of Shanghai Jiao Tong University, 2000. 34(11): 1594-1597 (in Chinese).

[14] M Lei and Z Z Wang, Study of the surrogate data method for nonlinearity of time series. Journal of Electronics and Information Technology, 2001. 23(3): 248-254 (in Chinese).

[15] M Lei, Z J Feng, and Z Z Wang, The Volterra-Wiener-Korenberg model nonlinear test method. Journal of Shanghai Jiao Tong University, 2003. 37(2): 269-272 (in Chinese).

[16] M Lei and G Meng, The influence of noise on nonlinear time series detection based on Volterra-Wiener-Korenberg model. Chaos, Solitons and Fractals, 2008. 36: 512-516.

[17] E N Lorenz, Determinstic nonperiodic flow. Journal of The Atmospheric Sciences, 1963. 20: 130-141.

[18] T Y Li and J A Yorke, Period three implies chaos. Amer Math Monthly, 1975. 82: 985-992.

[19] R M May, Simple mathematical models with very complicated dynamics. Nature, 1976. 261: 459-467.

[20] G U Yule., On a method of investigating periodicities in disturbed series with special reference to wolfer's sunspot numbers. Phil. Trans. R. Soc. London A, 1927. 226(636-646): 267-298

[21] F Takens, Detecting Strange Attractors in Turbulence. Dynamical Systems and Turbulence, 1980. 898: p. 366-381.

[22] N H Packard, J P Crutchfield, J D Farmer, et al., Geometry from a time series. Phys. Rev. Lett., 1980. 45: 712-716.

[23] K Vibe and J M Vesin, On chaos detection methods. International Journal of Bifurcation and Chaos, 1996. 6(3): 529-543.

[24] A M Fraser, Information and entropy in strange attractors. IEEE Trans. Inf. Theory, 1989. 35(2): 245-262.

[25] B Cheng and H Tong, Orthoggonal Projection, Embeding Dimension and Sample size in chaotic times series from a statistical perspective. Nonlinear time series and chaos, 1994. 2(15): 1-30.

[26] H S Kim, R Eykholt, and J D Salas, Nonlinear dynamics, delay times, and embedding windows. Physica D, 1999. 127: 48-60.

[27] D Kugiumtzis, State space reconstruction parameters in the analysis of chaotic time series — the role of the time window length. Physica D, 1996. 95(1): 13–28.

[28] M T Rosenstein, J J Collins, and C J D Luca, Reconstruction expansion as a geometry-based framework for choosing proper delay times. Physica D, 1994. 73: 82-98.

[29] J M Martinerie, A M Albano, A I Mees, et al., Mutual information, strange attractors, and the optimal estimation of dimension. Phys. Rev. A 1992. 45: 7058-7064.

[30] A M Fraser and H L Swinney, Independent coordinates for strange attractors from mutual information. Phys. Rev. A, 1986. 33(2): 1134-1140.

[31] D S Broomhead and G P King, Extracting qualitative dynamics from experimental data. Physica D, 1986. 20(2-3): 217–236.

[32] M Knennel, R Brown, and H Abarbanel., Determining embedding dimension for phase — space reconstruction using a geometrical construction. Phys. Rev. A, 1992. 45: 3403–3411.

[33] P Grassberger and I Procaccia, Measuring the strangeness of strange attractors. Physica D, 1983. 9(1-2): 189-208.

[34] A Galka, T Maaß, and P G., Estimating the dimension of high-dimensional attractors: a comparison between two algorithms. Physica D, 1998. 121: 237-251.

[35] K Judd and A Mees, Embedding as a modeling problem. Physica D, 1998. 120: 273-286.

[36] L Cao, Practical method for determining the minimum embedding dimension of a scalar time series. Physica D, 1997. 110(1-2): 43–50.

[37] M Palus and I Dvorak, Singular-value decomposition in attractor reconstruction: pitfalls and precautions. Physica D, 1992. 55: 221-234.

[38] K Judd, An improved estimator of dimension and some comments on providing confidence intervals. Physica D, 1992. 56: 216-228.

[39] P Grassberger, Generalized dimensions of strange attractors. Phys. Lett. A, 1983. 97: 227-234.

[40] P Grassberger and I Procaccia, Characterization of strange attractors. Phys. Rev. Lett., 1983. 50: 346–349.

[41] M Ding, C Grebogi, E Ott, et al., Plateau onset for correlation dimension: when does it occur? Phys. Rev. Lett. , 1993. 70: 3872–3875.

[42] M Small and K Judd, Detecting nonlinearity in experimental data. International Journal of Bifurcation and Chaos, 1998. 8(6): 1231-1244.

[43] A Wolf, J Swift, H Swinney, et al., Determining Lyapunov exponents from a time series. Physica D, 1985. 16: 285-317.

[44] M Sano and Y Sawada, Measurement of the Lyapunov spectrum from a chaotic time series. Phys. Rev. Lett., 1985. 55(10): 1082-1085.

[45] M T Rosenstein, J J Collins, and C J D Luca, A practical method for calculating largest lyapunov exponents from small data sets. Physica D, 1993. 65: 117-134.

[46] A I Mees, P E Rapp, and L S Jennings, Singular-value decomposition and embedding dimension. Phys. Rev. A, 1987. 36: 340–346.

[47] A M Fraser., Reconstructing attractors from scalar time series : a comparison of singular system and redundancy criteria. Physica D, 1989. 34: 391-404.

[48] A Brandsttater, H L Swinney, and G I Chapman, Characterizing turbulent channel flow. in: Dimensions and entropies in chaotic systems, G. Mayer-Kree(Ed.), Springer, Berlin 1986: 150.

[49] M Lei, Z Z Wang, and Z J Feng, A method of embedding dimension estimation based on symplectic geometry. Phys. Lett. A, 2002. 303(2-3): 179-189.

[50] X Lu and R Schmid, Symplectic integration of Sine-Gordon type systems. Mathematics and Computers in Simulation, 1999. 50: 255-263.

[51] Z G Ying and W Q Zhu, Exact stationary solutions of stochastically excited and dissipated gyroscopic systems. International Journal of Non-Linear Mechanics, 2000. 35: 837-848.

[52] A C J Luo and R P S Han, The resonance theory for stochastic layers in nonlinear dynamic systems. Chaos, Solitons and Fractals, 2001. 12: 2493-2508.

[53] K Feng, Proceeding of the 1984 Beijing Symposium on Differential Geometry and Differential Equations: Computation of partial differential equations, ed. F. Kang. 1985: Science Press, 42.

[54] C V Loan, A Symplectic Method for Approximating All the Elgenvalues of a Hamiltonian Matrix. Linear Algebra and Its Applications, 1984. 61: 233-251.

[55] M Lei, Z Z Wang, and Z J Feng, The application of symplectic geometry on nonlinear dynamics analysis of the experimental data. 14th International Conference on Digital Signal Processing Proceeding, 2002. 1-2: 1137-1140.

[56] M Lei and G Meng, Detecting nonlinearity of sunspot number. International Journal of Nonlinear Sciences and Numerical Simulation, 2004. 5(4): 321-326.

[57] X Niu, F Qu, and N Wang, Evaluating Sprinters' Surface EMG Signals Based on EMD and Symplectic Geometry. J of Ocean Univ. of Qingdao, 2005. 35(1): 125-129.(in Chinese).

[58] H Xie, Z Z Wang, and H Huang, Identification determinism in time series based on symplectic geometry spectra. Phys. Lett. A, 2005. 342(1-2): 156-161.

[59] M Lei and G Meng, Symplectic principal component analysis: a new method for time series analysis. Mathematical Problems in Engineering, 2011. 2011: Article ID 793429, 14pages.

[60] M Lei and G Meng, A noise reduction method for continuous chaotic systems based on symplectic geometry. The Seventh International Conference on Vibration Engineering and Technology of Machinery, 2011. 1: Article ID 173, 6pages.

[61] Y Gong and J Xu, Chaos signal and noise. Signal Processing, 1997. 13(2): 112-118 (in Chinese)

[62] J Yuan and X C Xiao, Higher-order singular-spectrum analysis of nonlinear time series. Acta Physica Sinica, 1998. 47(6): 897-905 (in Chinese).

[63] B B Mandelbrot, Self-affine fractals and fractal dimension. Physica Scripta, 1985. 32: 257-260.

[64] B B Mandelbrot, The fractal geometry of Nature. 1982: San Francisco: Freeman.

[65] K Falconer, Fractal Geometry: Mathematical Foundations and Applications. 2003: John Wiley &Sons Ltd. 337.

[66] B D Malamud and D L Turcotte, Self-affine time series: measures of weak and strong persistence. Journal of Statistical Planning and Inference, 1999. 80: 173-196.

[67] A N Pavlov and V S Anishchenko, Multifractal analysis of complex signals. Physics-Uspekhi, 2007. 50(8): 819-834.

[68] R H Riedi, M S Crouse, V J Ribeiro, et al., A multifractal wavelet model with application to network traffic. IEEE Trans. On Information Theory, 1999. 45(3): 992-1018.

[69] A Z R Langi, K Soemintapura, and W Kinsner. Multifractal processing of speech signals. in International Conference on Information, Communications and Signal Processing. 1997.

[70] Z Xu and S Xiao. Fractal dimension of surface EMG and its determinants. in Proceedings of the 19th Annual International Conference of the IEEE Engineerings in Medicine and Biology Society. 1997.

[71] O Adeyemi and G F Boudreaux-Bartels. Improved accuracy in the singularity spectrum of multifractal chaotic time series. in IEEE International Conference on Acoustics, Speech, and Signal Processing. 1997.

[72] C J Aumuth, Fractals dimension of electromyographic signals recorded with surface electrodes during isometric contractions with muscle activation. Muscle & Nerve, 1994. 17: 953-954.

[73] J Huang, The practical modeling method of static and dynamic mathematical model. 1988, Beijing: Mechanical Industry Press (in Chinese).

Chapter 7

Normalization of EMG Signals: To Normalize or Not to Normalize and What to Normalize to?

Mark Halaki and Karen Ginn

Additional information is available at the end of the chapter

http://dx.doi.org/10.5772/49957

1. Introduction

Electromyography (EMG) has been around since the 1600s [1]. It is a tool used to measure the action potentials of motor units in muscles [2]. The EMG electrodes are like little microphones which "listen" for muscle action potentials so having these microphones in different locations relative to the muscle or motor units affects the nature of the recording [3]. The amplitude and frequency characteristics of the raw electromyogram signal have been shown to be highly variable and sensitive to many factors. De Luca [4] provided a detailed account of these characteristics which have a "basic" or "elemental" effect on the signal dividing them into extrinsic and intrinsic sub-factors. Extrinsic factors are those which can be influenced by the experimenter, and include: electrode configuration (distance between electrodes as well as area and shape of the electrodes); electrode placement with respect to the motor points in the muscle and lateral edge of the muscle as well as the orientation to the muscle fibres; skin preparation and impedance [5, 6]; and perspiration and temperature [7]. Intrinsic factors include: physiological, anatomical and biochemical characteristics of the muscles such as the number of active motor units; fiber type composition of the muscles; blood flow in the muscle; muscle fiber diameter; the distance between the active fibers within the muscle with respect to the electrode; and the amount of tissue between the surface of the muscle and the electrode. These factors vary between individuals, between days within an individual and within a day in an individual if the electrode set up has been altered. Given that there are many factors that influence the EMG signal, voltage recorded from a muscle is difficult to describe in terms of level if there is no reference value to which it can be compared. Therefore, interpretation of the amplitude of the raw EMG signal is problematic unless some kind of normalization procedure is performed. Normalization refers to the conversion of the signal to a scale relative to a known and repeatable value. It has been reported [8] that normalized EMG signals were first presented by Eberhart, Inman & Bresler in 1954 [9]. Since then, there have been a number of methods used to normalize EMG signals with no consensus as to which method is most appropriate [8]. In this chapter, we will outline when the presentation of raw EMG is acceptable and when normalization is essential as well as the various methods used to normalize EMG signals. A discussion of the advantages and disadvantages of each method and examples of its uses will be provided.

2. Raw EMG signals (without normalization)

As indicated in the introduction, there are many factors that influence the EMG signal. However, it is generally accepted that within a data collection session and within an individual where no changes have been made to the configuration of the EMG set-up (electrode placement, amplification, filtering etc), under constant temperature and humidity conditions and within a short period of time, the raw EMG can be used for limited comparisons such as:

1. the analysis of the frequency content of the EMG signal. In this type of analysis, the power spectrum of the EMG signal can be obtained by applying a Fast Fourier Transform to the EMG signal. The power density function of the EMG provides a distribution of the signal power as a function of frequency. Changes in the shape of the power density function of the EMG is usually analysed and shifts in the power density to lower frequencies is associated with fatigue. Since the shape of the power spectra is what is important, the amplitude of the EMG signal is not critical and EMG normalization is not required.
2. the decomposition of the EMG into wavelets for an analysis of motor unit firing patterns, or cross talk between muscles. In this analysis, the EMG signal is decomposed into small wavelets (small waveforms). The wavelets are then used to identify and characterize motor unit action potentials by compressing and/or rescaling the wavelets and identifying them in the EMG signal. Again, the amplitude of the EMG signal is not critical and EMG normalization is not required.
3. the time of the initiation of muscle activation. This type of analysis does not require EMG normalization as the time of activation is usually identified from the raw signal e.g. when the raw EMG signal amplitude reaches 2 [10] or 3 [11] standard deviations of the mean above baseline levels.
4. amplitude comparisons of signals from a given muscle between short term interventions/movements within an individual in the same session under the same experimental conditions without changes to the EMG electrode set-up [12] e.g. when comparing the EMG signal between different interventions/movements in a given muscle in each individual [13-16]. Because the absolute amplitude of the signal is meaningless, one cannot evaluate the level of activity in the muscle, but only that it is more or less active in one intervention/movement compared to the other. Therefore, comparison of muscle activity levels between muscles or individuals is not valid.

3. Normalization of EMG signals

To be able to compare EMG activity in the same muscle on different days or in different individuals or to compare EMG activity between muscles, the EMG must be normalized [4,

17, 18]. Normalization of EMG signals is usually performed by dividing the EMG signals during a task by a reference EMG value obtained from the same muscle. By normalizing to a reference EMG value collected using the same electrode configuration, factors that affect the EMG signals during the task and the reference contraction are the same. Therefore, one can validly obtain a relative measure of the activation compared to the reference value.

The common consensus is that a "good" reference value to which to normalize EMG signals should have high repeatability, especially in the same subject in the same session, and be meaningful. By choosing a reference value repeatable within an individual, one can compare the levels obtained from any task to that reference value. The choice of reference value should allow comparisons between individuals and between muscles. To be able to do so, the reference value should have similar meaning between individuals and between muscles. The choice of normalization method is critical in the interpretation of the EMG signals as it will influence the amplitude and pattern of the EMG signals [8]. Unfortunately, there is no consensus as to a single "best" method for normalization of EMG data [8, 18] and a variety of methods have been used to obtain normalization reference values:

1. Maximum (peak) activation levels during maximum contractions
2. Peak or mean activation levels obtained during the task under investigation
3. Activation levels during submaximal isometric contractions
4. Peak to peak amplitude of the maximum M-wave (M-max)

3.1. Maximum (peak) activation levels during maximum contractions

3.1.1. Maximal voluntary isometric contractions

The most common method of normalizing EMG signals from a given muscle uses to the EMG recorded from the same muscle during a maximal voluntary isometric contraction (MVIC) as the reference value [19-23]. The process of normalization using MVICs is that a reference test (usually a manual muscle test) is identified which produces a maximum contraction in the muscle of interest. Based on the repeatability between tests measures, it is recommended that at least 3 repetitions of the test be performed separated by at least 2 minutes to reduce any fatigue effects [12]. The EMG signals are then processed either by high-pass filtering, rectifying and smoothing or by calculating the root mean square of the signal. The maximum value obtained [12] from the processed signals during all repetitions of the test is then used as the reference value for normalizing the EMG signals, processed in the same way, from the muscle of interest. This allows the assessment of the level of activity of the muscle of interest during the task under investigation compared to the maximal neural activation capacity of the muscle [24-26].

This method sounds simple enough. However, when trying to implement it, investigators are faced with an important question: *What test should be used to produce maximum neural activation in a given muscle?* The choice of MVIC should reflect the maximal neural activation capacity of the given muscle [27]. Unfortunately, there is no consensus as to which test produces maximal activation in all individuals in any given muscle. Table 1 provides some examples of different tests that have been used for the same muscle in different studies. Note the number of different reference tests used for each muscle indicating the lack of consensus as to what test generates maximum activity in any given muscle.

Muscles investigated	Manual muscle test
upper trapezius	• shoulder shrug [28, 29] • combined shoulder elevation/arm flexion/abduction in the scapular plane at 90° abduction [30] • shoulder abduction in scapular plane at 90° abduction [31, 32] • lumbar extension [33]
supraspinatus	• shoulder abduction at 90°, internal rotation (seated) [28] • shoulder abduction at 90°, elbow flexed to 90° (seated) [34] • shoulder external rotation and abduction, shoulder abducted to 20°, elbow flexed to 90°, no shoulder flexion [29]
infraspinatus	• shoulder external rotation, arm at side, elbow flexed to 90° (seated) [28, 31, 34] • shoulder external rotation, shoulder abducted to 45°, elbow flexed to 90°, no shoulder flexion [29]
subscapularis	• shoulder internal rotation, arm at side, elbow flexed to 90° (seated) [28, 34] • shoulder internal rotation, shoulder abducted to 45°, elbow flexed to 90°, no shoulder flexion [29]
latissimus dorsi	• shoulder depression with resistance or adduction and internal rotation, arm at side (seated) [28] • shoulder extension and internal rotation with arm straight, abducted to 30° in the coronal plane and internally rotated [29] • shoulder extension (prone lying) [35, 36]
serratus anterior	• scapular protraction, shoulder abducted to 90°-100° (seated) [28] • scapular protraction, elbow flexed to 45°, shoulder abducted to 75° and internally rotated to 45° [29]
upper rectus abdominis	• trunk flexion, hips and knees flexed to 90°, feet supported, trunk in full flexion (supine) [35, 36] • trunk flexion, legs bent at 45°,and secured, trunk position not mentioned (supine) [37]
internal oblique	• trunk flexion and lateral flexion, hips and knees flexed to 90°, feet supported, trunk in full flexion and rotated contra-laterally (supine) [35] • trunk flexion and lateral flexion, hips and knees flexed to 90°, feet supported, trunk in full flexion and rotated ipsi-laterally (supine) [36]
gluteus maximus	• hip extension, hip flexed 45° (prone) [38] • back extension, hip flexed 30° (seated) [39] • hip abduction at 10° abduction, leg fully extended (side lying) contra-lateral knee and hip flexed 30° [40]
gluteus medius	• hip abduction at 10° abduction, leg fully extended (side lying) contra-lateral knee and hip flexed 30° [40, 41] • hip abduction at 25° abduction, leg fully extended (side lying) [42]

Muscles investigated	Manual muscle test
vastus lateralis	• knee extension, knee flexed 90°, hip flexed 90° (sitting) [38, 43] • knee extension, knee flexed 60°, hip flexed 90° (sitting) [44, 45] • knee extension, knee flexed 45° (sitting) [37]
vastus medialis	• knee extension, knee flexed 60° (sitting) [44, 45] • knee extension, knee flexed 90°, hip flexed 90° (sitting) [43]
rectus femoris	• knee extension, knee flexed 90°, hip flexed 80° to 90° (sitting) [35, 36, 38, 43] • knee extension, knee flexed 60°, hip flexed 90° (sitting) [44-46]
lateral hamstring (biceps femoris) long head	• knee flexion, knee flexed 90°, hip flexed 90° (sitting) [38] • knee flexion, knee flexed 60° (sitting) [44, 46] • knee flexion, knee flexed 60° (prone) [45] • knee flexion, knee flexed 90°, hands clasped behind head (prone) [37]
gastrocnemius lateralis	• ankle plantar flexion, ankle -15°, knee flexed 30° [44] • ankle plantar flexion, mid ankle position (standing unilateral – body weight) [47] • ankle plantar flexion, ankle, knee and hip in neutral position (prone) [45]
gastrocnemius medialis	• ankle plantar flexion, ankle, knee and hip in neutral position (prone) [38, 45] • ankle plantar flexion, ankle -15°, knee flexed 30° [44] • ankle plantar flexion, mid ankle position (standing unilateral – body weight) [47] • ankle plantar flexion (supine) [33]
soleus	• ankle plantar flexion, mid ankle position (prone) [38] • ankle plantar flexion, ankle in neutral position; knee and hip flexed 90° (quadruped position) [45, 46]
tibialis anterior	• ankle dorsi flexion, ankle, knee and hip in neutral position (supine) [45] • ankle dorsi flexion, ankle in neutral position; knee and hip flexed 90° (quadruped position) [46]

Table 1. Examples of MVIC tests used to generate maximum activity levels in various muscles

Although the repeatability of the EMG recorded during MVICs within individuals on the same day has been questioned [34], the majority of studies indicate that the reliability of MVICs within individuals on the same day is high [42, 48, 49]. High repeatability requires proper guidance of the subjects to perform the tests identically with each repetition, familiarity of the subjects with the production of maximum effort and the avoidance of fatigue.

Because the test that will yield maximal activation in any given muscle is not known, many studies report EMG levels during various tasks that are >100% MVIC particularly during rapid, forceful contractions [18] or eccentric contractions [50]. For example, Jobe et al. [51] reported EMG signals from serratus anterior and triceps brachii during the acceleration phase of the over arm throw to be 226% and 212% respectively of the EMG from maximal manual muscle tests which were not described. Reported normalized EMG signals >100% indicate that the normalization test used to generate the MVIC is not accurately revealing the maximum muscle activation capacity. If maximum activity in each muscle is not obtained during the normalization contractions, a systematic error will be introduced which leads to an over estimation of activation levels [30]. This could lead to an incorrect interpretation of the intensity of the muscle activity required to perform a given task. In addition, if the activity in all muscles is not being referenced to the same activity level, e.g. maximum capacity, comparison of activity levels between muscles is not valid.

The problem of not eliciting maximum capacity in each muscle tested would be avoided if standard tests that reliably elicit maximum activation levels were identified [52]. A number of studies have attempted to identify voluntary isometric tests that produce maximum activation levels in various muscles. These studies have shown that multiple tests can produce maximum recording from any given muscle [52-56] and that no specific test produces maximum recording from a given muscle in all individuals tested [27, 53, 54, 56-63]. These findings indicate that the use of single MVIC test to identify maximum activity in a given muscle is not valid and that sets of tests are required in order to ensure maximum activity in a given muscle is recorded from all subjects. Table 2 summarizes the sets of MVIC tests that have been shown to produce maximum activity in face, trunk, shoulder and leg muscles.

Provided that maximum neural activation is achieved in all muscles and individuals tested, using MVICs is a highly reliable method to normalize EMG data and can be used to compare activity between muscles, between tasks and between individuals. To achieve the maximum neural activation in all muscles and individuals, sets of MVIC tests that produce maximum activation in each muscle need to be identified. The highest value recorded for each muscle from at least 3 attempts at these MVIC tests should be used as the normalization value to ensure that the recorded values reflect maximum neural activation levels.

Study	Muscles investigated	MVIC test	Isometric tests that produce maximum EMG in the muscles investigated
O'Dwyer et al (1981) [56]	levator labii superiori zygomaticus major buccinator risorius orbicularis oris superioris orbicularis oris inferioris depressor anguli oris depressor labii inferioris mentalis intrinsic tongue muscles anterior genioglossus styloglossus/hyoglossus geniohyoid mylohyoid digastric (anterior belly) internal (medial) pterygoid temporalis	Maximum EMG from each muscle across all tests	1. unilateral snarl 2. broad laugh 3. puff out cheeks, mouth closed 4. broad smile, mouth closed 5. compress upper lip against upper incisors 6. compress lower lip against lower incisors 7. depress comers of mouth 8. depress lower lip, jaw closed 9. raise and evert lower lip while wrinkling chin 10. curl sides of tongue up 11. saliva swallow 12. gentle tongue protrusion 13. lower jaw against resistance 14. intercuspal bite on hard object 15. clench jaw.

Study	Muscles investigated	MVIC test	Isometric tests that produce maximum EMG in the muscles investigated
McGill (1991) [59]	rectus abdominis external oblique internal oblique latissimus dorsi upper erector spinae (T9) lower erector spinae (L3)	1,2,6,7 1,2,5,6,7 1,3,5,6,7 2,3,6,7 3,4,7 4	1. resisted bent-knee sit-up (feet restrained trunk at 30º hands behind head). 2. standing pelvis fixed flexing forward 3. standing pelvis fixed lateral bend 4. hanging over the edge of the test table in a prone posture and extending upward against resistance 5. hanging over the edge of the test table supine and flexing upward against resistance 6. hanging over the edge of the test table on side and lateral bending upward against resistance 7. clockwise and anticlockwise trunk twist at 0º and pre-rotated at ± 30º
Nieminen et al (1993) [61]	supraspinatus infraspinatus upper trapezius middle trapezius lower trapezius anterior deltoid middle deltoid pectoralis major	5,6,7,8 2,5,6,7 5,6,7,8 2,3,4,6,7 1,2,5,6,8 3,5,6,7 2,3,5,6,7 1,4,5,9	1. internal rotation shoulder at 0º abduction, elbow at 90º flexion 2. external rotation shoulder at 0º abduction, elbow at 90º flexion 3. abduction shoulder at 0º abduction 4. shoulder elevation 5. flexion arm horizontal 6. flexion hand 25 cm above and 25 cm right of horizontal 7. flexion hand 25 cm above and 25 cm left of horizontal 8. flexion hand 25 cm below and 25 cm right of horizontal 9. flexion hand 25 cm below and 25 cm left of horizontal
Kelly et al 1996 [54]	supraspinatus infraspinatus subscapularis anterior deltoid middle deltoid posterior deltoid latissimus dorsi pectoralis major	7-9,12-14 10-12 16,17 1-9 7 12 16,17 15	Coded: Activity at shoulder abduction angle; humeral rotation angle 1. abduction at 0º; -45º 2. abduction at 0º; 0º 3. abduction at 0º; +45º 4. abduction at 45º; -45º 5. abduction at 45º; 0º 6. abduction at 45º; +45º 7. abduction at 90º; -45º 8. abduction at 90º; 0º 9. abduction at 90º; +45º 10. external rotation at 0º; -45º 11. external rotation at 45º; -45º 12. external rotation at 90º; -45º 13. external rotation at 90º; 0º 14. external rotation at 90º; +45º 15. internal rotation at 0º; 0º 16. internal rotation at 90º; -45º 17. internal rotation at 90º; 0º

Study	Muscles investigated	MVIC test	Isometric tests that produce maximum EMG in the muscles investigated
Ekstrom et al (2005) [27]	upper trapezius middle trapezius lower trapezius serratus anterior	1,2,3,4,5,7 5,6,7 1,2,3,5,7,8 1,2,3	1. shoulder flexion at 125º with scapula resistance 2. shoulder abducted to 125º scapular plane 3. shoulder abducted to 90º with the neck side bent, rotated to the opposite side, and extended 4. scapula elevated with the neck side bent, rotated to the opposite side, and extended 5. shoulder horizontally abducted and externally rotated 6. shoulder horizontally abducted and internally rotated 7. arm raised above the head in line with the lower trapezius muscle 8. shoulder externally rotated at 90º abduction
Hsu et al (2006) [45]	tibialis anterior lateral gastrocnemius medial gastrocnemius soleus vastus lateralis vastus medialis rectus femoris lateral hamstrings (biceps femoris) medial hamstrings (semitendinosus)	Maximum EMG from each muscle across all tests	1. entire leg flexion and extension, seated with backrest reclined 45º, hip flexed 110º, knee flexed 60º, ankle neutral. 2. knee flexion and extension, seated with backrest vertical, knee flexed 60º
Boettcher et al 2008 [53] and Ginn et al 2011 [57]	supraspinatus infraspinatus subscapularis lower subscapularis upper trapezius middle trapezius lower trapezius serratus anterior latissimus dorsi rhomboid major teres major anterior deltoid middle deltoid posterior deltoid pectoralis major (clavicular head)	Maximum EMG from each muscle across all 5 tests provides >95% chance of eliciting maximum for all muscles	1. shoulder extension seated with the arm at 30º abduction, elbow fully extended, and thumb toward the body; arm extended as resistance applied over the distal forearm. 2. shoulder abduction at 90º with internal rotation 3. shoulder internal rotation in 90º abduction 4. shoulder flexion at 125º with scapula resistance 5. shoulder horizontal adduction at 90º flexion
Chopp et al (2010) [52]	anterior deltoid middle deltoid pectoralis major (clavicular head) pectoralis major (sternal head)	1,4-6,10 2-6 7-12 7,8,10	1. Coded: force direction – shoulder flexion angle – horizontal abduction angle 2. UP-45-0 3. UP-45-45 4. UP-45-90 5. UP-90-0 6. UP-90-45 7. UP-90-90

Study	Muscles investigated	MVIC test	Isometric tests that produce maximum EMG in the muscles investigated
			8. IN-45-0 9. IN-45-45 10. IN-45-90 11. IN-90-0 12. IN-90-45 13. IN-90-90
Vera-Garcia et al (2010) [64]	upper rectus abdominis lower rectus abdominis lateral external oblique medial external oblique internal oblique latissimus dorsi (T9) erector spinae (T9) erector spinae (L5)	1,2,6 1,2,3,4 1,3,4,5,6,10 1,3,5,6 2,3,5,6 3,4,5,9 7,8,9 7,8	1. upper trunk flexion 2. lower trunk flexion 3. upper trunk twisting 4. lower trunk twisting 5. upper trunk bending 6. lower trunk bending 7. upper trunk extension 8. lower trunk extension 9. shoulder rotation and adduction 10. abdominal hollowing
Rutherford et al (2011) [58]	lateral gastrocnemius medial gastrocnemius vastus lateralis vastus medialis rectus femoris lateral hamstrings (biceps femoris) medial hamstrings (semitendinosus)	2,4,5,6,7,8 4,5,6,7,8 1,2,3,7,8 1,2,3,7,8 1,2,3 4,5,6 4,5,6	1. knee extension at 45º knee flexion in sitting 2. combined knee extension + hip flexion at 45º knee flexion in sitting 3. knee extension at 15º knee flexion in supine position 4. knee flexion at 15º knee flexion in supine position 5. knee flexion at 55º knee flexion in sitting 6. knee flexion at 55º knee flexion in prone position 7. plantar-flexion at neutral ankle, knee and hip in supine position 8. unilateral plantar-flexion in standing

Table 2. Examples of studies that have identified tests that produce maximum recordings from given muscles and recommend the use of multiple tests to make sure maximum activation is produced by all individuals tested.

3.1.2. The maximum activation obtained during the task under investigation performed at maximum effort

To reduce the possibility of obtaining normalized EMG levels during a task greater than 100%, investigators have used the EMG obtained during the task under investigation performed at maximum effort as the normalization value. For example, maximum EMG recorded during isometric shoulder abduction has been used to normalize the EMG during submaximal abduction [65], maximum crunch exercise for submaximal crunch exercise [66], maximum sprinting for normalizing the EMG during walking [44, 67] and maximum sprint cycling for normalizing the EMG during cycling [38].

This method of normalizing EMG data produces high reliability between trials [44, 67] and greatly reduces the possibility of obtaining EMG levels during the task of interest greater than the reference value. However, the maximum activation levels of muscles are unknown since maximum force production during the task under investigation does not necessarily produce a maximum activation level in any of the muscles under investigation [8]. In addition, different individuals may use different muscle control strategies to produce the same movement, resulting in different activation levels during the reference contraction in a given muscle between individuals. Therefore, although highly reliable, the use of this method to normalize EMG data to compare muscle activation levels between individuals and between muscles in the task being investigated is not valid. In addition, because this reference value is task dependent, it cannot be used to compare muscle activation levels between different tasks.

3.1.3. The maximum activation obtained at a range of joint angles under maximum effort during dynamic contraction

There is a debate about whether isometric contraction can be used to obtain reference EMG levels for use during dynamic tasks [25]. Some research has found that the EMG levels change with muscle length [68-71], while other studies indicate that joint angle has little effect on maximum EMG levels [72-74] or that there is no consistent pattern of change in the EMG levels with joint angle [74-76]. To address this potential problem, it has been recommended that maximum dynamic (usually isokinetic) contractions be used to obtain reference EMG levels in order to normalize EMG data obtained during movement [77]. In this method, the individual performs a maximum isokinetic contraction at a speed similar to the dynamic task under investigation. The activation levels vs joint angle curve generated from the maximum dynamic contraction is then used to normalize the EMG data [77].

This normalization method has been shown to have low within subject reliability [78] and, because EMG is depended on the velocity of movement for a given force level [79], normalization curves need to be generated for different speeds of movement.

The use of supramaximal stimulation to determine if voluntary contractions are being performed at maximum levels

Maximal voluntary activation can be assessed by interpolation of an electrical stimulus to all or part of the nerve supply to a muscle during maximum voluntary effort. Single electrical stimuli are delivered to the nerve that innervates the muscle during maximum voluntary contraction with increasing intensity until no additional increment in force can be seen. Then 2-4 electric stimuli trains (20 ms between stimuli) are delivered at that intensity as they produce substantially larger evoked responses [80-82]. If the stimulus fails to evoke an increment in force it can be deduced that all motoneurones innervating the muscle are recruited i.e. that the muscle is being maximally activated [83-85].

One criticism of this method of generating maximal activation in a given muscle is that the force output of a muscle during a synchronous activation of the motor neurons, due to the stimulation of a nerve, does not necessarily produce the same force as when the motor neurons are being asynchronously activated by the central nervous system [4].In addition, its use for some muscles will be problematic due to difficulty accessing the nerve/s supplying these muscles e.g. branches of the brachial plexus supplying shoulder muscles. It also has the disadvantage that strong contractions maintained for more than a few seconds will lead to muscle fatigue.

3.2. Peak or mean activation levels obtained during the task under investigation

The first report of normalized EMG signals [9] presented quadriceps EMG signals during walking as a percentage of the peak muscle activity that occurred during the gait cycle [8]. Since then, this method has been used to investigate muscle activation patterns during various activities e.g. walking [25, 86], cycling [87], biceps curl exercise [24] and kayaking [88]. In this method, the EMG data is normalized to the peak or mean activity obtained during the activity in each muscle for each individual separately.

Normalising to the peak or mean amplitude during the activity of interest has been shown to decrease the variability between individuals compared to using raw EMG data or when normalising to MVICs [24, 25, 86, 87]. Normalizing to the mean amplitude during the activity of interest has been reported to be either comparable to [34], or better than [24, 42, 89, 90], normalizing to the peak amplitude during the activity in reducing the variability between subjects. Although the within subject and within day reliability have been shown to be high for both peak and mean amplitude during an activity [42], it has also been shown that they may be less reliable between days in the same individuals compared to normalizing to MVICs [90].

However, the reduction in the variability between individuals by normalising to the peak or mean amplitude recorded during an activity is achieved by removing some real biological variation (e.g. strength difference) between individuals [24, 90]. The amount of muscle activity required to lift a given load, would vary according to each individual's strength. As the reference value used in this method is relative to the task and not to the maximum capacity of the muscle, muscle activity levels cannot be compared between muscles, tasks or individuals. This method, however, can be used to compare patterns of muscle activation between individuals over time [24, 25, 42, 90].

3.3. Activation levels during submaximal isometric contractions

The use of maximal contractions to obtain reference EMG levels has been questioned because of difficulty in getting subjects to mobilize their maximal potential especially in symptomatic subjects who cannot perform a maximum contraction because of pain, muscle inhibition [42, 91] or risk of injury [91]. As a result, the use of tests at submaximal contraction levels have been used to produce reference EMG levels for the purposes of normalizing the EMG signals. De Luca [4] encouraged the use of EMGs from contractions < 80% of MVIC. However, there is no consensus as to whether submaximal contractions have higher within-day reliability than [23], or similar reliability to [92], maximal contractions. Commonly used submaximal isometric contractions include holding a limb against gravity [24, 26, 48, 87, 92] or holding a given load, either an absolute load [24, 93-95] or a relative load determined as a percentage of each individual's maximum load [25]. The muscle activity recorded during the submaximal isometric contraction is then used to normalize the EMG in the same muscle while performing the task under investigation.

The main limitation of using submaximal isometric contractions is that comparisons of activity levels between muscles and individuals are not valid because, once again, the reference value used in this method is not relative to the maximum capacity of the muscle. Lifting an absolute load of say 1 kg mass might require 10% of the maximum muscle capacity in a strong individual compared to say 40% of the maximum muscle capacity in another person who is not as strong. It is not possible to estimate maximum muscle activity from a relative submaximal contraction by linear extrapolation because the torque/EMG relationship is nonlinear [96]. Additionally, the lengths of muscle moment arms in individuals vary and since the EMG signal is related to the force produced by the muscle and not the torque produced by the limb, the force required by the muscle to produce a given torque would be different between individuals. Another limitation is that the motor strategy may not be the same between individuals or between sides within the same individual [95] during the reference submaximal contraction. This is not a problem during maximal contractions as heightened central drive engages all possible muscle resources to achieve the maximum force possible. Therefore, using submaximal isometric contractions as the reference for normalizing EMG data is reliable but doesn't allow valid comparisons between muscles or individuals.

3.4. Peak to peak amplitude of the maximum M-wave (M-max)

This method of normalizing EMG signals involves external stimulation of α-motor neurons. When a peripheral motor nerve is stimulated at a point proximal to a muscle it activates the muscle to contract. This signal is called the M-wave and can be recorded using EMG electrodes placed on/in that muscle. To obtain maximum activation in the muscle and produce a maximum M-wave (M-max), the amplitude of stimulation is increased until the peak to peak amplitude of the M-wave does not increase further. To ensure maximum simulation, the amplitude of the stimulation is increased by an additional 30%. The amplitude of the M-max is then used to normalize EMG signals from the same muscle during the tasks of interest [97]. Currently, this normalization method is problematic as the repeatability of the M-max is questionable. It seems to be less reliable as the background contraction level increases [98], decreases with time [99], and is dependent on muscle length [100-102] and the task performed [98, 102]. If these factors that affect the M-max values could be controlled resulting in more reliable measurements, this method to normalize EMG data has the potential to facilitate comparisons between muscle, between tasks and between individuals.

4. Summary

In summary, only the normalization method that uses MVICs as the reference level can be validly used to compare muscle activity levels and activation patterns between muscles, tasks and individuals, provided that maximum neural activation is achieved in all muscles and individuals tested. The use of peak or mean activation levels obtained during the task under investigation as the reference EMG level can be used to compare patterns of muscle activation between individuals over time with high reliability but does not allow comparisons of activity levels between muscles, tasks or individuals. The normalization methods of submaximal isometric contractions or maximum activation during the task under investigation performed at maximum effort also do not allow valid comparisons of muscle activity levels between muscles or individuals, and in addition, muscle activation patterns between individuals are potentially more variable because different individual motor control strategies may be used. Finally, the use of maximum activation levels obtained under maximum effort during dynamic contraction and the M-max methods to normalize EMG signals are associated with low within subject reliability and cannot be recommended.

5. EMG Normalization in clinical populations

Studies use EMG to identify differences in the activation levels and patterns between normal subjects and those with neuro-musculo-skeletal dysfunction with the aim of understanding the cause of the dysfunction and developing improved rehabilitation programs to treat the dysfunction. Since the use of MVICs is the most valid method to normalize EMG data allowing comparison of activity levels between muscles in different individuals, it should be the normalization method of choice when evaluating muscle function in clinical populations provided symptomatic individuals can produce MVICs. Indeed recent studies have shown that individuals from some clinical populations (moderate knee osteoarthritis [58], following knee surgery [103], back pain [104, 105], cerebral palsy [106], stroke [45, 107]), are able to produce maximum activation levels using the same MVIC tests as healthy individuals [8]. If symptomatic individuals are unable to elicit maximal contractions, e.g. as a result of pain due to illness or injury, then comparisons between these clinical populations and normal subjects can only be made using normalization to peak or mean activation levels obtained during the task under investigation. Under these circumstances comparisons of activity levels between muscles, between tasks and between individuals are not valid. Only comparison of muscle activation patterns between normal and symptomatic individuals can be made.

Author details

Mark Halaki

Discipline of Exercise and Sport Science, Faculty of Health Science, The University of Sydney, Sydney, Australia

Karen Ginn

Discipline of Biomedical Sciences, Sydney Medical School, The University of Sydney, Sydney, Australia

6. References

[1] Cram JR, Kasman GS. (2011) The basics of surface electromyography. In: Criswell E, Cram JR, editors. Cram's introduction to surface electromyography. 2nd ed. Sudbury, MA: Jones and Bartlett. p. 1-170.

[2] Basmajian JV (1967) Muscles alive: their functions revealed by electromyography. 2d ed. Baltimore,: Williams & Wilkins; xi, 421 p.

[3] Cram JR (2003) The history of surface electromyography. Appl Psychophysiol Biofeedback. 28(2):81-91.

[4] De Luca C (1997) The use of surface electromyography in biomechanics. Journal of Applied Biomechanics. 13:135-63.

[5] Cram JR, Rommen D (1976) Effects of Skin Preparation on Data Collected Using an EMG Muscle-Scanning Procedure. Biofeedback and Self-Regulation. 14(1).

[6] Schanne FJ, Chaffin DB (1970) The effects of skin resistance and capacitance coupling on EMG amplitude and power spectra. Electromyography. 10(3):273-86.

[7] Winkel J, Jorgensen K (1991) Significance of skin temperature changes in surface electromyography. Eur J Appl Physiol Occup Physiol. 63(5):345-8.

[8] Burden A (2010) How should we normalize electromyograms obtained from healthy participants? What we have learned from over 25 years of research. J Electromyogr Kinesiol. 20(6):1023-35.

[9] Eberhart HD, Inman VT, Bresler B. (1954) The principal elements in human locomotion. In: Klopsteg PEW, P.D., editor. Human limbs and their substitutes. New York: McGraw-Hill. p. 437-71.

[10] Hodges PW, Richardson CA (1996) Inefficient muscular stabilization of the lumbar spine associated with low back pain. A motor control evaluation of transversus abdominis. Spine (Phila Pa 1976). 21(22):2640-50.

[11] Di Fabio RP (1987) Reliability of computerized surface electromyography for determining the onset of muscle activity. Phys Ther. 67(1):43-8.

[12] Mathiassen SE, Winkel J, Hagg GM (1995) Normalization of surface EMG amplitude from the upper trapezius muscle in ergonomic studies - A review. J Electromyogr Kinesiol. 5(4):197-226.

[13] Erdelyi A, Sihvonen T, Helin P, Hanninen O (1988) Shoulder strain in keyboard workers and its alleviation by arm supports. Int Arch Occup Environ Health. 60(2):119-24.

[14] Granstrom B, Kvarnstrom S, Tiefenbacher F (1985) Electromyography as an aid in the prevention of excessive shoulder strain. Appl Ergon. 16(1):49-54.

[15] Lundervold A (1951) Electromyographic investigations during sedentary work, especially typewriting. Br J Phys Med. 14(2):32-6.

[16] Lundervold AJ (1951) Electromyographic investigations of position and manner of working in typewriting. Acta Physiol Scand Suppl. 24(84):1-171.

[17] Cram JR, Kasman GS, Holtz J (1998) Introduction to surface electromyography. Gaithersburg, Md.: Aspen Publishers; xiv, 408 p.

[18] Perry J (1992) Gait analysis : normal and pathological function. Thorofare, NJ: SLACK; xxxii, 524 p.

[19] Arsenault AB, Winter DA, Marteniuk RG, Hayes KC (1986) How many strides are required for the analysis of electromyographic data in gait? Scand J Rehabil Med. 18(3):133-5.

[20] Neumann DA, Cook TM (1985) Effect of load and carrying position on the electromyographic activity of the gluteus medius muscle during walking. Phys Ther. 65(3):305-11.

[21] Soderberg GL, Cook TM, Rider SC, Stephenitch BL (1991) Electromyographic activity of selected leg musculature in subjects with normal and chronically sprained ankles performing on a BAPS board. Phys Ther. 71(7):514-22.

[22] Woods JJ, Bigland-Ritchie B (1983) Linear and non-linear surface EMG/force relationships in human muscles. An anatomical/functional argument for the existence of both. Am J Phys Med. 62(6):287-99.

[23] Yang JF, Winter DA (1983) Electromyography reliability in maximal and submaximal isometric contractions. Arch Phys Med Rehabil. 64(9):417-20.

[24] Allison GT, Marshall RN, Singer KP (1993) EMG signal amplitude normalization technique in stretch-shortening cycle movements. J Electromyogr Kinesiol. 3(4):236-44.

[25] Yang JF, Winter DA (1984) Electromyographic amplitude normalization methods: improving their sensitivity as diagnostic tools in gait analysis. Arch Phys Med Rehabil. 65(9):517-21.

[26] Allison GT, Godfrey P, Robinson G (1998) EMG signal amplitude assessment during abdominal bracing and hollowing. J Electromyogr Kinesiol. 8(1):51-7.

[27] Ekstrom RA, Soderberg GL, Donatelli RA (2005) Normalization procedures using maximum voluntary isometric contractions for the serratus anterior and trapezius muscles during surface EMG analysis. J Electromyogr Kinesiol. 15(4):418-28.

[28] Gowan ID, Jobe FW, Tibone JE, Perry J, Moynes DR (1987) A comparative electromyographic analysis of the shoulder during pitching. Professional versus amateur pitchers. Am J Sports Med. 15(6):586-90.

[29] Hintermeister RA, Lange GW, Schultheis JM, Bey MJ, Hawkins RJ (1998) Electromyographic activity and applied load during shoulder rehabilitation exercises using elastic resistance. Am J Sports Med. 26(2):210-20.

[30] Harms-Ringdahl K, Ekholm J, Schuldt K, Linder J, Ericson M (1996) Assessment of jet pilots' upper trapezius load calibrated to maximal voluntary contraction and a standardized load. J Electromyogr Kinesiol. 6(1):67-72.

[31] Nordander C, Balogh I, Mathiassen SE, Ohlsson K, Unge J, Skerfving S, et al. (2004) Precision of measurements of physical workload during standardised manual handling. Part I: surface electromyography of m. trapezius, m. infraspinatus and the forearm extensors. J Electromyogr Kinesiol. 14(4):443-54.

[32] Hansson GA, Nordander C, Asterland P, Ohlsson K, Stromberg U, Skerfving S, et al. (2000) Sensitivity of trapezius electromyography to differences between work tasks - influence of gap definition and normalisation methods. J Electromyogr Kinesiol. 10(2):103-15.

[33] Baldisserotto SM, Cosme DC, Loss JF, Shinkai RSA (2010) Reliability of EMG activity in complete denture users during simulation of activities of daily living. Rev odonto ciênc. 25(1):42-7.

[34] Morris AD, Kemp GJ, Lees A, Frostick SP (1998) A study of the reproducibility of three different normalisation methods in intramuscular dual fine wire electromyography of the shoulder. J Electromyogr Kinesiol. 8(5):317-22.

[35] Escamilla RF, McTaggart MS, Fricklas EJ, DeWitt R, Kelleher P, Taylor MK, et al. (2006) An electromyographic analysis of commercial and common abdominal exercises: implications for rehabilitation and training. J Orthop Sports Phys Ther. 36(2):45-57.

[36] Escamilla RF, Lewis C, Bell D, Bramblet G, Daffron J, Lambert S, et al. (2010) Core muscle activation during Swiss ball and traditional abdominal exercises. J Orthop Sports Phys Ther. 40(5):265-76.

[37] Burnett AF, Wee WK, Xie W, Oh PW, Lim JJ, Tan KW (2012) Levels of muscle activation in strength and conditioning exercises and dynamometer hiking in junior sailors. J Strength Cond Res. 26(4):1066-75.

[38] Rouffet DM, Hautier CA (2008) EMG normalization to study muscle activation in cycling. J Electromyogr Kinesiol. 18(5):866-78.

[39] Kankaanpaa M, Taimela S, Laaksonen D, Hanninen O, Airaksinen O (1998) Back and hip extensor fatigability in chronic low back pain patients and controls. Arch Phys Med Rehabil. 79(4):412-7.

[40] Boren K, Conrey C, Le Coguic J, Paprocki L, Voight M, Robinson TK (2011) Electromyographic analysis of gluteus medius and gluteus maximus during rehabilitation exercises. Int J Sports Phys Ther. 6(3):206-23.

[41] Widler KS, Glatthorn JF, Bizzini M, Impellizzeri FM, Munzinger U, Leunig M, et al. (2009) Assessment of hip abductor muscle strength. A validity and reliability study. J Bone Joint Surg Am. 91(11):2666-72.

[42] Bolgla LA, Uhl TL (2007) Reliability of electromyographic normalization methods for evaluating the hip musculature. J Electromyogr Kinesiol. 17(1):102-11.

[43] Purkayastha S, Cramer JT, Trowbridge CA, Fincher AL, Marek SM (2006) Surface electromyographic amplitude-to-work ratios during isokinetic and isotonic muscle actions. J Athl Train. 41(3):314-20.

[44] Albertus-Kajee Y, Tucker R, Derman W, Lamberts RP, Lambert MI (2011) Alternative methods of normalising EMG during running. J Electromyogr Kinesiol. 21(4):579-86.

[45] Hsu WL, Krishnamoorthy V, Scholz JP (2006) An alternative test of electromyographic normalization in patients. Muscle Nerve. 33(2):232-41.

[46] Sousa CO, Ferreira JJA, Veras Medeiros AC, Carvalho AH, Pereira RC, Guedes DT, et al. (2007) Electromyograhic activity in squatting at 40°, 60° and 90° knee flexion positions. Rev Bras Med Esporte. 13(5):280e-6e.

[47] Riemann BL, Limbaugh GK, Eitner JD, LeFavi RG (2011) Medial and lateral gastrocnemius activation differences during heel-raise exercise with three different foot positions. J Strength Cond Res. 25(3):634-9.

[48] Dankaerts W, O'Sullivan PB, Burnett AF, Straker LM, Danneels LA (2004) Reliability of EMG measurements for trunk muscles during maximal and sub-maximal voluntary isometric contractions in healthy controls and CLBP patients. J Electromyogr Kinesiol. 14(3):333-42.

[49] Viitasalo JT, Saukkonen S, Komi PV (1980) Reproducibility of measurements of selected neuromuscular performance variables in man. Electromyogr Clin Neurophysiol. 20(6):487-501.

[50] Winter DA. (1996) EMG interpretation. In: Kumar S, Mital A, editors. Electromyography in ergonomics. London ; Bristol, PA: Taylor & Francis. p. 109-25.

[51] Jobe FW, Moynes DR, Tibone JE, Perry J (1984) An EMG analysis of the shoulder in pitching. A second report. Am J Sports Med. 12(3):218-20.

[52] Chopp JN, Fischer SL, Dickerson CR (2010) On the feasibility of obtaining multiple muscular maximal voluntary excitation levels from test exertions: a shoulder example. J Electromyogr Kinesiol. 20(5):896-902.

[53] Boettcher CE, Ginn KA, Cathers I (2008) Standard maximum isometric voluntary contraction tests for normalizing shoulder muscle EMG. J Orthop Res. 26(12):1591-7.

[54] Kelly BT, Kadrmas WR, Kirkendall DT, Speer KP (1996) Optimal normalization tests for shoulder muscle activation: an electromyographic study. J Orthop Res. 14(4):647-53.

[55] Ekstrom RA, Donatelli RA, Soderberg GL (2003) Surface electromyographic analysis of exercises for the trapezius and serratus anterior muscles. J Orthop Sports Phys Ther. 33(5):247-58.

[56] O'Dwyer NJ, Quinn PT, Guitar BE, Andrews G, Neilson PD (1981) Procedures for verification of electrode placement in EMG studies of orofacial and mandibular muscles. J Speech Hear Res. 24(2):273-88.

[57] Ginn KA, Halaki M, Cathers I (2011) Revision of the Shoulder Normalization Tests is required to include rhomboid major and teres major. J Orthop Res. 29(12):1846-9.

[58] Rutherford DJ, Hubley-Kozey CL, Stanish WD (2011) Maximal voluntary isometric contraction exercises: a methodological investigation in moderate knee osteoarthritis. J Electromyogr Kinesiol. 21(1):154-60.

[59] McGill SM (1991) Electromyographic activity of the abdominal and low back musculature during the generation of isometric and dynamic axial trunk torque: implications for lumbar mechanics. J Orthop Res. 9(1):91-103.

[60] Smith J, Padgett DJ, Kaufman KR, Harrington SP, An KN, Irby SE (2004) Rhomboid muscle electromyography activity during 3 different manual muscle tests. Arch Phys Med Rehabil. 85(6):987-92.

[61] Nieminen H, Takala EP, Viikari-Juntura E (1993) Normalization of electromyogram in the neck-shoulder region. Eur J Appl Physiol Occup Physiol. 67(3):199-207.

[62] Hebert-Losier K, Schneiders AG, Garcia JA, Sullivan SJ, Simoneau GG (2011) Peak triceps surae muscle activity is not specific to knee flexion angles during MVIC. J Electromyogr Kinesiol. 21(5):819-26.

[63] Ekstrom RA, Osborn RW, Goehner HM, Moen AC, Ommen BM, Mefferd MJ, et al. (2012) Electromyographic normalization procedures for determining exercise intensity of closed chain exercises for strengthening the quadriceps femoris muscles. J Strength Cond Res. 26(3):766-71.

[64] Vera-Garcia FJ, Moreside JM, McGill SM (2010) MVC techniques to normalize trunk muscle EMG in healthy women. J Electromyogr Kinesiol. 20(1):10-6.

[65] Ringelberg JA (1985) EMG and force production of some human shoulder muscles during isometric abduction. J Biomech. 18(12):939-47.

[66] Moraes AC, Pinto RS, Valamatos MJ, Pezarat-Correia PL, Okano AH, Santos PM, et al. (2009) EMG activation of abdominal muscles in the crunch exercise performed with different external loads. Phys Ther Sport. 10(2):57-62.

[67] Fernandez-Pena E, Lucertini F, Ditroilo M (2009) A maximal isokinetic pedalling exercise for EMG normalization in cycling. J Electromyogr Kinesiol. 19(3):e162-70.

[68] Liberson WT, Dondey M, Asa MM (1962) Brief repeated isometric maximal exercises. An evaluation by integrative electromyography. Am J Phys Med. 41:3-14.

[69] Inman VT, Ralston HJ, Saunders JB, Feinstein B, Wright EW, Jr. (1952) Relation of human electromyogram to muscular tension. Electroencephalogr Clin Neurophysiol. 4(2):187-94.

[70] Lunnen JD, Yack J, LeVeau BF (1981) Relationship between muscle length, muscle activity, and torque of the hamstring muscles. Phys Ther. 61(2):190-5.

[71] Pincivero DM, Salfetnikov Y, Campy RM, Coelho AJ (2004) Angle- and gender-specific quadriceps femoris muscle recruitment and knee extensor torque. J Biomech. 37(11):1689-97.

[72] Kasprisin JE, Grabiner MD (1998) EMG variability during maximum voluntary isometric and anisometric contractions is reduced using spatial averaging. J Electromyogr Kinesiol. 8(1):45-50.

[73] Leedham JS, Dowling JJ (1995) Force-length, torque-angle and EMG-joint angle relationships of the human in vivo biceps brachii. Eur J Appl Physiol Occup Physiol. 70(5):421-6.

[74] Barr AE, Goldsheyder D, Ozkaya N, Nordin M (2001) Testing apparatus and experimental procedure for position specific normalization of electromyographic measurements of distal upper extremity musculature. Clin Biomech (Bristol, Avon). 16(7):576-85.

[75] Mohamed O, Perry J, Hislop H (2002) Relationship between wire EMG activity, muscle length, and torque of the hamstrings. Clin Biomech (Bristol, Avon). 17(8):569-79.

[76] Okada M (1987) Effect of muscle length on surface EMG wave forms in isometric contractions. Eur J Appl Physiol Occup Physiol. 56(4):482-6.

[77] Mirka GA (1991) The quantification of EMG normalization error. Ergonomics. 34(3):343-52.

[78] Burden AM, Trew M, Baltzopoulos V (2003) Normalisation of gait EMGs: a re-examination. J Electromyogr Kinesiol. 13(6):519-32.

[79] Heckathorne CW, Childress DS (1981) Relationships of the surface electromyogram to the force, length, velocity, and contraction rate of the cineplastic human biceps. Am J Phys Med. 60(1):1-19.

[80] Hales JP, Gandevia SC (1988) Assessment of maximal voluntary contraction with twitch interpolation: an instrument to measure twitch responses. J Neurosci Methods. 25(2):97-102.

[81] Gandevia SC, McKenzie DK (1985) Activation of the human diaphragm during maximal static efforts. J Physiol. 367:45-56.

[82] Gandevia SC, McKenzie DK (1988) Activation of human muscles at short muscle lengths during maximal static efforts. J Physiol. 407:599-613.
[83] Merton PA (1954) Voluntary strength and fatigue. J Physiol. 123(3):553-64.
[84] Belanger AY, McComas AJ (1981) Extent of motor unit activation during effort. J Appl Physiol. 51(5):1131-5.
[85] Bigland-Ritchie B, Woods JJ (1984) Changes in muscle contractile properties and neural control during human muscular fatigue. Muscle Nerve. 7(9):691-9.
[86] Winter DA, Yack HJ (1987) EMG profiles during normal human walking: stride-to-stride and inter-subject variability. Electroencephalogr Clin Neurophysiol. 67(5):402-11.
[87] Chapman AR, Vicenzino B, Blanch P, Knox JJ, Hodges PW (2010) Intramuscular fine-wire electromyography during cycling: repeatability, normalisation and a comparison to surface electromyography. J Electromyogr Kinesiol. 20(1):108-17.
[88] Trevithick BA, Ginn KA, Halaki M, Balnave R (2007) Shoulder muscle recruitment patterns during a kayak stroke performed on a paddling ergometer. J Electromyogr Kinesiol. 17(1):74-9.
[89] Burden A, Bartlett R (1999) Normalisation of EMG amplitude: an evaluation and comparison of old and new methods. Med Eng Phys. 21(4):247-57.
[90] Knutson LM, Soderberg GL, Ballantyne BT, Clarke WR (1994) A study of various normalization procedures for within day electromyographic data. J Electromyogr Kinesiol. 4(1):47-59.
[91] Veiersted KB (1991) The reproducibility of test contractions for calibration of electromyographic measurements. Eur J Appl Physiol Occup Physiol. 62(2):91-8.
[92] Bao S, Mathiassen SE, Winkel J (1995) Normalizing upper trapezius EMG amplitude: Comparison of different procedures. J Electromyogr Kinesiol. 5(4):251-7.
[93] Lehman GJ (2002) Clinical considerations in the use of surface electromyography: three experimental studies. J Manipulative Physiol Ther. 25(5):293-9.
[94] Mathiassen SE, Winkel J (1990) Electromyographic activity in the shoulder-neck region according to arm position and glenohumeral torque. Eur J Appl Physiol Occup Physiol. 61(5-6):370-9.
[95] Ounpuu S, Winter DA (1989) Bilateral electromyographical analysis of the lower limbs during walking in normal adults. Electroencephalogr Clin Neurophysiol. 72(5):429-38.
[96] Anders C, Bretschneider S, Bernsdorf A, Schneider W (2005) Activation characteristics of shoulder muscles during maximal and submaximal efforts. Eur J Appl Physiol. 93(5-6):540-6.
[97] Pucci AR, Griffin L, Cafarelli E (2006) Maximal motor unit firing rates during isometric resistance training in men. Exp Physiol. 91(1):171-8.
[98] Lee M, Carroll TJ (2005) The amplitude of Mmax in human wrist flexors varies during different muscle contractions despite constant posture. J Neurosci Methods. 149(2):95-100.
[99] Crone C, Johnsen LL, Hultborn H, Orsnes GB (1999) Amplitude of the maximum motor response (Mmax) in human muscles typically decreases during the course of an experiment. Exp Brain Res. 124(2):265-70.

[100] Maffiuletti NA, Lepers R (2003) Quadriceps femoris torque and EMG activity in seated versus supine position. Med Sci Sports Exerc. 35(9):1511-6.

[101] Cresswell AG, Loscher WN, Thorstensson A (1995) Influence of gastrocnemius muscle length on triceps surae torque development and electromyographic activity in man. Exp Brain Res. 105(2):283-90.

[102] Tucker KJ, Tuncer M, Turker KS (2005) A review of the H-reflex and M-wave in the human triceps surae. Hum Mov Sci. 24(5-6):667-88.

[103] Krebs DE (1989) Isokinetic, electrophysiologic, and clinical function relationships following tourniquet-aided knee arthrotomy. Phys Ther. 69(10):803-15.

[104] Ng JK, Richardson CA, Parnianpour M, Kippers V (2002) Fatigue-related changes in torque output and electromyographic parameters of trunk muscles during isometric axial rotation exertion: an investigation in patients with back pain and in healthy subjects. Spine (Phila Pa 1976). 27(6):637-46.

[105] Ng JK, Richardson CA, Parnianpour M, Kippers V (2002) EMG activity of trunk muscles and torque output during isometric axial rotation exertion: a comparison between back pain patients and matched controls. J Orthop Res. 20(1):112-21.

[106] Damiano DL, Martellotta TL, Sullivan DJ, Granata KP, Abel MF (2000) Muscle force production and functional performance in spastic cerebral palsy: relationship of cocontraction. Arch Phys Med Rehabil. 81(7):895-900.

[107] Mulroy S, Gronley J, Weiss W, Newsam C, Perry J (2003) Use of cluster analysis for gait pattern classification of patients in the early and late recovery phases following stroke. Gait Posture. 18(1):114-25.

Chapter 8

The Usefulness of Mean and Median Frequencies in Electromyography Analysis

Angkoon Phinyomark, Sirinee Thongpanja, Huosheng Hu,
Pornchai Phukpattaranont and Chusak Limsakul

Additional information is available at the end of the chapter

http://dx.doi.org/10.5772/50639

1. Introduction

Rich useful information can be obtained from the muscles and researchers can use such information in a wide class of clinical and engineering applications by measuring surface electromyography (EMG) signals (Merletti & Parker, 2004). Normally, EMG signals are acquired by surface electrodes that are placed on the skin superimposed on the targeted muscle. In order to use the EMG signal as a diagnosis signal or a control signal, a feature is often extracted before performing analysis or classification stage (Phinyomark et al., 2012a) because a lot of information, both useful information and noise (Phinyomark et al., 2012b), is contained in the raw EMG data. An EMG feature is a distinct characteristic of the signal that can be described or observed quantitatively, such as being large or small, spiky or smooth, and fast or slow. Generally, EMG features can be computed in numerical form from a finite length time interval and can change as a function of time, i.e. a voltage or a frequency. They can be computed in several domains, such as time domain, frequency domain, time-frequency and time-scale representations (Boostani & Moradi, 2003). However, frequency-domain features show the better performance than other-domain features in case of the assessing muscle fatigue (Al-Mulla et al., 2012). Mean frequency (MNF) and median frequency (MDF) are the most useful and popular frequency-domain features (Phinyomark et al., 2009) and frequently used for the assessment of muscle fatigue in surface EMG signals (Cifrek et al., 2009).

This chapter presents a usefulness of MNF and MDF in electromyography analysis. The successful muscular fatigue assessment based on MNF and MDF methods is presented together with the principle and theory of MNF and MDF in this chapter, and also up-to-date literature reviews of MNF and MDF in the analysis of EMG signals. In order to analyse the EMG signals during dynamic movements, the effects of muscle force and muscle geometry (joint angle) should have paid more attention (Cechetto et al., 2001; Doheny et al., 2008). In the literature, such effects on MNF and MDF have still been inconclusive (Doheny et al., 2008; Phinyomark et al., 2012c). A summary of the conflicting results mentioned in the literature is also presented. The possible reasons for the conflicting results in both effects are discussed. In addition to the clinical applications, the classification of EMG signals during upper-limb movements for using in the engineering applications (Oskoei & Hu, 2007) is proposed in this chapter.

The rest of this chapter is as follows: Section 2 presents the principle and theory of MNF and MDF, and the relations between MNF (and MDF) and other EMG frequency-domain features are also described and discussed. In Section 3, the extensive review and careful survey of the up-to-date experiments for the assessing muscle fatigue using MNF and MDF in numerous applications are summarized, and moreover, the recent trend of MNF and MDF in the assessment of muscle fatigue is discussed in this section. On the other hand, the effects of muscle force and muscle geometry are described respectively in Section 4 and Section 5, with the re-evaluating results for both effects using the new EMG data set. In addition, a number of techniques that are possible to make the consistent results for both effects are suggested. In Section 6, the usefulness of MNF and MDF in the EMG pattern classification is proposed with the related works. The modified MNF and MDF in order to improve the robustness property for the classifying EMG signals are also presented. Lastly, the conclusion and future trends of using MNF and MDF to analyse EMG signals are presented in Section 7.

2. Principle and theory of mean and median frequencies

Frequency-domain or spectral-domain features are usually used in the assessing muscle fatigue and analysing MU recruitment (Oskoei & Hu, 2008). To transform the EMG signal in the time-domain to the frequency-domain, a Fourier transform of the autocorrelation function of the EMG signal is employed to provide the power spectrum (PS) or the power spectral density (PSD). Although PSD can be estimated by different methods, i.e. modern, parametric or model-based, the most commonly used PSD estimator in the EMG signal analysis is the Periodogram. It is defined as the square of absolute value of the Fourier transform of EMG signal divided by the signal length. Another stable and accurate PSD estimator is the autoregressive (AR) model (Zhang et al., 2010). Different kinds of statistical variables are applied to the PSD of EMG signal and the two popular used variables of PSD are mean and median. However, there are several possible statistical variables that can be applied to the PSD of EMG signal, such as summation or total, and peak value. Definitions of other statistical variables are presented in Section 2.2.

2.1. The definition of mean and median frequencies

MNF is an average frequency which is calculated as the sum of product of the EMG power spectrum and the frequency divided by the total sum of the power spectrum (e.g. Oskoei & Hu, 2008; Phinyomark et al., 2012a). MNF has a similar definition as several features, i.e.

the central frequency (f_c), centroid and the spectral center of gravity, in a number of studies (Du & Vuskovic, 2004; Farina & Merletti, 2000). In addition, MNF is also called as mean power frequency and mean spectral frequency in several works. The definition of MNF is given by

$$MNF = \sum_{j=1}^{M} f_j P_j \Big/ \sum_{j=1}^{M} P_j \,, \tag{1}$$

where f_j is the frequency value of EMG power spectrum at the frequency bin j, P_j is the EMG power spectrum at the frequency bin j, and M is the length of frequency bin. In the analysis of EMG signal, M is usually defined as the next power of 2 from the length of EMG data in time-domain.

MDF is a frequency at which the EMG power spectrum is divided into two regions with equal amplitude (e.g. Oskoei & Hu, 2008; Phinyomark et al., 2012a). MDF is also defined as a half of the total power, or TTP (dividing the total power area into two equal parts). The definition of MDF is given by

$$\sum_{j=1}^{MDF} P_j = \sum_{j=MDF}^{M} P_j = \frac{1}{2}\sum_{j=1}^{M} P_j \,. \tag{2}$$

The behaviour of MNF and MDF is always similar. However, the performance of MNF in each of the applications is quite different compared to the performance of MDF, although both features are two kinds of averages in statistics. More details about the performance of both features are discussed in Section 3 to Section 6.

It should be noted that MNF is always slightly higher than MDF because of the skewed shape of EMG power spectrum (Knaflitz et al., 1990), whereas the variance of MNF is typically lower than that of MDF. In theory, the standard deviation of MDF is higher than that of MNF by a factor 1.253 (Balestra et al., 1988). However, the estimation of MDF is less affected by random noise, particularly in the case of noise located in the high frequency band of EMG power spectrum, and more affected by muscle fatigue (Stulen & De Luca, 1981).

2.2. The relations between mean and median frequencies and other EMG frequency-domain features

Other spectral variables that have been applied in the analysis of EMG signal are total power (TTP), mean power (MNP), peak frequency (PKF), the spectral moments (SM), frequency ratio (FR), power spectrum ratio (PSR), and variance of central frequency (VCF) (Phinyomark et al., 2012a). The definition of all variables is presented in the following.

1. TTP is an aggregate of EMG power spectrum (Phinyomark et al., 2012a). This feature is also defined as the energy and the zero spectral moment (SM0) (Du & Vuskovic, 2004). Its equation can be expressed as

$$TTP = \sum_{j=1}^{M} P_j = SM0 \,. \tag{3}$$

2. MNP is an average power of EMG power spectrum (Phinyomark et al., 2012a). It can be defined as

$$MNP = \sum_{j=1}^{M} P_j \Big/ M \,. \tag{4}$$

3. PKF is a frequency at which the maximum EMG power occurs (Phinyomark et al., 2012a). It can be expressed as

$$PKF = \max(P_j), \quad j=1, \ldots, M \,. \tag{5}$$

4. SM is an alternative statistical analysis way to extract feature from the power spectrum of EMG signal. Normally, the first three moments (SM1-SM3) are employed as the EMG features (Du & Vuskovic, 2004). Their equations can be defined as

$$SM1 = \sum_{j=1}^{M} P_j f_j; \; SM2 = \sum_{j=1}^{M} P_j f_j^2; \; SM3 = \sum_{j=1}^{M} P_j f_j^3 \,. \tag{6}$$

5. FR is used to discriminate between relaxation and contraction of the muscle using a ratio between low- and high-frequency components of EMG signal (Han et al., 2000; Phinyomark et al., 2012a). The equation is defined as

$$FR = \sum_{j=LLC}^{ULC} P_j \Big/ \sum_{j=LHC}^{UHC} P_j \,, \tag{7}$$

where *ULC* and *LLC* are respectively the upper- and the lower-cutoff frequency of low-frequency band, and *UHC* and *LHC* are respectively the upper- and the lower-cutoff frequency of high-frequency band. The cutoff frequency between low- and high-frequencies can be defined by two ways: the experiment (Han et al., 2000) and the MNF value (Oskoei & Hu, 2006).

6. PSR is a ratio between the energy P_0 which is nearby the maximum value of EMG power spectrum and the energy *P* which is the whole energy of EMG power spectrum (Qingju & Zhizeng, 2006). It can be seen as an extended version of PKF and FR. The equation can be expressed as

$$PSR = \frac{P_0}{P} = \sum_{j=f_0-n}^{f_0+n} P_j \Big/ \sum_{j=-\infty}^{\infty} P_j \,, \tag{8}$$

where f_0 is defined as the value of PKF and n is the integral limit.

7. VCF is defined by using a number of the spectral moments (SM0-SM2) and MNF. It can be computed by the following equation

$$VCF = \frac{1}{SM0}\sum_{j=1}^{M} P_j \left(f_j - MNF\right)^2 = \frac{SM2}{SM0} - \left(\frac{SM1}{SM0}\right)^2 . \tag{9}$$

TTP, MNP, and SM are frequency-domain features that extract the same information as time-domain features based on the energy information (Phinyomark et al., 2012a). Hence, the discriminant of TTP, MNP and SM in space has the similar pattern as the time-domain features based on the energy information, i.e. integrated EMG (IEMG), root mean square (RMS), mean absolute value (MAV), and variance of EMG (VAR). Due to the fact that muscle fatigue results in an increase of EMG signal amplitude, time-domain features based on energy information, i.e. IEMG, MAV and RMS, can track this behaviour. Thus, TTP, MNP and SM can also be used as an indicator of muscle fatigue, although EMG signal amplitude, itself, is rarely used to detect muscle fatigue. However, these features can be used in a combination with the spectral analysis i.e. MNF and MDF. On the other hand, all spectral features except PSR have the different discriminant patterns in feature space compared with MNF and MDF. In case of n = 20, the pattern of PSR is an inverse case of MNF and MDF patterns (Phinyomark et al., 2012a).

3. Assessing the muscle fatigue using mean and median frequencies

Muscle fatigue is generally defined as an activity induced loss of the ability to produce force with the muscle. Usually, the muscle fatigue is a result of prolonged or repetitive works (De Luca, 1984). It should be noted that the usual term "muscle fatigue" is generally meaning in fact "local muscle fatigue" (Chaffin, 1973). Undetected fatigue for a long-time can cause injury to the subject and is often irreversible. If an automated muscle fatigue detection system in wearable technology was feasible, it could be employed as an indicator to reduce the chances of work-place injury and aid sporting performance (Al-Mulla et al., 2012). Among a number of sources and techniques (Al-Mulla et al., 2011), e.g. acoustic-myography (AMG), mechano-myography (MMG), near-infrared spectroscopy (NIRS), sono-myography (SMG) and ultrasound, the EMG signal is used even more often and has several advantages, such as a non-invasiveness, an ability to monitor fatigue of a particular muscle and a real-time muscle fatigue monitoring during the performance of defined work (Petrofsky et al., 1982).

The assessment of muscle fatigue with surface EMG signals can be applied in a wide class of applications, such as muscle fatigue during repeated cycling sprints (Hautier et al., 2000), muscle fatigue in children with cerebral palsy (Leunkeu et al., 2010), muscle fatigue during playing the PC games (Oskoei et al., 2008), and the low back pain in helicopter pilots (Balasubramanian et al., 2011). Several classical and modern signal processing techniques have been applied (Cifrek et al., 2009), such as the RMS, the zero-crossing rate (ZCR), the averaged instantaneous frequency, wavelet analysis, fractal analysis, and also MNF and MDF.

Among such techniques, MNF and MDF so far have been hailed as the gold standard for muscle fatigue assessment with surface EMG signals due to the fact that muscle fatigue results in a downward shift of frequency spectrum of the EMG signal. Moreover, during the fatigue of muscle, several changes have been found, i.e. a relative decrease in signal power at high-frequency, a small increase in signal power at low-frequency, an increase in spectrum slope at high-frequency, and a decrease in spectrum slope at low-frequency (Petrofsky et al., 1982; Sato, 1982; Viitasalo & Komi, 1977). There are several possible reasons for the changes in the EMG signal, such as the modulation of recruitment firing rate, the grouping and slowing of CV, and synchronization of the signal (De Luca, 1979; Hermens et al., 1984; Viitasalo & Komi, 1977).

Using MNF and MDF to detect muscle fatigue in static contractions is clearly known because during static contraction the EMG signals may be assumed to be stationary during short-time intervals (0.5-2s). On the other hand, in dynamic contractions, the EMG signal information has been changed as a function of time that cannot be analyzed by simply applying FFT and most recently EMG studies have been applied to the study of dynamic contraction. The instantaneous mean and median frequency (IMNF and IMDF) are introduced to fulfill the requirement (Roy et al., 1998) by using time-frequency or time-scale approaches, such as short-time Fourier transform (STFT) (Cifrek et al., 2000; Thongpanja et al., 2010, 2011), Wigner distribution (WD), Choi-Williams distribution (CWD) (Knaflitz & Bonato, 1999), time-varying autoregressive approach (TVAR) (Zhang et al., 2010), and continuous wavelet transform (CWT) (Karlsson et al., 2000).

Further, there are several ways to use IMNF and IMDF to detect muscle fatigue. For example, Georgakis et al. (2003) demonstrated that the performance of the average of IMNF and IMDF is better than the traditional MNF and MDF. On the other hand, a slope of the regression line that fits the maximum values of IMNF and IMDF during cyclic contractions is used as a fatigue index in Cifrek et al. (2000).

Many research works reported on the effectiveness of MNF and MDF applied to EMG signal as a mean of identifying muscle fatigue. The experimental conditions for several studies (based on literature published between 1980-2011) are summarized in Table 1. Most of the studies have been performed MNF and MDF to detect the muscle fatigue in primarily static muscle contraction but also in dynamic muscle contraction.

In Table 1, most of the studies recorded EMG data from 10 subjects and the volunteers between 20 and 30 years of age (young subjects) are the main target. However, in Masuda et al. (1999), age of the subjects is ranged from 19 to 73 years (both young and older subjects). EMG signals obtained from young and older subjects are quite different, as mentioned in Tavakolan et al. (2011) that the difference in classification accuracy obtained from the young and older subjects is approximately 7%. Although Kalra et al. (2012) found that MDF of EMG is not significantly impacted by age at 50-100%MVC of the BB muscle, the effect of age needs to be carefully considered in future research. In addition to the effect of age, the effect of gender is another factor that should be paid more an interest (Kalra et al., 2012).

Reference	*N*	Age	Muscle	ID	Force levels	RT	Filter
Petrofsky & Lind (1980b)	10	23.2±2.3	BR	40	25, 40, 70%MVC	F	-
Gerdle et al. (1990)	9	30-40	BB	-	20, 40, 60, 80, 100%MVC	-	-
Merletti & Roy (1996)	6	-	TA	-	50, 60, 70, 80%MVC	90-170	-
Mannion & Dolan (1996)	10	-	RF, VL	-	20, 30, 40, 50, 60%MVC	F	-
Potvin (1997)	15	24±3	BB	30	7kg	F	15-450
Masuda et al. (1999)	19	19-73	VL	5	50%MVC	F	5-1000
Rainoldi et al. (1999)	10	30.2±6.1	BB	10	10, 30, 50, 70%MVC	30	10-450
Cifrek et al. (2000)	10	22.9±1.5	RF, VL, VM	30	50%MVC	F	20-480
Bonato et al. (2001)	-	-	FDI	5	10%MVC	150	8-450
MacIsaac et al. (2001)	7	26±7	BB	40	20-30%MVC	F	1-1000
Arnall et al. (2002)	10	-	PS	-	40, 50, 60%MVC	60	-
Allison & Fujiwara (2002)	10	29.4±4.8	BB	25	60%MVC	C1	20-500
Bilodeau et al. (2003)	14	22-43	RF, VL, VM	20	100%MVC	C2	15-4000
Georgakis et al. (2003)	30	-	RF, VL, VM	20	60%MVC	60	10-500
Clancy et al. (2005)	12	31.4±11.1	FDS, ECR	-	10, 20, 30, 40, 50, 60, 70, 80, 90%MVC	F	25-1350
Ravier et al. (2005)	10	24±1.5	BB	75	70%MVC	F	2-600
Zaman et al. (2011)	11	24±4	BB	5	40%MVC	F	-
Soares et al. (2011)	10	24±2.8	BB	5	40%MVC	90	-

Table 1. A survey of the experimental conditions in related works about muscle fatigue assessment with surface EMG signals using MNF and MDF in chronological order. Note that *N* is the number of subjects; ID is the inter-electrode distance (mm); RT is the recording time (s); Filter is the specification of filtering (Hz); MVC is maximum voluntary contraction; F is the EMG data is recorded until the subject cannot support the required force level; C1 is the EMG data is recorded until force is below 35%MVC; C2 is the EMG data is recorded until force is below 50%MVC; BR is brachioradialis; BB is biceps brachii; TA is tibialis anterior; RF is rectus femoris; VL is vastus lateralis; VM is vastus medialis; FDI is first dorsal interossrous; PS is paraspinal; FDS is flexor digitorum superficialis; ECR is extensor carpi radialis.

The next interested factor in Table 1 is the recording time. Because in the analysis of muscle fatigue, the EMG signals recorded during the fatigue of muscle are needed. Most of the studies used a level of force as the threshold to finish the recording. In other words, the EMG data have been recorded until the subject cannot maintain the required force level. However, several studies define the specific recording times that range from 30s to 170s.

Other factors are varied, such as the inter-electrode distance (5-75 mm), the levels of force (10-100%MVC), and the specification of filtering (1-1350 Hz). However, most of the studies paid more an interest to the study of biceps brachii muscle. The evaluating performance between each pair of the methods and the muscles should be done in future study.

4. Effect of muscle force on mean and median frequencies

In order to make a reliably automate the muscle fatigue determination, the knowledge of the effects of time-varying factors on MNF and MDF is very important. Two time-varying factors, muscle force and muscle geometry, are the major factors due to the activities that involve dynamic muscle contractions (muscle force and/or geometry are changing) (Cechetto et al., 2001). It should be noted that the number and firing rate of active motor units (MUs) do not significantly affect MNF and MDF in both experimental and theoretical studies (Englehart & Parker, 1994; Solomonow et al., 1990).

The individual effects of muscle force and muscle geometry on MNF and MDF have been investigated in many previous researches. The effect of muscle force is discussed in this section, while the effect of muscle geometry will be discussed in the next section.

At present, the conflicting results of MNF and MDF with the muscle force effect exist in the literature. The difference in the experimental conditions for most of the studies is presented in Table 2. Maybe it is the possible reasons for the conflicting results of MNF and MDF on muscle force effect. It can be observed from the table that three different cases exist for the effect of muscle force on MNF and MDF.

- In the first case (CF1), MNF and MDF are unaffected or only weakly affected by changes in muscle force or load levels (Bilodeau et al., 1991; Cechetto et al., 2001; Hagberg & Ericsson, 1982; Inbar et al., 1986; Merletti et al., 1984; Petrofsky & Lind, 1980a, 1980b; Viitasalo & Komi, 1978).
- In the second case (CF2), MNF and MDF increase as muscle force levels increase (Doheny et al., 2008; Gander & Hudgins, 1985; Gerdle et al., 1990; Hagberg & Ericsson, 1982; Hagberg & Hagberg, 1989; Moritani & Muro, 1987; Muro et al., 1982; Van Boxtel & Schomaker, 1984).
- In the third case (CF3), MNF and MDF decrease as muscle force levels increase (Kaplanis et al., 2009; Rainoldi et al., 1999).

Each of the first two cases is found in eight publications, while the third case exists only in two publications. However, the third case is found in the most recent study (Kaplanis et al., 2009) which used the EMG data recorded from 94 subjects (the largest EMG data compared with other publications).

Reference	N	Age	Muscle	ID	Force levels	RT	Filter	CF
Viitasalo & Komi (1978)	7	-	RF,VL,VM	-	-	-	-	1
Petrofsky & Lind (1980a)	8	22-52	FCR	40	5-100%MVC	3	-	1
Petrofsky & Lind (1980b)	10	23.2±2.3	BR	40	10, 20, 40, 60, 80, 100%MVC	3	-	1
Hagberg & Ericsson (1982)	4	21-24	BB,BR,BL	20	5, 10, 15, 20, 25, 30, 40, 50, 80%MVC	3-5	0.2-2000	1,2
Muro et al. (1982)	5	32.5±8.2	BB	-	0.25, 0.5, 1, 2, 3kg	10	-	2
Merletti et al. (1984)	26	22.6±6.4	FDI	10	20, 80%MVC	3-5	30-350	1
Van Boxtel & Schomaker (1984)	19	18-32	FL,CS	15	20, 40, 60, 80%MA	3	3-520	2
Gander & Hudgins (1985)	6	20-40	BB	-	1-10Nm	8.2	-	2
Inbar et al. (1986)	9	30-40	BB,ED	35	30, 50, 70, 90%MVC	6	1-1000	1
Moritani & Muro (1987)	12	26.3±2.5	BB	6	0-80%MVC	5	< 520	2
Hagberg & Hagberg (1989)	14	36±8	TZ	30	0-100%MVC	10-15	5-500	2
Gerdle et al. (1990)	9	30-40	BB	-	20, 40, 60, 80, 100%MVC	1-2	-	2
Bilodeau et al. (1991)	14	30.2±7.8	TB,AN	6	10, 20, 40, 60, 80%MVC	3	16-800	1
Rainoldi et al. (1999)	10	30.2±6.1	BB	10	10, 30, 50, 70%MVC	30	10-450	3
Cechetto et al. (2001)	12	31.1±10	BB	40	20, 30, 40, 50, 60%MVC	5	0.1-3000	1
Doheny et al. (2008)	12	24.8±2.8	BB,BR,TB	10	10, 20, 30, 40, 50, 60, 70%MVC	8	20-450	2
Kaplanis et al. (2009)	94	5-69	BB	10	10, 30, 50, 70, 100%MVC	5	20-500	3

Table 2. A survey of the experimental conditions in related works about the effect of muscle force on MNF and MDF in chronological order. Note that CF is one of three conflicting cases for muscle force effect; MA is maximum amplitude; FCR is flexor carpi radialis; BL is brachialis; FL is frontalis; CS is corrugator supercilii; ED is extensor digitorum; TZ is trapezius; TB is triceps brachii; AN is anconeus.

There are several possible reasons for the conflicting results presented above.

Firstly, the different muscles studied have the different muscle fibre composition and distribution, and also the different tissue filter effects (Farina et al., 2002). The EMG power spectrum can be changed by both of which. Moreover, the difference of subject gender can produce the differences in fibre diameters and types (Sabbahi et al., 1981). Hence, the difference in the type and distribution of muscle fibres should be one of the major reasons, although the conflicting results exist in the same muscle i.e. the biceps brachii.

Secondly, the electrode locations over the muscle are different in the experiments. Komi and Viitasalo (1976) mentioned that MNF increase with muscle force levels unless the electrodes were located over the motor point area.

Thirdly, the inter-electrode distance (ID) of the bipolar surface electrodes may be the possible reason for the conflicting results. However, based on the observation throughout Table 2, the different inter-electrode distances are also found in the same case (all cases).

Fourthly, Bilodeau et al. (1992) found the different results between two genders for MDF but not for MNF. The difference in skinfold layer is the main contributor for the differences between two genders in that study. On the other hand, Kaplanis et al. (2009) found that no significant differences exist between values based on gender and age.

Other possible reasons are the limited and different number of subjects (i.e. 4–94 subjects), the level of force exhibited (i.e. %MVC or weight in kg), the range of joint angle exhibited (i.e. 0-150 degrees of extension), the difference in recording time (i.e. 1–30s), the existence of fatigue that resulting from the longer recording times (Lariviere et al., 2001), and the method of statistical analysis used.

To confirm the effect of muscle force on MNF and MDF, the relationship between MNF (and also MDF) and muscle force level was re-evaluated by the new EMG data (Phinyomark et al., 2012c). Figs. 1(a), 1(c) and 1(e) illustrate the relationship between muscle force level and MNF at the constant angle, while Figs. 1(b), 1(d) and 1(f) display the relationship between muscle load level and MDF at the same condition.

Three conflicting cases were found in our experiments for the effect of muscle force on MNF and MDF. The results are the subject-dependent. It is similar as the three conflicting cases which were found in the literature. To answer the question "why's the subject-dependent?", several related anthropometric variables obtained from the volunteers should be intended to find the possible reasons (Phinyomark et al., 2012c). The preliminary study showed that a number of anthropometric variables have a correlation with the conflicting results, such as standing height, hand breadth, body mass, and forward grip reach.

In order to modify MNF and MDF to have the consistent results (the same case), a modification of traditional MNF and MDF should be done. In one of our previous works (Thongpanja et al., 2010), we found that if a concept of using consecutive fast Fourier transform (FFT) is used instead of using a whole signal FFT, a certain relationship between MNF (and MDF) and muscle force level (the third case) can be found in the middle range of consecutive feature series for all trials and subjects, as an example is shown in Fig. 2. This is not found for traditional MNF and MDF. This finding can be applied for the EMG signals recorded from the biceps brachii (Thongpanja et al., 2010, 2011) and also the flexor pollicis longus (Thongpanja et al., 2012). To easily observe and use in applications, five statistical variables consisting mean, median, variance, the RMS and kurtosis are used to apply with the selected efficient range of consecutive feature series. The results showed that the consistent results exist across the subjects (subject-independent) by applying mean and median variables (Thongpanja et al., 2011, 2013). The optimization of such techniques can be found more details in Thongpanja et al. (2013).

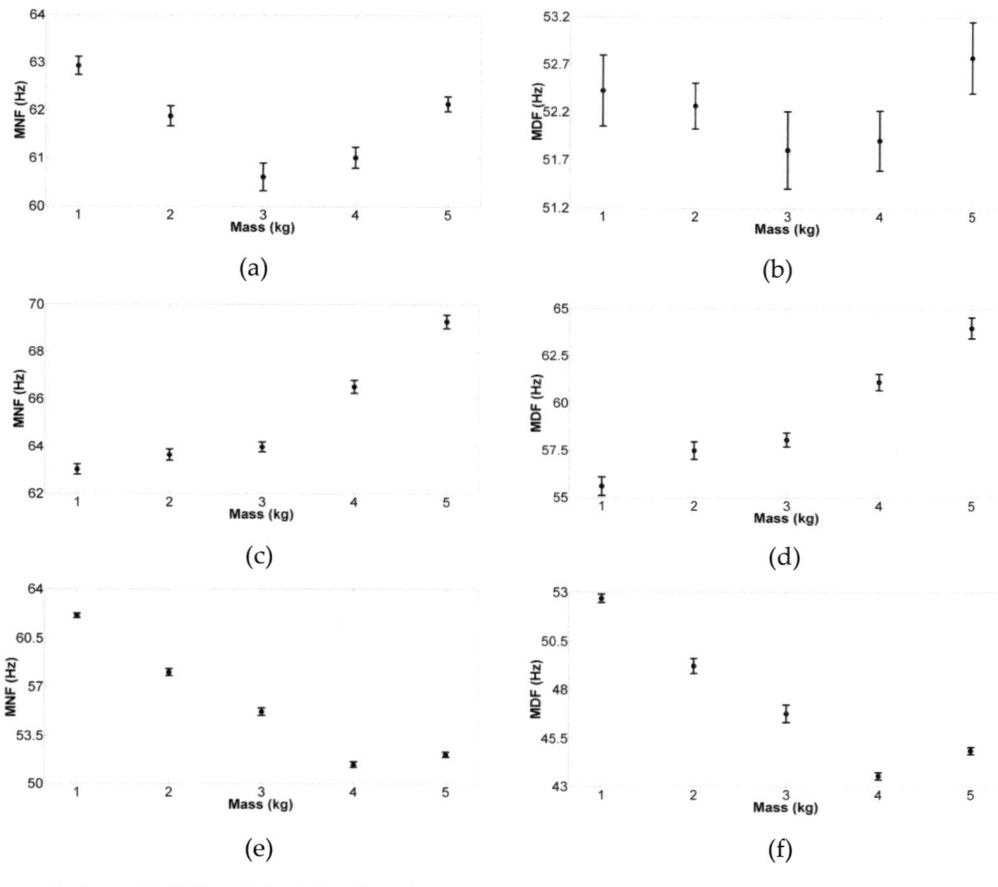

Figure 1. (a, c, e) MNF and (b, d, f) MDF of EMG signals recorded at a constant joint angle (90º) as a function of muscle force (1-5 kg) for three subjects. (a-b) the first case in muscle force effect or CF1 (c-d) the second case in muscle force effect or CF2 (e-f) the third case in muscle force effect or CF3. The error bars shown are given by the standard deviation of the mean value.

5. Effect of muscle geometry on mean and median frequencies

Muscle geometry is another main factor that does significantly affect MNF and MDF. Generally, the effect of muscle geometry including electrode configuration, fibre diameter and subcutaneous tissue thickness has been evaluated by the resulting from changes in joint

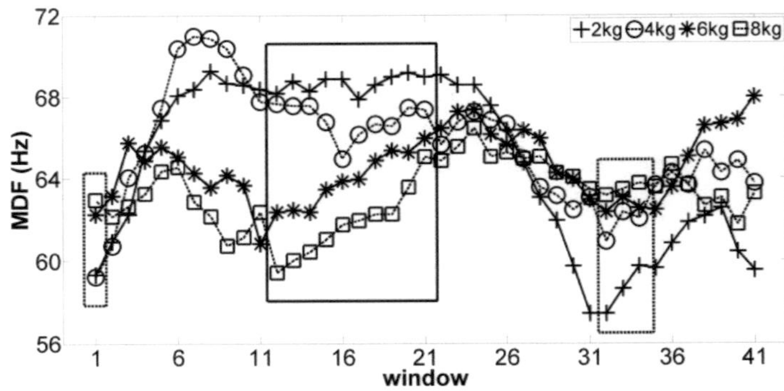

Figure 2. The consecutive MDF feature series computed from the EMG signals recorded from the biceps brachii during dynamic muscle contractions (0-150 degrees of extension). Four load levels are applied: 2, 4, 6 and 8 kg. The FFT is computed using the window size of 512 samples and window overlapping of 64 samples. Note that the second case exists in the beginning and the end ranges (the dashed line boxes) and the third case exists in the middle range (the solid line box).

angle or muscle length (Merletti et al., 1999). Changing in such factors can vary producing a time-varying EMG spectrum. In the literature, two different cases exist for the effect of muscle geometry on MNF and MDF.

In the first case (CG1), MNF and MDF are unaffected by changes in joint angle or muscle length (Sato, 1976). A number of the studies showed no significant change in the power spectrum of EMG signals acquired from the biceps brachii under constant load while joint angle varied. It is also found for the EMG signals recorded from the trapezius, deltoid and the infraspinatus (Gerdle et al., 1988).

In the second case (CG2), MNF (and MDF) increases as muscle length or joint angle (degrees of extension) decreases (Inbar et al., 1987; Shankar et al., 1989). This case exists in most of the studies for EMG signals acquired from the biceps brachii (Cechetto et al., 2001; Doheny et al., 2008; Moritani et al., 1988; Okada, 1987; Potvin, 1997), and is also found for EMG signals acquired from other muscles, such as the tibialis anterior (Merletti et al., 1993), the brachioradialis (Doheny et al., 2008), and the triceps brachii (Doheny et al., 2008; Okada, 1987). The second case, however, is found frequently in the recent studies compared to the first case.

The experimental conditions for several studies are summarized in Table 3. The difference in the experimental conditions may be the reasons for the conflicting results presented in the literature.

Firstly, muscle types and electrode locations over the muscle are different in the experiments. Doheny et al. (2008) mentioned that this factor is one of the reasons for the second case effect. However, the conflicting results are also found in the same muscle i.e. the biceps brachii.

Secondly, Cechetto et al. (2001) proposed that the inter-electrode distance (ID) may be the possible reason for the conflicting results. However, based on the observation through Table 3, three different inter-electrode distances (10, 30 and 40 mm) are found in the same case (the second case).

Thirdly, it can be observed that the frequency band of EMG signals does not affect MNF and MDF.

Reference	*N*	Age	Muscle	ID	Force levels	Joint angles	Filter	CG
Gerdle et al. (1988)	23	20-30	TZ,DT, IF,BB	-	-	45º, 65º, 90º	-	1
Moritani et al. (1988)	12	-	BB	-	-	30º-150º	-	2
Merletti et al. (1993)	10	-	TA	-	-	0º, 15º, 30º, 45º	-	2
Potvin (1997)	15	24±3	BB	30	7kg	0º-140º	15-450	2
Cechetto et al. (2001)	12	31.1±10	BB	40	20, 30, 40, 50, 60%MVC	50º, 70º, 90º, 110º, 130º	0.1-3000	2
Doheny et al. (2008)	12	24.8±2.8	BB,BR, TB	10	10, 20, 30, 40, 50, 60, 70%MVC	45º, 60º, 75º, 90º, 105º, 120º	20-450	2

Table 3. A survey of the experimental conditions in related works about the effect of muscle geometry (joint angle) on MNF and MDF in chronological order. Note that CF is one of the two conflicting cases for the muscle geometry effect; DT is Deltoid; IF is infraspinatus.

Due to the incompleteness of captured information in the literature, in future study, a request to complete all interested information to the first author or the corresponding author should be done.

As the possible reasons mentioned above that are inconclusive, the main reason for the conflicting results should be the changes of muscle force with the muscle length. The same weight was used at all angles in most of the studies, therefore the changes in MNF and MDF were not due to changes in the muscle length, or joint angle, only but also to changes in the muscle force. In future work, EMG signals should be measured from the muscle under a constant force (varying loads) while joint angles varied.

To confirm the effect of muscle geometry on MNF and MDF, the relationship between MNF (and also MDF) and elbow joint angle was re-evaluated by the similar EMG data as used in Section 4. Figs. 3(a), 3(c) and 3(e) illustrate the relationship between joint angle and MNF at the constant load, while Figs. 3(b), 3(d) and 3(f) display the relationship between joint angle and MDF at the same condition.

Three conflicting cases were found in our experiments for the effect of elbow joint angle on MNF and MDF. The results are the subject-dependent. It is similar as the three conflicting cases which were found in the effect of muscle force on MNF and MDF. In the third case or CG3, MNF (and MDF) increases as muscle length or joint angle (degrees of flexion) increases, as can be observed in Figs. 3(e) and 3(f). In future work, several related anthropometric variables obtained from the volunteers should be intended to find the possible reasons, as mentioned in Section 4.

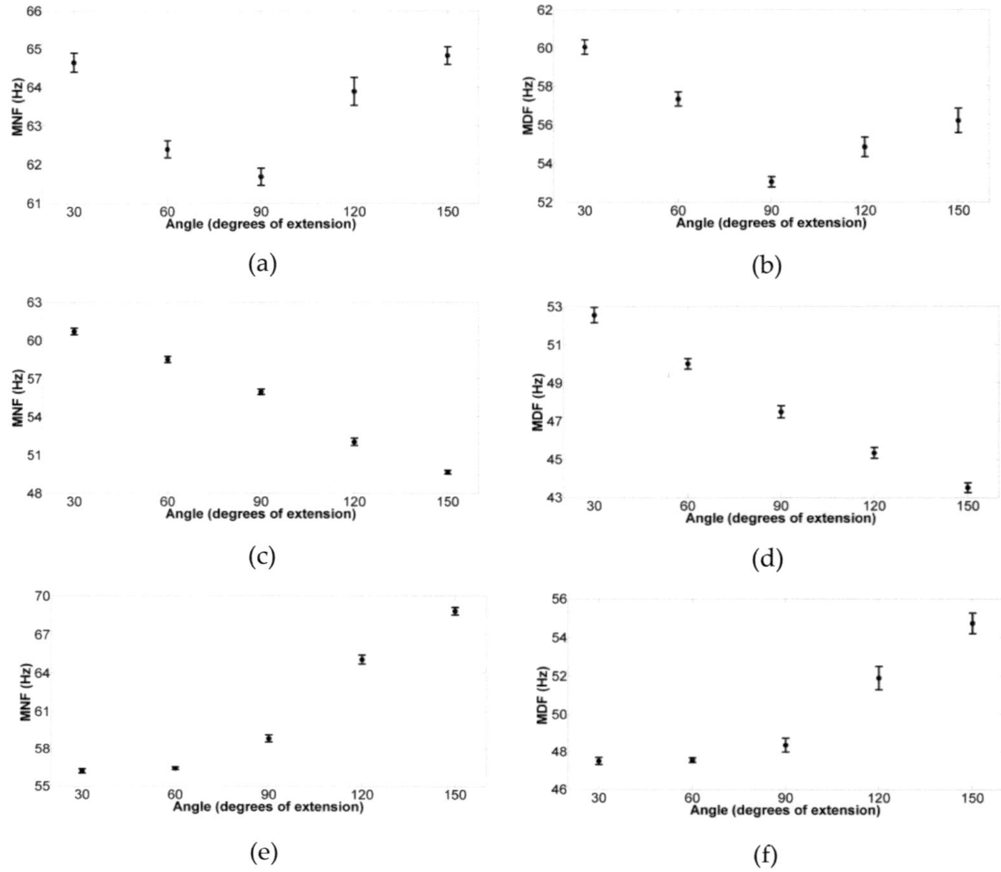

Figure 3. (a, c, e) MNF and (b, d, f) MDF of EMG signals recorded at a constant muscle force (3 kg) as a function of elbow joint angles (30-150 degrees of extension) for three subjects. (a-b) the first case in muscle geometry effect or CG1 (c-d) the second case in muscle geometry effect or CG2 (e-f) the third case in muscle geometry effect or CG3. The error bars shown are given by the standard deviation of the mean value.

In order to modify MNF and MDF to have the consistent results (the same case), a modification of traditional MNF and MDF should be done. Figs. 4(a) and 4(b) show the sample in time-domain of EMG signals measured at the same constant force level with the elbow joint angles at 30º and 150º of extension, respectively. It was found that at narrow elbow joint angles, i.e. 30º of extension, the distribution of positive and negative amplitudes is asymmetry, but at wide elbow joint angles, i.e. 150º of extension, the distribution of positive and negative amplitude is symmetry. The power spectrum of each of the samples is respectively shown in Figs. 4(c) and 4(d). Based on the observation of the distribution, if the EMG signal is normalized by setting the highest value to 1 and the lowest value to -1 for an asymmetric signal, the EMG baseline should be shifted away from the true zero line, as can be observed in Fig. 5(a). On the other hand, the EMG baseline should not be shifted away from the true zero line in the case of normalized symmetric signal, as can be observed in Fig. 5(b). Hence, the values of MNF and MDF that are calculated from the normalized EMG signals measured at the narrow joint angles should decrease, while the values of MNF and MDF that are computed from the normalized EMG signals measured at wide joint angles should be same as the old one. It can be observed throughout Figs. 5(c) and 5(d). As a result, the consistent results should exist across the subjects (subject-independent). The consistent case is the second case. In future work, the evaluation of this finding should be done with the large EMG data set.

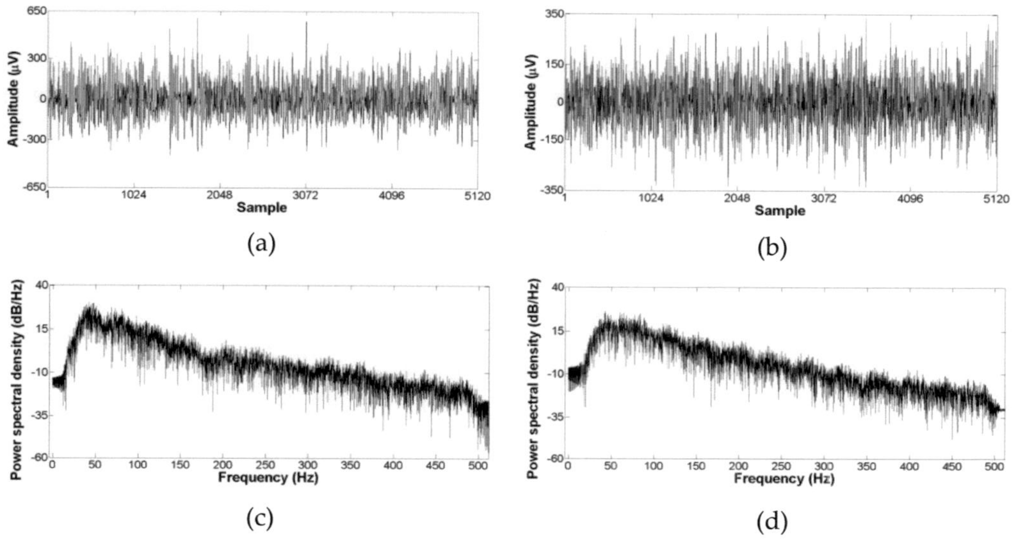

Figure 4. Samples of raw EMG signals recorded from the biceps brachii at (a) 30º and (b) 150º of extension in time-domain, and their power spectrum at (c) 30º and (d) 150º of extension. Note that a constant force (3kg) is performed for each angle.

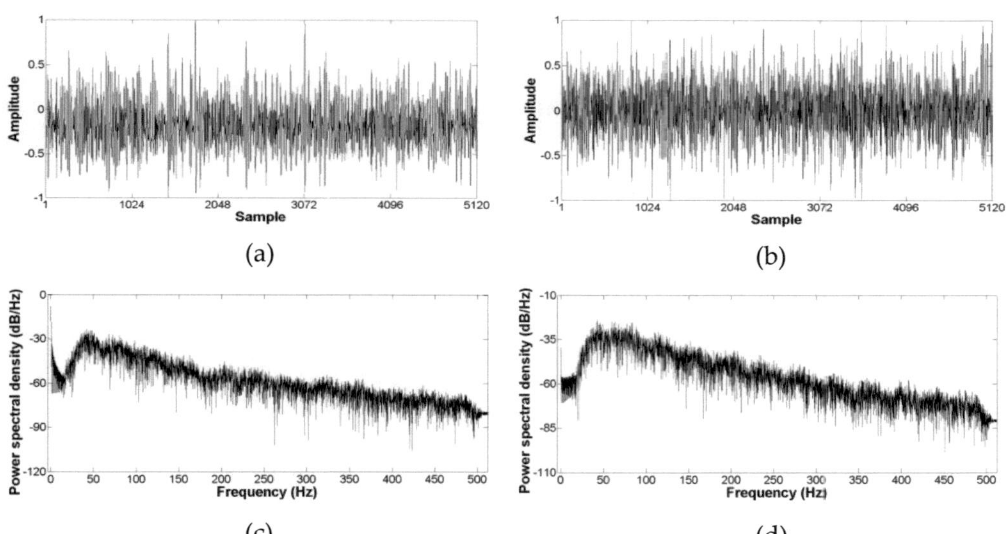

Figure 5. Samples of normalized EMG signals recorded from the biceps brachii at (a) 30º and (b) 150º of extension in time-domain, and their power spectrum at (c) 30º and (d) 150º of extension. Note that a constant force (3kg) is performed for each angle.

6. EMG pattern classification using mean and median frequencies

EMG pattern classification is applied in several potential applications, particularly in the engineering context. The multifunction myoelectric control system (MMCS) is a main engineering application (Oskoei & Hu, 2007; Zecca et al., 2002) consisting the control of prosthesis, industrial robot arms, electric wheelchairs, virtual keyboard and virtual mouse. To be successful in the classification of EMG signals, three main cascaded modules should be carefully considered: data-preprocessing, feature extraction, and classification methods, especially the selection of feature extraction methods (Boostani & Moradi, 2003; Phinyomark et al., 2012a).

Three criteria: maximum class separability, robustness and complexity, have been suggested and generally used to evaluate the EMG features for MMCS. Time-domain features have been usually used to make an optimal feature vector. However, only one feature per EMG channel is obtained from most of the frequency-domain methods (Boostani & Moradi, 2003), and their discriminant patterns in feature space are different from that of time-domain features (Phinyomark et al., 2012a). For a more powerful feature vector, an optimal frequency-domain feature should be combined with other successful time-domain features, such as the waveform length or WL (Oskoei & Hu, 2008), the RMS (Phinyomark et al., 2010), and the Willison amplitude or WAMP (Phinyomark et al., 2011).

First, the classification performance of the MNF and MDF features is discussed. Both features have the similar discriminant patterns, as can be observed from the scatter plots in Figs. 6(a) and 6(b). However, the MNF feature showed (a bit) better performance in class separation than the MDF feature. This can be confirmed by the classification accuracy obtained from the linear discriminant (LD) classifier. Mean and standard deviation of the classification accuracy obtained from MNF and MDF are 75.56±11.8% and 70.54±10.4%, respectively (Phinyomark et al., 2012a). Such classification accuracies are computed based on the classification of six upper-limb movements (hand open or HO, hand close or HC, wrist extension or WE, wrist flexion or WF, forearm pronation or FP, and forearm supination or FS) and five EMG channels (the extensor carpi radialis longus, the extensor carpi ulnaris, the extensor digitorum communis, the flexor carpi radialis, and the biceps brachii) from twenty healthy subjects (ten men and ten women).

For other frequency-domain features, five features consisting TTP, MNP, SM1, SM2 and SM3 have the same discriminant patterns in feature space as features in time-domain i.e. the RMS and the WL (Phinyomark et al., 2012a). Therefore, these features are not recommended to be one of the optimal features due to their higher computational cost. Moreover, the discriminant pattern of PSR is an inverse case of MNF and MDF, but the classification accuracy of PSR is less than that of MNF and MDF.

On the other hand, three features consisting PKF, VCF, and FR have the different discriminant patterns by comparing with MNF, MDF, and also time-domain features. The classification accuracies obtained from the classifier of PKF and VCF are very low (<50%), while the classification accuracy of FR (69.81%) is a bit less than that of MNF and MDF (Phinyomark et al., 2012a). Based on the results mentioned above, it can be concluded that MNF is an optimal frequency-domain feature for the EMG pattern classification.

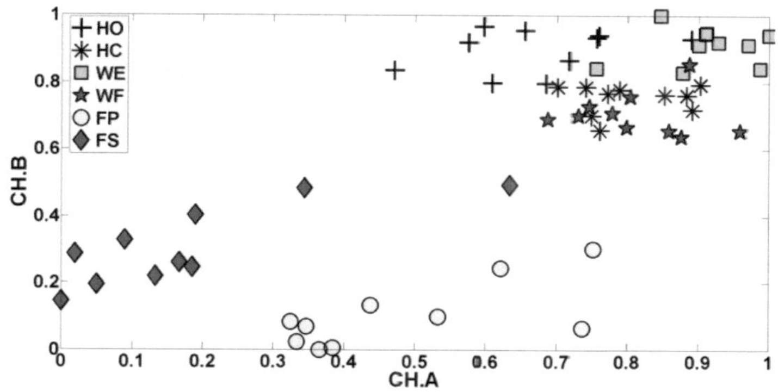

(a)

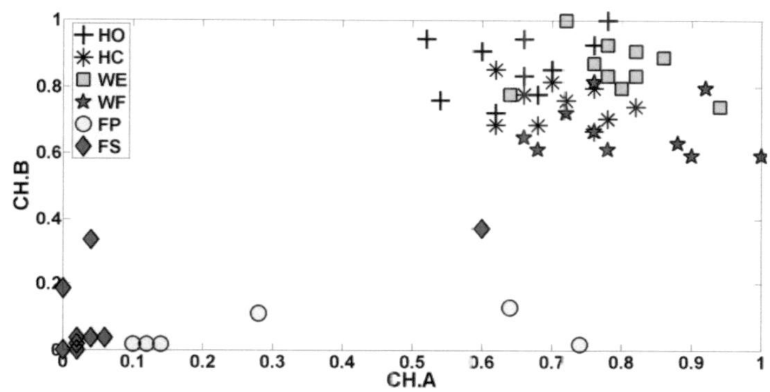

(b)

Figure 6. Scatter plots of (a) MNF and (b) MDF for 2 EMG channels (CH.A and CH.B) and 6 upper-limb movements (HO, HC, WE, WF, FP and FS) of a healthy subject. Note that CH.A is flexor carpi radialis muscle; CH.B is extensor carpi radialis longus muscle.

Further, in order to increase the robustness property of the MNF and MDF features, a modification of the MNF and MDF methods was proposed in one of our previous works (Phinyomark et al., 2009). The statistical variables (mean and median) were applied to the amplitude spectrum instead of the power spectrum, as used in the traditional methods, because the variation of the amplitude spectrum is less than that of the power spectrum. As a result, the variation of the modified MNF and MDF features is less than that of the traditional MNF and MDF features. These findings are confirmed using the real EMG data as presented in Phinyomark et al. (2009).

7. Conclusion and future trends

Mean frequency (MNF) and median frequency (MDF) are two useful and popular frequency-domain features for electromyography analysis both in clinical and engineering applications. MNF and MDF are frequently used as the gold standard tool to detect fatigue in the target muscles using EMG signals. The effectiveness of MNF and MDF under many experimental conditions is presented and confirmed in this chapter, although the effects of muscle force and muscle geometry on MNF and MDF are inconclusive. However, the possible reasons for the conflicting results in both effects have been described and discussed in detail together with the possible techniques to make the consistent results for MNF and MDF with the both effects, as mentioned in the following.

- For the effect of muscle force, the selection of time-dependent MNF and MDF should be applied to the raw EMG data. As a result, MNF and MDF should increase as the muscle force or load increases.
- For the effect of muscle geometry or joint angle, the normalization technique should be applied to the raw EMG data. As a result, MNF and MDF should increase as the muscle length or joint angle (degrees of extension) decreases.

However, the question remains whether the conflicting results, i.e. subject dependent, are found for the effect of both muscle force and muscle geometry on MNF and MDF. To address this question, two further works should be investigated: (1) finding the correlation between related anthropometric variables obtained from the subjects and MNF (or MDF), and (2) requesting all interested information to complete all components in Tables 2 and 3, and finding the possible reasons from the complete experimental conditions.

In total, MNF and MDF features extracted from the EMG signal are the optimal variables to identify muscle fatigue, particularly for static muscle contraction. However, for dynamic muscle contraction, applying instantaneous MNF and MDF are recommended.

The recommendations above can be useful to apply for most electromyography applications, such as human-computer interaction (HCI), ergonomics, occupational therapy and sport science. In addition, applying both techniques can make the MNF and MDF features to be the universal indices than can identify all factors including muscle force, muscle geometry, and muscle fatigue.

Author details

Angkoon Phinyomark, Sirinee Thongpanja, Pornchai Phukpattaranont
and Chusak Limsakul
Department of Electrical Engineering, Prince of Songkla University, Songkhla, Thailand

Huosheng Hu
School of Computer Science & Electronic Engineering, University of Essex, Colchester, United Kingdom

8. References

Allison, G. T. & Fujiwara, T. (2002). The Relationship between EMG Median Frequency and Low Frequency Band Amplitude Changes at Different Levels of Muscle Capacity. *Clinical Biomechanics*, Vol.17, No.6, pp. 464-469, ISSN 0268-0033

Al-Mulla, M. R.; Sepulveda, F. and Colley, M. (2011). A Review of Non-invasive Techniques to Detect and Predict localised Muscle Fatigue. *Sensors*, Vol.11, No.4, pp. 3545-3594, ISSN 1424-8220

Al-Mulla, M. R.; Sepulveda, F. and Colley, M. (2012b). sEMG Techniques to Detect and Predict Localised Muscle Fatigue, In: *EMG Methods for Evaluating Muscle and Nerve Function*, Mark Schwartz, pp. 157-186, InTech, ISBN 978-953-307-793-2, Rijeka, Croatia

Arnall, F. A.; Koumantakis, G. A.; Oldham, J. A. & Cooper, R. G. (2002). Between-days Reliability of Electromyographic Measures of Paraspinal Muscle Fatigue at 40, 50 and 60% Levels of Maximal Voluntary Contractile Force. *Clinical Rehabilitation*, Vol.16, No.7, pp. 761-771, ISSN 0269-2155

Balasubramanian, V.; Dutt, A. & Rai, S. (2011). Analysis of Muscle Fatigue in Helicopter Pilots. *Applied Ergonomics*, Vol.42, No.6, pp. 913-918, ISSN 0003-6870

Balestra, G.; Knaflitz, M. & Merletti, R. (1988). Comparison between Myoelectric Signal Mean and Median Frequency Estimated. *Proceedings of EMBC 1988 Annual International Conference of the IEEE Engineering in Medicine and Biology Society*, pp. 1708-1709, ISBN 0-7803-0785-2, New Orleans, LA, USA, November 4-7, 1988

Bilodeau, M.; Arsenault, A. B.; Gravel, D. & Bourbonnais, D. (1991). EMG Power Spectra of Elbow Extensors during Ramp and Step Isometric Contractions. *European Journal of Applied Physiology and Occupational Physiology*, Vol.63, No.1, pp. 24-28, ISSN 0301-5548

Bilodeau, M.; Arsenault, A. B.; Gravel, D. & Bourbonnais, D. (1992). Influence of Gender on the EMG Power Spectrum during an Increasing Force Level. *Journal of Electromyography and Kinesiology*, Vol.2, No.3, pp. 121-129, ISSN 1050-6411

Bilodeau, M.; Schindler-Ivens, S.; Williams, D. M.; Chandran, R. & Sharma, S. S. (2003). EMG Frequency Content Changes with Increasing Force and during Fatigue in the Quadriceps Femoris Muscle of Men and Women. *Journal of Electromyography and Kinesiology*, Vol.13, No.1, pp. 83-92, ISSN 1050-6411

Bonato, P.; Roy, S. H.; Knaflitz, M. & De Luca, C. J. (2001). Time Frequency Parameters of the Surface Myoelectric Signal for Assessing Muscle Fatigue during Cyclic Dynamic Contractions. *IEEE Transactions on Biomedical Engineering*, Vol.48, No.7, pp. 745-753, ISSN 0018-9294

Boostani, R. & Moradi, M. H. (2003). Evaluation of the Forearm EMG Signal Features for the Control of a Prosthetic Hand. *Physiological Measurement*, Vol.24, No.2, pp. 309-319, ISSN 0967-3334

Cechetto, A. D.; Parker, P. A. & Scott, R. N. (2001). The Effects of Four Time-varying Factors on the Mean Frequency of a Myoelectric Signal. *Journal of Electromyography and Kinesiology*, Vol.11, No.5, pp. 347-354, ISSN 1050-6411

Cifrek, M.; Medved, V.; Tonković, S. & Ostojić, S. (2009). Surface EMG based Muscle Fatigue Evaluation in Biomechanics. *Clinical Biomechanics*, Vol.24, No.4, pp. 327-340, ISSN 0268-0033

Cifrek, M.; Tonković, S. & Medved, V. (2000). Measurement and Analysis of Surface Myoelectric Signals during Fatigued Cyclic Dynamic Contractions. *Measurement*, Vol.27, No.2, pp. 85-92, ISSN 0263-2241

Chaffin, D. B. (1973). Localized Muscle Fatigue-definition and Measurement. *Journal of Occupational Medicine*, Vol.15, No.4, pp. 346-354, ISSN 0096-1736

Clancy, E. A.; Farina, D. & Merletti, R. (2005). Cross-comparison of Time- and Frequency-domain Methods for Monitoring the Myoelectric Signal during a Cyclic, Force-varying, Fatiguing Hand-grip Task. *Journal of Electromyography and Kinesiology*, Vol.15, No.3, pp. 256-265, ISSN 1050-6411

De Luca, C. J. (1979). Physiology and Mathematics of Myoelectric Signals. *IEEE Transactions on Biomedical Engineering*, Vol.26, No.6, pp. 313-325, ISSN 0018-9294

De Luca, C. J. (1984). Myoelectric Manifestations of Localized Muscular Fatigue in Humans. *Critical Reviews in Biomedical Engineering*, Vol.11, No.4, pp. 251-279, ISSN 0278-940X

Doheny, E. P.; Lowery, M. M.; FitzPatrick, D. P. & O'Malley, M. J. (2008). Effect of Elbow Joint Angle on Force–EMG Relationships in Human Elbow Flexor and Extensor Muscles. *Journal of Electromyography and Kinesiology*, Vol.18, No.5, pp. 760-770, ISSN 1050-6411

Du, S. & Vuskovic, M. (2004). Temporal vs. Spectral Approach to Feature Extraction from Prehensile EMG Signals. *Proceedings of IRI 2004 IEEE International Conference on Information Reuse and Integration*, pp. 344-350, ISBN 0-7803-8819-4, Las Vegas, NV, USA, November 8-10, 2004

Englehart, K. B. & Parker, P. A. (1994). Single Motor Unit Myoelectric Signal Analysis with Nonstationary Data. *IEEE Transactions on Biomedical Engineering*, Vol.41, No.2, pp. 168-180, ISSN 0018-9294

Farina, D.; Fosci, M. & Merletti, R. (2002). Motor Unit Recruitment Strategies Investigated by Surface EMG Variables. *Journal of Applied Physiology*, Vol.92, No.1, pp. 235-247, ISSN 8750-7587

Farina, D. & Merletti, R. (2000). Comparison of Algorithms for Estimation of EMG Variables during Voluntary Isometric Contractions. *Journal of Electromyography and Kinesiology*, Vol.10, No.5, pp. 337-349, ISSN 1050-6411

Gander, R. E. & Hudgins, R. E. (1985). Power Spectral Density of the Surface Myoelectric Signal of the Biceps Brachii as a Function of Static Load. *Electromyography and Clinical Neurophysiology*, Vol.25, No.7-8, pp. 469-478, ISSN 0301-150X

Georgakis, A., Stergioulas, L. K. & Giakas, G. (2003). Fatigue Analysis of the Surface EMG Signal in Isometric Constant Force Contractions Using the Averaged Instantaneous Frequency. *IEEE Transactions on Biomedical Engineering*, Vol.50, No.2, pp. 262-265, ISSN 0018-9294

Gerdle, B.; Eriksson, N. E.; Brundin, L. & Edstrom, M. (1988). Surface EMG Recordings during Maximum Static Shoulder Forward Flexion in Different Positions. *European Journal of Applied Physiology and Occupational Physiology*, Vol.57, No.4, pp. 415-419, ISSN 0301-5548

Gerdle, B.; Eriksson, N. E. & Brundin, L. (1990). The Behaviour of Mean Power Frequency of the Surface Electromyogram in Biceps Brachii with Increasing Force and during Fatigue. With Special regard to the Electrode Distance. *Electromyography and Clinical Neurophysiology*, Vol.30, No.8, pp. 483-489, ISSN 0301-150X

Hagberg, M. & Ericsson, B. E. (1982). Myoelectric Power Spectrum Dependence on Muscular Contraction Level of Elbow Flexors. *European Journal of Applied Physiology and Occupational Physiology*, Vol.48, No.2, pp. 147-156, ISSN 0301-5548

Hagberg, C. & Hagberg, M. (1989). Surface EMG Amplitude and Frequency Dependence on Exerted Force for the Upper Trapezius Muscle: A Comparison between Right and Left Sides. *European Journal of Applied Physiology and Occupational Physiology*, Vol.58, No.6, pp. 641-645, ISSN 0301-5548

Han, J. -S.; Song, W. -K.; Kim, J. -S.; Bang, W. -C.; Lee, H. & Bien, Z. (2000). New EMG Pattern Recognition Based on Soft Computing Techniques and its Application to Control a Rehabilitation Robotic Arm. *Proceedings of IIZUKA 2000 6th International Conference on Soft Computing*, pp. 890-897, Fukuoka, Japan, October 1-4, 2000

Hautier, C. A.; Arsac, L. M.; Deghdegh, K.; Souquet, J.; Belli, A. & Lacour, J. R. (2000). Influence of Fatigue on EMG/Force Ratio and Cocontraction in Cycling. *Medicine and Science in Sports and Exercise*, Vol.32, No.4, pp. 839-843, ISSN 0195-9131

Hermens, H. J.; Boon, K. L. & Zilvold, G. (1984). The Clinical Use of Surface EMG. *Electromyography and Clinical Neurophysiology*, Vol.24, No.4, pp. 243-265, ISSN 0301-150X

Inbar, G. F.; Allin, J. & Kranz, H. (1987). Surface EMG Spectral Changes with Muscle Length. *Medical and Biological Engineering and Computing*, Vol.25, No.6, pp. 683-689, ISSN 0140-0118

Inbar, G. F.; Allin, J.; Paiss, O. & Kranz, H. (1986). Monitoring Surface EMG Spectral Changes by the Zero Crossing Rate. *Medical and Biological Engineering and Computing*, Vol.24, No.1, pp. 10-18, ISSN 0140-0118

Kalra, C. ; Kumar, D. K. & Arjunan, S. (2012). Age and Gender Related Differences on Surface Electromyogram During Various Levels of Contraction. *Journal of Medical and Biological Engineering*, in press, ISSN 1609-0985

Kaplanis, P. A.; Pattichis, C. S.; Hadjileontiadis, L. J. & Roberts, V. C. (2009). Surface EMG Analysis on Normal Subjects Based on Isometric Voluntary Contraction. *Journal of Electromyography and Kinesiology*, Vol.19, No.1, pp. 157-171, ISSN 1050-6411

Karlsson, S.; Yu, J. & Akay, M. (2000). Time-frequency Analysis of Myoelectric Signals during Dynamic Contractions: A Comparative Study. *IEEE Transactions on Biomedical Engineering*, Vol.47, No.2, pp. 228-238, ISSN 0018-9294

Knaflitz, M. and Bonato, P. (1999). Time-frequency Methods Applied to Muscle Fatigue Assessment during Dynamic Contractions. *Journal of Electromyography and Kinesiology*, Vol.9, No.5, pp. 337-350, ISSN 1050-6411

Knaflitz, M.; Merletti, R. & De Luca, C. J. (1990). Inference of Motor Unit Recruitment Order in Voluntary and Electrically Elicited Contractions. *Journal of Applied Physiology*, Vol.68, No.4, pp. 1657-1667, ISSN 8750-7587

Lariviere, C.; Arsenault, A. B.; Gravel, D.; Gagnon, D. & Loisel, P. (2001). Median Frequency of the Electromyographic Signal: Effect of Time-window Location on Brief Step Contractions. *Journal of Electromyography and Kinesiology*, Vol.11, No.1, pp. 65-71, ISSN 1050-6411

Leunkeu, A. N.; Keefer, D. J.; Imed, M. & Ahmaidi, S. (2010). Electromyographic (EMG) Analysis of Quadriceps Muscle Fatigue in Children with Cerebral Palsy during a Sustained Isometric Contraction. *Journal of Child Neurology*, Vol.25, No.3, pp. 287-293, ISSN 0883-0738

MacIsaac, D.; Parker, P. A. & Scott, R. N. (2001). The Short-time Fourier Transform and Muscle Fatigue Assessment in Dynamic Contractions. *Journal of Electromyography and Kinesiology*, Vol.11, No.6, pp. 439-449, ISSN 1050-6411

Mannion, A. F. & Dolan, P. (1996). Relationship between Myoelectric and Mechanical Manifestations of Fatigue in the Quadriceps Femoris Muscle Group. *European Journal of Applied Physiology and Occupational Physiology*, Vol.74, No., pp. 411-419, ISSN 0301-5548

Masuda, K.; Masuda, T.; Sadoyama, T.; Mitsuharu, I. & Katsuta, S. (1999). Changes in Surface EMG Parameters during Static and Dynamic Fatiguing Contractions. *Journal of Electromyography and Kinesiology*, Vol.9, No.1, pp. 39-46, ISSN 1050-6411

Merletti, R.; Lo Conte, L. R.; Avignone, E. & Guglielminotti, P. (1999). Modeling of Surface Myoelectric Signals - Part I : Model Implementation. *IEEE Transactions on Biomedical Engineering*, Vol.46, No.7, pp. 810-820, ISSN 0018-9294

Merletti, R.; Lo Conte, L. R.; Cisari, C. & Massazza, U. (1993). Effect of Ankle Joint Position on Electrically Evoked Surface Myoelectric Signals of the Tibialis Anterior Muscle. *Archives of Physical Medicine and Rehabilitation*, Vol.74, No.5, pp. 501-506, ISSN 0003-9993

Merletti, R. & Parker, P. (2004). *ELECTROMYOGRAPHY Physiology, Engineering, and Noninvasive Applications*, John Wiley & Sons, ISBN 0-471-67580-6, USA

Merletti, R. & Roy, S. (1996). Myoelectric and Mechanical Manifestations of Muscle Fatigue in Voluntary Contractions. *Journal of Orthopaedic and Sports Physical Therapy*, Vol.24, No.6, pp. 342-353, ISSN 0190-6011

Merletti, R.; Sabbahi, M. A. & De Luca, C. J. (1984). Median Frequency of the Myoelectric Signal: Effects of Muscle Ischemia and Cooling. *European Journal of Applied Physiology and Occupational Physiology*, Vol.52, No.3, pp. 258-265, ISSN 0301-5548

Moritani, T.; Muramatsu, S. & Muro, M. (1988). Activity of Motor Units during Concentric and Eccentric Contractions. *American Journal of Physical Medicine*, Vol.66, No.6, pp. 338-350, ISSN 0002-9491

Moritani, T. & Muro, M. (1987). Motor Unit Activity and Surface Electromyogram Power Spectrum during Increasing Force of Contraction. *European Journal of Applied Physiology and Occupational Physiology*, Vol.56, No.3, pp. 260-265, ISSN 0301-5548

Muro, M. ; Nagata, A.; Murakami, K. & Moritani, T. (1982). Surface EMG Power Spectral Analysis of Neuromuscular Disorders during Isometric and Isotonic Contraction. *American Journal of Physical Medicine*, Vol.61, No.5, pp. 244-254, ISSN 0894-9115

Okada, M. (1987). Effect of Muscle Length on Surface EMG Wave Forms in Isometric Contractions. *European Journal of Applied Physiology and Occupational Physiology*, Vol.56, No.4, pp. 482-486, ISSN 1439-6319

Oskoei, M. A. & Hu, H. (2006). GA-based Feature Subset Selection for Myoelectric Classification. *Proceedings of ROBIO 2006 IEEE International Conference on Robotics and Biomimetics*, pp. 1465-1470, ISBN 1-4244-0570-X, Kunming, China, December 17-20, 2006

Oskoei, M. A. & Hu, H. (2007). Myoelectric Control Systems—A Survey. *Biomedical Signal Processing and Control*, Vol.2, No.4, pp. 275-294, ISSN 1746-8094

Oskoei, M. A. & Hu, H. (2008). Support Vector Machine based Classification Scheme for Myoelectric Control Applied to Upper Limb. *IEEE Transactions on Biomedical Engineering*, Vol.55, No.8, pp. 1956-1965, ISSN 0018-9294

Oskoei, M. A.; Hu, H. & Gan, J. Q. (2008). Manifestation of Fatigue in Myoelectric Signals of Dynamic Contractions Produced during Playing PC Games. *Proceedings of EMBS 2008 30th Annual International Conference of the IEEE Engineering in Medicine and Biology Society*, pp. 315-318, ISBN 978-1-4244-1814-5, Vancouver, BC, Canada, August 20-25, 2008

Petrofsky, J. S.; Glaser, R. M.; Philips, C. A.; Lind, A. R. & Williams, C. (1982). Evaluation of Amplitude and Frequency Components of the Surface EMG as an Index of Muscle Fatigue. *Ergonomics*, Vol.25, No.3, pp. 213-223, ISSN 0014-0139

Petrofsky, J. S. & Lind, A. R. (1980a). Frequency Analysis of the Surface Electromyogram during Sustained Isometric Contractions. *European Journal of Applied Physiology and Occupational Physiology*, Vol.43, No.2, pp. 173-182, ISSN 0301-5548

Petrofsky, J. S. & Lind, A. R. (1980b). The Influence of Temperature on the Amplitude and Frequency Components of the EMG during Brief and Sustained Isometric Contractions. *European Journal of Applied Physiology and Occupational Physiology*, Vol.44, No.2, pp. 189-200, ISSN 0301-5548

Phinyomark, A.; Limsakul, C. & Phukpattaranont, P. (2009). A Novel Feature Extraction for Robust EMG Pattern Recognition. *Journal of Computing*, Vol.1, No.1, pp. 71-80, ISSN 2151-9617

Phinyomark, A.; Hirunviriya, S.; Phukpattaranont, P. & Limsakul, C. (2010). Evaluation of EMG Feature Extraction for Hand Movement Recognition Based on Euclidean Distance and Standard Deviation. *Proceedings of ECTI-CON 2010 7th International Conference on Electrical Engineering/Electronics, Computer, Telecommunications and Information Technology*, pp. 856-860, ISBN 978-1-4244-5606-2, Chiang Mai, Thailand, May 19-21, 2010

Phinyomark, A.; Hirunviriya, S.; Nuidod, A.; Phukpattaranont, P. & Limsakul, C. (2011). Evaluation of EMG Feature Extraction for Movement Control of Upper Limb Prostheses Based on Class Separation Index. *IFMBE Proceedings*, Vol. 35, Part 8, pp. 750-754, ISSN 1680-0737

Phinyomark, A.; Phukpattaranont, P. & Limsakul, C. (2012a). Feature Reduction and Selection for EMG Signal Classification. *Expert Systems with Applications*, Vol.39, No.8, pp. 7420-7431, ISSN 0957-4174

Phinyomark, A.; Phukpattaranont, P. & Limsakul, C. (2012b). The Usefulness of Wavelet Transform to Reduce Noise in the SEMG Signal, In: *EMG Methods for Evaluating Muscle and Nerve Function*, Mark Schwartz, pp. 107-132, InTech, ISBN 978-953-307-793-2, Rijeka, Croatia

Phinyomark, A.; Thongpanja, S.; Phukpattaranont, P. & Limsakul, C. (2012c). Investigation of Conflicting Results of Muscle Force Effect on Mean and Median Frequencies. *Australasian Physical and Engineering Sciences in Medicine*, in submitted, ISSN 0158-9938

Potvin, J. R. (1997). Effects of Muscle Kinematics on Surface EMG Amplitude and Frequency during Fatiguing Dynamic Contractions. *Journal of Applied Physiology*, Vol.82, No.1, pp. 144-151, ISSN 0021-8987

Qingju, Z. & Zhizeng, L. (2006). Wavelet De-noising of Electromyography. *Proceedings of ICMA 2006 IEEE International Conference on Mechatronics Automation*, pp. 1553–1558, ISBN 1-4244-0465-7, Luoyang, Henan, China, June 25-28, 2006

Rainoldi, A.; Galardi, G.; Maderna, L.; Comi, G.; Conte, L. L. & Merletti, R. (1999). Repeatability of Surface EMG Variables during Voluntary Isometric Contraction of the Biceps Brachii Muscle. *Journal of Electromyography and Kinesiology*, Vol.9, No.2, pp. 105-119, ISSN 1050-6411

Ravier, P.; Buttelli, O.; Jennane, R. & Couratier, P. (2005). An EMG Fractal Indicator Having Different Sensitivities to Changes in Force and Muscle Fatigue during Voluntary Static Muscle Contractions. *Journal of Electromyography and Kinesiology*, Vol.15, No.2, pp. 210-221, ISSN 1050-6411

Roy, S. H., Bonato, P. & Knaflitz, M. (1998). EMG Assessment of Back Muscle Function during Cyclical Lifting. *Journal of Electromyography and Kinesiology*, Vol.8, No.4, pp. 233-245, ISSN 1050-6411

Sabbahi, M. A.; Merletti, R.; De Luca, C. J. & Rosenthal, R. G. (1981). How Handidness, Sexa md Force Level Affect the Median Frequency of the Myoelectric Signal. *Proceedings of 1981 4th Annual Conference on Rehabilitation Engineering*, pp. 232-234, Washington, D.C., USA, August 30-September 3, 1981

Sato, H. (1976). Some Factors Affecting the Power Spectra of Surface Electromyograms in Isometric Contractions. *Journal of Anthropology of the Nippon Society*, Vol.84, No.2, pp. 105-113, ISSN 0918-7960

Sato, H. (1982). Functional Characteristics of Human Skeletal Muscle Revealed by Spectral Analysis of the Surface Electromyogram. *Electromyography and Clinical Neurophysiology*, Vol.22, No.6, pp. 459-516, ISSN 0301-150X

Shankar, S.; Gander, R. E. & Brandell, B. R. (1989). Changes in the Myoelectric Signal (MES) Power Spectra during Dynamic Contractions. *Electroencephalography and Clinical Neurophysiology*, Vol.73, No.2, pp. 142-150, ISSN 0013-4694

Soares, F. A.; Salomoni, S. E.; Veneziano, W. H.; De Carvalho, J. L. A.; Nascimento, F. A. D. O.; Pires, K. F. & Da Rocha, A. F. (2011). On the Behavior of Surface Electromyographic Variables during the Menstrual Cycle. *Physiological Measurement*, Vol.32, No.5, pp. 543-557, ISSN 0967-3334

Solomonow, M.; Baten, C.; Smit, J.; Baratta, R.; Hermens, H.; D'Ambrosia, R. & Shoji, H. (1990). Electromyogram Power Spectra Frequencies Associated with Motor Unit Recruitment Strategies. *Journal of Applied Physiology*, Vol.68, No.3, pp. 1177-1185, ISSN 0021-8987

Stulen, F. B. & De Luca, C. J. (1981). Frequency Parameters of the Myoelectric Signal as a Measure of Muscle Conduction Velocity. *IEEE Transactions on Biomedical Engineering*, Vol.28, No.7, pp. 515-523, ISSN 0018-9294

Tavakolan, M.; Xiao, Z. G. & Menon, C. (2011). A Preliminary Investigation Assessing the Viability of Classifying Hand Postures in Seniors. *Biomedical Engineering* Online, Vol.10, No.79, ISSN 1475-925X

Thongpanja, S.; Phinyomark, A.; Phukpattaranont, P. & Limsakul, C. (2010). Time-dependent EMG Power Spectrum Features of Biceps Brachii During Isotonic Exercise. *Journal of Sports Science and Technology*, Vol.10, No.2S, pp. 314-318, ISSN 1513-7201

Thongpanja, S.; Phinyomark, A.; Phukpattaranont, P. & Limsakul, C. (2011). Time-dependent EMG Power Spectrum Parameters of Biceps Brachii During Cyclic Dynamic Contraction. *IFMBE Proceedings*, Vol.35, No.8, pp. 233-236, ISSN 1680-0737

Thongpanja, S.; Phinyomark, A.; Phukpattaranont, P. & Limsakul, C. (2012). A Feasibility Study of Fatigue and Muscle Contraction Indices Based on EMG Time-dependent Spectral Analysis. *Procedia Engineering*, Vol.32, pp. 239-245, ISSN 1877-7058

Thongpanja, S.; Phinyomark, A.; Phukpattaranont, P. & Limsakul, C. (2013). Mean and Median Frequency of EMG Signal to Determine Muscle Force Based on Time-Dependent Power Spectrum. *Electronics and Electrical Engineering*, Vol.129, No.3, ISSN 2029-5731

Van Boxtel, A. & Schomaker, L. R. B. (1984). Influence of Motor Unit Firing Statistics on the Median Frequency of the EMG Power Spectrum. *European Journal of Applied Physiology and Occupational Physiology*, Vol.52, No.2, pp. 207-213, ISSN 0301-5548

Viitasalo, J. T. & Komi, P. V. (1977). Signal Characteristics of EMG during Fatigue. *European Journal of Applied Physiology and Occupational Physiology*, Vol.37, No.2, pp. 111-121, ISSN 0301-5548

Viitasalo, J. T. & Komi, P. V. (1978). Interrelationships of EMG Signal Characteristics at Different Levels of Muscle Tension and during Fatigue. *Electromyography and Clinical Neurophysiology*, Vol.18, No.3-4, pp. 167-178, ISSN 0301-150X

Zaman, S. A.; MacIsaac, D. T. & Parker, P. A. (2011). Repeatability of Surface EMG-based Single Parameter Muscle Fatigue Assessment Strategies in Static and Cyclic Contractions. *Proceedings of EMBC 2011 33rd Annual International Conference of the IEEE Engineering in Medicine and Biology Society*, pp. 3857-3860, ISBN 978-142444121-1, Boston, MA, USA, August 30-September 3, 2011

Zecca, M.; Micera, S.; Carrozza, M. C. & Dario, P. (2002). Control of Multifunctional Prosthetic Hands by Processing the Electromyographic Signal. *Critical Reviews in Biomedical Engineering*, Vol.30, No.4-6, pp. 459-485, ISSN 0278-940X

Zhang, Z. G.; Liu, H. T.; Chan, S. C.; Luk, K. D. & Hu, Y. (2010). Time-dependent Power Spectral Density Estimation of Surface Electromyograhy during Isometric Muscle Contraction : Methods and Comparisons. *Journal of Electromyography and Kinesiology*, Vol.20, No.1, pp. 89-101, ISSN 1050-6411

Chapter 9

Feature Extraction Methods for Studying Surface Electromyography and Kinematic Measurements in Parkinson's Disease

Saara M. Rissanen, Markku Kankaanpää,
Mika P. Tarvainen and Pasi A. Karjalainen

Additional information is available at the end of the chapter

http://dx.doi.org/10.5772/48820

1. Introduction

1.1. Parkinson's disease (PD)

Parkinson's disease is a progressive neurodegenerative disease that affects 1 % of people over 60 years of age [9]. In PD, there is a dopaminergic neuronal loss in the substantia nigra in the basal ganglia of the cerebra [48]. It has been observed that the basal ganglia has a specific effect on the temporal organization of motor cortical activity during muscle contractions. In this way, the dysfunction of the basal ganglia may lead to motor symptoms of PD. [37] The primary symptoms of PD include tremor, muscle rigidity and slowness of movements. The diagnosis is based on the presence of the primary symptoms and on the response to medication. [17, 18]. However, the diagnosis can be problematic. Clinicopathological studies from the UK and Canada have shown that the disease is diagnosed incorrectly in about 25 % of patients [48]. The pre-motor period before diagnosis may be long (5–20 years) and at the time of the diagnosis already 50–60 % of the dopaminergic neurons may be lost [22, 38].

Although there is no cure for PD, the symptoms can be relieved reasonably with medication or with the deep brain stimulation (DBS) [17]. The motor impairment, the disease progression and the efficacy of treatment are commonly evaluated subjectively using standardized rating scales such as the Unified Parkinson's disease rating scale (UPDRS) [12, 15]. No objectively measured characteristics and methods are widely used for quantifying motor symptoms of PD [2].

Several objective methods have been proposed for improving the diagnostic accuracy of PD, for enabling earlier diagnosis, and for quantifying the disease severity, progression and the efficacy of treatment. These methods include: kinematic measurements of motor tasks (e.g. finger tapping), testing of olfactory loss, imaging techniques (e.g. magnetic resonance imaging and positron emission tomography), and biochemical tests of blood and cerebrospinal fluid.

However, none of the proposed methods is widely used for PD. The validation of new methods for clinical use takes time. In order to be more sensitive than the traditional methods it is probable that a combination of several methods will be needed for PD. [2, 11, 24]

1.2. Surface electromyography and kinematic measurements in PD

Surface electromyography (EMG) and kinematic measurements are non-invasive and relatively simple and cost-effective methods for quantifying neuromuscular function and movement. Therefore, these methods may be suitable for quantifying objectively the motor impairment in PD and the effects of treatment. A few new technologies based on kinematic sensors have been recently commercialized for measuring motor symptoms of PD. The kinematic measurements provide information about human movements. However, it is possible that surface EMG provides earlier or more direct information about PD than the sole kinematic measures based on movement.

Several studies have analyzed the surface EMG and kinematic signals of PD patients in comparison to the signals of healthy subjects and aimed to correlate the most significant findings with the clinical rating scales. Differences between patients and healthy subjects have been observed in the tremor-EMG coherence [50], in the cortico-muscular coherence [37] and in the muscle activation patterns during limb movements [13, 26, 35]. In the gait characteristics, differences have been observed in the gait speed and stride length, in the arm and leg swing and in the muscle activation patterns of gait [5–7, 36, 43].

Several studies have evaluated effects of PD treatment (medication and DBS) on the basis of EMG and kinematic measurements. It has been observed that the medication and DBS may modify the tremor amplitude, regularity and frequency [4, 41, 42], movement speed [3, 8, 34, 40, 44, 49, 51, 52], joint kinetics and muscle activation during movements [55], EMG burst patterns during movement [34, 51, 52] and the cortico-muscular coherence [25, 37]. There is currently a lot of interest for characterizing EMG and kinematic signals of PD patients. However, many studies have analyzed the EMG signals of PD patients by using conventional amplitude- and spectral based methods. More information about PD could be extracted from the EMG signals by using also more modern methods of signal analysis, by analyzing sets of signal features and by analyzing the signal characteristics also on individual level.

EMG signals are impulse-like waveforms because they consist of motor unit (MU) action potentials. The level of MU synchronization is increased in PD [14, 50], which appears as an increased number of recurring spikes and bursts in the EMG signals. Therefore, there is important information about PD in the morphology of the EMG signal and in the recurring signal patterns. It has been observed that the conventional EMG signal parameters (amplitudes and the mean and median frequencies) are not effective in capturing impulse-like structures [23]. Therefore, more modern methods of signal analysis are needed for analyzing the EMG signals of PD patients.

1.3. Our approach for studying surface EMG and kinematic measurements in PD

In order to extract PD-related information from the surface EMG signals effectively, we proposed specific methods based on signal morphology, nonlinear dynamics and wavelets for analyzing the EMG signals of PD patients in [28–32]. One aim of those studies was to develop objective methods for discriminating between PD patients and healthy subjects on the basis of surface EMG signal morphology [32] and on the basis of simultaneous EMG and acceleration (ACC) recordings during isometric [28] and dynamic muscle contractions [29]. Another aim was to develop methods based on surface EMG and kinematic measurements and analysis for quantifying effects of PD treatment (medication and DBS) on individual level. All of those studies presented an innovative approach, that combines a principal component (PC) -based method with a set of effective signal features, for analyzing the EMG and acceleration signals in PD. In the following sections 2, 3 and 4, we describe the methods that were developed and used for feature extraction and discrimination between subjects in [28–32]. All methods were tested with the measured data. In total, the measurement data from 62 PD patients and 72 healthy subjects were analyzed. The main findings of those studies are also described.

2. Analysis EMG signal morphology in PD

EMG signal is a sum of MU action potentials at a given location and therefore it is an impulse-like waveform. The EMG signals of PD patients are characterized by recurring spikes and bursts (see Figure 1) that are likely caused by the increased level of MU synchronization. Important information about PD is in the EMG signal morphology and in the recurring signal patters.

In [32], the EMG signal morphology of 25 PD patients and 22 healthy subjects was analyzed by using sample histograms and crossing rate (CR) expansions. The analyzed EMG signals were measured during the isometric contraction of biceps brachii (BB) muscles. During the task, subjects were asked to hold their elbows at a 90° angle with their palms up. The measurements were performed by using the ME6000 -biosignal monitor (Mega Electronics Ltd., Kuopio, Finland) and disposable Ag/AgCl electrodes (Medicotest, model M-00-S, Ølstykke, Denmark) in bipolar connection. The sampling rate was 1000 Hz.

Typical EMG signals of one healthy subject and one PD patient are presented in Figure 1. One can observe that the EMG signal of the patient contains recurring EMG bursts while the EMG signal of the healthy subject does not.

2.1. Feature extraction by using sample histograms and CR expansions

Sample histograms were extracted from the scaled (between -1 and 1) EMG signals with 200 bins and the CR expansions from the scaled EMGs as the number of crossings at given threshold levels (201 threshold levels). An example of the sample histogram and the CR expansion for the healthy subject and for the PD patient are presented in Figure 1. One can observe that the sample histogram of the patient is sharper and the CR expansion narrower than those of the healthy subject.

2.2. Discrimination analysis between subjects

The calculated sample histograms and CR expansions of PD patients (with medication on) and healthy subjects were used as high-dimensional feature vectors for discrimination analysis between subjects. The PC-based approach was used for decreasing the dimensionality of the

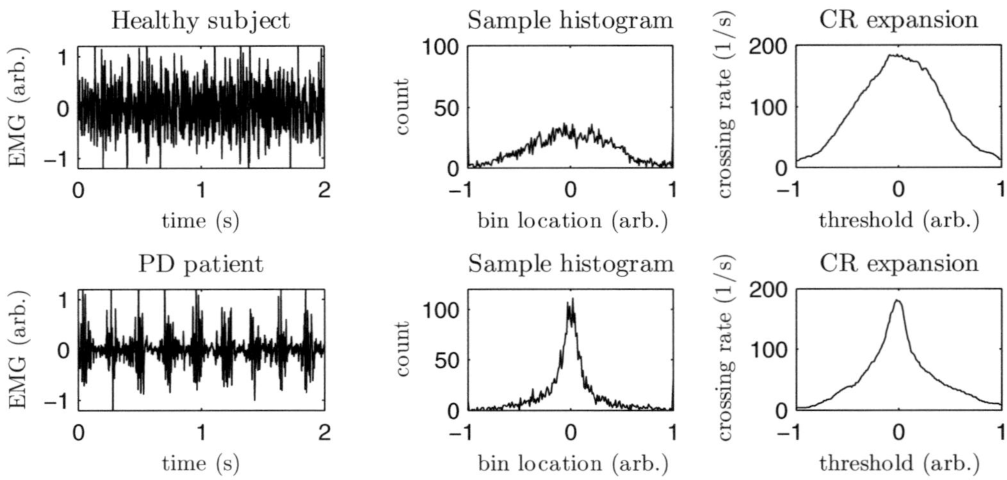

Figure 1. EMG signals of one healthy subject (top) and one PD patient (bottom). The sample histograms and crossing rate expansions of the healthy subject and the PD patient.

feature vectors and the discriminant analysis of subjects was performed in a two-dimensional feature space.

In the PC-based approach [19], each feature vector $z_j \in \mathbb{R}^{N_p}$ is modeled with a linear model

$$z_j = H\theta_j + v_j. \tag{1}$$

In the linear model, $H = [\phi_1 \ \phi_2 \ \ldots \ \phi_K] \in \mathbb{R}^{N_p \times K}$ is the model matrix that contains the basis vectors $\phi_k \in \mathbb{R}^{N_p}$ in its columns. Vector $\theta_j \in \mathbb{R}^K$ contains the model weights and $v_j \in \mathbb{R}^{N_p}$ the model error for the j'th feature vector. The basis vectors ϕ_k are selected to be the eigenvectors of the data correlation matrix

$$R_z = \frac{1}{M}\sum_{j=1}^{M} z_j z_j^T, \tag{2}$$

where M is the total number of feature vectors and $(\cdot)^T$ denotes the transpose. Because the eigenvectors are orthonormal, the least squares solution for the model weights θ_j is of the form

$$\hat{\theta}_j = (H^T H)^{-1} H^T z_j = H^T z_j. \tag{3}$$

These weights are called the principal components. By choosing K ($K < N_p$) eigenvectors corresponding to K largest eigenvalues for modeling, the best K-dimensional orthogonal approximation for the data set is obtained. The PCs are the new uncorrelated features and they can be used for discriminating between subjects in a low-dimensional feature space.

In [32], three feature vectors were formed for each subject: one containing the EMG sample histogram, one containing the CR expansion and one containing both of them (augmented PC approach). Thus, the original dimensionality of the feature vectors was reasonably high ($N_p \geq 200$). The feature vectors of one PD patient and one healthy subject in the augmented

PC approach are illustrated in Figure 2. In addition, the correlation matrix and the three eigenvectors corresponding to the three largest eigenvalues are presented in the same figure.

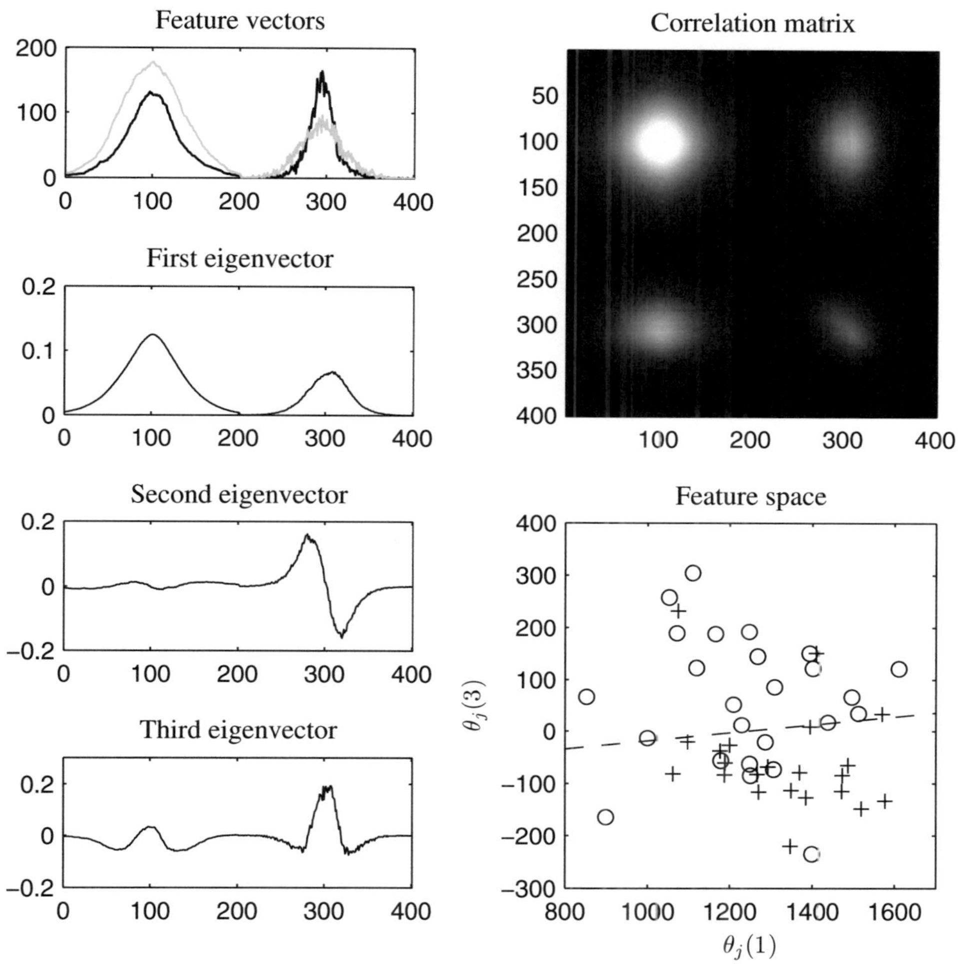

Figure 2. The feature vectors of one PD patient (black) and one healthy subject (gray) in the augmented PC approach (top left). Three eigenvectors corresponding to the three largest eigenvalues (left). The data correlation matrix (top right). The third PCs $\theta_j(3)$ with respect to the first PCs $\theta_j(1)$ of 22 healthy subjects (+) and 25 PD patients (○) (bottom right).

The correlation matrix in Figure 2 contains four white areas with high correlation. The white area in the top left corner describes correlations between the CR expansion values. The white area in the bottom right corner describes correlations between the sample histogram values. The non-diagonal white areas describe cross-correlations between the CR expansion values and the sample histogram values.

The eigenvectors in Figure 2 can be interpreted as follows:

- The first eigenvector is the best mean-square fit for the feature vectors of all subjects. Thus, it is similar to the mean of all feature vectors. Therefore, the first PC describes the amplitude of the histogram and the CR expansion with respect to the mean of all subjects.
- The second eigenvector is the best mean-square fit for the residual of the first fit. The second eigenvector describes variations in the peaks (modes) of the histograms and CR expansions of all subjects.
- The third eigenvector models variations in the heights and widths of the histograms and CR expansions in the whole data set.

The rest of the eigenvectors contain information about higher frequencies of the data and do not interest us in this case. The biggest differences between patients and healthy subjects were found in the third PC and some differences were observed in the first PC. Therefore, the discrimination between subjects was performed with respect to the third and the first PC.

2.3. Results

A linear discriminant was used in [32] for discriminating between the subjects in the two-dimensional feature space that was spanned by the third and the first PCs. The best discrimination results were obtained by using the augmented PC approach (see results in Figure 2). According to the results, 72 % of PD patients can be discriminated from 86 % of healthy subjects on the basis of EMG signal morphology.

3. Analysis of simultaneous EMG and acceleration recordings in PD

3.1. EMG and acceleration measurements

We analyzed simultaneous EMG and acceleration measurements of PD patients and healthy subjects in [28, 29] and aimed to develop methods for discriminating between the patients and the healthy subjects on the basis of the measured signals. The signals were measured during isometric contraction of BB muscles [28] and during dynamic elbow flexion-extension movements [29].

During the isometric task, the subjects were asked to hold their elbows at a 90° angle with their palms up. During the dynamic task, the subjects were asked to flex and extend their both elbows vertically and freely in two-second cycles with their palms up. Surface EMGs were registered continuously from the BB muscles and the accelerations of forearms simultaneously from the palmar side of subject's wrists. All measurements were performed by using the ME6000 -biosignal monitor (Mega Electronics Ltd., Kuopio, Finland), disposable Ag/AgCl electrodes (Medicotest, model M-00-S, Ølstykke, Denmark) in bipolar connection and tri-axial accelerometers (Meac-x, Mega Electronics Ltd., range ± 10 g). Signals were sampled with the rate of 1000 Hz. The resultant of the acceleration was used in the analysis. Low-frequency trends were removed from both signals by using the smoothness priors method [46]. The high-pass cut-off frequencies were 10 Hz for EMG and 2 Hz for acceleration.

Typical EMG and acceleration signals of one PD patient and one healthy subject during the isometric and dynamic task are presented in Figure 3. It is observed in the isometric

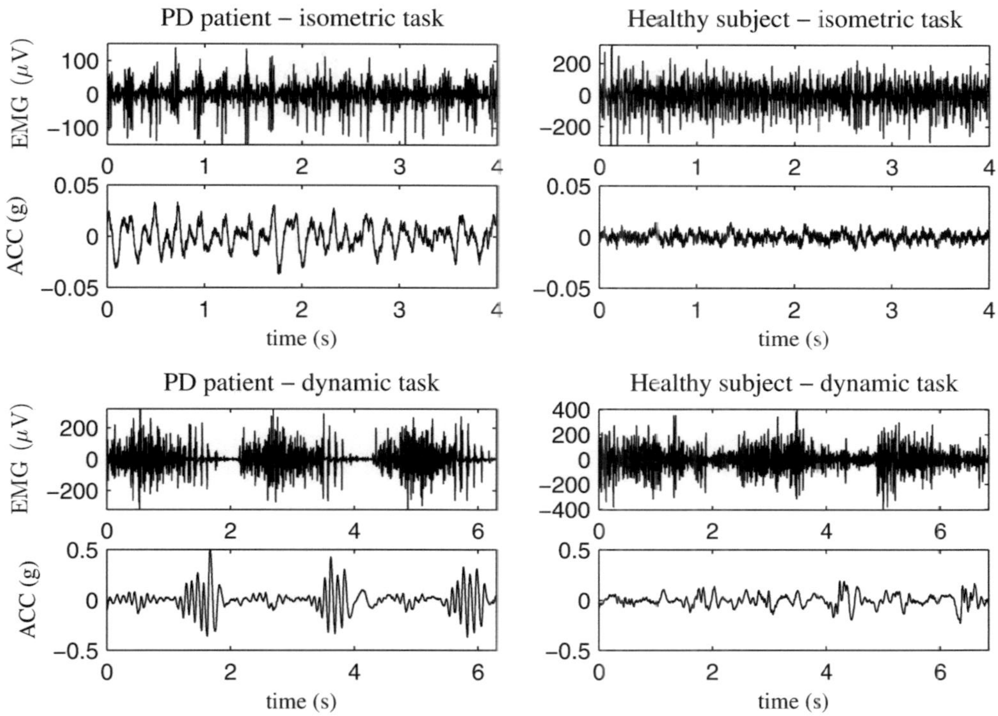

Figure 3. EMG and acceleration recordings of one PD patient (left) and one healthy subject (right) during the isometric and the dynamic task.

recording, that the EMG signal of the PD patient differs from the EMG signal of the healthy subject by containing recurring EMG bursts and the acceleration signal by containing regular high-amplitude oscillation. This oscillation is likely due to the resting and postural tremor. It is observed in the dynamic recording, that the EMG signal of the PD patient is characterized by recurring spikes and the acceleration recording by containing high-amplitude oscillation during the extension phases of the movement. The oscillation in the acceleration signal (which was high-pass-filtered with 2 Hz as cut-off frequency) is likely due to muscle rigidity and kinetic tremor (tremor that occurs during movement). In the flexion phases of the movement, the differences between the patient and the healthy subject are not as pronounced.

3.2. Feature extraction from EMG and acceleration signals

It was observed in [23] and [28, 29] that the conventional amplitude- and spectral-based EMG parameters (root mean square value and median frequency) are not effective in characterizing the EMG signals of PD patients in comparison to the signals of the healthy subjects. Therefore, we extracted a set of other PD characteristic signal features from the isometric [28] and dynamic EMG and acceleration recordings [29]. These parameters are detailed in Table 1 and they were calculated as epoch averages from the isometric EMG and acceleration signals and as time-varying from the dynamic signals.

Task type	Signal features	Notations
Isometric	sample kurtosis of EMG	k_r and k_l
	crossing rate variable of EMG	cr_r and cr_l
	correlation dimension of EMG	$D_{2,r}$ and $D_{2,l}$
	recurrence rate of EMG	%REC$_r$ and %REC$_l$
	sample entropy of ACC	SampEn$_r$ and SampEn$_l$
	coherence between EMG and ACC	Coh$_r$ and Coh$_l$
Dynamic	recurrence rate of EMG	%REC$_r$ and %REC$_l$
	cross-recurrence rate of EMG	%REC$_{r,l}$
	wavelet variable of EMG	$W_{max,r}$ and $W_{max,l}$
	cross-wavelet variable of EMG	$W_{max,rl}$
	power of ACC	$P_{acc,r}$ and $P_{acc,l}$
	sample entropy of ACC	SampEn$_r$ and SampEn$_l$

Table 1. PD characteristic signal features and their notations. The subscripts r and l in the notations stand for the side of the body.

3.2.1. *Parameters of surface EMG signal morphology*

In [28], we used two parameters (k and cr) for measuring the peakedness of EMG signals. The sample kurtosis was calculated as the fourth centered moment of the time series x (length N):

$$k = \frac{\frac{1}{N}\sum_{i=1}^{N}(x_i - \mu_x)^4}{\sigma_x^4}, \tag{4}$$

where μ_x is the mean and σ_x the standard deviation (SD) of the sample values. Parameter k is higher for more peaked signals.

The parameter cr was calculated as the width/height of the CR expansion. The width of the CR expansion was defined at the level of 50 crossings/second and the height as the maximum value of the CR expansion. Parameter cr is lower for more peaked signals.

3.2.2. *EMG parameters of nonlinear dynamics*

In [28, 29], we used parameters of nonlinear dynamics (correlation dimension, recurrence rate and cross-recurrence rate) for analyzing the EMG signal complexity and recurring EMG patterns. In nonlinear dynamics, the original time series (EMG signal) x is used to form embedding vectors u_i

$$u_i = [x_i \; x_{i+\lambda} \; x_{i+2\lambda} \; \cdots \; x_{i+(m-1)\lambda}], \tag{5}$$

where λ is the delay parameter and m the embedding dimension [45]. The number of different embedding vectors is $N_m = N_e - (m-1)\lambda$ for each epoch (length N_e) of the time series x.

The correlation dimension [16] describes the complexity of the time series and it can be calculated from the embedding vectors as follows. First, the Euclidean distances between each pair of embedding vectors u_i and u_j in (5) are quantified as

$$d_e(u_i, u_j) = \sqrt{\sum_{k=0}^{m-1} |x_{i+k\lambda} - x_{j+k\lambda}|^2}. \tag{6}$$

The correlation sum is then calculated as

$$C^m(r) = \frac{1}{N_m^2} \sum_{i,j=1}^{N_m} \Theta(r - d_e(u_i, u_j)) \tag{7}$$

$$\Theta(s) = \begin{cases} 0, & s < 0 \\ 1, & s \geq 0, \end{cases}$$

where r is the threshold distance. The correlation dimension is formally defined as

$$D_2(m) = \lim_{r \to 0} \lim_{N_m \to \infty} \frac{\log C^m(r)}{\log r}. \tag{8}$$

Practically, D_2 is calculated as the slope of the regression curve in the log-log-representation.

Recurrence rate [53] measures the percentage of recurring patterns in the EMG signal. It can be calculated from the embedding vector distances in (6) as a percentage of distances that are below of the threshold distance r. The binary image, that contains a value 1 in the cells (i, j) where $d_e(u_i, u_j) < r$, is called the recurrence plot. The recurrence plots of one healthy subject and one PD patient are illustrated in Figure 4. One can observe that the recurrence plot of the patient contains more cells with the value 1 (white cells) than the recurrence plot of the healthy subject. It means that the EMG signal of the patient contains more recurring patterns than the EMG signal of the healthy subject. In the cross-recurrence rate, the embedding vectors in (5) are formed for two time series and the Euclidean distances in (6) are evaluated between the embedding vectors of the two different time series.

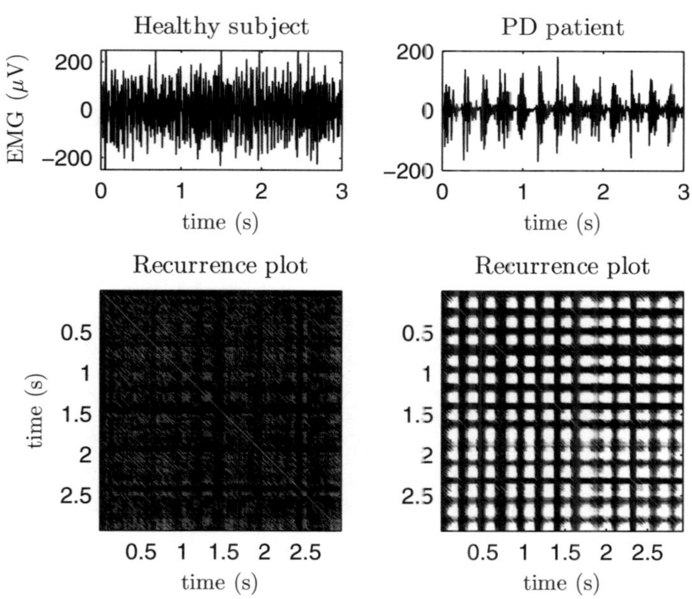

Figure 4. EMG signals and recurrence plots of one healthy subject and one PD patient.

3.2.3. Spectral-based parameters

In spectral analysis, the aim is to present the signal in the frequency-domain by estimating its power spectral density (PSD). The PSD estimation can be based on a Fourier transform or wavelet transform or on parametric modeling. In [28, 29], the Fourier- and wavelet-based approaches were used for analyzing the EMG and acceleration signals of PD patients and healthy subjects.

The coherence was used in [28] for quantifying similarities in the power spectra of the EMG and acceleration signals. It was calculated from the PSDs of the EMG and acceleration signals ($P_x(f)$ and $P_y(f)$) and from the cross-spectral density $P_{xy}(f)$, which were estimated by using the Welch's averaged periodogram method [54]. The magnitude-squared coherence is defined as

$$C_{xy}(f) = \frac{|P_{xy}(f)|^2}{P_x(f)P_y(f)} \tag{9}$$

and it gives values between 0 and 1. Variable Coh was calculated as the area of the coherence spectrum above a threshold value in the frequency range 0–50 Hz. The magnitude-squared coherence estimates of one healthy subject and one PD patient are presented in Figure 5. One can observe that the area of the coherence spectrum is larger for the PD patient than for the healthy subject.

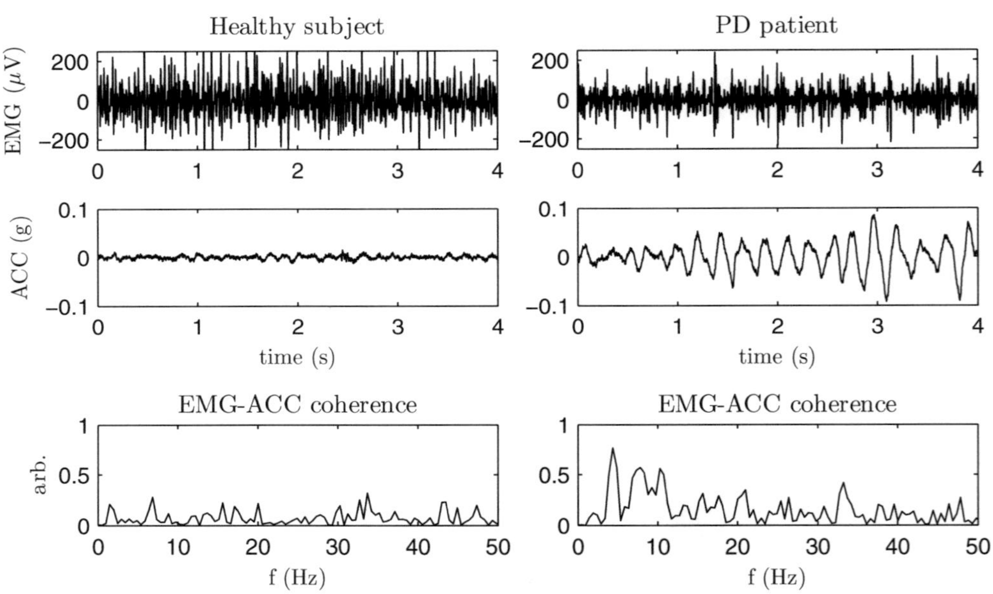

Figure 5. EMG and acceleration signals and magnitude-squared coherence estimates of one healthy subject and one PD patient.

While in Fourier approach the basis functions in the spectral decomposition are global functions, in wavelet approach [1] the functions are local. Therefore, the wavelet-based methods can be more effective than the Fourier-based method in detecting time varying features in the spectrum [10]. The basic idea in the wavelet transform is to decompose the signal into a set of basis functions, which are obtained by scaling and shifting the wavelet function $\psi(t)$. In continuous form, the wavelet transform of the signal $x(t)$ is defined as

$$W_x(a,b) = \frac{1}{\sqrt{a}} \int_{-\infty}^{\infty} x(t)\psi^* \left(\frac{t-b}{a}\right) dt, \tag{10}$$

where a is the scale, b is the shift, and $(\cdot)^*$ denotes the complex conjugate operator. Different kinds of wavelet functions have been defined for analysis. For discrete signals one must use discrete wavelets. The magnitude-squared wavelet transform is called the scalogram

$$P_x^W(a,b) = |W_x(a,b)W_x^*(a,b)|. \tag{11}$$

If the wavelet transforms of two signals x and y are denoted with $W_x(a,b)$ and $W_y(a,b)$, the wavelet cross-scalogram is defined as

$$P_{xy}^W(a,b) = |W_x(a,b)W_y^*(a,b)|. \tag{12}$$

In [29], the discrete Morlet wavelet was used for analysis as in many other EMG studies [10, 20, 40]. The scalograms (11) were calculated from the EMG signals of both sides of the body and the cross-scalogram (12) between the right and left side signals. The scalograms and cross-scalograms were scaled to present the percentage of energy for each wavelet coefficient as a function of time. The wavelet parameter W_{max} was calculated as the maximum energy of all wavelet coefficients from both the scalograms and the cross-scalograms as a function of time. The wavelet cross-scalograms and parameters $W_{\text{max,rl}}$ are presented for one healthy subject and one PD patient in Figure 6. One can observe that in the wavelet cross-scalogram of the patient the energy is more spread into different wavelet coefficients than in the cross-scalogram of the healthy subject. Parameter $W_{\text{max,rl}}$ is lower for the patient.

3.2.4. **Acceleration signal features**

Sample entropy is a parameter of nonlinear dynamics and it can be used for quantifying the regularity of acceleration signals in PD when compared to the healthy subjects. It was calculated in [28, 29] from the embedding vectors in (5) as described in [27]. In [29], the power of the acceleration signal was extracted from the dynamic acceleration recordings for quantifying kinetic tremor and rigidity during movement.

3.3. Cluster analysis of subjects

The aim in [28, 29] was to develop a method for discriminating between PD patients and healthy subjects on the basis of EMG and accelerations signal features. In total, the data from 42 PD patients and 59 healthy subjects were analyzed in [28] and the data from 49 PD patients and 59 healthy subjects were analyzed in [29].

In [28, 29], there were many parameters that could capture essential information in the measured signals. These original signal features p_j ($j = 1, 2, ..., N_p$) (detailed in Table 1) were used to form feature vectors $z_j \in \mathbb{R}^{N_p}$ for each subject.

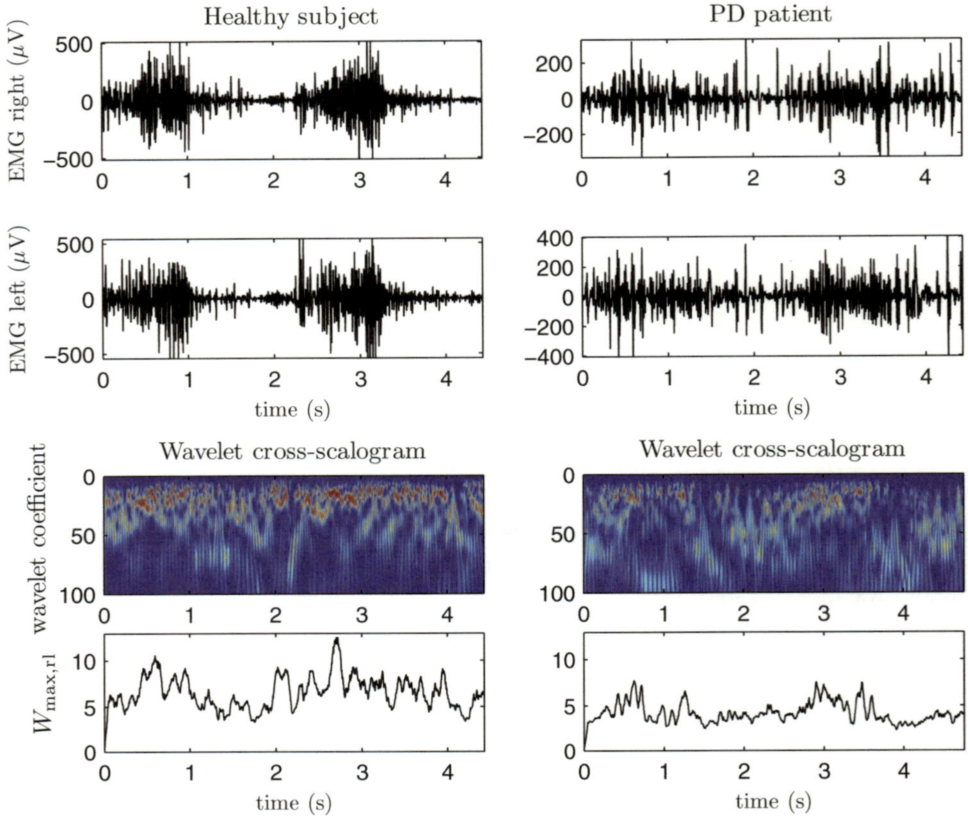

Figure 6. Right and left side EMG signals of one healthy subject and one PD patient. Wavelet cross-scalograms and $W_{max,rl}$ parameters for the healthy subject and the PD patient.

$$z_j = [p_1 \, p_2 \ldots p_{N_p}]^T \tag{13}$$

The PC-based approach [19] was used in both studies for reducing the number signal features and for transforming the original possibly correlated parameters into uncorrelated parameters.

In [28], one feature vector was formed for each healthy subject, for each patient with medication on (MED on) and for 13 patients also with medication off (MED off, no medication 24 hours before the measurement) by using the twelve EMG and acceleration parameters (six parameters from each body side) that are detailed in Table 1. The original signal parameters were normalized (to zero mean and unit SD of all subjects) before applying the PC approach. The PC approach was applied once as described in section 2.2. In [29], two feature vectors were formed for each patient and for each healthy subject of the ten EMG and acceleration parameters that are detailed in Table 1. One of the feature vectors was formed by using the mean parameter values during flexion and the other by using the mean parameter values during extension. The signal variables were normalized and the PC approach was applied separately for the flexion and extension phases of the movement as described in section 2.2.

Cluster analysis was used in [28, 29] for grouping subjects with similar EMG and acceleration signal features into groups. This could be done by clustering the model weights (PCs) in the sum (1). An iterative k-means algorithm [47] was used for clustering the feature vectors of subjects in a two-dimensional feature space. In k-means algorithm, the only parameter given to the algorithm is the number of clusters. The algorithm begins by choosing initial estimates for each cluster center point. In each iteration step, it is determined to which cluster the feature vectors belong. The feature vector belongs to that cluster for which the squared Euclidean distance between the vector and the cluster center point in the two-dimensional feature space is minimized. The cluster center points are updated to be the mean of the feature vectors in each cluster in the two-dimensional feature space. The iteration continues until the sum of vector-to-center point distances summed over all clusters is minimized.

The validation of the clustering results was performed by using the leave-one-out method. In the method, the eigenvectors and PCs are solved for each combination of $M - 1$ feature vectors, where M means the total number of feature vectors. That is, one feature vector is left out of the group each time the eigenvectors and PCs are computed. The clustering is then performed for each combination of $M - 1$ feature vectors, and in each case, it is tested to which cluster the feature vector that was left out belongs. In [28, 29], the correct ratings of clustering were defined as the percentage (mean$\pm$SD values) of healthy subjects that belong to the healthy subject cluster and the percentage of patients that belong to the patient clusters.

3.4. Discrimination results

In [28], twelve features were extracted from the isometric EMG and acceleration signals of 59 healthy subjects and 42 PD patients. The normalized signal features (mean$\pm$SD values) for the healthy subject group and for the PD patient group are presented in Figure 7. The results show that the parameters SampEn, cr and D_2 seem to be lower and the parameters k, Coh and %REC higher for the patients than for the healthy subjects. That is, the EMGs of the patients tend to be less complex and contain more recurring patterns than the EMGs of the healthy subjects. The acceleration signals of the patients tend to be more regular and more coherent with the EMGs than the acceleration signals of the healthy subjects.

The cluster analysis of subjects was performed in a two-dimensional feature space, that was spanned by the PC sum $\theta_j(2) + \theta_j(5)$ and the first PC $\theta_j(1)$ by using the k-means algorithm. This PC sum was used, because it works better in discrimination than the single PCs. The results in Figure 7 show that 90 % of the healthy subjects belong to the cluster O_1 and 76 % of the patients in two other clusters O_2 and O_3. Seven patients with severe motor symptoms are distinguished in O_3. The ten patients in the healthy subject cluster O_1 have only little or no tremor at all in their hands. The validation by using the leave-one-out method resulted in correct discrimination rates of 90 $\pm$ 1 % for the healthy subjects and 74 $\pm$ 6 % for the patients.

In [29], ten features were extracted from the EMG and acceleration signals of 59 healthy subjects and 49 PD patients and used to form feature vectors for subjects. The normalized signal features (mean$\pm$SD values) for the healthy subject group and for the PD patient group

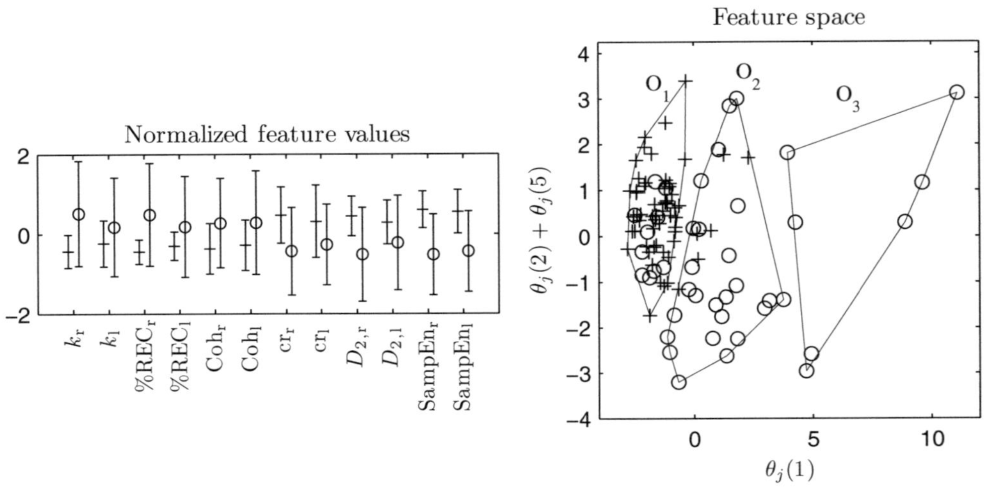

Figure 7. Mean ± SD values of normalized signal features for the patient group (○) and for the healthy subject group (+) (left). The cluster analysis of 42 PD patients (○) and 59 healthy subjects (+) in the feature space ($\theta_j(2)$+$\theta_j(5)$ with respect to $\theta_j(1)$). The three clusters O_1, O_2 and O_3.

in flexion and in extension are presented in Figure 8. The results show that parameters %REC and P_{acc} tend to be higher and parameters SampEn and W_{max} lower for patients than for healthy subjects both in flexion and in extension. That is, the EMGs of the patients tend to contain more recurring patterns than the EMGs of the healthy subjects and the EMG wavelet power tends to be more spread for patients. The acceleration signals of the patients tend to be of higher amplitude and more regular than the acceleration signals of the healthy subjects.

The cluster analysis of subjects was performed in a two-dimensional feature space that was spanned by the second PC and the first PC by using the k-means algorithm. The results are presented in Figure 8. According to the results, the method can discriminate 80 ± 1 % of the patient extension movements from 87 ± 1 % of the extension movements of healthy subjects, and 73 ± 1 % of the patient flexion movements from 82 ± 1 % of the flexion movements of healthy subjects. The leave-one-out method was used for validation. The patients, that could not be discriminated from the healthy subjects, had mild motor symptoms of PD.

4. PC-based approaches for quantifying effects of treatment

In addition to the discrimination analysis between subjects, the principal component -based approach can be used for quantifying the effects of treatment. In [30, 31], we aimed to develop objective methods for quantifying effects of PD treatment (DBS and medication) on the basis of surface EMG and acceleration measurements and analysis.

4.1. EMG and acceleration measurements for quantifying effects of treatment

In [30], the PC-based approach was used for quantifying the effects of DBS treatment on the basis of a set of EMG and acceleration signal features. In total, the measurement data from 13 PD patients with DBS and 13 healthy subjects were analyzed. Measurements were performed

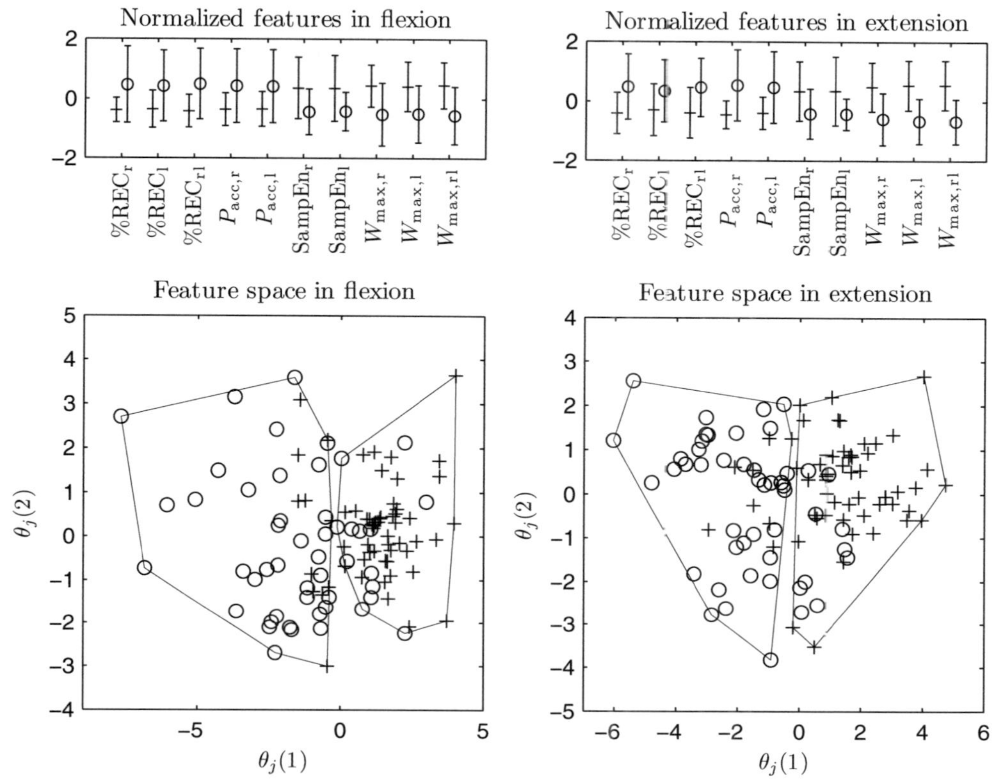

Figure 8. Mean ± SD values of normalized signal features for the patient group (∘) and for the healthy subject group (+) in flexion and in extension (top). The cluster analysis of 49 PD patients (∘) and 59 healthy subjects (+) in the feature space ($\theta_j(2)$ with respect to $\theta_j(1)$).

during the isometric contraction of BB muscles (see section 3.1) and they were performed once for the healthy subjects and twice for the patients: with DBS on (stimulator was turned on) and with DBS off (stimulator was turned off). Ninth order Butterworth low-pass filter with 110 Hz cutoff was used for removing the DBS artifact from the EMG signals. The low-pass filtering was performed similarly for all subjects (patients and healthy subjects). The UPDRS -motor examination was performed for each patient with DBS on and with DBS off. The measured signals of one PD patient with DBS on and off are presented in Figure 9. One can observe that the EMG signal of the patient contains recurring EMG bursts and the acceleration signal high-amplitude tremor with DBS off but not with DBS on.

In [31], the PC-based approach was used for quantifying the effects of anti-parkinsonian medication on the basis of a set of EMG and acceleration signal features. In total, the measurement data from nine PD patients were analyzed. The subjects were measured in four different medication conditions: off-medication, and two and three and four hours after taking the medication. The isometric task (described in section 3.1) was analyzed. The UPDRS -motor examination was performed for each patient in each medication condition. The EMG and acceleration signals of one PD patient in each medication condition are presented in Figure

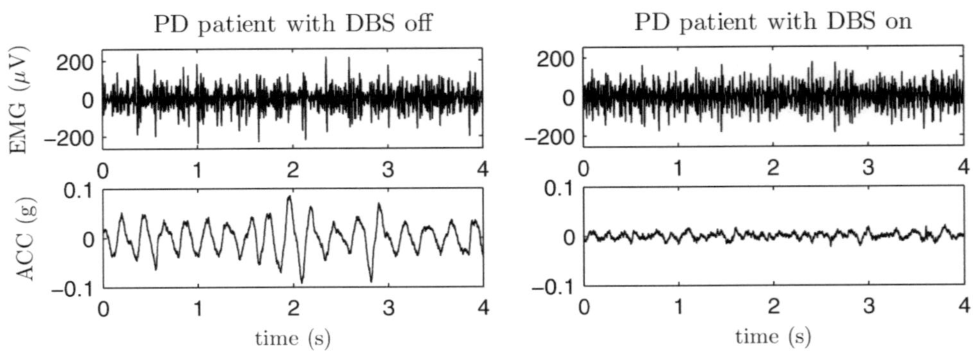

Figure 9. The EMG and acceleration signals of one PD patient with DBS on and with DBS off.

10. It is observed that the number of recurring EMG bursts and the amplitude of tremor decrease with medication and start to increase three hours after taking the medication.

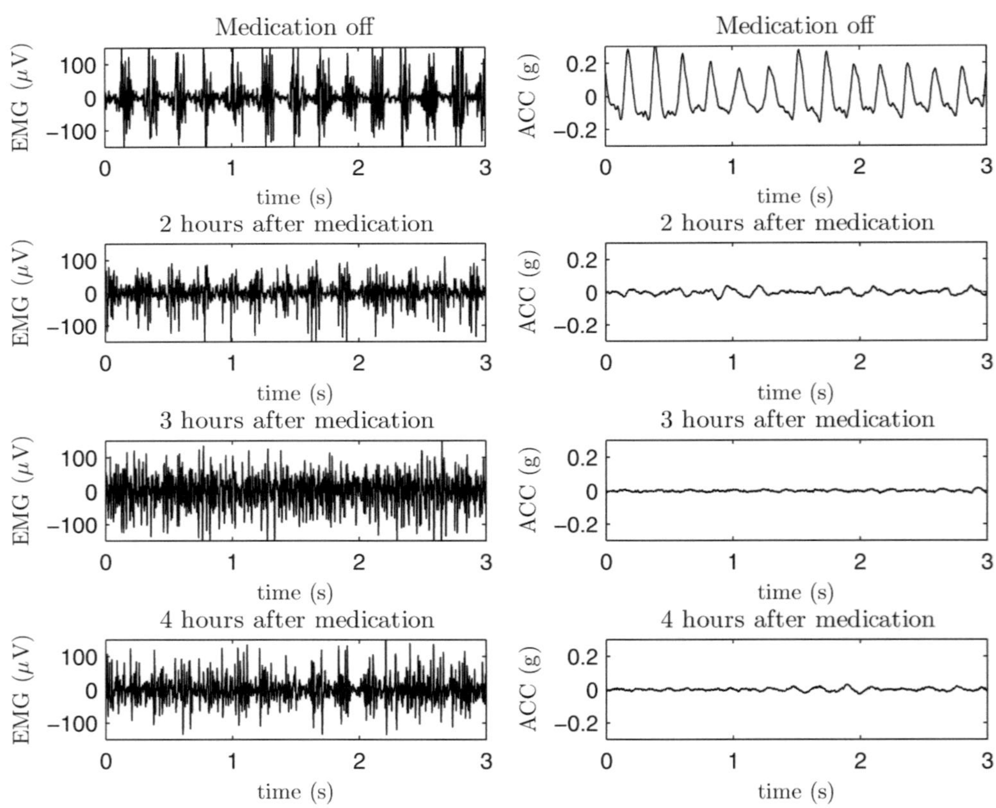

Figure 10. The EMG and acceleration signals of one PD patient in four medication conditions: with medication off, and two and three and four hours after taking the medication.

4.2. EMG and acceleration signal features for characterizing effects of treatment

Several EMG and acceleration signal features were observed to be effective in characterizing the effects of treatment on PD patients in [30, 31]. These features are detailed in Table 2.

Treatment	Signal features	Notations
DBS	correlation dimension of EMG	$D_{2,r}$ and $D_{2,l}$
	recurrence rate of EMG	$\%REC_r$ and $\%REC_l$
	root mean square amplitude of ACC	RMS_r and RMS_l
	sample entropy of ACC	$SampEn_r$ and $SampEn_l$
	coherence between EMG and ACC	Coh_r and Coh_l
Medication	sample kurtosis of EMG	k_r and k_l
	recurrence rate of EMG	$\%REC_r$ and $\%REC_l$
	root mean square amplitude of ACC	RMS_r and RMS_l
	sample entropy of ACC	$SampEn_r$ and $SampEn_l$

Table 2. PD characteristic signal features for quantifying effects of treatment. The subscripts r and l in the notations stand for the side of the body.

The parameters were calculated as described in section 3.2. The root mean square amplitude of acceleration was calculated for quantifying tremor amplitude.

4.3. Principal components in quantifying the effects of treatment

In [30], the ten signal features (five features from each body side) in Table 2 were normalized (to zero mean and unit SD of healthy subjects) and used to form feature vectors for subjects. One feature vector was formed for each healthy subject and two feature vectors for each patient: one with DBS on and one with DBS off. The PC approach (see section 2.2) was applied once. The eigenvectors were solved by using the feature vectors of healthy subjects. In this way, the healthy subject group formed the normal group for later comparison.

In [31], the eight signal parameters in Table 2 were normalized (to zero mean and unit SD of all patients) and used to form feature vectors for PD patients. Four feature vectors were formed for each patient (one feature vector in each medication condition). The PC approach (see section 2.2) was applied once.

4.4. Results

In [30], the group mean values of the parameters D_2 and SampEn increased and the group mean values of the parameters %REC, RMS and Coh decreased with DBS for the patient group. However, the SDs of the parameters were very high for the patient group because of its heterogeneity. Therefore, the patient measurements were studied individually. The first and the third PCs worked best in characterizing effects of DBS and differences between patients and healthy subjects. According to the results in Figure 11, 12 out of 13 patients are closer to the center point of healthy subjects with DBS on than with DBS off in the two-dimensional feature space ($\theta_3(j)$ with respect to $\theta_1(j)$). That is, the EMG and acceleration signals of PD patients are more similar with the signals of the healthy subjects with DBS on than with DBS off. The distances of the patients from the center of healthy subjects and the clinical UPDRS -motor scores are highly individual (see Table 3). It was observed in a more detailed analysis that the method is most sensitive to PD with associated tremor. In Figure 11, one patient is farther from the healthy subjects with DBS on than with DBS off. This patient has higher tremor (acceleration signal) amplitude and regularity and less complex EMG recordings (higher %REC and lower D_2) with DBS on than with DBS off. For that patient, the measurement results contradict the subjective clinical scores.

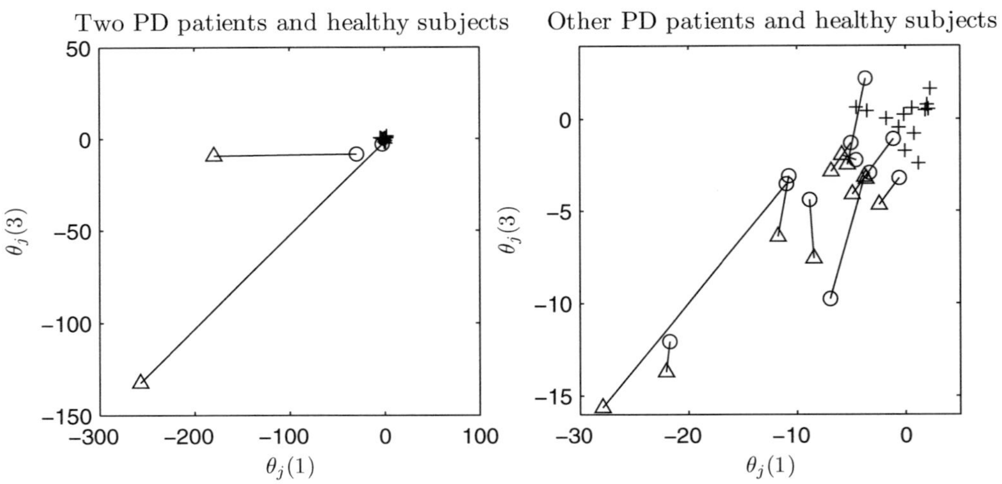

Figure 11. The third PCs $\theta_j(3)$ with respect to the first PCs $\theta_j(1)$ of 13 healthy subjects (+) and 13 PD patients with DBS on (○) and off (△). The patients are divided into two figures, but the healthy subjects are the same in both figures. The DBS on- and off-states of each patient are connected with a line.

In [31], the first PC worked best in characterizing the effects of medication. The first PCs and the total UPDRS -motor scores in each medication condition for each patient are presented in Figure 12. One can observe that the total UPDRS -motor scores decrease (motor symptoms are relieved) with medication for all patients. Correspondingly the first PCs decrease with medication for eight out of nine patients. By examining the first eigenvector in Figure 12 one can realize that the reduction in the first PC indicates reduction in the parameters k (less spiky EMG), %REC (less recurring patterns) and RMS (lower tremor amplitude), and increase in the parameter SampEn (more complex tremor). The severity of motor symptoms (UPDRS -motor score) starts to increase 2–3 hours after medication for all patients, which indicates that the efficacy of medication starts to weaken 2–3 hours after medication. Correspondingly, the first PCs start to increase 2–3 hours after medication for seven out of nine patients. The UPDRS -motor scores and the first PCs do not start to increase at the same time for all patients, which indicates that these scores do not measure exactly the same thing.

5. Discussion

There is a need for finding objective methods for Parkinson's disease for improving the diagnostic accuracy, for enabling earlier diagnosis, and for quantifying the disease progression and the efficacy of treatment [2, 11, 24]. Surface EMG and the kinematic measurements may be potentially useful methods for quantifying the motor impairment in PD and the effects of

Patient no.	UPDRS off	UPDRS on	Distance off	Distance on
1	56	43	26	25
2	64	48	32	12
3	59	40	7	5
4	34	14	180	30
5	71	42	289	4
6	38	31	5	12
7	47	28	6	2
8	57	33	6	4
9	43	34	13	11
10	43	24	11	10
11	44	30	6	5
12	62	38	5	4
13	43	30	5	3

Table 3. Total UPDRS -motor scores and the distances from the center of healthy subjects with DBS on and off.

treatment. However, the EMG signals of PD patients are characterized by spikes and bursts that are not effectively captured with conventional amplitude- and spectral-based parameters of EMG. Therefore, more novel methods of EMG analysis are needed for PD.

5.1. Discrimination between patients and healthy subjects

We have developed methods for discriminating between PD patients and healthy subjects on the basis of surface EMG and kinematic measurements and analysis in [28, 29, 32]. One developed approach was based on analyzing the surface EMG signal morphology [32]. One approach was based on analyzing isometric [28] and one approach on analyzing dynamic muscle contractions [29]. Principal components were used in each approach for discrimination between subjects. All methods were tested with the measured data. The obtained discrimination rates were 72 % for patients and 86 % for healthy subjects on the basis of surface EMG signal morphology, 76 % for patients and 90 % for healthy subjects on the basis of isometric EMG and acceleration recordings, 73 % for patients and 82 % for healthy subjects on the basis of elbow flexion movements, and 80 % for patients and 87 % for healthy subjects on the basis of elbow extension movements. These percentages predict the sensitivities and specificities of the methods in the subject groups that were studied.

The best discrimination rates between patients and healthy subjects were obtained by analyzing the EMG and acceleration signals measured during the isometric contraction and elbow extension movements [28, 29]. In fact, it has been observed previously, that the elbow extension movements are more impaired than the flexion movements of PD patients [33]. The isometric approach was most sensitive to patients with associated tremor [28] and the dynamic approach to patients with various motor symptoms (rigidity, bradykinesia and tremor) and

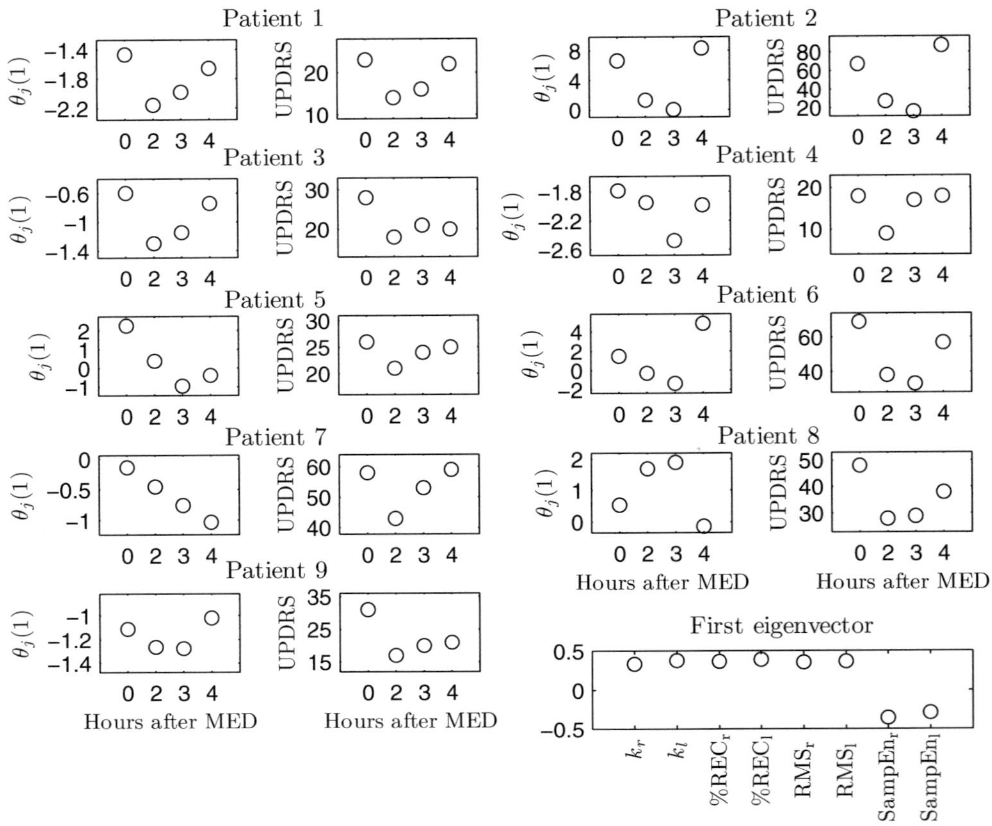

Figure 12. The first PCs ($\theta_j(1)$) and UPDRS -motor scores of nine PD patients with medication off, and two and three and hour hours after taking the medication. The first eigenvector (bottom right).

especially to patients with problems in performing movement tasks [29]. Therefore, the analysis of both kind of muscle contractions is essential when quantifying motor impairment in PD.

5.2. Quantification of the effects of treatment

In studies [30, 31], we developed methods for quantifying the effects of treatment in PD on the basis of surface EMG and kinematic measurements and analysis. The results of the study [30] show that the measured EMG and acceleration signals of 12 out of 13 PD patients were more similar with the signals of the healthy subjects with DBS on than with DBS off. This result indicates that it is possible to detect DBS-induced improvements in the neuromuscular and motor function of PD patients by using the developed analysis approach.

In [31], the EMG signals of eight out of nine PD patients changed into less spiky and the acceleration recordings into more complex after taking the medication. A reverse phenomenon in the signal characteristics was observed 3–4 hours after taking the medication for seven out of nine patients. This result indicates that it is possible to detect medication-induced changes in the neuromuscular and motor function of PD patients by using the developed methods.

5.3. Methods of signal analysis

We extracted a large number of features from the EMG and acceleration signals of PD patients and healthy subjects in [28–32] and chose the most effective features for characterizing PD and the effects of treatment into the feature vectors for deeper analysis. The chosen EMG features were not conventional EMG parameters but they were based on nonlinear dynamics, signal morphology, wavelets and EMG-acceleration coherence. Previously, there have been only one [14] or few other studies, in which a method of nonlinear dynamics has been used for studying EMGs of PD patients. Our studies [30, 31] are the only studies that have analyzed the effects of PD treatment (DBS and medication) by using methods of nonlinear dynamics for EMG.

All of the studies [28–32] were based on an innovative way of combining the PC-based approach with the selection of feature vectors instead of analyzing the statistics of single signal parameters. The PC-based approach provided a better discrimination between the subjects by capturing essential information in the combination of variables. With the PC-based approach, it was possible to examine the effects of treatment in a feature space on an individual level.

Few things about signal quality and electrode placement should be kept in mind when analyzing the EMG signals with the proposed analysis methods. First, the EMG signal amplitude is relatively low and the signal is sensitive to noise that is coming from other electrical sources. This noise may affect the calculated signal parameters. Therefore, the noise should be eliminated already during the measurements whenever it is possible. Another thing is that sometimes a large MU is firing constantly and dominantly in the proximity of the recording electrode causing recurring impulse-like patterns into the EMG signal. In that case, a better placement of recording electrodes would be advisable.

In PD patients with DBS, the stimulator causes artifacts into the EMG signal. The DBS artifact and its filtering may affect the calculated signal parameters. Previously, the DBS artifact has been removed from the EMG signal by low-pass filtering the rectified signal with a low (20–60 Hz) cut-off frequency [21, 41, 42, 51, 52]. In our study [30], we low-pass filtered the EMG signal with the 110 Hz cut-off frequency. Our aim was to remove the DBS artifact from the EMG as effectively as possible without removing important information and to perform the filtering in the same way for all subjects in order to get comparable results.

5.4. Conclusions

In this chapter, we presented several approaches for feature extraction from surface EMG and acceleration signals and for discrimination between PD patients and healthy subjects on the basis of the extracted signal features. The presented discrimination approaches were developed in our studies [28, 29, 32]. By using the developed approaches, we could discriminate 72-80 % of PD patients from 82-90 % of healthy subjects depending on the analyzed signal features and the muscle contraction type. These percentages can be regarded as promising because it is known that the PD diagnostics can be difficult. Clinicopathological studies from the UK and Canada have shown that the disease is diagnosed incorrectly in about 25 % of cases [48]. On the basis of our discrimination results, further research and clinical studies are suggested for evaluating the sensitivity of the developed approaches in patients with different types of PD and in patients with early stages of PD. In addition, the ability of EMG and acceleration signal features in discriminating between PD patients and other patients with similar symptoms should be studied.

In this chapter, we presented two approaches for quantifying the effects of PD treatment (medication and DBS) on the basis of the extracted EMG and acceleration signal features. The presented approaches were developed in our studies [30, 31]. By using the developed approaches, we could detect DBS- and medication-induced improvements in the neuromuscular and motor function of PD patients. This result is encouraging because the widely used method for evaluating the efficacy of PD treatment is subjective. However, the sensitivity of the developed approaches should be quantified with a larger number of PD patients.

The need for finding objective methods for PD diagnosis and for quantifying the disease progression and the efficacy of treatment is well known [2, 11, 24]. We hope that our results [28–32] can help in creating a practical method for quantifying motor impairment in PD and the effects of treatment on individual PD patients. However, in order to be more sensitive than the traditional methods, it is probable that a combination of several objective methods will be needed for PD.

5.5. Future directions

There is currently a lot of effort for determining objective methods and characteristics for PD [2, 11, 24]. One important goal of current research is to determine criteria for the pre-motor and pre-clinical phases of PD [39]. In surface EMG studies, the sensitivity of surface EMG signal features in detecting PD patients before the actual diagnosis of PD should be studied. It will be important to analyze differences in the signal characteristics between PD patients and other patients with similar symptoms. These other similar diseases form currently a significant reason for the wrong diagnosis of PD [17]. It has been observed that surface EMG and kinematic measurements can provide information about the effects of PD treatments (medication and DBS). The ability of these measurements in helping the optimal adjustment of these treatments should be evaluated.

Acknowledgments

This work was supported by the Academy of Finland under Project 252748.

Author details

Rissanen Saara M., Tarvainen Mika P. and Karjalainen Pasi A.
Department of Applied Physics, University of Eastern Finland, Kuopio, Finland

Kankaanpää Markku
Department of Physical and Rehabilitation Medicine, Tampere University Hospital, Tampere, Finland

6. References

[1] Akay, M. [1998]. *Time frequency and wavelets in biomedical signal processing*, IEEE Press series in biomedical engineering, IEEE Press, New York.

[2] Antoniades, C. & Barker, R. [2008]. The search for biomarkers in Parkinson's disease: a critical review, *Expert Rev. Neurother.* 8(12): 1841–1852.

[3] Bastian, A., Kelly, V., Revilla, F., Perlmutter, J. & Mink, J. [2003]. Different effects of unilateral versus bilateral subthalamic nucleus stimulation on walking and reaching in Parkinson's disease, *Mov. Disord.* 18(9): 1000–1007.

[4] Blahak, C., Wöhrle, J., Capelle, H.-H., Bäzner, H., Grips, E., Weigel, R., Hennerici, M. & Krauss, J. [2007]. Tremor reduction by subthalamic nucleus stimulation and medication in advanced Parkinson's disease, *J. Neurol.* 254(2): 169–178.

[5] Carpinella, I., Crenna, P., Calabrese, E., Rabuffetti, M., Mazzoleni, P., Nemni, R. & Ferrarin, M. [2007]. Locomotor function in the early stage of Parkinson's disease, *IEEE Trans. Neural. Syst. Rehabil. Eng.* 15(4): 543–551.

[6] Carpinella, I., Crenna, P., Marzegan, A., Rabuffetti, M., Rizzone, M., Lopiano, L. & Ferrarin [2007]. Effect of l-dopa and subthalamic nucleus stimulation on arm and leg swing during gait in Parkinson's disease, *Conf. Proc. IEEE Eng. Med. Biol. Soc.*, pp. 6665–6668.

[7] Chastan, N., Westby, G., Yelnik, J., Bardinet, E., Do, M., Agid, Y. & Welter, M. [2009]. Effects of nigral stimulation on locomotion and postural stability in patients with Parkinson's disease, *Brain* 132(1): 172–184.

[8] Dafotakis, M., Fink, G., Allert, N. & Nowak, D. [2008]. The impact of subthalamic deep brain stimulation on bradykinesia of proximal and distal upper limb muscles in Parkinson's disease, *J. Neurol.* 255(3): 429–437.

[9] de Lau, L. & Breteler, M. [2006]. Epidemiology of Parkinson's disease, *Lancet Neurol.* 5(6): 525–535.

[10] de Michele, G., Sello, S., Carboncini, M., Rossi, B. & Strambi, S.-K. [2003]. Cross-correlation time-frequency analysis for multiple EMG signals in Parkinson's disease: a wavelet approach, *Med. Eng. Phys.* 25(5): 361–369.

[11] Dorsey, E., Holloway, R. & Ravina, B. [2008]. Status of biological markers, *in* S. Factor & W. Weiner (eds), *Parkinson's disease: diagnosis and clinical management (2nd Edition)*, Demos Medical Publishing, Inc., New York, chapter 24, pp. 277–284.

[12] Fahn, S. & Elton, R. [1987]. The Unified Parkinson's disease rating scale, *in* S. Fahn, C. Marsden, D. Calne & M. Goldstein (eds), *Recent developments in Parkinson's disease*, Macmillan Healthcare Information, Florham Park, N.J., pp. 153–63.

[13] Farley, B., Sherman, S. & Koshland, G. [2004]. Shoulder muscle activity in Parkinson's disease during multijoint arm movements across a range of speeds, *Exp. Brain Res.* 154(2): 160–175.

[14] Fattorini, L., Felici, F., Filligoi, G., Traballesi, M. & Farina, D. [2005]. Influence of high motor unit synchronization levels on non-linear and spectral variables of the surface EMG, *J. Neurosci. Methods* 143(2): 133–139.

[15] Gancher, S. [2008]. Clinical rating scales, *in* S. Factor & W. Weiner (eds), *Parkinson's disease: diagnosis and clinical management (2nd Edition)*, Demos Medical Publishing, Inc., New York, chapter 14, pp. 135–143.

[16] Grassberger, P. & Procaccia, I. [1983]. Characterization of strange attractors, *Phys. Rev. Lett.* 50(5): 346–349.

[17] Grosset, D., Grosset, K., Okun, M. & Fernandez, H. [2009]. *Parkinson's disease - Clinician's desk reference*, Manson Publishing Ltd., London.

[18] Jankovic, J. [2008]. Parkinson's disease: clinical features and diagnosis, *J. Neurol. Neurosurg. Psychiatry* 79(4): 368–376.

[19] Jolliffe, I. [2002]. *Principal Component Analysis*, Springer-Verlag, New York.

[20] Karlsson, S., Yu, J. & Akay, M. [2000]. Time-frequency analysis of myoelectric signals during dynamic contractions: A comparative study, *IEEE Trans. Biomed. Eng.* 47(2): 228–238.

[21] Levin, J., Krafczyk, S., Valkovič, P., Eggert, T., Claassen, J. & Bötzel, K. [2009]. Objective measurement of muscle rigidity in parkinsonian patients treated with subthalamic stimulation, *Mov. Disord.* 24(1): 57–63.

[22] Marek, K., Jennings, D., Tamagnan, G. & Seibyl, J. [2008]. Biomarkers for Parkinson's disease: tools to assess Parkinson's disease onset and progression, *Ann. Neurol.* 64 (suppl. 2): S111–S121.

[23] Meigal, A., Rissanen, S., Tarvainen, M., Karjalainen, P., Iudina-Vassel, I., Airaksinen, O. & Kankaanpää, M. [2009]. Novel parameters of surface EMG in patients with Parkinson's disease and healthy young and old controls, *J. Electromyogr. Kinesiol.* 19(3): e206–e213.

[24] Morgan, J., Mehta, S. & Sethi, K. [2010]. Biomarkers in Parkinson's disease, *Curr. Neurol. Neurosci. Rep.* 10(6): 423–430.

[25] Park, H., Kim, J., Paek, S., Jeon, B., Lee, J. & Chung, C. [2009]. Cortico-muscular coherence increases with tremor improvement after deep brain stimulation in Parkinson's disease, *Neuroreport* 20(16): 1444–1449.

[26] Pfann, K., Buchman, A., Comella, C. & Corcos, D. [2001]. Control of movement distance in Parkinson's disease, *Mov. Disord.* 16(6): 1048–1065.

[27] Richman, J. & Moorman, J. [2000]. Physiological time-series analysis using approximate entropy and sample entropy, *Am. J. Physiol. Heart Circ. Physiol.* 278(6): H2039–H2049.

[28] Rissanen, S., Kankaanpää, M., Meigal, A., Tarvainen, M., Nuutinen, J., Tarkka, I., Airaksinen, O. & Karjalainen, P. [2008]. Surface EMG and acceleration signals in Parkinson's disease: feature extraction and cluster analysis, *Med. Biol. Eng. Comput.* 46(9): 849–858.

[29] Rissanen, S., Kankaanpää, M., Tarvainen, M., Meigal, A., Nuutinen, J., Tarkka, I., Airaksinen, O. & Karjalainen, P. [2009]. Analysis of dynamic voluntary muscle contractions in Parkinson's disease, *IEEE Trans. Biomed. Eng.* 56(9): 2280–2288.

[30] Rissanen, S., Kankaanpää, M., Tarvainen, M., Novak, V., Novak, P., Hu, K., Manor, B., Airaksinen, O. & Karjalainen, P. [2011]. Analysis of EMG and acceleration signals for quantifying the effects of deep brain stimulation in Parkinson's disease, *IEEE Trans. Biomed. Eng.* 58(9): 2545–2553.

[31] Rissanen, S., Kankaanpää, M., Tarvainen, M., Nuutinen, J., Airaksinen, O. & Karjalainen, P. [2011]. EMG and acceleration signal analysis for quantifying the effects of medication in Parkinson's disease, *Conf. Proc. IEEE Eng. Med. Biol. Soc.*, pp. 7496–7499.

[32] Rissanen, S., Kankaanpää, M., Tarvainen, M., Nuutinen, J., Tarkka, I., Airaksinen, O. & Karjalainen, P. [2007]. Analysis of surface EMG signal morphology in Parkinson's disease, *Physiol. Meas.* 28(12): 1507–1521.

[33] Robichaud, J., Pfann, K., Comella, C., Brandabur, M. & Corcos, D. [2004]. Greater impairment of extension movements as compared to flexion movements in Parkinson's disease, *Exp. Brain Res.* 156(2): 240–254.

[34] Robichaud, J., Pfann, K., Comella, C. & Corcos, D. [2002]. Effect of medication on EMG patterns in individuals with Parkinson's disease, *Mov. Disord.* 17(5): 950–960.

[35] Robichaud, J., Pfann, K., Leurgans, S., Vaillancourt, D., Comella, C. & Corcos, D. [2009]. Variability of EMG patterns: a potential neurophysiological marker of Parkinson's disease, *Clin. Neurophysiol.* 120(2): 390–397.

[36] Roiz, R., Cacho, E., Pazinatto, M., Reis, J., Cliquet, A. & Barasnevicius-Quagliato, E. [2010]. Gait analysis comparing Parkinson's disease with healthy elderly subjects., *Arq. Neuropsiquiatr.* 68(1): 81–86.

[37] Salenius, S., Avikainen, S., Kaakkola, S., Hari, R. & Brown, P. [2002]. Defective cortical drive to muscle in Parkinson's disease and its improvement with levodopa, *Brain* 125(3): 491–500.

[38] Savica, R., Rocca, W. & Ahlskog, J. [2010]. When does Parkinson disease start?, *Arch. Neurol.* 67(7): 798–801.

[39] Stern, M., Lang, A. & Poewe, W. [2012]. Toward a redefinition of Parkinson's disease?, *Mov. Disord.* 27(1): 54–60.

[40] Strambi, S., Rossi, B., de Michele, G. & Sello, S. [2004]. Effect of medication in Parkinson's disease: a wavelet analysis of EMG signals, *Med. Eng. Phys.* 26(4): 279–290.

[41] Sturman, M., Vaillancourt, D., Metman, L., Bakay, R. & Corcos, D. [2004]. Effects of subthalamic nucleus stimulation and medication on resting and postural tremor in Parkinson's disease, *Brain* 127(9): 2131–2143.

[42] Sturman, M., Vaillancourt, D., Metman, L., Sierens, D., Bakay, R. & Corcos, D. [2007]. Deep brain stimulation and medication for parkinsonian tremor during secondary tasks, *Mov. Disord.* 22(8): 1157–1163.

[43] Svehlík, M., Zwick, E., Steinwender, G., Linhart, W., Schwingenschuh, P., Katschnig, P., Ott, E. & Enzinger, C. [2009]. Gait analysis in patients with Parkinson's disease off dopaminergic therapy, *Arch. Phys. Med. Rehabil.* 90(11): 1880–1886.

[44] Tabbal, S., Ushe, M., Mink, J., Revilla, F., Wernle, A., Hong, M., Karimi, M. & Perlmutter, J. [2008]. Unilateral subthalamic nucleus stimulation has a measurable ipsilateral effect on rigidity and bradykinesia in Parkinson disease, *Exp. Neurol.* 211(1): 234–242.

[45] Takens, F. [1981]. Detecting strange attractors in turbulence, *in* D. Rand & L.-S. Young (eds), *Dynamical Systems and Turbulence, Warwick 1980*, Vol. 898 of *Lecture Notes in Mathematics*, Springer Berlin / Heidelberg, pp. 366–381.

[46] Tarvainen, M., Ranta-aho, P. & Karjalainen, P. [2002]. An advanced detrending method with application to HRV analysis, *IEEE Trans. Biomed. Eng.* 49(2): 172–175.

[47] Theodoridis, S. & Koutroumbas, K. [2006]. *Pattern recognition*, Elsevier/Academic Press, USA.

[48] Tolosa, E., Wenning, G. & Poewe, W. [2006]. The diagnosis of Parkinson's disease, *Lancet Neurol.* 5(1): 75–86.

[49] Tucha, O., Mecklinger, L., Thome, J., Reiter, A., Alders, G., Sartor, H., Naumann, M. & Lange, K. [2006]. Kinematic analysis of dopaminergic effects on skilled handwriting movements in Parkinson's disease, *J. Neural. Transm.* 113(5): 609–623.

[50] Vaillancourt, D. & Newell, K. [2000]. The dynamics of resting and postural tremor in Parkinson's disease, *Clin. Neurophysiol.* 111(11): 2046–2056.

[51] Vaillancourt, D., Prodoehl, J., Metman, L., Bakay, R. & Corcos, D. [2004]. Effects of deep brain stimulation and medication on bradykinesia and muscle activation in Parkinson's disease, *Brain* 127(3): 491–504.

[52] Vaillancourt, D., Prodoehl, J., Sturman, M., Bakay, R., Metman, L. & Corcos, D. [2006]. Effects of deep brain stimulation and medication on strength, bradykinesia, and electromyographic patterns of the ankle joint in Parkinson's disease, *Mov. Disord.* 21(1): 50–58.

[53] Webber, C. & Zbilut, J. [1994]. Dynamical assessment of physiological systems and states using recurrence plot strategies, *J. Appl. Physiol.* 76(2): 965–973.

[54] Welch, P. [1967]. The used of FFT for estimation of power spectra:a method based on time averaging over short modified periodograms, *IEEE Trans. Audio Electroacoust.* 15: 70–73.

[55] Xia, R. & Rymer, W. [2004]. The role of shortening reaction in mediating rigidity in Parkinson's disease, *Exp. Brain Res.* 156(4): 524–528.

Chapter 10

Distinction of Abnormality of Surgical Operation on the Basis of Surface EMG Signals

Chiharu Ishii

Additional information is available at the end of the chapter

http://dx.doi.org/10.5772/50601

1. Introduction

Recently, minimally invasive surgery such as endoscopic surgery is taking the place of laparotomy. In the field of minimally invasive surgery, a typical commercial surgical robot, such as the da Vinci system produced by Intuitive Surgical Inc., is currently in clinical use. In the robot supported surgery, master-slave system is employed. In such master-slave systems, usually motions of the master device are detected by sensors, and the slave device is controlled to follow the behavior of the master device based on the measured information by those sensors. Therefore, even the mistaken operation will be reflected.

To perform a robotic surgery, a surgeon must have considerable skill. Operation by an unskilled surgeon may result in serious malpractice. Therefore, development of a system which urges an appropriate operation to the unskilled surgeon is in demand. As described in (Tanoue et al., 2007), for training of the robotic surgery, training box or simulator has been generally used.

Recently, in order to help surgeon's dexterity, force feedback to a surgeon through the master device of a surgical robot has been studied in (Ishii et al., 2011). In order to perform safe surgery, (Ikuta et al., 2007) proposed safe operation strategies, called "Safety operation space" and "Variable compliance system" for the surgical robot. The former can prevent collision between the forceps and organs. The latter can reduce the collision force between the forceps and organs.

In addition, training systems to practice operation of surgical robot through simulation using virtual reality environment (e.g. Tokuda et al., 2009), and navigation systems which guide a surgical instrument to the targeted location during the robotic surgery (e.g. Krupa et al., 2003), have been studied.

To the best of our knowledge, however, a system that recognizes and points out any singularity in a surgical operation because of the inexpertness of an unskilled surgeon has not been established yet.

In this study, to detect any singularity in a surgical operation, surface electromyography (SEMG) is employed. Our final goal is to develop such a system that recognizes and points out any singularity in a surgical operation because of the inexpertness of the unskilled surgeon on the basis of operator's SEMG signals during the operation of the surgical robot.

To this end, a novel method for automatic identification of a surgical operation and on-line distinction of any singularity of the identified surgical operation on the basis of the SEMG measurements of an operator and movement of the forceps, is proposed.

Use of the SEMG has attracted an attention of researchers as a method of interaction between human and machines. The amplitude property of waveform and the power spectrum based on frequency analysis are typical information which can be extracted from the SEMG signal.

In (Harada et al., 2010), to control a thumb and index finger of a myoelectric prosthetic hand independently, identification of four finger motions was executed using neural networks on the basis of the SEMG measurements.

In such SEMG based interaction systems, hand gestures are identified by measuring the activities of the musculature system using the SEMG sensors. It is well known that by measuring SEMG signals, not only hand gestures but also distinction between skilled person and unskilled person, and fatigue of the muscle can be recognized (e.g. Sadoyama et al., 1981, and Kizuka et al., 2006).

In (Chen et al., 2007), recognition of 25 kinds of hand gestures consisting of various motions of wrist and fingers, was performed using only two electrodes, and the high recognition rate was successfully obtained. On the other hand, (Nakaya et al., 2010) proposed a hand gesture identification method and a distinction method of any singularity in the identified hand gesture on the basis of the SEMG measurements.

(Kita et al., 2010) proposed a self-organizing approach with level of proficiency to perform stable classification of operation. (Tada et al., 2006) proposed a distinction method of unusual manipulation of a driver when driving an automobile, using the degree of deviation on the basis of the acceleration measurements.

On the other hand, as for the surgical operation, (Hayama et al., 2009) proposed an automatic classification method of four basic surgical operations using a sensing forceps made of a forceps and strain gauges. (Kumagai et al., 2008, and Yamashita, 2009) reported that in surgical operations, a difference arises between skilled surgeon and unskilled surgeon in the following points; the magnitude and direction of the handling force of the object, the manner of having surgical instrument, and surgeon's posture. (Rosen et al., 2006) proposed an evaluation method for the state transition of the forceps operation in cholecystectomy based on comparison of skilled operator and unskilled operator.

In this chapter, a novel method for automatic identification of a surgical operation and on-line distinction of the singularity of the identified surgical operation is proposed. Suturing is divided into six operations. The features of the operation are extracted from the measurements of the movement of the forceps, and then, on the basis of the threshold criteria for the six operations, a surgical operation is identified as one of the six operations.

Next, the features of any singularity of operation are extracted from operator's surface electromyogram signals, and the identified surgical operation is classified as either normal or singular using a self-organizing map: SOM (Kohonen, 2000).

Using the built laparoscopic-surgery simulation box with two forceps, the identification of each surgical operation and the distinction of the singularity of the identified surgical operation were carried out for a specific surgical operation, namely, insertion of a needle during suturing. Each surgical operation in suturing could be identified with more than 80% accuracy, and the singularity of the surgical operation of insertion could be distinguished with approximately 80% accuracy on an average. The experimental results showed the effectiveness of the proposed method.

2. Experimental system

2.1. Simulation box

Laparoscopic-surgery simulation box is shown in Fig.1. Inside of the mannequin, a rubber sheet of 1mm thickness is installed. The image of inside of the simulation box taken by the digital video camera is projected on a central monitor. An operator performs surgical operation using the two forceps, a needle driver (right hand side) and assistant forceps (left hand side) inserted into inside of a mannequin through the trocar, by looking at the monitor. The distance between the two forceps was determined based on the spatial relationship called "triangle formation" recommended in (Hashizume et al., 2005).

In this study, an operator simulates the suturing performed in a laparoscopic surgery using the simulation box.

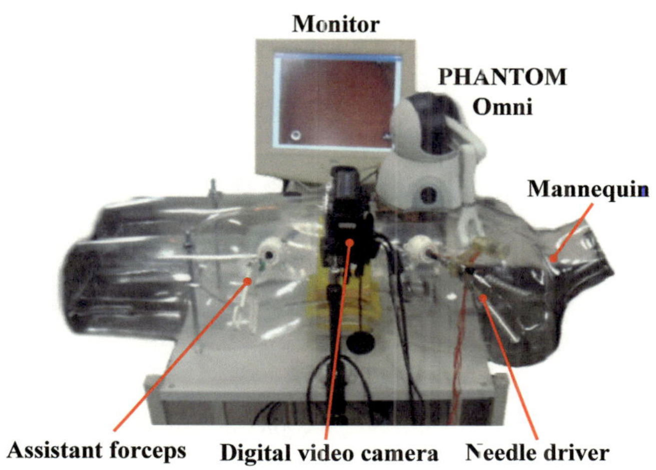

Figure 1. Simulation box

As shown in Fig.2, the movement of the needle driver is measured by the haptics device PHANTOM Omni and attached four strain gauges.

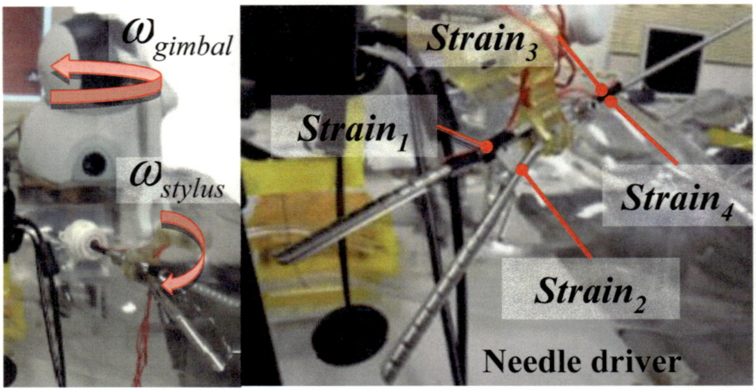

Figure 2. Sensor allocation for needle driver

2.2. Measurement of surface electromyography

The SEMG signals are measured by three electrodes stuck on the forearm of the operator as shown in Fig.3. The electrode 1 was stuck on the musculus flexor carpi radialis, the electrode 2 was stuck on the musculus extensor carpi ulnaris, the electrode 3 was stuck on the musculus extensor carpi radialis longus, and the earth electrode was stuck on the wrist.

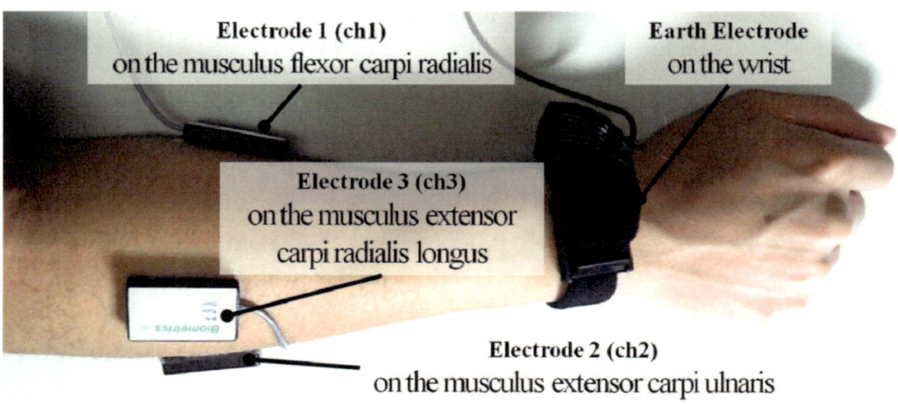

Figure 3. Allocation of surface electrode

3. Distinction of singularity of surgical operation

In this study, suturing is chosen as the objective surgical operation for automatic identification, and especially "insertion of a needle" in suturing is selected as the objective surgical operation for distinction of singularity. The flow for distinction of the singularity of the surgical operation "insertion of a needle" is explained as follows.

3.1. Features of the operation

From measurements of the SEMG signals by three electrodes, the amount of distortion by four strain gauges, and the angular velocity of gimbal and stylus by haptic device, the features are defined as follows.

For identifying the surgical operation, the features of the operation are extracted from the measurements of the movement of the needle driver. Define the features as follows.

$$St_{ch} = \frac{1}{N}\sum_{n=1}^{N} strain_{ch(n)} \tag{1}$$

$$\Omega_{gimbal} = \frac{1}{N}\sum_{n=1}^{N} \omega_{gimbal(n)} \tag{2}$$

$$\Omega_{stylus} = \frac{1}{N}\sum_{n=1}^{N} \omega_{stylusl(n)} \tag{3}$$

where $strain_{ch(n)}$ (ch=1,2…4) is measured value from each strain gauge, $\omega_{gimbel(n)}$ and $\omega_{stylus(n)}$ are measured angular velocity from the haptic device, and n represents the number of the sampled signals.

The features of any singularity of operation are extracted from operator's SEMG signals. The SEMG signals are measured by sampling frequency Fs=2 kHz, and Fast Fourier Transform (FFT) is performed to each SEMG signal for every N=512 sampled data, which is equivalent to perform FFT every 0.256 seconds.

After filtering the SEMG signals by the fourth order Butterworth type band pass filter with 10 Hz to 1 kHz range, the full wave rectification is carried out. In addition, for normalization, the measured SEMG signal of each electrode is divided by the maximum value of the pre-measured SEMG for each operation. Define the features as follows.

Average absolute value: In order to perform pattern recognition, average absolute value of each electrode is often used, which is given as follows.

$$MAV_{ch} = \frac{1}{N}\sum_{n=1}^{N} \left| EMG_{ch(n)} \right| \tag{4}$$

where $EMG_{ch(n)}$ (ch=1,2,3) is SEMG signal of each electrode, and n represents the number of the sampled signals.

Center-of-gravity: In the case where the singular operation is performed, it is expected that change of the waveform can be observed in the SEMG signal. Therefore, as a value representing change of the waveform of the SEMG signal, the value of center-of-gravity is employed, which is defined as follows.

$$cog_{ch} = \sum_{n=1}^{N}\left(n \cdot \left|EMG_{ch(n)}\right|\right) \Big/ \sum_{n=1}^{N}\left|EMG_{ch(n)}\right| \tag{5}$$

Spectrum ratio: Also, in the case where the singular operation is performed, it is expected that change of distribution of the power spectrum can be observed in the SEMG signal. Therefore, ratio of distribution of the power spectrum of the SEMG signal is also employed.

It is well known that the SEMG signal is distributed in the frequency band between 5 Hz to 500 Hz. Therefore, to see the ratio of the spectrum, frequency band is divided into 5 to 250 Hz and 250 to 500 Hz. Thus, the value of spectrum ratio is defined as follows.

$$Fr_{ch} = Fh_{ch} / Fl_{ch} \tag{6}$$

where

$$\begin{cases} Fl_{ch} = \sum_{kf=2}^{N/8} \left|F_{ch(kf)}\right|^2 & 5 \sim 250Hz \\ Fh_{ch} = \sum_{kf=N/8+1}^{N/4} \left|F_{ch(kf)}\right|^2 & 250 \sim 500Hz \end{cases} \tag{7}$$

and $|F_{ch(kf)}|$ is spectrum value in frequency *kf* obtained by Fast Fourier Transform (FFT).

3.2. Automatic identification of surgical operation

The suturing is divided into six operations as shown in Fig.4.

1. Grasping: the grasping state by closing the gripper of the needle driver.
2. Touch: the state where the needle driver touches the objects.
3. Haulage: the state where the needle driver touches the object with grasping the needle disposable.
4. Insertion: the state where the needle disposable is inserted.
5. Extraction: the state where the needle disposable is extracted.
6. Neutral: the state where nothing is operating.

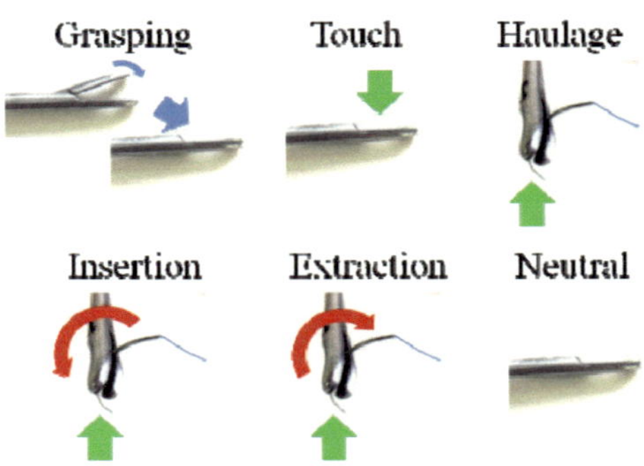

Figure 4. Surgical operations for suturing

In addition, to identify the state of operation of the needle driver using a threshold value, the following new features are defined using the features (1) to (3).

$$V_1 = St_1 \cdot St_2 \tag{8}$$

$$V_2 = \sqrt{St_3^2 + St_4^2} \tag{9}$$

$$V_3 = \Omega_{gimbal} \cdot \Omega_{stylus} \tag{10}$$

For identifying the surgical operation, the following values are defined.

$$T_i = \begin{cases} 1 & V_i > TH_i \\ 0 & else \end{cases}, \quad (i\text{=}1,2) \tag{11}$$

$$T_3 = \begin{cases} 1 & (CW) \quad V_3 > TH_{3H} \\ -1 & (CCW) \quad V_3 < TH_{3L} \\ 0 & \qquad else \end{cases} \tag{12}$$

where TH_i (i=1,2,3H, 3L) is threshold value for each new feature determined through trial and error. On the basis of the threshold criteria for the six operations, a surgical operation is identified as one of the six operations as shown in Table 1.

Discriminant value /Operation	T_1	T_2	T_3
1.Grasping	1	0	0
2.Touch	0	1	0
3.Haulage	1	1	0
4.Insertion	1	1	1(CW)
5.Extraction	1	1	-1(CCW)
6.Neutral	Else		

Table 1. Logical definition of needle driver operation

3.3. Distinction of singularity of surgical operation

In this study, (a)a normal operation and a (b)singular operation are defined as follows. A normal operation is a surgical operation performed in the expected manner. The singular operation is assumed to be the following surgical operations: (b-1)the surgical operation performed at a posture in which the operator's elbow is raised, denoted as "Posture", (b-2)the surgical operation performed in the state in which the operator is straining, denoted as "Straining", and (b-3)rough surgical operation performed suddenly by the operator, denoted as "Sudden". These are illustrated in Fig.5.

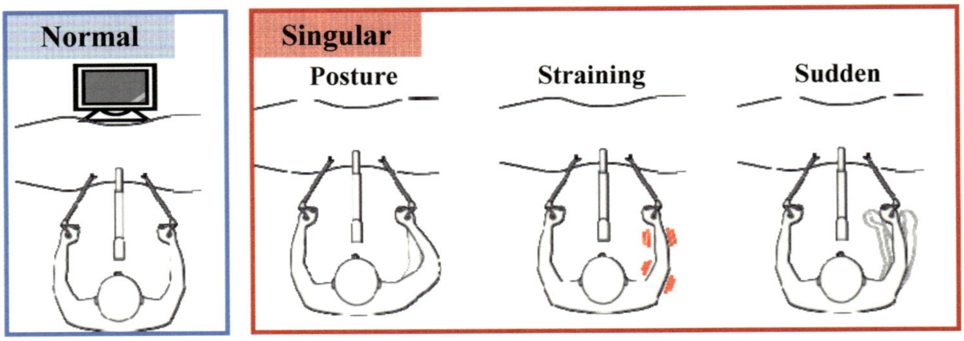

Figure 5. Experimental situations for surgical operation

The surgical operation of (4) insertion of a needle in suturing is classified as either normal or singular by using a self-organizing map: SOM. For classifying the surgical operation, the feature vector which is input to the SOM, is defined as follows using the features (4) to (6).

$$Xs = \left(\frac{MAV_1}{\overline{MAV}}, \frac{MAV_2}{\overline{MAV}}, \frac{MAV_3}{\overline{MAV}}, \frac{cog_2}{cog_1}, \frac{cog_3}{cog_1}, \frac{cog_3}{cog_2}, Fr_1, Fr_2, Fr_3 \right)^T \tag{13}$$

Where $\overline{MAV}$ is an average of MAV_{ch} (ch=1,2,3).

In each state shown in Fig.5, 20 features for normal operation and 60 features for singular operation (20 features for each singular operation) were pre-measured, and total 80 feature vectors defined by (13) are used for batch learning of the SOM. The size of the SOM was determined as hexagon lattice type of 10 x 10.

In addition, k-means method was employed to divide the map into four fields, namely, (a)Normal, (b-1)Posture, (b-2)Straining and (b-3)Sudden.

A feature vector extracted from on-line surgical operation is mapped on the map of the learned SOM, and singular operation is recognized by the distribution on the map. In addition, SOM was built using SOM Toolbox.

4. Experiments and results

The one healthy 20th generation adult man was chosen as an operator, and identification of surgical operation for "suturing" and distinction of the singularity of the identified surgical operation "insertion" were performed.

4.1. Method of experiments

In the experiment, the operator repeatedly performed the suturing process (1) to (6) classified in section 3.2, under the four situations (a)Normal, (b-1)Posture, (b-2)Straining and (b-3)Sudden. The surgical operation "suturing" performed in the experiment is shown in Fig.6. Then, rate of identification of each surgical operation in suturing and rate of distinction of the singularity in the case of (4) insertion were examined.

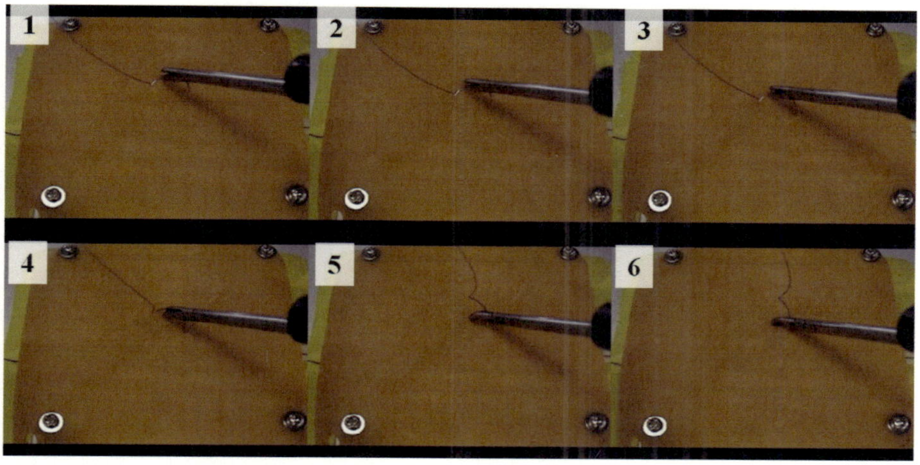

Figure 6. Suturing performed in experiment

4.2. Result for automatic identification

Recognition rate for insertion is shown in Table 2.

A: Actual operation times	19 times
B: Recognition count	21 times
Times which was not counted although operation was performed.	0
Times which was counted although operation was not performed.	2
Difference: ∣A-B∣	2
False recognition rate: ∣A-B∣/A*100	10.5%
Recognition rate	89.5%

Table 2. Recognition rate for insertion operation

Recognition rate for other operations is shown in Table 3.

Operation	A: Actual operation times	B: Recognition count	Recognition rate
1.Grasping	8 times	9 times	87.5%
2.Touch	Non		
3.Haulage	30 times	36 times	80.0%
4.Insertion	19 times	21 times	89.5%
5.Extraction	19 times	22 times	84.2%
6.Neutral	6 times	6 times	100%

Table 3. Recognition rate for automatic identification

The threshold value TH_i (i=1,2,3H, 3L) determined through trial and error is shown in Table 4.

Threshold	Value
TH_1	0.045
TH_2	0.5×10^{-9}
TH_{3H}	0.25
TH_{3L}	0.2

Table 4. Threshold values

As shown in Table 3, each surgical operation could be identified with more than 80% accuracy.

4.3. Result for singularity distinction

In order to classify the singularity of the surgical operation of (4) insertion, a SOM was used. The SOM was constructed by batch learning using the feature vectors of any singularity of operation pre-extracted from SEMG in the case of insertion. Fig.7 shows the constructed SOM and distribution of the mapping of the feature vectors extracted on-line from SEMG for each experimental operation of insertion. The domain of the SOM is roughly divided into two fields, which include the domain for the normal operation denoted as "Normal" and the domain for the singular operation denoted as "Singular." In addition, the domain for the singular operation is divided into three fields, namely, "Posture," "Straining," and "Sudden."

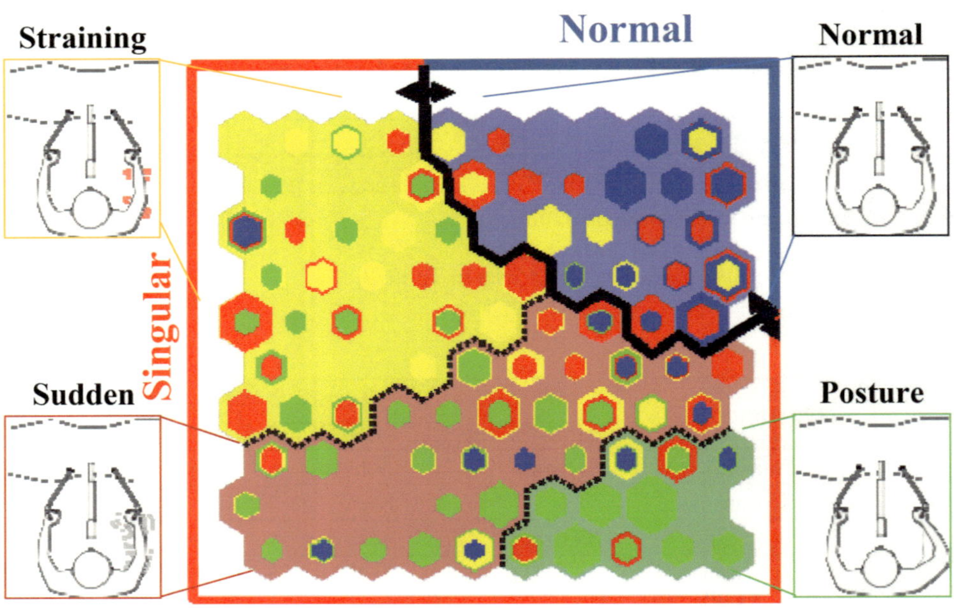

Figure 7. Distribution of experimental operation on SOM

The number of the hexagon counted in each field on the map is shown in Table 5.

	Situation			
	Normal	Posture	Straining	Sudden
Normal field	39	1	14	28
Posture field	2	24	4	7
Straining field	2	20	23	31
Sudden field	8	33	28	23
Total count	51	78	69	89

Table 5. The number of hexagon counted in each field on SOM

Recognition rate for singularity distinction is shown in Table 6.

	Recognition rate[%]	
Normal	76.5	(39/51)
Singular	81.8	(193/236)
Posture	30.8	(24/78)
Straining	33.3	(23/69)
Sudden	25.8	(23/89)

Table 6. Recognition rate for singularity distinction

As shown in Table 5, the normal and the singular operation of insertion could be distinguished with 76.5% and 81.8% accuracy, respectively. However, the accuracy of recognition of the singularity (i.e., "Posture," "Straining," or "Sudden") of the operation is approximately 30%.

As one of the reasons of this low recognition rate in the singularity distinction, the following cause is considered. In the states of "Posture", "Straining" and "Sudden", the singular operation is similar, and the difference does not appear easily in the feature vector.

In order to examine efficiency of each feature, namely average absolute value, center-of-gravity and spectrum ratio, in the feature vector defined by equation (13), singular operation was recognized by SOM using the three-dimensional feature vector which consists of each feature only. Singularity recognition rate for each feature is shown in Table 7.

From Table 7, it turns out that the average absolute value contributes to distinction of normal operation compared with the center-of-gravity and the spectrum ratio, and conversely, the center-of-gravity and the spectrum ratio contribute to the whole singularity distinction compared with the average absolute value.

Based on the above result, to raise the singularity recognition rate in each state (Posture, Straining, and Sudden), singularity distinction was performed repeatedly by combining three kinds of features in the feature vector (Average absolute value, Center-of-gravity, and Spectrum ratio) through trial and error.

As a result, the best singularity recognition rate was obtained for the following six-dimensional feature vector removing the spectrum ratio.

$$Xs = \left(\frac{MAV_1}{MAV}, \frac{MAV_2}{MAV}, \frac{MAV_3}{MAV}, \frac{cog_2}{cog_1}, \frac{cog_3}{cog_1}, \frac{cog_3}{cog_2} \right)^T \tag{14}$$

Then, two operators were added and the singularity distinction was performed by SOM using the feature vector defined by (14). Recognition rate for singularity distinction using the feature vector given by (14) is shown in Table 8.

	Recognition rate[%]		
	Average absolute value	Center-of-gravity	Spectrum ratio
Normal	76.5	78.4	37.3
Singular	80.9	85.2	84.7
Posture	35.9	24.4	59.0
Straining	42.0	39.1	24.6
Sudden	31.5	30.3	24.7

Table 7. Singularity recognition rate for each feature

	Recognition rate[%]					
	Operator A		Operator B		Operator C	
Normal	76.5	(39/51)	72.0	(36/50)	86.0	(43/50)
Singular	81.4	(192/236)	89.3	(134/150)	72.0	(108/150)
Posture	25.6	(20/78)	74.0	(37/50)	44.0	(22/50)
Straining	31.9	(22/69)	96.0	(48/50)	82.0	(41/50)
Sudden	25.8	(23/89)	56.0	(28/50)	32.0	(16/50)

Table 8. Modified recognition rate for singularity distinction

From Table 8, for the operators B and C, the singularity recognition rate for "Posture" and "Straining" was improved.

5. Conclusion

In this study, a novel method for automatic identification of a surgical operation and on-line distinction of the singularity of the identified surgical operation was proposed. The surgical operation "suturing" was performed using two forceps, namely a needle driver and assistant forceps, in the built simulation box for laparoscopic-surgery. Then, the identification of the surgical operation for "suturing" and the singularity distinction of the identified surgical operation "insertion of a needle" were carried out.

As for the identification of the surgical operation, suturing was divided into six operations. The features of the operation are extracted from the measurements of the movement of the forceps, namely the amount of distortion measured by four strain gauges and the angular velocity of gimbal and stylus measured by haptic device PHANTOM Omni. Then, on the basis of the threshold criteria for the six operations, the surgical operation was identified as one of the six operations. Each surgical operation in suturing could be identified with more than 80% accuracy.

As for the singularity distinction of the identified surgical operation, when the surgical operation was identified as "insertion of a needle", general distinction of normal operation or singular operation and distinction of three kinds of the states, namely "Posture", "Straining" or "Sudden" in the singular operation, were performed by the SOM using the 6-dimensional feature vector which extracted the features from SEMG. Then, the singularity of the surgical operation of insertion could be distinguished with approximately 80% accuracy on an average.

On the other hand, recognition rate of each state in the singular operation was approximately 30% to 90% accuracy depending on the individual difference. Therefore, it is difficult to distinguish three kinds of the states in the singular operation with sufficient accuracy.

However, in a complicated surgical operation such as insertion of a needle, it can be said that general distinction of normal operation or singular operation was able to be recognized with high accuracy.

6. Future directions

In this study, operator for the experiments was only three persons. In order to demonstrate the reliability of the proposed automatic identification and singularity distinction method, it is necessary to perform verification of the proposed method by many operators. However, since SEMG depends on the individuals, it is considered that learning of the SOM for singularity distinction for every operator is required.

In addition, it is also necessary to extend the proposed identification and singularity distinction method for a surgical operation performed with not only a right hand but also both hands. As for this point, we are now applying the proposed identification method to a surgical operation of ligation performed with both hands, and the singularity distinction method to a thread knotting also performed with both hands.

Furthermore, construction of the system to avoid malpractice by presenting recognition of the singular operation to the operator and to provide safe endoscopic-surgery is left as future work.

Author details

Chiharu Ishii
Hosei University, Japan

Acknowledgement

The part of this work was supported by Grant-in-Aid for Scientific Research (23650100). The author thanks Y. Nakaya for his assistance in experimental works.

7. References

Chen, X.; Zhang, X.; Zhao, Z.Y. & Yang, J.H. (2007). Multiple Hand Gesture Recognition based on Surface EMG Signal, *Proceedings of International Conference on Bioinformatics and Biomedical Engineering*, pp. 506-509

Harada, A.; Ishii, C.; Nakakuki, T. & Hikita, M. (2010). Robot Finger Design for Myoelectric Prosthetic Hand and Recognition of Finger Motions via Surface EMG, *Proceedings of 2010 IEEE International Conference on Automation and Logistics*, pp. 273-278

Hashizume, M.; Konishi, K.; Okazaki, K. & Tanoue, K. (2005). Fundamental Training for safe Endoscopic Surgery, Daidogakkan Press (in Japanese)

Hayama, Y.; Kurita, Y.; Kawahara, T.; Okajima, M. & Ogasawara, T. (2009). Automatic Measurement of Forceps Manipulation Logs for Laparoscopic Surgery, Journal of Japan Society of Computer Aided Surgery, Vol.11, No.3, pp. 328-329 (in Japanese)

Ikuta, K.; Hasegawa, M. & Goto, H. (2007). Total System of Hyper Finger for Remote Minimally Invasive Surgery (The 9th Report) Proposal and Experimental Verification of Safety Operation Strategies, *Proceedings of the 16th Annual Meeting of The Japan Society of Computer Aided Surgery*, pp. 43-44

Ishii, C.; Mikami, H.; Nakakuki, T. & Hashimoto, H. (2011). Bilateral Control for Remote Controlled Robotic Forceps System with Time Varying Delay, *Proceedings of IEEE International Conference on Human System Interaction*, pp. 330-335

Kita, K.; Kato, R. & Yokoi, H. (2010). EMG-to-Motion Classification for Prosthetic Applications ? A Self-Organizing Approach with Level of Proficiency -, Journal of the Robotics Society of Japan, Vol.28, No.7, pp. 783-791 (in Japanese)

Kizuka, T.; Masuda, T.; Kiryu, T & Sadoyama, T. (2006). Biomechanism Library Practical Usage of Surface Electromyogram, Tokyo Denki University Press (in Japanese)

Kohonen, T. (2000). Self-Organizing Maps, *Springer*

Krupa, A.; Gangloff, J.; Doignon, C.; de Mathelin, M. F.; Morel, G.; Leroy, J.; Soler, L. & Marescaux, J. (2003). Autonomous 3-D Positioning of Surgical Instruments in Robotized Laparoscopic Surgery Using Visual Servoing, IEEE Transactions on Robotics and Automation, Vol.19, No.5, pp. 842-853

Kumagai, T.; Yamashita, J.; Morikawa, O.; Yokoyama, K.; Fujimaki, S.; Konishi, T.; Ishimasa, H.; Murata, H. & Tomoda. K. (2008). Distance Education System for Teaching Manual Skills in Endoscopic Paranasal Sinus Surgery Using "HyperMirror" Telecommunication Interface, Proceedings of IEEE Virtual Reality 08, pp. 233-236

Nakaya, Y.; Ishii, C.; Nakakuki, T. & Hikita, M. (2010). A Practical Approach for Recognition of Hand Gesture and Distinction of Its Singularity, *Proceedings of 2010 IEEE International Conference on Automation and Logistics*, pp. 474-479

Rosen, J.; Brown, J. D.; Chang, L.; Sinanan, M. N. & Hannaford, B. (2006). Generalized Approach for Modeling Minimally Invasive Surgery as a Stochastic Process Using a Discrete Markov Model, IEEE Transactions on Biomedical Engineering, Vol.53, No.3, pp. 399-413

Sadoyama, T. & Miyano, H. (1981). Frequency analysis of surface EMG to evaluation of muscle fatigue, European Journal of Applied Physiology and Occupational Physiology, Vol.47, No.3, pp. 239-246

Tada, M.; Omura, R.; Naya, F.; Noma, H.; Toriyama, T. & Kogure, K. (2006). Analysis of Steering Control Behavior Using 3D-Accelerometers, IPSJ SIG Technical Report, SIG-CVIM-93, pp. 233-240 (in Japanese)

Tanoue, K. & Hashizume, M. (2007). Advanced medicine and innovative technology, Fukuoka Acta Medica, Vol.98, No.4, pp. 100-105 (in Japanese)

Tokuda, J.; Fischer, G. S.; Papademetris, X.; Yaniv, Z.; Ibanez, L.; Cheng, P.; Liu, H.; Blevins, J.; Arata, J.; Golby, A. J.; Kapur, T.; Pieper, S.; Burdette, E. C.; Fichtinger, G.; Tempany, C. M. & Hata, N. (2009). OpenIGTLink: an open network protocol for image-guided therapy environment, The International Journal of Medical Robotics and Computer Assisted Surgery, Vol.5, No.4, pp. 423-434

Yamashita, J. (2009). A distance- and Self-Education System to Learn Experts' Postures for Technical Skills Training in Endoscopic Sinus Surgery, Journal of Japan Society of Computer Aided Surgery, Vol.11, No.3, pp. 170-171 (in Japanese)

Chapter 11

EMG Decomposition and Artefact Removal

Adriano O. Andrade, Alcimar B. Soares,
Slawomir J. Nasuto and Peter J. Kyberd

Additional information is available at the end of the chapter

http://dx.doi.org/10.5772/50819

1. Introduction

Traditionally, in clinical electromyography (EMG), neurophysiologists assess the state of the muscle by studying basic units of an EMG signal, which are referred to as motor unit action potentials (MUAPs). Information regarding the morphology and rate of occurrence of MUAPs is often used for diagnosis of neuromuscular disorders. In addition, recent studies have shown that the analysis of the energy content of MUAPs is a possible way for discriminating among normal, neurogenic, and myopathic MUAPs [38], illustrating, thus, the clinical value of the interpretation of MUAP information.

A common way of obtaining such information is by observing MUAP activities on an oscilloscope and listening to their audio characteristics over the speakers. When doing this, the researcher is implicitly performing a time and frequency analysis of MUAPs. However, the results of this analysis are dependent on the experience of the investigator and on his ability to extract relevant information from the visual and auditory analysis. Furthermore, this procedure is time-consuming and prone to error.

The drawbacks related to the procedure described above have motivated the use of computer-based techniques for extraction of MUAPs from EMG signals [3, 19, 22, 27, 29, 32, 40]. Such methods, also known as EMG decomposition techniques, aim at classifying MUAPs generated by a common source into the same group. The results of this classification may provide information regarding the orchestration of the neuromuscular system, and therefore of the state of the muscle. A similar problem, often referred to as spike sorting, is found in the study of neuronal activities [25]. In this case, neuronal action potentials from the same source are classified into a common group.

Originally, the investigation of MUAP activities belonged to needle electromyographic (NEMG) studies, mainly because surface electrodes may easily produce an integration of many potentials, which precludes accurate study of their individual form. However, some recent studies have shown that the use of surface electrodes may be successfully applied for detection of MUAPs from superficial muscles [8]. This advancement has received widespread support among researchers and clinicians because of the ease of use, reduced risk of infection, and the greater number of motor unit action potential trains obtained compared to needle sensor techniques [47].

Currently, computer-based EMG has become an indispensable tool for investigations seeking to explain the state of the muscle. Different methodologies, ranging from simple quantitative measures to automatic systems that enable the assessment of neuromuscular disorders, have been developed [30]. Such tools are important for standardization of results and also they may reveal important features in the signals, which might be barely perceived from a manual analysis [35].

A typical system for extraction of MUAPs from EMG signals may require several stages of signal processing, for instance, signal detection and filtering (i.e., artefact removal) [45], feature extraction or selection [36], data clustering or classification [23]. Specific research may be carried out in each of these steps.

2. Strategies for EMG decomposition

One of the most rudimentary strategies for isolation of MUAPs belonging to a common group is by means of a thresholding scheme. The central idea of this technique is to use a voltage threshold trigger for detection of MUAPs that have similar height, which is represented by the amplitude of the highest peak of a MUAP. In this method the experimenter positions the recording electrode so that MUAPs of interest are maximally separated from the background activity (noise). MUAP activities are then measured with a hardware threshold trigger, which generates a pulse whenever the measured voltage crosses the threshold. Such pulses may be used for triggering data collection and further storage of MUAPs or their occurrence time in a computer. The main advantages of this method are that: (i) It is easy to apply since it requires minimal hardware and software; (ii) It is a good starting point for detection of the strongest MUAPs. The main drawbacks of this technique are that: (i) The threshold level, mainly dependent on the signal-to-noise ratio, determines the trade-off between missed spikes (false negatives) and the number of background events that cross the threshold (false positives); (ii) Only a single feature (the MUAP highest peak) is used for data classification. As a consequence of this strategy two MUAPs with different shapes might be grouped together because they have similar peak amplitude.

The drawbacks related to the technique discussed above highlight the importance of a pre-processing stage prior to grouping MUAPs. The presence of high levels of background activity in the signal suggests that the use of a filter for reduction of the background activity is necessary. Different digital filters may be used for this purpose. Typically high band-pass filters are used for attenuation of very low frequency components in the signal related to noise, which can be either inherent from the hardware used for data acquisition or the contribution of distant MUAPs from the detection point.

Another common approach is the use of differential filters. Such filters are low-pass filters and have been used in many investigations. The main drawback of such filters is that they may generate artificial spikes and modify the shape of MUAPs. This has motivated the use of alternative filtering procedures, for instance, wavelets and a spatial filter, known as a Laplacian filter. The implementation of these filters as well as the introduction of an alternative method for EMG signal filtering is further discussed in the chapter.

Another relevant pre-processing step is the one that segments the EMG signal into windows containing active and inactive segments. This is a signal detection stage which aims to identify the activities of single MUAPs or their combinations, which is known as MUAP overlaps. Furthermore, this step separates noise in inactive segments from useful information in active segments. The detection of active and inactive segments may be performed visually or manually, i.e. the researcher may classify regions of an electromyographic signal into one of those categories, however such a method is time-consuming and requires concentration, which may introduce inconsistency in the signal analysis.

Different approaches may be employed for automation of this pre-processing stage: (i) The use of the root-mean square of the EMG signal together with a pre-defined threshold; (ii) A threshold proportional to the maximum peak in the signal; (iii) A threshold which is manually adjusted; (iv) Wavelets. The main assumption of this method is that there might be similarity between the mother wavelet and action potentials, and when the correlation between an active window and the mother wavelet is high an active segment is detected.

As one may note there exists a variety of strategies that could be considered for automation of the detection of active and inactive segments. Techniques that make an assumption about a pre-defined height and width of MUAPs may be more susceptible to failures, i.e. active regions that do not fit the predefined window will not be detected. Note also that the level of the background activity in the signal will also influence the determination of the beginning and end of active segments. The detection of active regions is further discussed in this chapter.

After detection of active regions it is possible to group them into logical units (clusters), however, it is very common to obtain features from those regions prior to data clustering. For example, morphological features of MUAPs, i.e. duration, amplitude, area, number of phases (number of baseline crossings) and number of turns (number of positive and negative peaks) have been employed. Other successful approaches include the use of coefficients of the Fourier transform, the coefficients of the Wavelet transform, the use of time samples of the band-pass filtered signal and low-pass differentiated signal, and the use of autoregressive and cepstral coefficients. Some other approaches, known as feature extraction and selection procedures, try to obtain features that maximize cluster separability. Examples of the use of such techniques include the application of Principal Component Analysis (PCA) and Independent Component Analysis (ICA).

The grouping of MUAPs is commonly performed by means of at least three distinct strategies: (i) Template matching: raw MUAPs, referred to as MUAP templates, are first classified or identified, and then used for classification of new MUAPs. The initial MUAP templates may be manually selected from the EMG signal or be chosen automatically from a clustering procedure. During data classification, usually MUAP templates are modified by an update rule, which takes into account the variability of MUAP shapes in the data set; (ii) Clustering: a clustering technique is used for grouping patterns represented by features selected from active regions; (iii) Hybrid: in this approach, first a clustering technique is used for grouping part of the data set (normally the first 3 to 5 seconds), and then the non-classified data set is grouped into one of the classes defined in the first step.

Both the template matching and hybrid techniques require a priori identification of patterns in the data set before classification of the entire data set. The main disadvantage of these methods is that if new MUAP classes appear they will not be identified. The main advantage is that extra information regarding MUAP activities, e.g. the study of the firing time of MUAPs, may be taken into account in the final classification. The clustering approach has the advantage that it makes no assumptions about the data set to be grouped.

The main processing steps discussed so far form the basis of a complete EMG decomposition system. When the final application of such system is to study the firing behaviour of sources that generate MUAPs, it may be necessary to include an extra stage that deals with a problem known as MUAP overlaps. Overlapping spikes occur when two or more spikes fire simultaneously. When using the clustering technique for grouping active segments it may be possible to detect such overlaps as outliers. There are at least three strategies for dealing with overlaps: (i) Once a spike is classified it is subtracted from the active segment, in the hope that this will improve the classification of subsequent spikes. This approach requires a template of the spike. It yields reasonable results when two spikes are separated well enough so that the first can be accurately classified, but fails when the spikes are close together. Another problem with this approach is that the subtraction can introduce more noise into the waveform if the spike model (template) is not accurate. Also subtraction-based approaches may introduce spurious spike-like shapes if the spike occurrence is not accurately estimated; (ii) Another approach is to compare all possible combinations of two or more spike models. However, for some applications the computation time for performing this comparison may be prohibitive; (iii) The use of multiple electrodes or an array of electrodes may reduce the problem of overlapping spikes, because what appears as an overlap on one channel might be an isolated unit on another. Since the main aim of solving the overlapping problem is to increase the accuracy of estimators (e.g. mean) obtained from the firing of motor units, an alternative option might be to work directly with a precise estimate of the estimator considering missing data points (i.e that some MUAPs are missing).

Finally, once the system is designed and implemented it is important to test its accuracy. At least three methods are well accepted for this purpose: (i) Synthetic signals: artificial EMG signals are generated and employed for testing the stages of the system. The main advantage of this approach is that the characteristics of the analyzed signal are totally known; (ii) Manual classification of MUAPs: MUAPs are visually classified by the researcher and the results of this classification are used as reference for evaluation of the automatic classification; (iii) Comparison between MUAP activities from different channels: the consistency of the decomposition data of the same units from two different electrodes provides an indirect measure of the accuracy in real data decomposition.

3. Artefact removal from EMG signals

The detection of electromyographic signals is a very complex process, which is affected not only by the muscle anatomy and the physiological process responsible for the signal generation but also by external factors, for instance, the inherent noise of the hardware employed in the signal amplification and digitalization. As a result EMG signals are often corrupted by noise.

It may be very difficult, if possible at all, to extract useful information from very poor signal-to-noise ratio EMG signals. In some applications, for example, the decomposition of electromyographic signals, a high level of background activity could impede the accurate segmentation of the signal into regions of activity that may represent the activity of single motor unit action potentials, influencing thus the final results of the EMG decomposition.

3.1. Conventional methods for EMG signal noise removal

3.1.1. Low-pass differential filter

Since its introduction, the low-pass differential filter (LPD) [44] has been widely employed in EMG signal processing [15, 19, 32, 40–42]. This filter is implemented in the time-domain as:

$$y_k = \sum_{n=1}^{N} (x_{k+n} - x_{k-n}), \tag{1}$$

where x_k is the discrete input time-series and y_k is the filtered output. N is the window width to adjust the cut-off frequency. Increasing N will reduce the cut-off frequency of the filter. This may be easily perceived if Equation 1 is studied in the frequency domain.

For this, consider the following difference equation obtained from Equation 1:

$$y[k] = \sum_{n=1}^{N} x[k+n] - \sum_{n=1}^{N} x[k-n]. \tag{2}$$

Its representation in the frequency domain may be obtained via its Z transform as follows,

$$\begin{aligned}
Z(y[k]) &= Z\left(\sum_{n=1}^{N} x[k+n]\right) - Z\left(\sum_{n=1}^{N} x[k-n]\right)\\
Z(y[k]) &= \sum_{n=1}^{N} Z(x[k+n]) - \sum_{n=1}^{N} Z(x[k-n])\\
Z(y[k]) = Y(z) &= \sum_{n=1}^{N} z^{n} X(z) - \sum_{n=1}^{N} z^{-n} X(z)\\
Y(z) &= X(z)\left(\sum_{n=1}^{N} (z^{n} - z^{-n})\right)\Bigg|_{z=e^{\frac{j2\pi f}{f_{sr}}}}
\end{aligned}$$

where the ratio $Y(z)/X(z)$ is the filter transfer function $H(z)$, f is the frequency in Hz and f_{sr} is the sampling frequency in Hz.

Figure 1 presents the results of the estimate of the filter transfer function with different sizes of windows, $N = 40$ and $N = 20$. Note how the cut-off frequency is shifted to a higher frequency when the window size is reduced.

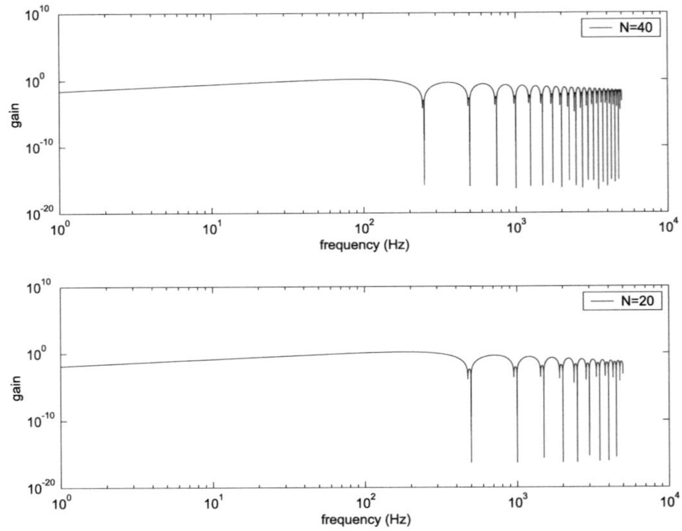

Figure 1. Frequency response of an LPD filter with window width 20 and 40.

The main advantages of using the LPD filter are that it is very easy to implement, and it is considerably fast for real-time applications, but some drawbacks regarding this filter are discussed in [46]:

- Under conditions of low signal-to-noise ratio the relatively strong high frequency noise (background activity) may be accentuated;
- Since the LPD filter is not an ideal low-pass filter, there will exist severe Gibbs phenomenon, that is, the leakage of energy frequency out of the filter pass-band as illustrated in the Bode diagrams shown in Figure 1. As a result, many high frequency noise components will pass through the filter.

3.1.2. *Weighted low-pass differential filter*

The weighted low-pass differential filter (WLPD) was proposed in [46] as an alternative to the LPD filter. The main difference is that an appropriately weighted window is included in Equation 2 for reduction of the Gibbs effect. The WLPD filter is implemented in the time-domain as:

$$y_k = \sum_{n=1}^{N} w(n)(x_{k+n} - x_{k-n}), \tag{3}$$

where $w(n)$ is an N point windowing function. Several windows such as Barlett, Hamming and Hanning may be employed. If a rectangular window is used then Equation 3 is an LPD filter. Similarly to the LPD filter the WLPD is very easy to implement and considerably fast for real-time applications, but results presented in [17, 46] show that phase distortion may

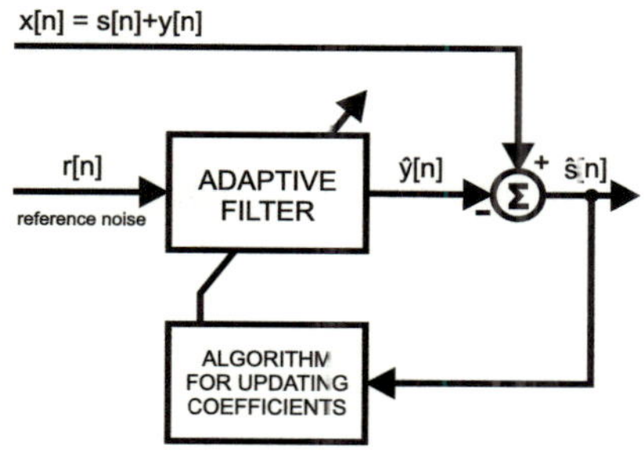

Figure 2. Adaptive noise canceller. $x[n]$ is the noise corrupted signal, $s[n]$ is the noise free signal, $y[n]$ the noise and $r[n]$ the reference noise. $\hat{y}[n]$ is the estimated noise, whereas $\hat{s}[n]$ the estimated signal.

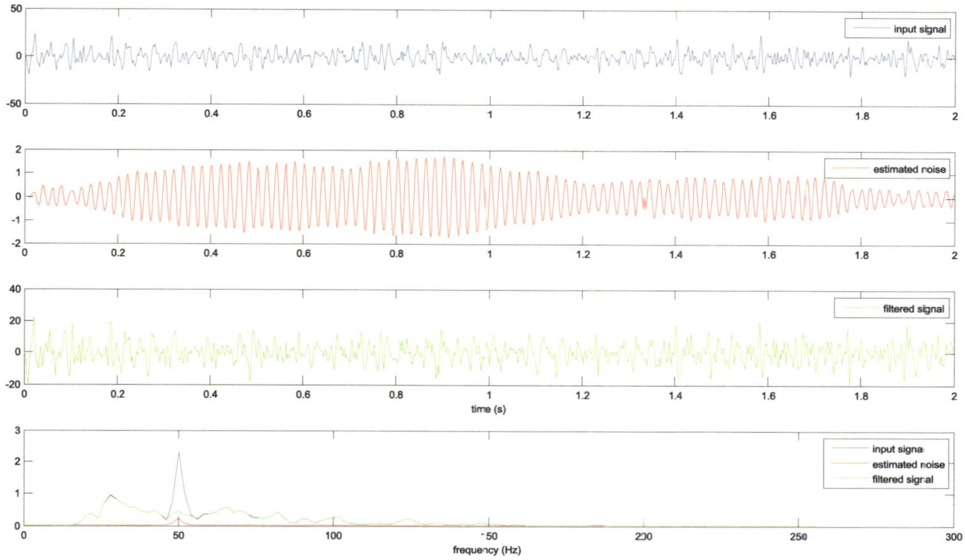

Figure 3. Example of application of the adaptive noise cancelling on a sample of EMG signal. The corrupted signal (top) is contrasted with the cleaned signal. The power spectra of the signals are shown at the bottom and illustrate the effect of the application of the filter on the 50 Hz component.

be present in the filtered signal and depending on the level of noise false spikes may be generated.

3.1.3. Adaptive 50/60 Hz noise cancellation

When the source of noise is well known it is possible to employ methods for adaptively reduce its influence over the desired signal. This is, for instance, the aim of adaptive 50/60 Hz noise cancellation based on the least mean square (LMS) algorithm [2].

The block diagram shown in Figure 2 depicts the main idea of the adaptive noise cancelling algorithm. The signal $s[n]$ is corrupted by the noise $y[n]$ yielding the corrupted signal $x[n]$. The adaptive algorithm will estimate parameters for a filter capable of attenuating the desired components and maintaining relevant information from the signal. The piece of code below is a Matlab function created for attenuating 50 Hz noise from signals. It was used to illustrate the application of the technique on an EMG signal which was strongly corrupted by 50 Hz noise. The plots given in Figure 3 show the input signal, the estimated noise and the filtered signal. The power spectra of these signals are given in the graph at the bottom. Their analysis allows us to conclude that the application of the adaptive filter attenuated the undesired 50 Hz component. Note that the 50 Hz component is also part of the EMG signal, therefore its complete elimination is not desired.

```
function [EstimatedNoise,filteredSig50Hz] = NoiseRemoval(x,fs)
%% Function name....: NoiseRemoval
% Description......:
%                    This function estimates a filtered signal based on a
%                    50Hz noise optimal filter (LMS algorithm)
% Parameters.......:
%                    x ......-> input time-series
%                    fs......-> sampling frequency (Hz)
% Return...........:
%                    EstimatedNoise... -> estimated 50 Hz noise
%                    filteredSig50Hz.. -> filtered signal (50 Hz noise free signal)

mu = 0.001; %constant of convergence of the LMS algorithm
taps = 10; %filter order
t = [0:1:length(x)-1]/fs;
d  = sin(2*pi*t*50);  % reference noise (component to be removed from the input signal)
ha = adaptfilt.lms(taps,mu);
[y,e] = filter(ha,d,y);
[EstimatedNoise,filteredSig50Hz] = filter(ha,d,e);
```

3.1.4. Signal filtering based on wavelets

One of the main applications of wavelets is noise removal from corrupted signals. A general procedure for signal de-noising involves the following three steps that have been successfully applied [14, 16, 33]:

1. Signal decomposition;
2. Detail coefficients thresholding;
3. Signal reconstruction.

In the first step, both a wavelet prototype and the decomposition level (N) are chosen, and the wavelet decomposition of the signal at level N is performed. In the next step, for each level from 1 to N, a threshold, t_N, is selected and soft-thresholding is applied to detail coefficients as shown in Equation 4.

$$Y_N = sign(D_N)(|D_N| - t_N)_+ \tag{4}$$

where Y_N is the de-noised version of the Nth detail coefficients and the function $(x)_+$ is defined as

$$(x)_+ = \begin{cases} 0, & x < 0 \\ x, & x >= 0. \end{cases} \tag{5}$$

Finally, in the third step the denoised signal is estimated by using the original approximation coefficients of level N and the modified detail coefficients of levels from 1 to N. The application of this procedure is illustrated in the following example.

3.1.5. Example of application

The procedure for noise removal based on wavelets is applied to an experimental surface EMG signal in this section. The main aim is to attenuate the background activity present in the signal and at the same time to preserve its shape.

The Matlab Wavelet Toolbox[1] is used for data processing (see Figure 4). The EMG signal is decomposed into three levels ($N = 5$) and the *db*5 wavelet prototype is employed. The choice for the decomposition level may be justified by the fact that this signal is mostly contaminated by high frequency noise that will be highlighted by short time-scale components (e.g. detail coefficients of the first and second level) and therefore further decomposition would not contribute significantly to the final form of the filtered signal. The criteria for selection of the wavelet family (Daubechies) is mainly because of its reported success in removing/attenuating noise from EMG signals, and in its use for feature extraction from MUAPs [18, 37, 48].

The results of the signal decomposition are depicted in Figure 4. A window of the input EMG signal together with its filtered version are presented in Figure 5.

3.2. EMG signal filtering based on Empirical Mode Decomposition

In this section a novel algorithm for signal de-noising based on the Empirical Mode Decomposition (EMD) method is presented [7]. The developed filter may be employed as an alternative to the approach based on wavelets described above.

3.2.1. The Empirical Mode Decomposition method

Huang *et al.* (1998) [21] described a new technique for analyzing nonlinear and non-stationary data. The key part of the method is the Empirical Mode Decomposition (EMD) method, in which any complicated data set can be adaptively decomposed into a finite, and often small, number of Intrinsic Mode Functions (IMFs). The name Intrinsic Mode Function is adopted because those components represent the oscillation modes embedded in the data. In the case of Fourier analysis, oscillation modes (i.e. components) in a signal are defined in terms of sine and cosine waves. The EMD thus defines oscillation modes in terms of IMFs, which are functions that satisfy two conditions [21]:

1. In the whole time-series, the number of extrema and the number of zero crossings must be either equal or differ at most by one. Note that extrema are either local minima or local maxima. Furthermore, a sample g_i in a time-series is a local maximum if $g_i > g_{i-1}$ and $g_i > g_{i+1}$, and a sample q_i is a local minimum if $q_i < q_{i-1}$ and $q_i < q_{i+1}$, where i is a discrete time.

[1] This toolbox can be invoked by typing *wavemenu* in the Matlab command environment.

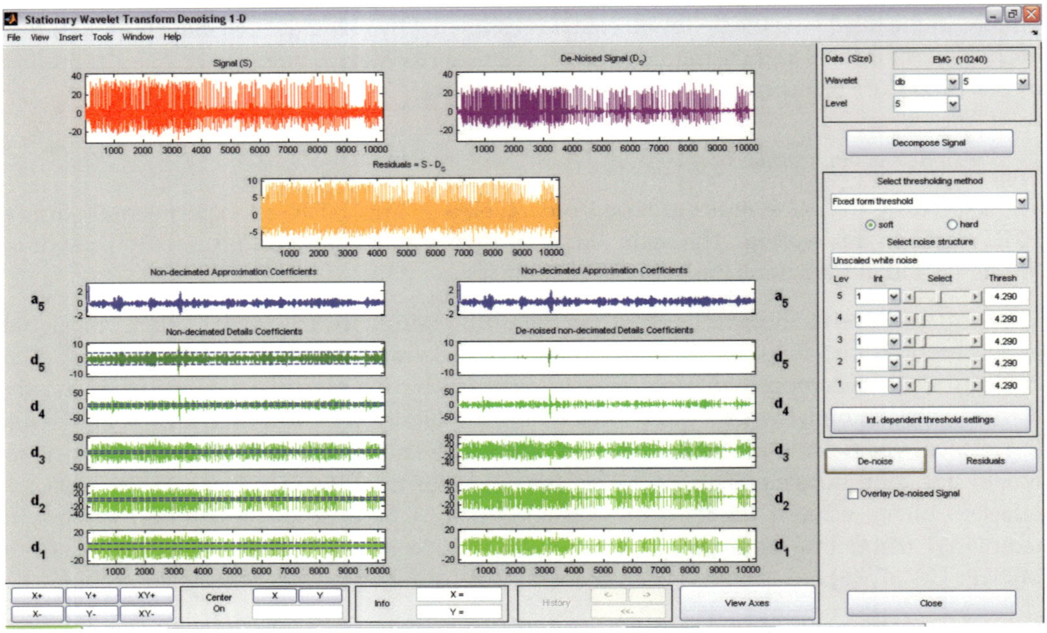

Figure 4. Graphical user interface of the Wavelet Matlab Toolbox used for signal denoising. The EMG signal and its denoised version are shown. The wavelet components are individually denoised by using a thresholding scheme.

2. At any point in the time-series, the mean value of the envelopes, one defined by the local maxima (upper envelope) and the other by the local minima (lower envelope), is zero.

The definition above is empirical and currently there is no explicit equation for estimating IMFs, thus any arbitrary time-series that satisfies conditions 1 and 2 is an IMF. Furthermore, by means of the analysis of the power spectra of IMFs it is possible to verify that these functions represent the original signal decomposed into different time-scales (or frequency bandwidths). This is illustrated in [4, 6]. Thus, both wavelets and the Empirical Mode Decomposition provide the decomposition of a signal into different time-scales. The main difference is that one method performs the signal decomposition adaptively and based solely on the available data, whereas the other normally uses a set of pre-fixed filters.

3.2.2. The algorithm for signal filtering based on the EMD

The success of the general procedure for noise removal using wavelets is based on the fact that it is possible to filter signal components individually instead of filtering the original signal. This is desirable because some components may highlight the noise and thus it may be easier to attenuate its presence.

Similarly, the Empirical Mode Decomposition also provides the decomposition of a signal into different time-scales or IMFs. This means that it is also possible to filter signal components individually instead of the original signal. This suggests that the strategy for signal de-noising

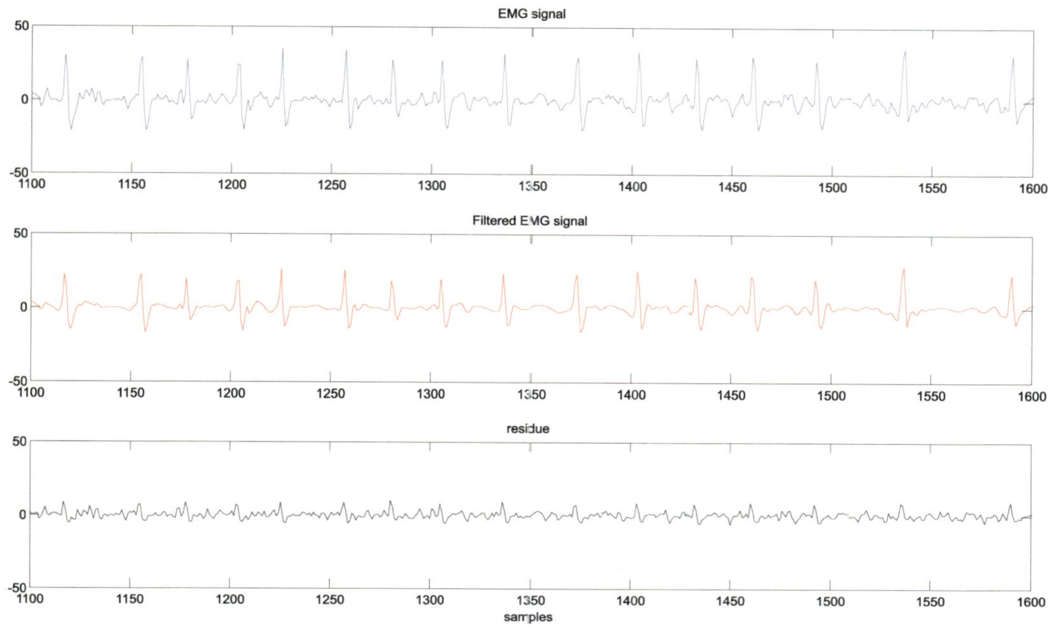

Figure 5. Segment of the EMG signal shown in Figure 4. The filtered signal and the residue is also presented.

based on wavelets may also be applied to intrinsic mode functions. Thus the following procedure was proposed for EMG signal filtering [3, 7]:

1. Decompose the signal into IMFs;
2. Threshold the estimated IMFs;
3. Reconstruct the signal.

This procedure is practical, mainly due to the empirical nature of the EMD method, and it may be applied to any signal as the EMD does not make any assumption about the input time-series. A block diagram describing the steps for its application is shown in Figure 6. First, the EMD method is used for decomposing the input signal into intrinsic mode functions, $IMF_1, \ldots, IMF_N$, where N is the number of IMFs. These IMFs are then soft-thresholded, yielding $tIMF_1, \ldots, tIMF_N$, which are thresholded versions of the original components. The filtered signal is obtained as a linear summation of thresholded IMFs.

A very common strategy used in the filtering procedure based on wavelets is to use the soft-thresholding technique described in [14]. The same idea is used for thresholding IMFs. For each IMF from 1 to N a threshold, $t_n, n = 1, \ldots, N$, is selected and soft-thresholding is applied to individual IMFs.

The threshold t_n is estimated by using the following strategy: a window of noise is selected from the original signal and then the boundaries of this window are used to extract regions of noise from IMFs. The standard deviation of each of those regions is then estimated, and

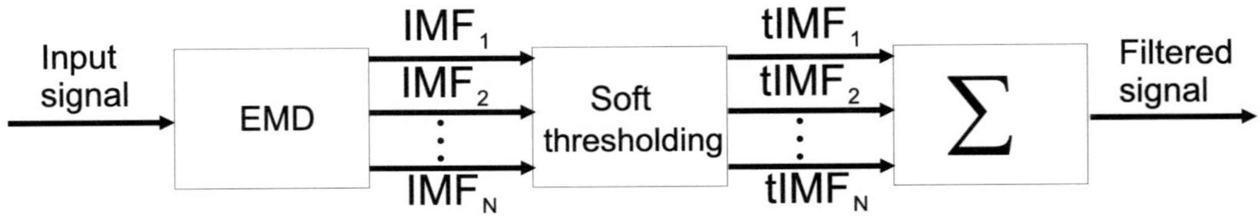

Figure 6. The EMD method is employed for decomposing the input signal into IMFs ($IMF_1, \ldots, IMF_N$, where N is the number of IMFs). These IMFs are soft-thresholded, yielding $tIMF_1, \ldots, tIMF_N$, which are thresholded versions of the original components. The filtered signal is obtained as a linear summation of thresholded IMFs.

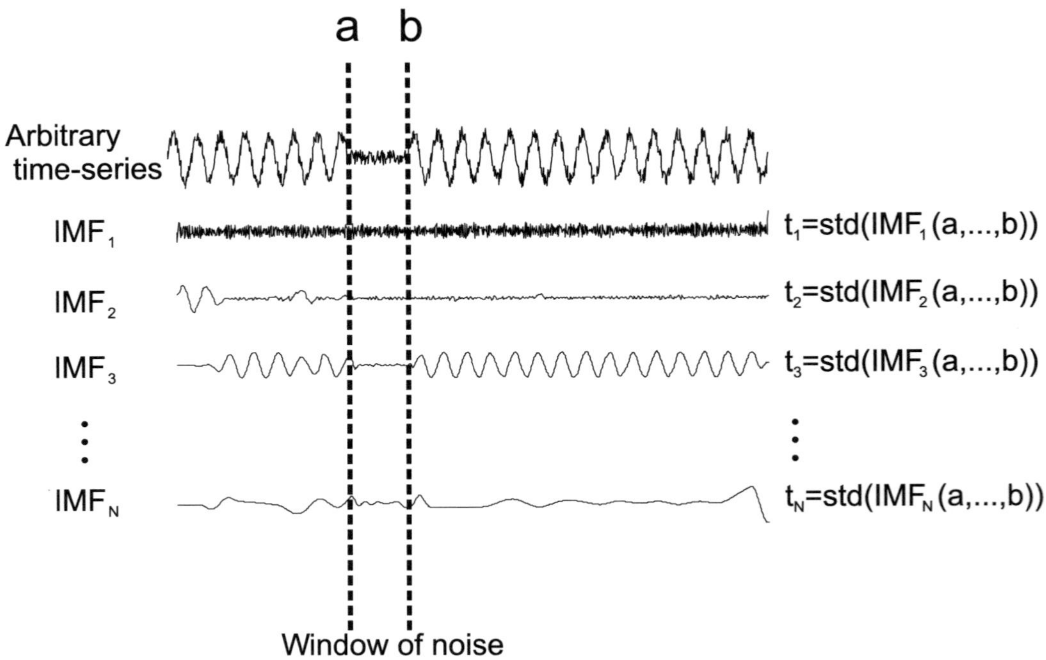

Figure 7. Illustrative example showing the estimate of thresholds t_n. First, a window of noise (i.e. samples within the interval [a,b]) is selected from the arbitrary time-series. The interval [a,b] is employed for selection of noise in the IMFs, and then from each IMF, thresholds $t_1, \ldots, t_N$ are defined. Note that *std* is the standard deviation.

these are regarded as the required thresholds ($t_1, ..., t_N$). Figure 7 illustrates the procedure for estimating t_n.

3.2.3. An example of application of the filter based on the EMD method

In this section, an example illustrating the application of the procedure for filtering EMG signals based on the EMD is provided. For this, the experimental surface electromyographic signal shown in Figure 8 is used.

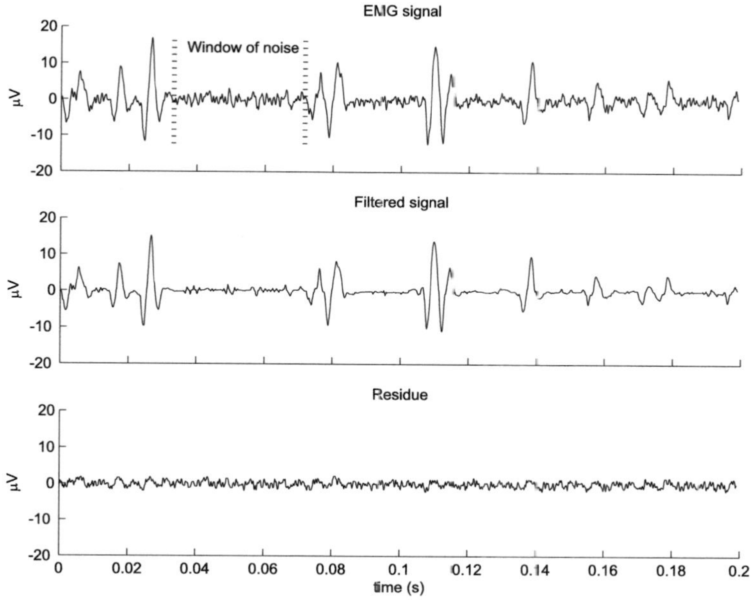

Figure 8. EMG signal and its filtered version. The residue, which is the difference between those signals is also shown.

The first step of the algorithm is to use the EMD (or sifting process) to decompose the experimental signal into intrinsic mode functions. Eight IMFs ($IMF1, \ldots, IMF8$) are obtained and they are presented in Figure 9(a).

The subsequent step is to threshold the components $IMF1, \ldots, IMF8$. Equation 4 was employed for denoising individual IMFs. The results of this procedure are shown in Figure 9(b). Note that in order to estimate thresholds for IMFs the boundaries of the window of noise (0.03 s and 0.07 s) indicated in Figure 8 were selected.

In the last step, the resulting (de-noised) components were combined to generate a filtered version of the original signal as shown in Figure 8. In the same figure, the residue, which is the difference between the original and filtered signals, is also presented. The random nature of this component and the attenuation of the noise in the EMG signal is apparent.

4. A system for extraction and visualization of MUAPs

The visual inspection of data is an important stage in signal analysis. It may help the investigator to identify relevant features, outliers and noise in the signal. Although visualization is an important and basic stage in data processing, in practice, its execution may be rather complex, specially when performed manually and the data lie in a high dimensional manifold.

In this context tools or systems that allow for an automatic visualization of signals play an important role. First, they significantly reduce the overall processing time of data, and

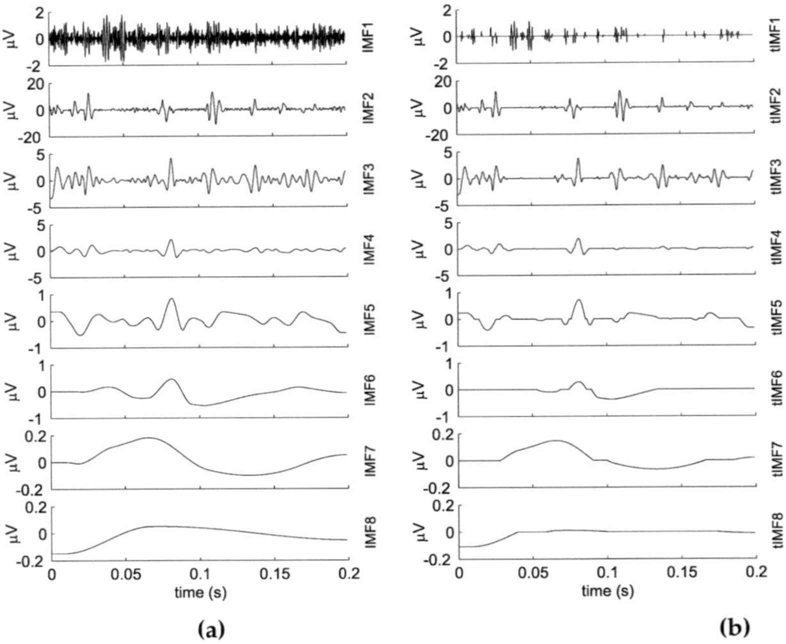

Figure 9. (a) Intrinsic mode functions ($IMF1, \ldots, IMF8$) obtained from the EMG signal presented in Figure 8. (b) De-noised intrinsic mode functions.

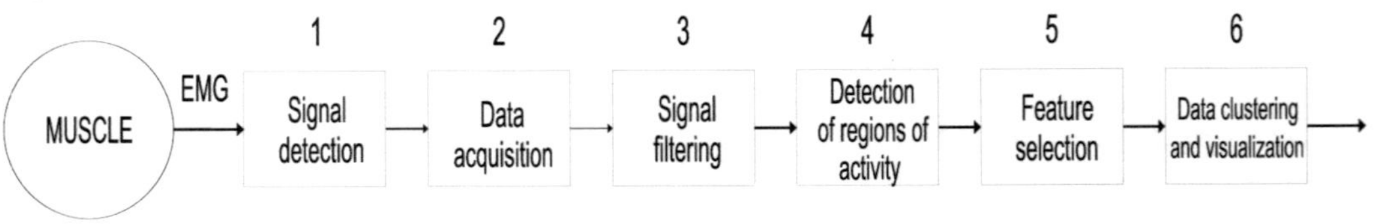

Figure 10. Block diagram of the system for extraction and visualization of MUAPs. After detection (1) and acquisition (2) the EMG signal is filtered (3), and signal windows, designated as regions of activity (RA), are extracted from it (4). In (5) features are selected from RA and then employed for their clustering and visualization.

secondly they may reveal information present in the signal which might be barely perceived in a manual analysis.

This section describes a system that can be used for the extraction and visualization of motor unit action potentials from electromyographic signals. It is formed by several basic units which are illustrated in Figure 10. Its input is a raw electromyographic signal, and its output is the visualization of MUAPs or any other information (e.g. noise) present in the signal grouped into logical units (clusters). This visualization allows the researcher to identify outliers, noise and groups of MUAPs. Each of the stages of this system is described below.

Once the EMG signal is detected it is amplified and digitized. An EMG amplifier[2] and data acquisition board[3] are important elements that contribute to the correct collection of data.

[2] Typical requirements of the signal conditioner are CMRR > 80 dB, input impedance $> 10^{15}$ Ω, noise level < 1.2 μV.
[3] A possible model would be PC-card DAS 16/16 Measurement Computing

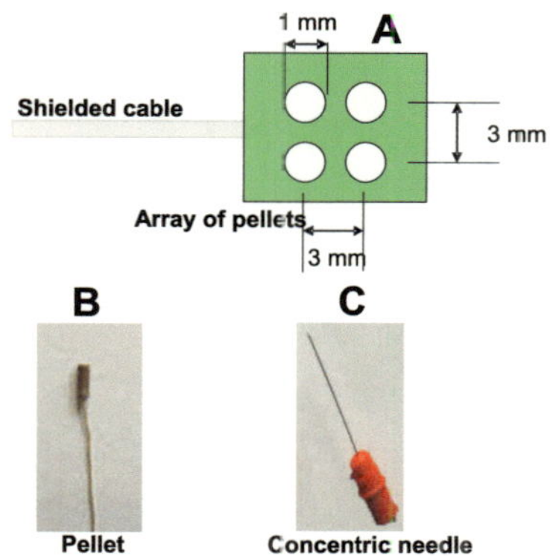

Figure 11. Types of electrodes for EMG signal detection. (A) A customized array of pellet electrodes. (B) Example of a single pellet electrode. (C) Concentric needle electrode.

Other relevant units include force sensors for monitoring the level of muscle contraction and biofeedback systems that provide a stimulus and information for subjects about the required task to be executed during the experiment.

4.1. System description

4.1.1. Signal detection and acquisition

The stage of signal detection will convert current generated by movement of ions (a physiological process) into current generated by movement of electrons (an electrical process). The choice of the type of electrode to be employed is dependent on the aim of the investigation. For instance, if the interest is to extract and visualize activity of motor unit action potentials from EMG signals, then needle electrodes are traditionally employed, mainly because of the high spatial resolution offered by these sensors. In fact, when studying the state of deep muscles this is the only possible choice. However, many studies [5, 11, 17, 43, 49] have shown that surface EMG electrodes with a sufficiently small contact surface may be successfully applied to the detection of MUAP activity in superficial muscles.

The system depicted in Figure 10 has been tested with two types of electrodes for signal detection. They are shown in Figure 11. One is a concentric needle electrode and the other is a customized array of pellet(surface) electrodes whose dimensions follow specifications provided in [43]. Both electrodes are passive and leads connecting them to the amplifier are shielded in order to attenuate the presence of spurious noise activity.

The use of pellet electrodes was a very cheap and simple solution for high spatial resolution signal detection, which yielded outstanding results and consistent detection of EMG signals.

4.1.2. Signal filtering

The main aim of this stage is to reduce the background activity present in electromyographic signals. This is relevant because high levels of background activity (noise) may affect the

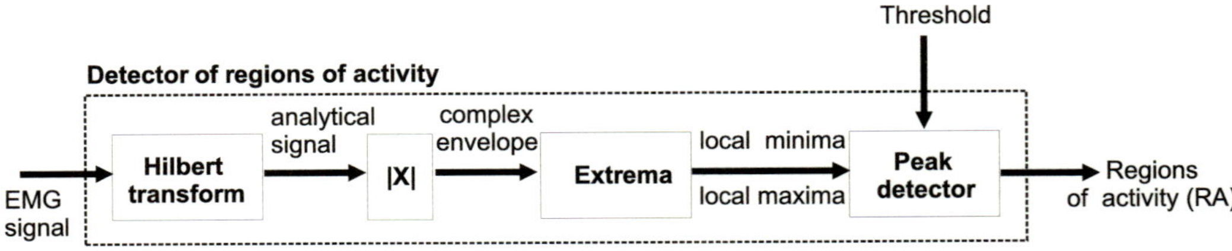

Figure 12. Block diagram of the detector of regions of activity.

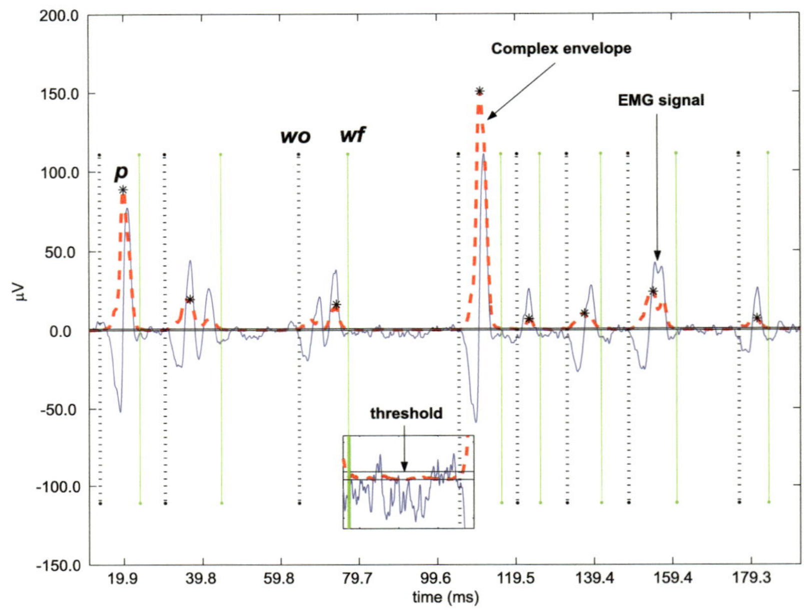

Figure 13. Example of detection of regions of activity. The experimental surface EMG signal and its complex envelope are shown. w_o and w_f are respectively the beginning and end of a region of activity. The peak (p) within each RA is marked with $*$ and it is used as a reference point for feature selection. The inset shows a window of noise with the pre-defined threshold level.

detection of useful information (e.g. MUAPs). This stage may be performed by the filtering procedure based on the Empirical Mode Decomposition described above.

4.1.3. Detection of regions of activity

Following the stage of signal filtering the EMG signal is segmented into small windows, so-called regions of activity (RA), that may contain the activity of single MUAPs, MUAP overlaps or noise. A detector of RA was devised for extraction of RA from EMG signals. The block diagram of this is shown in Figure 12 and an example of its application is provided in Figure 13. Its input may be either a raw or filtered EMG signal and the output is a set of regions of activity.

Basically, this system will estimate the signal envelope and it will select from it reference points which define the beginnings and ends of RAs. Intuitively, the envelope is the overall shape of the amplitude of the signal and its use instead of the raw signal may simplify, in terms of practical implementation, the solution for this problem, mainly because the signal envelope is positive. For instance, a unique positive threshold may be employed for selection of RAs which are above it.

The envelope of time domain signals can be computed by low pass filtering and curve fitting techniques [21], or by using the Hilbert transform to compute the analytic signal [13]. The signal envelope generated from the first two methods is dependent on the choice of parameters like the filter order and the method for data fitting, whereas in the latter strategy no a priori parameters should be set before calculation of the signal envelope. For this reason this is the method implemented in this system, that is, the absolute value of the complex analytic signal (also known as the complex envelope [13]) is used to estimate the signal envelope.

From the signal envelope, local minima and local maxima points are estimated. This will reduce the number of candidate points to be searched by the peak detector. As a consequence, the processing time will also be reduced, which may be relevant for the analysis of either long or oversampled time-series. Another benefit of this stage is that noise activity may be eliminated.

The role of the peak detector is to search for extrema points which are above or below a threshold. Once a maximum (w_o) is found, the mean of the small window, $h_o = w_o + u$, is estimated and only if this mean is above the pre-defined threshold, w_o will be selected as the beginning of an RA. In this system u is set to 1 ms. Note that the analysis of the mean of h_o may avert the selection of spurious activity (e.g. noise). The end of an RA is detected when a minimum (w_f) is found. In this case, w_f is considered to be valid only if the mean of the window $h_o = w_o - u$ is below the threshold.

The threshold, th, is estimated as $th = k \times std(W_{noise})$, where W_{noise} is a window of noise directly selected from the analysed signal, $std(W_{noise})$ is the standard deviation of W_{noise}, and k is a user-defined constant which controls the threshold level. A typical value for k is 5. It is supported by the Chebyshev theorem [26]. This theorem states that, for any distribution, if $k > 1$ then the fraction of observations that fall within a range of $\pm k \times std(W_{noise})$ around the mean is at least $F = 1 - (1/k^2)$. For instance, $F = 0.96$ for $k = 5$, which means in practice that any sample within the interval $[mean(W_{noise}) - k \times std(W_{noise}), mean(W_{noise}) + k \times std(W_{noise})]$ has a 96% chance of really being noise.

4.1.4. Feature selection

In the feature selection stage, features will be selected for use in data clustering from a window within the region of activity. Figure 14 shows reference points in time (w_o, p_o, p, p_f, w_f) for definition of this window.

w_o and w_f are respectively the time when the region of activity starts and ends. These points are estimated by the detector of regions of activity. p is the time when the highest peak in the

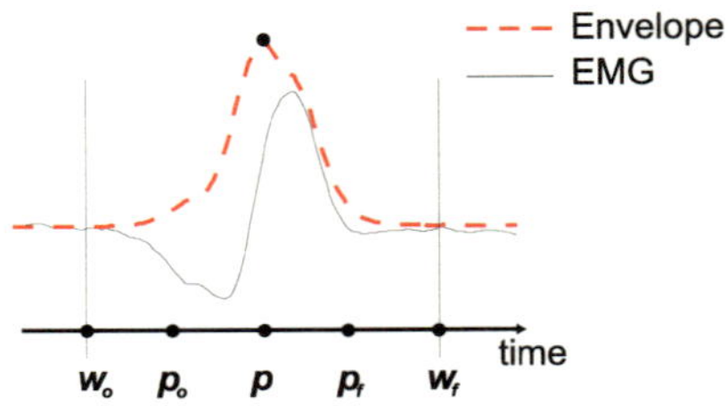

Figure 14. Identification of reference points in time for feature selection. w_o and w_f indicate the beginning and end of the region of activity. p is the time when the highest peak in the envelope and within the interval $[w_o, w_f]$ occurs, and p_o and p_f define the boundaries of a rectangular window for feature selection.

envelope of the RA occurs. This point is also the point where the variation in amplitude of the signal is maximal within the RA. This is illustrated in Figure 13.

p_o and p_f are respectively the beginning and end of the window to be selected for analysis. These points are defined as follows: $p_o = p - min\{t_o, p - w_o\}$ and $p_f = p + min\{t_o, w_f - p\}$, with t_o set to 2 ms. Note that the width of the window defined by p_o and p_f may vary for different RAs. Therefore, interpolation (splines) was employed for selection of 40 samples from each window defined in the interval $[p_o, p_f]$. This means that after feature selection each pattern is represented by a 40D vector with samples obtained via an interpolation procedure.

4.1.5. Data visualization and clustering

In order to ease the application of the sequence of steps detailed in Figure 10 a graphical user interface (GUI) was devised. The main GUI is shown in Figure 15. The system is capable of importing EMG data organized in columns of a text file and storing them in user-defined variables which are available in a list box. The main interface is organized into four logical sections (tabs) that should be accessed sequentially.

Figure 16 shows the module which allows the user to filter the EMG signal. The filtering procedure based on the Empirical Mode Decomposition is available here. The result of the automatic detection of regions activity is given in the interface shown in Figure 17.

The results of the data clustering and visualization step are presented in the GUI shown in Figure 18. At this stage patterns are clustered by means of Generative Topographic Mapping (GTM) and data visualization is performed with the GTM grid [3, 9]. For generation of the GTM grid, a GTM model with 25 Gaussian functions and 16 basis functions with a width of 1 is fitted to the data. The data can also be projected onto the two-dimensional space so that the user can visualize the distances of distinct groups of MUAPs (see Figure 19).

5. The application of EMG decomposition in the treatment of neuromuscular disorders triggered by stroke

Stroke, or cerebrovascular accident (CVA), affects a great number of individuals, and is the leading cause of disability among adults [10, 24]. After the event, most individuals must deal with severe reduction of motor functionality [31].

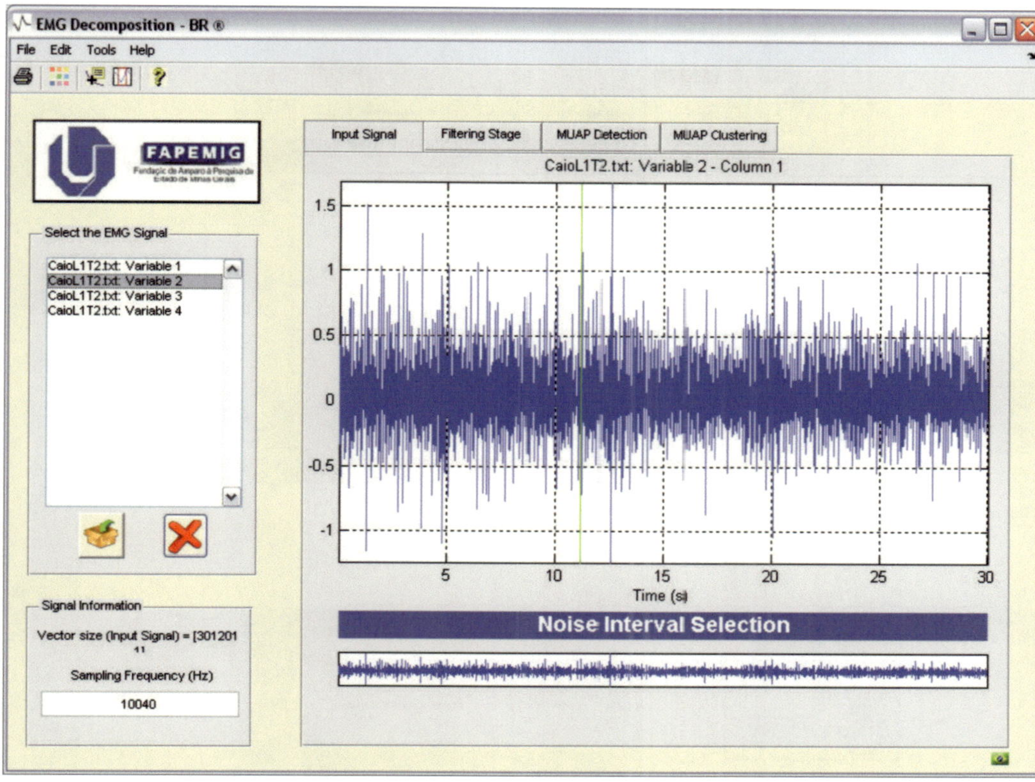

Figure 15. Main graphical user interface of a software that implements the sequence of steps detailed in Figure 10.

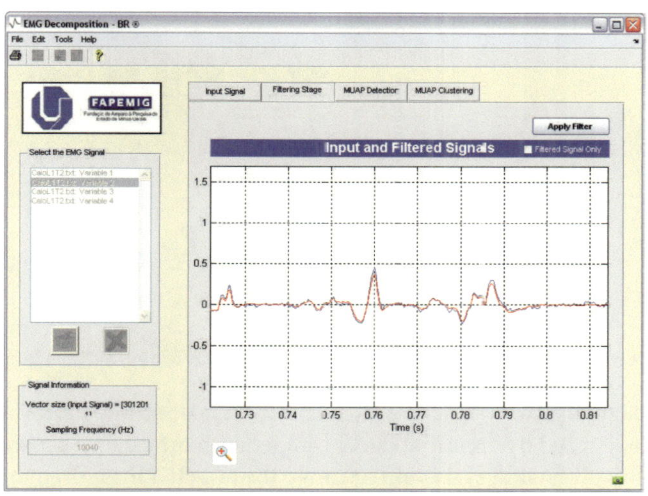

Figure 16. Graphical user interface which allows the user to filter the input signal.

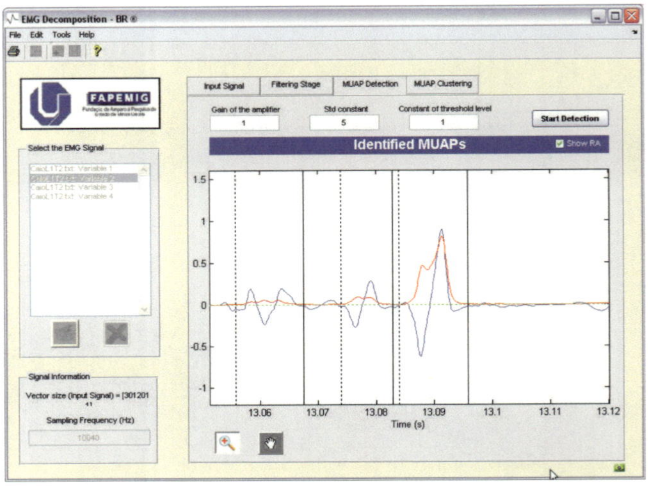

Figure 17. Automatic detection of regions of activity.

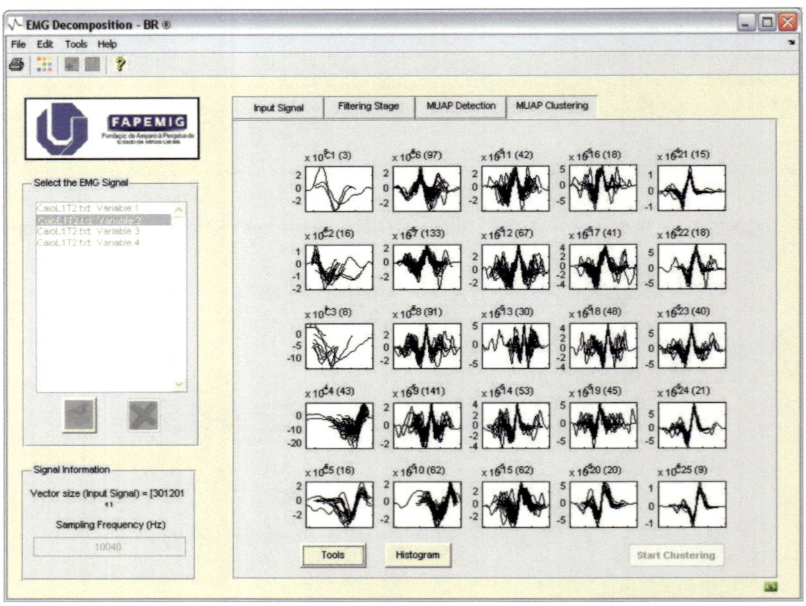

Figure 18. Data clustering and visualization based on Generative Topographic Mapping [3, 9].

Hemiplegia and spasticity are among the most common post-stroke motor deficits. In general, hemiplegia is characterized by an initial flaccid stage, with motor and sensory losses, in which the patient finds himself unable to sustain or move the affected limb. In many cases, the motor sequel evolves into spasticity, a stage characterized by muscle hypertonia. Hemiplegia and spasticity are closely related to the disuse of the affected limb and to secondary changes in muscles, such as: selective atrophy of fast twitch type II muscle fibers, abnormal recruitment

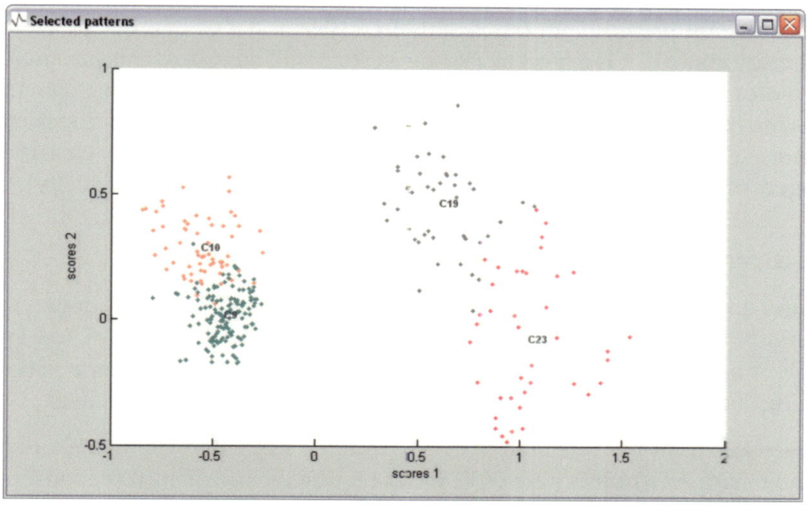

Figure 19. Two-dimensional visualization of groups of MUAPs obtained from the application of Principal Component Analysis.

of motor units, muscle contractures, and decreased cortical representation, due to disuse of the affected limb [28].

Several rehabilitation therapies have been used in an attempt to recover motor functionality, especially for upper limbs. The majority is based on the premise that the neural system can be retrained [20, 34]. The ability of the neural system to adapt to a new structural and functional condition, as well as its response to a traumatic destructive injury or to subtle changes resulting from the processes of learning and memory, is called 'neuroplasticity" [1, 12].

Recent studies have shown that behavioral experiments, important tools used in rehabilitation strategies based biofeedback techniques, have a strong impact on the motor cortical representation post-stroke. In this sense, we can also infer that it is possible to use biofeedback strategies for the modulation of neural plasticity, seeking the recovery of motor skills in rehabilitation protocols. The question is: how can we generate the appropriate information for feedback in a situation where the encephalic damage is manifested by an uncontrolled recruitment, or the lack of recruitment, of muscle fibers - leading to involuntary muscle hypotonia or hypertonia? Looking for a solution to this problem, a novel strategy, based in the assessment of the recruitment rate of motor units, is under test (see [39]), to generate control information for a multimodal biofeedback system. In this approach, instead of simply evaluating the process of muscle contraction, the researches decided to focus on the neural control over the muscles. However, the information regarding the recruitment of motor units are not readily available through standard surface EMG. Hence, the biofeedback relies heavily on a robust EMG decomposition system.

The strategy addressed by [39] is based on the discrimination and feature extraction of EMG signals (Motor Unit Action Potential) in order to control a virtual device. The biofeedback protocol immerses the patient in a virtual reality environment in which a representation of the affected limb will be presented. This virtual member is controlled according to the pattern of motor unit recruitment. Thus, although the spastic or hemiplegic patient lacks of proper voluntary control, it is expected that the system will be able to capture small voluntary changes in motor recruitment, as a result of his desire to do so. These changes can then be used to guide the movements of the virtual member. In so doing, the virtual feedback operates as a guide, indicating that the current mental strategy (neuromotor control) is correct and should be encouraged, reinforcing the process of neural reorganization (neuroplasticity).

6. Future directions

The widespread use of automatic tools for decomposing EMG signals is dependent on how easy is to detect MUAPs from the surface of the skin, on the identification of new applications, either online or offline, which might employ the results of the EMG decomposition, and also on the sharing and availability of developed tools to clinicians and researchers.

Ideally the sensors used for detecting MUAPs from the surface of the skin should be easy of applying and using. As a number of applications require the use of multiple sensors organized on an array the solution to this issue becomes more complex. Therefore, further research on this area, with the aim of developing sensors that allow for the reproduction of experiments is required.

Most applications found in the area of EMG decomposition are solely focused on the development of the automatic tool for decomposing the EMG signal, or in the classification and discrimination of MUAPs. Therefore, the identification of new useful applications are required in order to disseminate the relevance of the technique to other areas. For instance, the use of motor unit information could be employed in robotics, myofeedback, and human-machine interface development.

A major limitation of the results in the area of EMG decomposition is that the developed tools are not shared by researchers. The sharing of these tools together with EMG signal databases could be beneficial to the widespread use of the tools. Furthermore, this would allow researchers to objectively compare distinct solutions.

Considering the application of artefact removal from biomedical signals, the development of algorithms for reducing the influence of noise over signals in real time, without a priori knowledge about the origins and characteristics of the noise, are required. In this way the application of adaptive techniques such as Empirical Mode Decomposition should be further exploited.

It is also expected that the use of these filters can be part of the solution of the problem of EMG decomposition by directly decomposing the raw EMG signal into its motor unit action potential trains. If such filters are developed, EMG decomposition tools could be embedded in hardware speeding up the results from multichannel data.

Acknowledgements

The authors would like to express their gratitude to the Research Foundation of the State of Minas Gerais (FAPEMIG), The National Council for Scientific and Technological Development (CNPq) and the Coordination for the Improvement of Higher Education Personnel (CAPES).

Author details

Adriano O. Andrade and Alcimar B. Soares
Faculty of Electrical Engineering, Laboratory of Biomedical Engineering, Federal University of Uberlândia, Uberlândia, Brazil

Slawomir J. Nasuto
School of Systems Engineering, University of Reading, Reading, United Kingdom

Peter J. Kyberd
Institute of Biomedical Engineering, University of New Brunswick, Fredericton, Canada

7. References

[1] I Adams. Comparison of synaptic changes in the precentral and postcentral cerebral cortex of aging humans: a quantitative ultrastructural study. *Neurobiology of Aging*, 8:203–12, 1987.

[2] Metin Akay. *Biomedical signal processing*. Academic Press, Inc, San Diego, California, 1st edition, 1994.

[3] Adriano O Andrade. *Decomposition and Analysis of Electromyographic Signals*. PhD thesis, University of Reading, Reading, UK, 2005.

[4] Adriano O Andrade, Peter J Kyberd, and Slawomir J Nasuto. Time-frequency analysis of surface electromyographic signals via Hilbert spectrum. In Serge H Roy, Paolo Bonato, and Jens Meyer, editors, *XVth ISEK Congress - An Invitation to Innovation*, page 68.

[5] Adriano O Andrade, Peter J Kyberd, and Slawomir J Nasuto. The application of the Hilbert spectrum to the analysis of electromyographic signals. *Information Sciences*, 178(9):2176–2193, 2008.

[6] Adriano O Andrade, Peter J Kyberd, and Sean D Taffler. A novel spectral representation of electromyographic signals. In Ron S. Leder, editor, *Engineering in Medicine and Biology Society - 25th Annual International Conference*, volume 1, pages 2598–2601. IEEE.

[7] Adriano O Andrade, Slawomir J Nasuto, and Peter J Kyberd. EMG signal filtering based on empirical mode decomposition. *Biomedical Signal Processing and Control*, 1(1):44–55, 2006.

[8] Adriano O Andrade, Slawomir J Nasuto, and Peter J Kyberd. Extraction of motor unit action potentials from electromyographic signals through generative topographic mapping. *Journal of the Franklin Institute*, 344(3-4 (May-July)):154–179, 2007.

[9] Adriano O Andrade, Slawomir J Nasuto, Peter J Kyberd, and Catherine M Sweeney-Reed. Generative topographic mapping applied to clustering and visualization of motor unit action potentials. *Biosystems*, 82(3):273–84, 2005.

[10] American Heart Association. Heart disease and stroke statistics — 2011 update: a report from the american heart association. *Circulation*, 123:e18–e209, 2011.

[11] Alfredo Avellido and Adriano O Andrade. Determination of feature relevance for the grouping of motor unit action potentials through a generative mixture model. *Biomedical Signal Processing and Control*, 2:111–121, 2007.

[12] S N Burke and C A Barnes. Neural plasticity in the ageing brain. *Nature Reviews Neuroscience*, (7):30–40, 2006.

[13] Lokenath Debnath and Piotr Mikusinski. *Introduction to Hilbert Spaces with applications*. Academic Press, San Diego, CA, second edition, 1999.

[14] David L Donoho. De-noising by soft-thresholding. *IEEE Transactions on Information Theory*, 41(3):613–627, 1995.

[15] H Etawil and Daniel W Stashuk. Resolving superimposed motor unit action potentials. *Medical and Biological Engineering and Computing*, 34(1):33–40, 1996.

[16] Jianjun Fang, Gyan C Agarwal, and Bhagwan T Shahani. Decomposition of multiunit electromyographic signals. *IEEE Transactions on Biomedical Engineering*, 46(6):685–697, 1999.

[17] Gonzalo A. Garcia, Kenzo Akazawa, and Ryuhei Okuno. Decomposition of surface electrode-array electromyogram of biceps brachii muscle in voluntary isometric contraction. In *Engineering in Medicine and Biology Society - 25th Annual International Conference*, pages 2483–2486. IEEE.

[18] Tamara Grujic and Ana Kuzmanic. Denoising of surface emg signals: a comparison of wavelet and classical digital filtering procedures. *Technology and Healthcare*, 12(2):130–135, 2004.

[19] Mohamed H Hassoun, Chuanming Wang, and A Robert Spitzer. NNERVE: Neural network extraction of repetitive vectors for electromyography - part I: Algorithm. *IEEE Transactions on Biomedical Engineering*, 41(11):1039 – 1051, 1994.

[20] Koichi Hiraoka. Rehabilitation effort to improve upper extremity function in post-stroke patients: A meta-analysis. *Journal of Physical Therapy Science*, 13:5–9, 2001.

[21] Norden E Huang, Zheng Shen, Steven R Long, Manli C Wu, Hsing H Shih, Quanan Zheng, Nai-Chyuan Yen, Chi Chao Tung, and Henry H Liu. The empirical mode decomposition and the Hilbert spectrum for nonlinear and non-stationary time series analysis. *Proceedings of Royal Society of London*, 454:903–995, 1998.

[22] R S LeFever and Carlo J De Luca. A procedure for decomposing the myoelectric signal into its constituent action potentials–part I: Technique, theory, and implementation. *IEEE Transactions on Biomedical Engineering*, 29(3):149–57, 1982.

[23] M. Lei and G. Meng. Classification of the action surface emg signals based on the dirichlet process mixtures method. volume 7101 LNAI of *4th International Conference on Intelligent Robotics and Applications, ICIRA 2011*, pages 212–220. Aachen, 2011.

[24] I Lessa. Epidemiologia das doenças cerebrovasculares no brasil. *Revista da Sociedade de Cardiologia do Estado de Sao Paulo*, 4:509–518, 1999.

[25] Michael S Lewicki. A review of methods for spike sorting: the detection and classification of neural action potentials. *Comput. Neural Syst.*, 9:R53 – R78, 1998.

[26] H Lohninger. *Teach/Me Data Analysis*. Springer-Verlag, Berlin, Germany, 1999.

[27] Carlos J De Luca. Decomposition of the EMG signal into constituent motor unit action potentials. *Muscle Nerve*, 18(12):1492–4, 1995.

[28] L Lundy-Ekman. *Neurociencias: fundamentos para reabilitaçao*, pages 155–199. Elsevier, Rio de Janeiro, 2008.

[29] Bruno Mambrito and Carlo J. De Luca. A technique for the detection, decomposition and analysis of the EMG signal. *Electroencephalography and clinical neurophysiology*, 58:175–188, 1984.

[30] H. R. Marateb, S. Muceli, K. C. McGill, R. Merletti, and D. Farina. Robust decomposition of single-channel intramuscular emg signals at low force levels. *Journal of Neural Engineering*, 8(6), 2011.

[31] N E Mayo, S Wood-Dauphinee, S Ahmed, C Gordon, J Higgins, S McEwen, and N Salbach. Disablement following stroke. *Disabil. Rehabil.*, 21(5-6):258–268, 1999.

[32] Kevin C. McGill, Kenneth L. Cummins, and Leslie J. Dorfman. Automatic decomposition of the clinical electromyogram. *IEEE Transactions on Biomedical Engineering*, BME-32(7):470–477, 1985.

[33] Michel Misiti, Yves Misiti, Georges Oppenheim, and Jean-Michel Poggi. *Wavelet toolbox user's guide*. The Mathworks, Inc, third edition, 2004.

[34] Susan O'Sullivan and Thomas Schmitz. *Fisioterapia: Avaliaçao e Tratamento*. Manole, 2010.

[35] H. Parsaei and D. W. Stashuk. A method for detecting and editing mupts contaminated by false classification errors during EMG signal decomposition. 33rd Annual International Conference of the IEEE Engineering in Medicine and Biology Society, EMBS 2011, pages 4394–4397.

[36] H. Parsaei and D. W. Stashuk. SVM-based validation of motor unit potential trains extracted by EMG signal decomposition. *IEEE transactions on biomedical engineering*, 59(1):183–191, 2012.

[37] Constantinos S Pattichis and Marios S Pattichis. Time-scale analysis of motor unit action potentials. *IEEE Transactions on Biomedical Engineering*, 46(11):1320 – 1329, 1999.

[38] G. L. Sheean. Quantification of motor unit action potential energy. *Clinical Neurophysiology*, 123(3):621–625, 2012.

[39] M B Silva, D Viera, Ângela A R de Sá, and Alcimar Barbosa Soares. Proposta de treinamento com biofeedback eletromiográfico em ambiente de realidade virtual como apoio a reabilitaçao motora após acidente vascular encefálico. In *2o Congresso Brasileiro de Eletromiografia e Cinesiologia, COBEC 2012*, pages 1–3.

[40] Daniel W Stashuk. Decomposition and quantitative analysis of clinical electromyographic signals. *Med Eng Phys*, 21(6-7):389–404, 1999.

[41] Daniel W Stashuk and G M Paoli. Robust supervised classification of motor unit action potentials. *Medical and Biological Engineering and Computing*, 36:75–82, 1998.

[42] Daniel W Stashuk and Y Qu. Adaptive motor unit action potential clustering using shape and temporal information. *Medical and Biological Engineering and Computing*, 34(1):41–9, 1996.

[43] Tzyh-Yi Sun, Thy-Sheng Lin, and Jia-Jin Chen. Multielectrode surface EMG for noninvasive estimation of motor unit size. *Muscle and Nerve*, 22:1063 – 1070, 1999.

[44] S Usui and I Amidor. Digital low-pass differentiation for biological signal processing. *IEEE Transactions on Biomedical Engineering*, 29:686–693, 1982.

[45] N. W. Willigenburg, A. Daffertshofer, I. Kingma, and J. H. van Dieën. Removing ecg contamination from emg recordings: A comparison of ica-based and other filtering procedures. *Journal of electromyography and kinesiology*, 2012.

[46] Zhengquan Xu and Shaojun Xiao. Digital filter design for peak detection of surface EMG. *Journal of Electromyography and Kinesiology*, 10:275–281, 2000.

[47] F. Zaheer, S. H. Roy, and C. J. De Luca. Preferred sensor sites for surface emg signal decomposition. *Physiological Measurement*, 33(2):195–206, 2012.

[48] Daniel Zennaro, Peter Wellig, Volker M. Koch, George S. Moschytz, and Thomas Laubli. A software package for the decomposition of long-term multichannel EMG signals using wavelet coefficients. *IEEE Transactions on Biomedical Engineering*, 50(1):58–69, 2003.

[49] Ping Zhou, Zeynep Erim, and W Z Rymer. Motor unit action potential counts in surface electrode array EMG. In *Engineering in Medicine and Biology Society - 25th Annual International Conference*, pages 2067–2070. IEEE.

Chapter 12

Sphincter EMG for Diagnosing Multiple System Atrophy and Related Disorders

Ryuji Sakakibara, Tomoyuki Uchiyama, Tatsuya Yamamoto, Fuyuki Tateno, Tomonori Yamanishi, Masahiko Kishi and Yohei Tsuyusaki

Additional information is available at the end of the chapter

http://dx.doi.org/10.5772/45880

1. Introduction

One of the hallmarks in the pathology of multiple system atrophy (MSA) is neuronal loss in the sacral Onuf's nucleus[11,33,37]. Onuf's nucleus plays a key role in urinary and fecal continence[12]. Neurons in this nucleus receive not only cortical inputs, but also noradrenergic and serotonergic facilitatory inputs via interneurons from various brainstem structures, including the pontine urine-storage center[57,68]. External anal sphincter (EAS)-electromyography (EMG) is an established method to detect neurogenic change in motor unit potentials (MUP), which mostly reflects denervation and reinnervation of the sphincter muscle[30]. The significance of the EAS-EMG in MSA has been well known[30,69,74]. Physiologically, external urethral sphincter (EUS) and EAS share sacral pudendal innervation from Onuf's nucleus[20]. In this article, we review the normal physiology and pathophysiology of the lower urinary tract and the lower gastrointestinal tract briefly, the current methods and interpretations of EAS or EUS-EMG, and sphincter EMG in autonomic disorders.

2. Physiology and pathophysiology of the lower urinary tract

The lower urinary tract consists of two major components, the bladder and urethra. The bladder is abundant with muscarinic M2,3 receptors (contraction) and adrenergic beta 3 receptors (relaxation)[12]. The urethra is abundant with adrenergic alpha 1A/D receptors (contraction) and nicotinic receptors (contraction) **(Fig. 1)**. The storage and emptying functions need an intact neuraxis that involves almost all parts of the nervous system[48]. This is in contrast to postural hypotension, which arises due to lesions below the medullary circulation center[56].

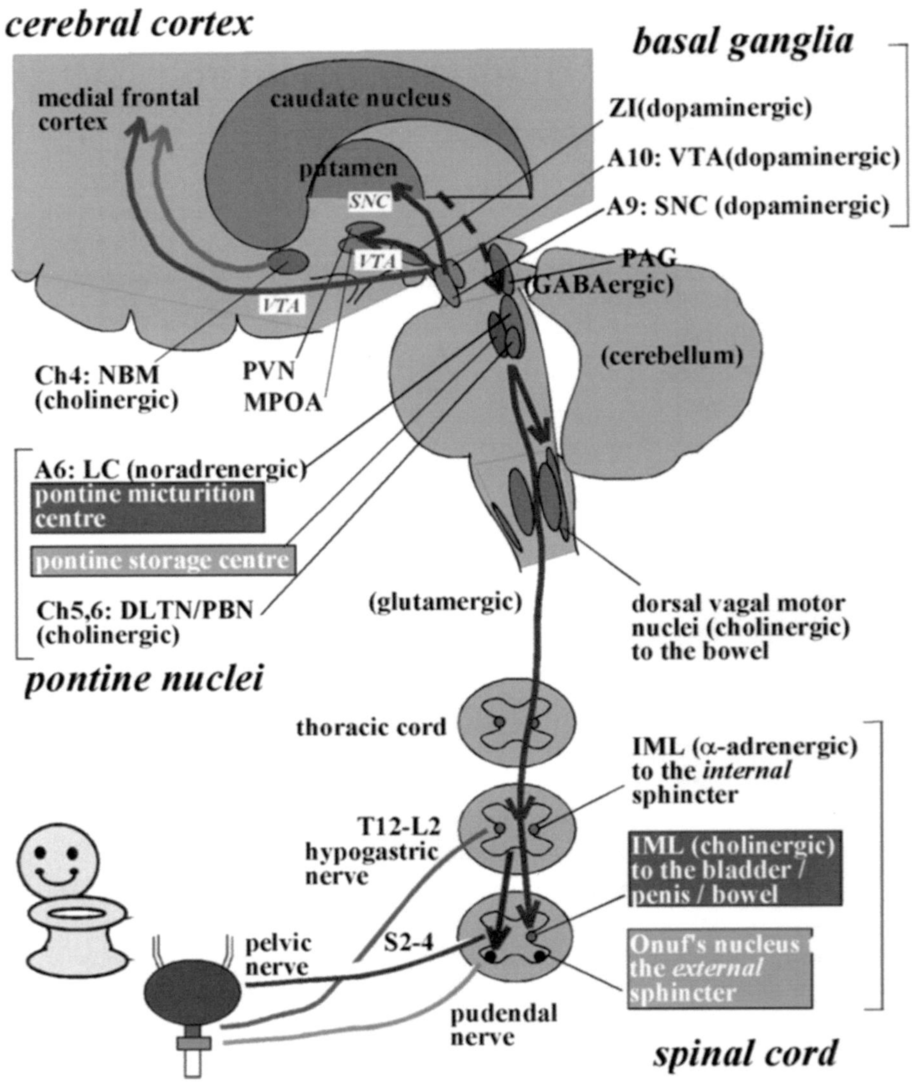

The lower urinary tract consists of two major components, the bladder and the urethra. The bladder is mainly innervated by the parasympathetic pelvic nerve. The urethra is innervated by the sympathetic hypogastric nerve and somatic pudendal nerve, respectively. Urinary storage is dependent on the reflex arc of the sacral spinal cord. The storage reflex is thought to be tonically facilitated by the brain, particularly the pontine storage center. The storage function is thought to be further facilitated by the hypothalamus, cerebellum, basal ganglia, and frontal cortex. Central cholinergic fibers from the nucleus basalis Meynert (NBM, also called the Ch4 cell group) seem to facilitate urinary storage. Micturition is dependent on the reflex arc of the brainstem and spinal cord, which involves the midbrain periaqueductal gray (PAG) and the pontine micturition center (located in or adjacent to the locus coeruleus [LC]). The voiding function is thought to be initiated by the hypothalamus and prefrontal cortex, which overlap the storage-facilitating area.
PVN: paraventricular nucleus, MPOA: medial preoptic area, A: adrenergic/noradrenergic, ZI: zona incerta, VTA: ventral tegmental area, SNC: substantia nigra pars compacta, DLTN: dorsolateral tegmental nucleus, PBN: parabrachial nucleus, IML: IML cell column, GABA: γ-aminobutyric acid, T: thoracic, L: lumbar, S: sacral
(cited from ref. 41)

Figure 1. Neural circuitry relevant to micturition.

Urinary storage is dependent on the autonomic reflex arc of the sacral cord[12]. This reflex is tonically facilitated by the brain, particularly the pontine storage center,[7,57] hypothalamus, cerebellum, basal ganglia, and frontal cortex[25]. In contrast, micturition is dependent on the autonomic reflex arc of the brainstem and spinal cord[12]. This reflex involves the periaqueductal gray[12,32,78] and the pontine micturition center (PMC)[6,7,12,54,63]. The PMC facilitates the sacral bladder preganglionic nucleus by glutamate[35], while inhibiting the sacral Onuf's nucleus by γ-amino-butyric acid (GABA) and glycine[8]. This reflex is regulated by the hypothalamus and prefrontal cortex[16,25].

Bladder (detrusor) overactivity is the major cause of urinary urgency/frequency and urgency incontinence[66]. In lesions above the brainstem, detrusor overactivity is considered an exaggerated micturition reflex[66]. This is in line with the fact that detrusor overactivity appearing after experimental stroke requires mRNA synthesis in the PMC[83]. The exaggeration of the micturition reflex might be brought about not only by decreased inhibition of the brain (by central cholinergic and D1 dopaminergic mechanisms); that is, it might be further facilitated by glutamatergic and D2 dopaminergic mechanisms[82]. Underactive detrusor (or bladder weakness) is the major cause of voiding difficulty in autonomic disorders. Underactive detrusor results from lesions in either upper or lower neurons innervating the bladder muscles, but typically occurs from lower neuron lesions.[1,48]

Urinary urgency incontinence and voiding difficulty in MSA result mostly from detrusor overactivity and underactive detrusor, respectively.[1,48] Patients with MSA often have a combination of detrusor overactivity in the filling phase and underactive detrusor in the voiding phase; this is called detrusor hyperactivity with impaired contractile function (DHIC). DHIC presumably reflects multiple lesions in both the storage-facilitating areas (the basal ganglia, pontine storage center) and the voiding-facilitating areas (the PMC, sacral preganglionic neurons in the intermediolateral [IML] cell columns) of this disorder.[23,79] In MSA, incomplete emptying is thought to be secondary to IML involvement.

Sphincter dysfunction contributes to voiding difficulty and urinary incontinence in autonomic disorders, although less commonly than over- or underactive detrusor does. When the urethral sphincter does not relax properly during voiding bladder contraction, it is called detrusor-sphincter dyssynergia.[1] Since a coordinated micturition reflex (bladder contraction with sphincter relaxation) needs an intact brainstem–sacral cord axis,[12] disruption of the axis (such as lesions affecting the cervical/thoracic spinal cord) may lead to detrusor–sphincter dyssynergia. Sphincter weakness is a cause of urinary incontinence. Sphincter weakness occurs from lesions in the sacral motoneurons (Onuf's nucleus), and typically appears in women with MSA as severe stress incontinence[49] or continuous urinary incontinence[34].

3. Physiology and pathophysiology of the lower gastrointestinal tract

The enteric nervous system plays the most important role in regulating the peristaltic reflex of the lower gastrointestinal tract[20]. Two types of myoelectrical activity or pressure changes in the colon are documented. Slow phasic pressure waves are the most common manometric phenomenon[26], and in humans are measured as spontaneous phasic rectal contraction[9,22]. The peristaltic reflex can be evoked by surface stroking or by circumferential stretching.[20] The reflex consists of two components: ascending contraction (mediated by cholinergic fibers) oral to the stimulus site, and descending relaxation (mediated by non-adrenergic, non-cholinergic fibers) caudal to the stimulus site[2].

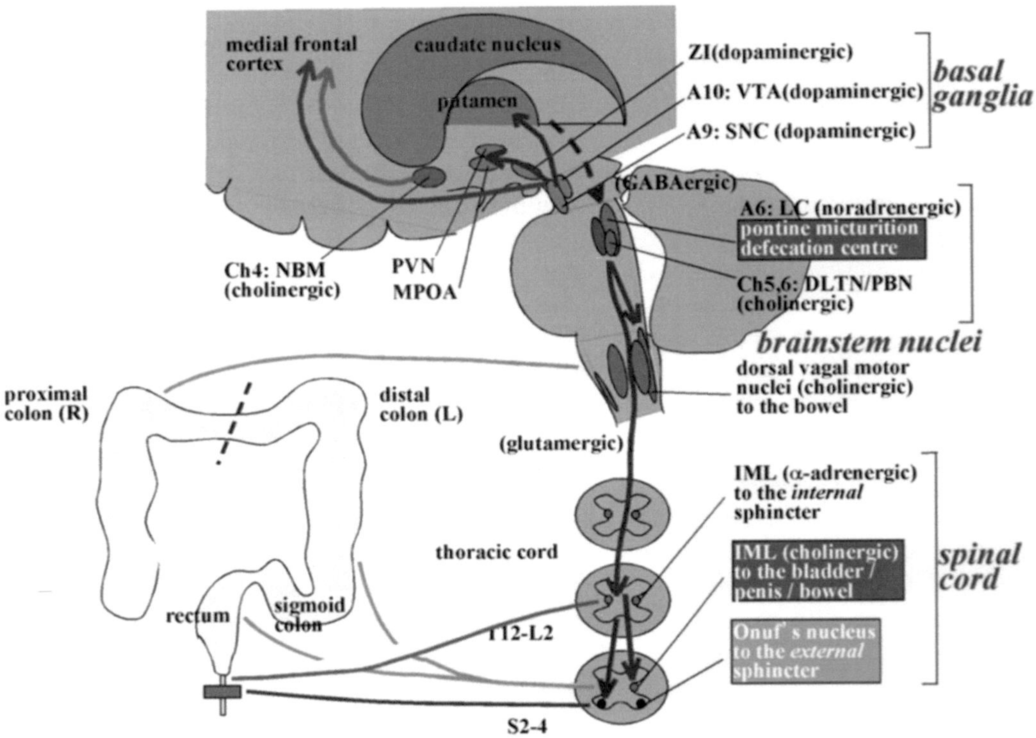

The function of the lower gastrointestinal tract is thought to depend on the brain and spinal cord, although less significantly than the lower urinary tract (LUT) does. Whereas the small intestine and ascending colon are innervated by the vagus nerves originating in the medulla, the descending colon, sigmoid colon, and rectum primarily share sacral innervation of the LUT (Figure 1). Both the sacral cord and the vagus nuclei receive projecting fibers from Barrington's nucleus (the pontine micturition/defecation center). Bowel function seems to be modulated by the higher brain structures, including the frontal lobe, the hypothalamus, and the basal ganglia; the main action of the latter on the bowel seems to be inhibitory.

NBM: nucleus basalis Meynert, Ch: cholinergic, PVN: paraventricular nucleus, MPOA: medial preoptic area, ZI: zona incerta, A: adrenergic/noradrenergic, VTA: ventral tegmental area, SNC: substantia nigra pars compacta, LC: locus ceruleus, DLTN: dorsolateral tegmental nucleus, PBN: parabrachial nucleus, PAG: periaqueductal gray, IML: IML cell column, GABA: γ-aminobutyric acid, T: thoracic, L: lumbar, S: sacral

(cited from ref. 41)

Figure 2. Neural circuitry relevant to defecation.

Other types of pressure changes in the colon include giant motor complexes[20]. A giant motor complex is a cyclic contractile activity with a periodicity of 20 to 30 min, and is perhaps analogous to the migrating motor complex of the small intestine[26]. A combination of slow waves and giant motor complexes is thought to promote bowel transport, which in humans is measured by colonic transit time[4]. The strength of cholinergic transmission in the enteric nervous system is thought to be regulated by opposing receptors; serotonin 5-HT4 receptor-mediating excitation[31,73] and dopamine D2 receptor-mediating inhibition[76].

Whereas the rostral lower gastrointestinal tract is innervated by the vagus nerves originating in the medulla, extra-enteric innervation of the caudal lower gastrointestinal tract primarily shares the innervation of the lower urinary tract **(Fig. 2)**[12,22]. The lower urinary tract and lower gastrointestinal tracts perform similar functions of storage and emptying. However, they differ profoundly with regard to anatomy (closed bag versus open-ended tube, respectively), luminal contents (liquid versus half-solid), and physiology (dysfunctional transport, rare ureter versus common bowel; smooth muscle contraction, bladder contraction only on emptying versus persistent spontaneous phasic rectal contraction; abdominal strain, minimal on urination versus strong on defecation)[22]. In addition, while the lower urinary tract requires an intact neuraxis for storage and emptying[12], it has not been entirely clear to what extent the lower gastrointestinal tract needs the extra-enteric nervous system.

Constipation in MSA most probably results from slow colonic transit, decreased phasic rectal contraction, and weak abdominal strain.[58] Some patients also have paradoxical sphincter contraction on defecation (PSCD).[58] The sites responsible for this dysfunction seem to be both the central and peripheral nervous systems, which regulate the lower gastrointestinal tract. Slow colonic transit and decreased phasic rectal contraction most probably reflect peripheral enteric nervous system lesions, whereas weak abdominal strain and PSCD may reflect central lesions.[61] In contrast, fecal incontinence results mostly from a weak anal sphincter due to denervation.[58]

4. Physiology and pathophysiology of the genital organ

The genital organ primarily shares lumbosacral innervation with the lower urinary tract. Erection is a vascular event[3]; occurring secondarily after dilatation of the cavernous helical artery and compression of the cavernous vein to the tunica albuginea[3]. Helical artery dilatation is brought about by activation of cholinergic and nitrergic nerves; this activation facilitates nitric oxide secretion from the vascular endothelium. Ejaculation is brought about by contraction of the vas deferens and the bladder neck, in order to prevent retrograde ejaculation, by activation of adrenergic nerves **(Fig. 3)**. Sacral Onuf's nucleus innervates the bulbocavernosus muscle; and is thought to participate in erection and ejaculation. Sexual intercourse in healthy men can be divided into 3 phases[65]: a) desire (libido), b) excitement and erection, and c) orgasm, seminal emission from the vas deferens, and ejaculation from the penis. Erection can be further classified into 3 types by the relevant stimulation: 1) psychogenic erection (by audiovisual stimulation), 2) reflexive erection (by somatosensory stimulation), and 3) nocturnal penile tumescence (NPT) (associated with rapid eye movement [REM]-sleep). 'Morning erection' is considered the last NPT in the nighttime.

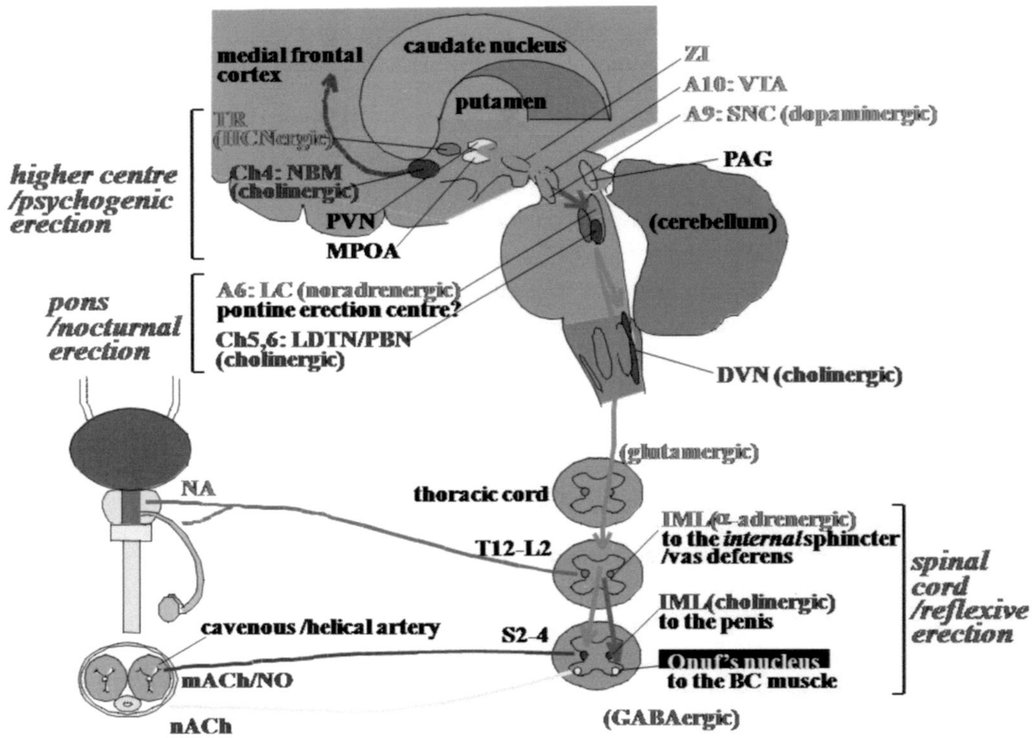

PAG, periaqueductal gray; LC, locus coeruleus; NBM, nucleus basalis Meynert; PVN, paraventricular nucleus; MPOA, medial preoptic area; A, adrenergic/noradrenergic; ZI, zona incerta; VTA, ventral tegmental area; SNC, substantia nigra pars compacta; DLTN, dorsolateral tegmental nucleus; PBN, parabrachial nucleus; IML, intermediolateral nucleus; GABA, γ-aminobutyric acid; T, thoracic; L, lumbar; S, sacral; NA, noradrenaline; Ach, acetylcholine; NO, nitric oxide. See text.

Figure 3. Neural circuitry relevant to erection.

Among the 3 types of erection, reflexive erection requires an intact sacral cord, particularly the intermediolateral (IML) cell columns. Pathology studies have shown that involvement of the IML nucleus is common in MSA, whereas it is uncommon in Parkinson's disease. Therefore, reflexive erection can be affected in patients with MSA. In patients with a supra-sacral spinal cord lesion, reflexive erection might be preserved, whereas psychogenic erection is severely disturbed because of a lesion in the spinal pathways to the sacral cord. Libido and erection are thought to be regulated by the hypothalamus; particularly the medial preoptic area (MPOA) and the paraventricular nucleus (PVN).[13,72] Recent neuroimaging studies have shown that penile stimulation or watching pornography activated these areas in humans[70]. NPT[15] seems to be regulated by the hypothalamic lateral preoptic area,[21] raphe nucleus, and locus ceruleus. Oxytocinergic neurons in the hypothalamic PVN are thought to facilitate erection by projecting directly to the sacral cord, and by projecting to the midbrain periaqueductal gray and the Barrington's nucleus (identical to the PMC).

In experimental animals, dopamine is known to facilitate erection and mating behaviors[13]. The MPOA/PVN receives projections from the nigral dopaminergic neurons. Prolactinergic neurons are thought to be inhibitory in sexual function. Prolactin-producing pituitary tumors often cause gynecomastia and erectile dysfunction in male patients. Hyperprolactinemia occurs after the use of sulpiride, metoclopramide, and chlorpromazine (all dopamine receptor antagonists). Therefore, dopaminergic neurons seem to facilitate oxytocinergic neurons whereas they inhibit prolactinergic neurons.

5. Methods and interpretations of sphincter EMG

In humans, the EUS and EAS share sacral pudendal innervation from Onuf's nucleus.[12,20] The EAS lies around the anal canal and forms an 8-shaped sphincter system on the pelvic floor **(Fig. 4)**. Although injury to the peripheral nerves may lead to the dysfunction of the EUS alone, lesions of the sacral Onuf's nucleus affect both the EAS and EUS. For this reason, we use EAS-EMG to assess urinary incontinence, as it is easier to perform and less painful than EUS-EMG. For the same reason, few studies have utilized EUS-EMG.[14,17] In women, the EUS muscle can be examined using a perineal approach. Examination of this muscle is more difficult in men; we can approach it with the fingers by feeling for the prostate within the rectum. However, EUS should be chosen in cases exhibiting a decelerating burst ('whale noise') with complex repetitive discharge in Fowler's syndrome.[24]

The EAS can be divided into a deep part (thick; around the rectal neck to the anal canal) and a subcutaneous part (thin; around the anus). The deep EAS is a major constituent in the generation of anal pressure to hold feces in when the rectum is full. The normal range of static anal pressure is more than 40 cmH_2O, and that of anal squeeze pressure is more than 50 cmH_2O.[22] The former is thought to reflect hypogastric adrenergic innervation, whereas the latter reflects somatic Onuf's nucleus innervation.[22] The subcutaneous EAS is easy to examine. It is reached by inserting a needle about 1 cm from the anal orifice, to a depth of 3–6 mm.[43]

Although the EAS is a skeletal muscle, it usually fires continuously during both waking and sleeping states. To assess EAS, an EMG computer with quantitative, template-operated MUP analysis software is recommended. The commonly used amplifier filter setting is 5–10 kHz. The tip of a concentric needle usually monitors an area approximately 500 micrometers in diameter, which includes approximately 20 MUPs. To assess acute denervation, insertion and spontaneous activities are checked as with the evaluation of other skeletal muscles. When the muscle is completely denervated, the EMG becomes silent. After an interval of 10–20 days, the insertion potentials become prolonged and abnormal spontaneous muscle activities, e.g., fibrillation potentials and positive sharp waves, appear. However, in the EAS, due to the continuous firing activities, it is not easy to see denervation potentials. In such cases, examination of the bulbocavernosus muscle has been recommended[44].

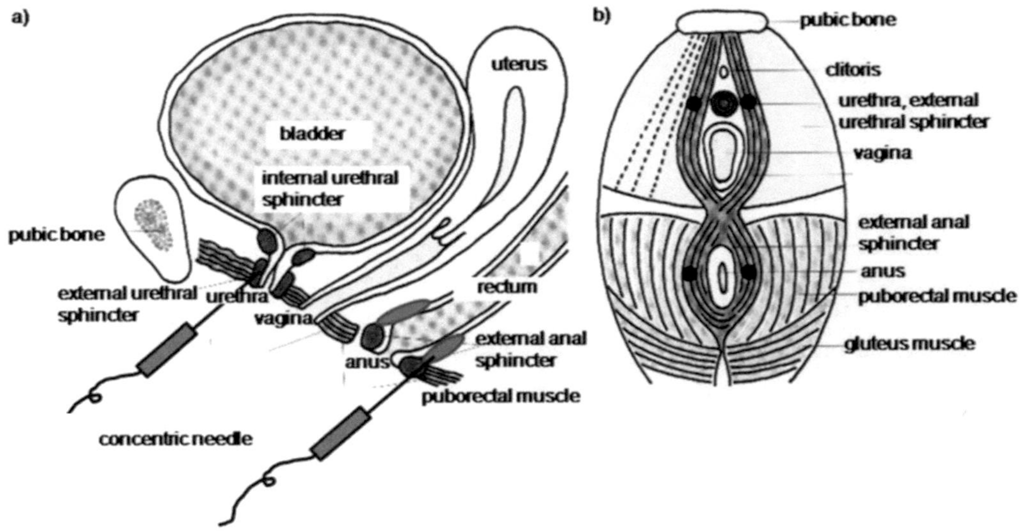

This figure illustrates where to insert concentric needles to measure external sphincter EMG.

Figure 4. The external anal sphincter and the external urethral sphincter.

A normal MUP usually has a 50–500 microV amplitude, a 3–8 msec duration, and 2–4 phases. In order to assess reinnervation, usually 10–20 single MUPs are recorded, which are automatically provided by an EMG computer. To ascertain single MUP, we still check each wave manually and adjust the onset and offset of each wave. It is particularly important to include late components (satellite potentials) to measure the duration of each unit.[42] When the muscle is chronically denervated, an intact nerve tends to innervate the adjacent denervated muscle fibers. As a result, MUPs become of high amplitude, of long duration, and polyphasic. Among various EMG parameters, the use of duration, MUP area, and number of turns is recommended for optimal diagnostic power (sensitivity and specificity) in the EAS muscle.[45] In addition, the results are dependent on the methods used; e.g., including or excluding late components. Palace et al. proposed that either of two criteria is sufficient to diagnose neurogenic changes in the EAS-EMG: (*a*) more than 20% of MUPs have a duration > 10 msec, or (*b*) the average duration of MUPs > 10 msec, particularly including the late components.[38] When satellite potentials were excluded, the duration of MUPs did not differ significantly between Parkinson's disease and MSA.[48] When lower motor neuron-type abnormalities are not apparent, it is reported that abnormal MUP recruitment pattern suggests pyramidal tract involvement.[18] In addition to MUP analysis in the external sphincter muscles, other neurophysiologic tests, e.g., pudendal nerve conduction, sacral reflexes, somatosensory evoked potentials and cranial magnetic stimulation, and urodynamic studies, can be of particular value in the study of autonomic patients.[29,40,41]

6. Sphincter EMG in autonomic disorders

6.1. MSA

Cardiovascular autonomic failure in MSA is thought to derive from neuron loss in the thoracolumbar intermediolateral (IML) cell columns of the spinal cord and the medullary circulation center. In contrast, lower urinary tract disorder in MSA is thought to reflect multiple lesions in the basal ganglia and the pontine storage center (storage-facilitating areas), as well as in the pontine micturition center in or adjacent to the locus ceruleus and the sacral IML cell columns (voiding-facilitating areas).[11] In addition, a distinguishing pathology in MSA is neuronal cell loss in the sacral Onuf nucleus.[33,37]

The first reports on neurogenic changes of EAS-EMG in MSA are attributed to Sakuta et al. (1978).[62] Since then, EAS-EMG results for over 500 MSA patients have been reported, with abnormality rates of more than 70% in many studies[5,30,36,38,47,53,62,64,71]. EAS-EMG is better tolerated and yields identical results to those from EUS investigation[5]. Abnormalities have also been recorded in the bulbocavernosus muscles in MSA.[67] In a larger study, Beck et al. (1994) reported that all (100%) 62 MSA patients with urological symptoms had abnormalities in both EAS and EUS-EMG.[5] Palace et al. (1997) reported abnormal EAS-EMG in 103 (82%) of 126 patients with MSA[38]. Chandiramani et al. (1997) found abnormal EAS-EMG in 49 (94%) of 52 patients with MSA[10]. Kirchhof et al. (1999) found abnormal EAS-EMG in 89 (91%) of 98 patients with MSA[28]. Sakakibara et al. (2000) found an abnormal EAS-EMG in 53 (74%) of 71 MSA patients[52]. These abnormalities correspond to selective loss of ventral horn cells and astrogliosis; the loss is particularly severe in the second and third sacral segments (Onuf's nucleus) in MSA[11]. Sphincter EMG has been proposed as a means of distinguishing between MSA and idiopathic Parkinson's disease (as described below), since the anterior horn cells of Onuf's nucleus are not affected in idiopathic Parkinson's disease.[10] In contrast, there have been debates about whether or not sphincter EMG can be used to distinguish MSA from idiopathic Parkinson's disease. In a study of 13 patients with idiopathic Parkinson's disease and 10 patients with MSA, Giladi et al. (2000) found significant overlap in all EMG parameters (presence of fibrillation potentials, MUP duration, presence of satellite potentials, percentage of polyphasic potentials)[19]. However, the durations of MUPs in both the MSA and Parkinson's disease groups were longer than in other studies.

It is reported that EAS-MUP abnormalities can distinguish MSA from idiopathic Parkinson's disease in the first 5 years after disease onset.[30,69,74] However, the prevalence of such abnormalities in the early stages of MSA has not been well known. In our recent study of 84 probable MSA cases, 62% exhibited neurogenic change.[80] The prevalence was relatively low presumably because up to 25% of our patients had a disease duration of 1 year or less. In such early cases, the diagnosis of MSA should be made with extreme caution. In addition to the clinical diagnostic criteria, we usually add an imaging study and we perform gene analysis to the extent possible. The prevalence of neurogenic change was 52% in the first year after disease onset, which increased to 83% by the fifth year (p<0.05) **(Fig. 5)**. Among the patients who underwent repeated studies, many had normal to mild abnormality at the initial examination, which turned into marked abnormality during the course of illness **(Fig. 6)**. Therefore, as expected, it is apparent that the involvement of Onuf's nucleus in MSA is time-dependent. In the early stages of illness, the prevalence of neurogenic change in MSA does not seem to be high. In 2 patients who underwent repeated studies, the EAS-EMG findings tended to remain normal. We do not know whether some MSA patients never develop neurogenic change during the course of their illness. However, Wenning et al. (1994) reported 3 patients with normal EAS-EMG and a postmortem confirmation of MSA.[77] Therefore, a negative result cannot exclude a diagnosis of MSA. More recently, Paviour et al. (2005) reported that among 30 sets of clinical data and postmortem confirmation in MSA cases with a duration of more than 5 years, 24 (80%) had abnormal EAS-EMG, 5 (17%) had a borderline result, and only 1 had a normal EMG.[39]

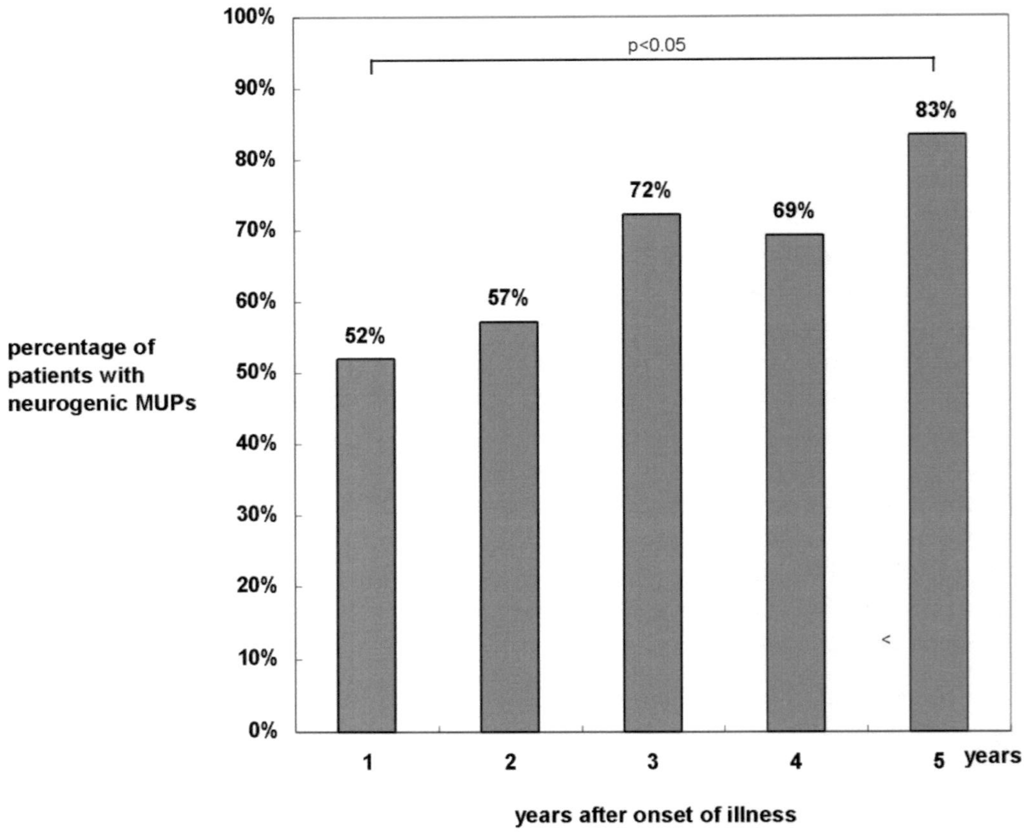

The prevalence of neurogenic sphincter EMG increased during the course of illness.
MUP: motor unit potential
(cited from ref. 74)

Figure 5. Neurogenic sphincter EMG and duration of illness.

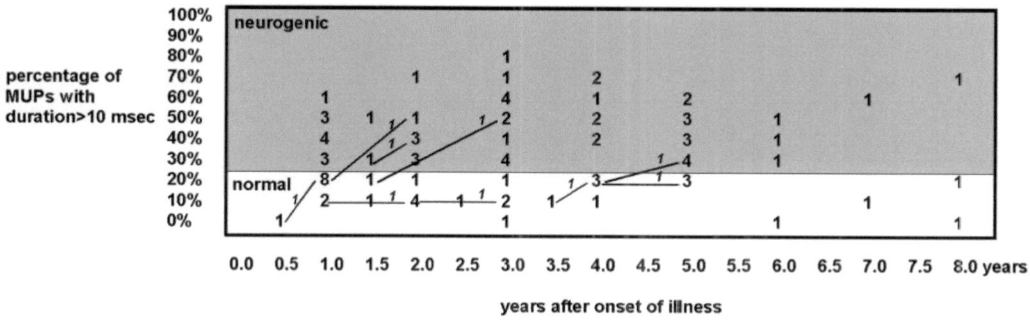

Percentage of MUPs with duration > 10 msec: one of two categories for neurogenic sphincter EMG.
straight figures: the number of patients
oblique figures: the number of patients who underwent the study repeatedly
MUP: motor unit potential
(cited from ref. 74)

Figure 6. Percentage of MUPs with duration > 10 msec and duration of illness.

The prevalence of neurogenic change also increased with the severity of gait disturbance ($p<0.05$) in our study. However, neurogenic change was not related to postural hypotension (reflecting adrenergic nerve dysfunction); erectile dysfunction in men (presumably reflecting cholinergic and nitrate oxidergic nerve dysfunction); detrusor overactivity (reflecting the central type of detrusor dysfunction); constipation (presumably reflecting both peripheral and central types of autonomic and somatic dysfunction); or gender **(Table 1)**. The neurogenic change in EAS-MUP was slightly more common in those with detrusor-sphincter dyssynergia (reflecting the central type of sphincter dysfunction). It has been reported that neurogenic change does not correlate directly with a clinically obvious functional deficit.[74] Patients with marked abnormalities in EAS-MUP may have no faecal incontinence,[77] although, in such patients, anal sphincter weakness is not uncommon.[58] In our study, the prevalence of neurogenic change slightly increased with the severity of storage disorder (incontinence). The most common type of urinary incontinence in MSA is urgency incontinence, which results mostly from detrusor (bladder) overactivity. However, we noted urinary incontinence in 17 patients without detrusor overactivity or low-compliance detrusor; in those cases, the urinary incontinence may have had a sphincter etiology. Urinary incontinence was more severe in the patients with neurogenic change than in those without it ($p<0.05$).

We recently retrospectively analysed 445 case records of EMG cystometry with pressure flow studies, single motor unit potential (MUP) analysis in patients with parkinsonian syndrome, e.g., MSA: n=267, Parkinson's disease (PD): n=129, Dementia with Lewy bodies (DLB): n=25, and progressive supranuclear palsy (PSP): n=24. We carried out receiver operating characteristics (ROC) analysis, revealing that an area under the ROC curve (AUC) in differentiating MSA from other parkinsonian syndrome was 0.70 in duration, 0.62 in phase and 0.51 in amplitude, respectively, with statistically significance. Therefore, duration of MUPs is most sensitive for the differentiation of MSA among MUPs parameters.

	Patients with neurogenic sphincter EMG No	%		Patients with neurogenic sphincter EMG No	%	
Male	27/42	65	Female	25/42	59	NS
Age <60 years	22/39	56	Age >60 years	30/45	66	NS
MSA-C	29/50	58	MSA-P	23/34	68	NS
Independent walking (1–3*)	11/23	48	Wheelchair bound(6–7*)	9/11	82	p<0.05
Postural hypotension −	30/48	63	Postural hypotension +	22/36	60	NS
Constipation −	40/66	61	Constipation +	12/18	67	NS
Erectile dysfunction −	4/5	80	Erectile dysfunction +	19/30	63	NS
Continent	15/25	59	Incontinent	37/59	63	NS
RU <200 ml	36/62	58	RU >200 ml	16/22	73	NS
Detrusor overactivity −	14/26	55	Detrusor overactivity +	38/58	65	NS
UD/AD −	29/52	56	UD/AD +	20/32	63	NS
DSD −	44/73	60	DSD +	8/11	73	NS

*International cooperative ataxia rating scale, walking capacities subscale.
AD, acontractile detrusor; DSD, detrusor sphincter dyssynergy; MSA, multiple system atrophy; RU, residual urine volume; UD, underactive detrusor.

MSA: multiple system atrophy, RU: residual urine volume, UD: underactive detrusor, AD: acontractile detrusor
DSD: detrusor-sphincter dyssynergia
*: International Cooperative Ataxia Rating Scale, walking capacities subscale
(cited from ref. 74)

Table 1. Neurogenic sphincter EMG and clinical variables other than duration of illness.

6.2. Lewy body diseases

6.2.1. Idiopathic Parkinson's disease (IPD)

Several reports of "supposed IPD" have shown severe bladder dysfunctions, e.g., large post-void residuals or neurogenic change in the EAS-EMG. However, some of these reports were published before a definition of MSA was established. Recent studies have reported almost normal EAS-EMG in patients with typical IPD[38,47,53,67]. Stocchi's study (1997) is important, since EMG in patients with IPD and MSA was performed by researchers blinded to the diagnosis.[67] Pathological studies of IPD have shown a degenerative lesion in the spinal parasympathetic PGN[75], although the lesions are much less developed than those in MSA. No Lewy bodies were found in Onuf's nucleus innervating the anal sphincter in IPD.[75] In contrast, Libelius and Johansson (2000) described neurogenic change in EAS-EMG in PD after a disease duration of more than 5 years.[30] This remains a matter of controversy; on the other hand, some patients with DLB may show abnormal EAS-EMG, as described below.

6.2.2. Dementia with Lewy bodies (DLB)

DLB is characterized as dementia with fluctuating cognition and visual hallucination, with (sometimes atypical) parkinsonism. Cardiovascular and urinary autonomic failure is another feature. We performed urodynamic studies in 7 patients with DLB, and performed EAS-EMG in 3. Two of those 3 patients exhibited neurogenic changes in MUPs.[55]

6.2.3. Autonomic failure with Parkinson's disease (AFPD)

AFPD is an intermediate entity that describes a combination of autonomic failure and IPD, but without dementia. We performed urodynamic studies in 7 patients with AFPD and performed EAS-EMG in 4. Three of those 4 patients exhibited neurogenic changes in MUPs[55].

6.2.4. Pure autonomic failure (PAF)

Earlier studies reported normal EAS-EMG in small groups of patients with PAF. However, Ravits et al. (1996)[46] found abnormal EAS-EMG in 2 of 7 patients with PAF, although both of them were multiparous women. Sakakibara et al. performed urodynamic studies in 6 patients with PAF and EAS-EMG in 4. Three of those 4 patients exhibited neurogenic changes in MUPs.[51] In PAF, parkinsonism may appear after a 10-year interval.[81] Therefore PAF can be listed in the differential diagnosis of degenerative parkinsonism. To sum up, in all three Lewy body diseases (DLB, AFPD, PAF), the frequency of neurogenic changes seemed higher in EAS-EMG than in IPD but lower than in MSA. This suggests the involvement of the sacral Onuf's nucleus or its fibers in the external sphincter in these diseases. The prevalence of neurogenic changes in EAS-EMG seems to be: **MSA >> DLB = AFPD = PAF >> PD (Table 2)**. However, these assumptions require confirmation with a larger study. The results seem to be in accordance with the fact that 29% of the DLB patients undergoing EMG-cystometry had a low-compliance detrusor, indicating a pre-ganglionic lesion of the pelvic nerves. The bethanechol test showed that both of these patients had denervation supersensitivity of the detrusor, indicating a post-ganglionic lesion of the pelvic nerves. The results of physiological studies and metaiodobenzylguanidine (MIBG) cardiac scintigraphy suggested post-ganglionic abnormalities in DLB.

Disease	LUT symptoms	Urinary incontinence (storage dysfunction)	PVR> 100 ml (voiding dysfunction)	No. of patients	Reference	Detrusor overactivity (central type)	Low compliance (preGGL type)	Bethanechol supersensitivity (denervation) (postGGL type)	Neurogenic change of sphincter MUPs (denervation) (Onuf's nucleus)	No. of patients	Reference
MSA	96%	63%	52%	121	9	56%	31%	19%	93%	121	9, 11
DLB	100%	91%	27%	11	-	71%	29%	2/2	2/3	7	-
AFPD	100%	43%	29%	7	19	86%	14%	1/3	4/4	7	19
PAF	100%	33%	33%	6	17	67%	33%	2/3	¾	6	17
PD	53–70%	25–28%	0%	115	18	81%	0%	Not performed	5%	21	11

AFPD, autonomic failure with Parkinson's disease; DLB, dementia of Lewy body type; GGL, ganglion; LUT, lower urinary tract; MSA, multiple system atrophy; MUP, motor unit potential; PAF, pure autonomic failure; PD, Parkinson's disease; PVR, post-void residual.

MSA: multiple system atrophy, DLB: Dementia with Lewy bodies, AFPD: Autonomic failure with Parkinson's disease
PAF: Pure autonomic failure, PD: Parkinson's disease, GGL: ganglionic
(cited from ref. 78)

Table 2. Comparison of lower urinary tract function in DLB, AFPD, PAF, PD and MSA. See text.

6.3. Other parkinsonian disorders

6.3.1. Progressive supranuclear palsy (PSP)

We performed urodynamic studies in 9 patients with PSP and performed EAS-EMG in 4. Two of these 4 patients exhibited neurogenic changes in MUPs.[50] Abnormal sphincter EMG was also reported in 5 of 12 patients by Valldeoriola et al. (1995)[71], and in 2 of 8 patients by Palace et al. (1997)[38]. Libelius and Johansson (2000) also described anal sphincter EMG abnormalities in 2 of 3 patients with PSP.[30]

6.3.2. Corticobasal degeneration (CBD)

We performed urodynamic studies in 6 patients with CBD and EAS-EMG in 5 of them. However, none of the 5 patients showed neurogenic changes in the MUPs.[60] There is a considerable overlap in the clinical presentation of the parkinsonian form of MSA (MSA-P) and that of PSP. Therefore, we should be cautious in interpreting sphincter EMG in these disorders.

6.4. Cerebellar ataxia

6.4.1. Spinocerebellar ataxia 3 (SCA3)/Machado-Joseph disease

We performed urodynamic studies in 11 patients with spinocerebellar ataxia 3 (SCA3) and performed EAS-EMG in 9. Six of the 9 patients showed neurogenic changes in MUPs.[59]

6.4.2. Late cortical cerebellar atrophy (LCCA):

We performed urodynamic studies in 7 patients with LCCA, which is a pure cerebellar ataxia without heredity, and EAS-EMG in 3 of them. However, none of the 3 patients exhibited neurogenic changes in the MUPs.

6.4.3. Spinocerebellar ataxia 6 (SCA6)

We performed urodynamic studies in 9 patients with spinocerebellar ataxia 6 (SCA6) and performed EAS-EMG in 8. Five of the 8 patients showed neurogenic changes in MUPs.

6.5. Other diseases

Sakuta et al. performed EAS-EMG in 30 patients with amyotrophic lateral sclerosis (ALS).[62] None of them exhibited neurogenic changes in the MUPs, which contrasted with common neurogenic changes in the limb muscles in this disorder. These EMG findings correspond to the postmortem selective sparing of sacral Onuf's nucleus, which contrasts with severe loss of anterior horn cells innervating the limbs, tongue, and bulbar muscles[2]. Neurons in Onuf's nucleus demonstrate some morphological differences from the anterior horn cells innervating limb muscle [33]. However, more recent studies have shown abnormalities in the

Onuf's nucleus in most advanced cases with ALS[27], particularly in patients under mechanical ventilation.

7. Conclusions

We have reviewed the normal physiology and pathophysiology of the lower urinary tract and the lower gastrointestinal tract, the current methods and interpretations of sphincter EMG, and the application of this technique to various autonomic disorders. Sphincter EMG makes it easier to distinguish MSA from idiopathic Parkinson's disease in the first 5 years after disease onset, reflecting the significant involvement of the sacral spinal cord in MSA. However, abnormal sphincter EMG is also seen in some, though not many, patients with DLB or PSP. It is noteworthy that sphincter denervation leads to severe urinary and fecal incontinence in some female patients with MSA, which severely affects their quality of life. Sphincter EMG and relevant sacral autonomic tests are good diagnostic tools in autonomic disorders.

Author details

Ryuji Sakakibara*, Fuyuki Tateno, Masahiko Kishi and Yohei Tsuyusaki
Neurology, Internal Medicine, Sakura Medical Center, Toho University, Sakura, Japan

Tomoyuki Uchiyama and Tatsuya Yamamoto
Neurology, Chiba University, Chiba, Japan

Tomonori Yamanishi
Urology, Dokkyo Medical College, Tochigi, Japan

8. References

[1] Abrams P, Cardozo L, Fall M, Griffiths D, Rosier P, Ulmsten U, van Kerrebrock P, Victor A, Wein A (2002) The standardization of terminology of lower urinary tract function: report from the standardization sub-committee of the international continence society. Neurourol Urodynam 21: 167-178

[2] Amborova P, Hubkal P, Ulkova I, Hulin I (2003) The pacemaker activity of interstitial cells of cajal and gastric electrical activity. Physiol Res 52: 275-284

[3] Argiolas A, Melis MR (2005). Central control of penile erection: role of the paraventricular nucleus of the hypothalamus. Prog Neurobiol 76: 1-21.

[4] Bassotti G, Maggio D, Battaglia E, Giulietti O, Spinozzi F, Reboldi G, Serra AM, Emanuelli G, Chiarioni G (2000) Manometric investigation of anorectal function in early and late stage Parkinson's disease. J Neurol Neurosurg Psychiatry 68; 768-770

[5] Beck RO, Betts CD, Fowler CJ (1994) Genitourinary dysfunction in multiple system atrophy: clinical features and treatment in 62 cases. J Urol 151: 1336-1341.

* Corresponding Author

[6] Betts CD, Kapoor R, Fowler CJ (1992) Pontine pathology and voiding dysfunction. Br J Urol. 70: 100-102

[7] Blok BF, Holstege G (1999) The central control of micturition and continence: implications for urology. Br J Urol Int 83 Suppl 2: 1-6

[8] Blok BF, de Weerd H, Holstege G (1997) The pontine micturition center projects to sacral cord GABA immunoreactive neurons in the cat. Neurosci Lett 233: 109-112

[9] Broens P, Vanbeckevoort D, Bellon E, Penninckx F (2002) Combined radiographic and manometric study of rectal filling sensation. Dis Colon Rectum 45: 1016-1022

[10] Chandiramani VA, Palace J, Fowler CJ (1997) How to recognize patients with parkinsonism who should not have urological surgery. Br J Urol 80: 100 –104.

[11] Daniel SE (1992) The neuropathology and neurochemistry of multiple system atrophy. In Autonomic Failure, 3rd ed., R Bannister and CJ Mathias, eds. Oxford Medical Publications, Oxford, UK, 564-585

[12] de Groat WC (2006) Integrative control of the lower urinary tract: preclinical perspective. BJP 147: S25-S40

[13] Dominguez JM, Hull EM (2005). Dopamine, the medial preoptic area, and male sexual behavior. Physiol Behavior 86: 356-368.

[14] Eardley I, Quinn NP, Fowler CJ, Kirby RS, Parkhouse HF, Marsden CD, Bannister R. (1989) The value of urethral sphincter electromyography in the differential diagnosis of parkinsonism. Br J Urol 64: 360 –362

[15] Fisher C, Gross J, Zuch AJ (1965). Cycle of penile erection synchronous with dreaming (REM) sleep. Arch Gen Psychiatry; 12: 29-45.

[16] Fowler CJ (2006) Integrated control of lower urinary tract: clinical perspective. BJP 147: S14-S24

[17] Fowler CJ, Kirby RS, Harrison MJ, Milroy EJ, Turner-Warwick R. (1984) Individual motor unit analysis in the diagnosis of disorders of urethral sphincter innervation. J Neurol Neurosurg Psychiatry 47: 637-641

[18] Gilad R, Giladi N, Korczyn AD, Gurevich T, Sadeh M (2001). Quantitative anal sphincter EMG in multisystem atrophy and 100 controls. J Neurol Neurosurg Psychiatry. 71: 596-599.

[19] Giladi N, Simon ES, Korczyn AD, Groozman GB, Orlov Y, Shabtai H, Drory VE (2000) Anal sphincter EMG does not distinguish between multiple system atrophy and Parkinson's disease. Muscle Nerve 23: 731–734.

[20] Hansen MB (2003) Neurohumoral control of GI motility. Physiol Res 52: 1-30

[21] Hirschkowitz M, Schmidt MH (2005). Sleep-related erections: clinical perspectives and neural mechanisms. Sleep Med Rev 9: 311-329.

[22] Ito T, Sakakibara R, Uchiyama T, Liu Z, Yamamoto T, Hattori T (2006b) Videomanometry of the pelvic organs; a comparison of the normal lower urinary and GI tracts. Int J Urol 13: 29-35

[23] Ito T., Sakakibara R, Yasuda K, Yamamoto T, Uchiyama T, Liu Z, Yamanishi T, Awa Y, Yamamoto K, Hattori T (2006) Incomplete emptying and urinary retention in multiple system atrophy: when does it occur and how do we manage it? Mov Disord 21: 816-823

[24] Kavia RB, Datta SN, Dasgupta R, Elneil S, Fowler CJ. (2006) Urinary retention in women: its causes and management. BJU Int 97: 281-287

[25] Kavia RBC, Dasgupta R, Fowler CJ (2005) Functional imaging and the central control of the bladder. J Comp Neurol 493: 27-32

[26] Kellow JE, Delvaux M, Azpiroz F, Camilleri M, Quigley EMM, Thompson DG (1999) Principles of applied neurogastroenterology: physiology/motility-sensation. Gut 45; 17-24

[27] Kihira T, Yoshida S, Yoshimasu F, Wakayama I, Yase Y. (1997) Involvement of Onuf's nucleus in amyotrophic lateral sclerosis. J Neurol Sci 147: 81-88.

[28] Kirchhof K, Mathias CJ, Fowler CJ (1999) The relationship of uro-genital dysfunction to other features of autonomic failure in MSA. Clin Auton Res 9: 1–28.

[29] Lefaucheur JP (2006). Neurophysiological testing in ancrectal disorders. Muscle Nerve. 33: 324-333.

[30] Libelius R, Johansson F (2000) Quantitative electromyography of the external anal sphincter in Parkinson's disease and multiple system atrophy. Muscle Nerve 23: 1250-1256

[31] Liu MT, Rayport S, Jiang L, Murphy DL, Gershon MD (2002) Expression and function of 5-HT3 receptors in the enteric neurons of mice lacking the serotonin transporter. Am J Physiol Gastrointest Liver Physiol 283: G1398-G1411

[32] Liu Z, Sakakibara R, Nakazawa K, Uchiyama T, Yamamoto T, Ito T, Hattori T (2004) Micturition-related neuronal firing in the periaqueductal gray area in cats. Neuroscience 126: 1075-1082

[33] Mannen T, Iwata M, Toyokura Y, Nagashima K (1982) The Onuf's nucleus and the external anal sphincter muscles in amyotrophic lateral sclerosis and Shy-Drager syndrome. Acta Neuropathol 58: 255-260

[34] Mashidori T, Yamanishi T, Yoshida K, Sakakibara R, Sakurai K, Hirata K. Continuous urinary incontinence presenting as the initial symptoms demonstrating acontractile detrusor and intrinsic sphincter deficiency in multiple system atrophy. Int J Urol. 14: 10; 972-974 2007

[35] Matsumoto G, Hisamitsu T, De Groat WC (1995) Role of glutamate and NMDA receptors in the descending limb of the spinobulbospinal micturition reflex pathway of the rat. Neurosci Lett 183: 58-61

[36] Nahm F, Freeman R (2003) Sphincter electromyography and multiple system atrophy. Muscle Nerve 28: 18-26.

[37] Onufrowicz B (1899) Notes on the arrangement and function of the cell groups in the sacral region of the spinal cord. J Nerv Ment Dis 26: 498-504

[38] Palace J, Chandiramani VA, Fowler CJ. (1997) Value of sphincter electromyography in the diagnosis of multiple system atrophy. Muscle Nerve 20: 1396-1403

[39] Paviour DC, Williams DC, Fowler CJ, Quinn NP, Lees AJ (2005) Is sphincter electromyography a helpful investigation in the diagnosis of multiple system atrophy? A retrospective study with pathological diagnosis. Mov Disord 20: 1425–1430.

[40] Pellegrinetti A, Moscato G, Siciliano G, Bonuccelli U, Orlandi G, Maritato P, Sartucci F (2003). Electrophysiological evaluation of genito-sphincteric dysfunction in multiple system atrophy. Int J Neurosci. 113: 1353-1369.

[41] Podnar S (2007). Neurophysiology of the neurogenic lower urinary tract disorders. Clin Neurophysiol. 118: 1423-1437.

[42] Podnar S, Fowler CJ. (2004) Sphincter electromyography in diagnosis of multiple system atrophy: technical issues. Muscle Nerve 29: 151–156

[43] Podnar S, Rodi Z, Lukanovic A, Trsinar B, Vodusek DB. (1999) Standardization of anal sphincter EMG: technique of needle examination. Muscle Nerve 22: 400-403

[44] Podnar S, Vodusek DB. (2001) Protocol for clinical neurophysiologic examination of the pelvic floor. Neurourol Urodyn 20: 669-682

[45] Podnar S. (2007) Neurophysiology of the neurogenic lower urinary tract disorders. Clin Neurophysiol. 118: 1423-1437

[46] Ravits J, Hallett M, Nilsson J, Polinsky R, Dambrosia J (1996). Electrophysiological tests of autonomic function in patients with idiopathic autonomic failure syndromes. Muscle Nerve. 19: 758-763.

[47] Rodi Z, Denislic M, Vodusek D (1996) External anal sphincter electromyography in the differential diagnosis of parkinsonism. J Neurol Neurosurg Psychiatry 60: 460-461.

[48] Sakakibara R, Fowler CJ (2001) Brain disease (Chapter 9). In: Seminars in Clinical Neurology (by World Federation of Neurology). Neurologic bladder, bowel, and sexual function. Edited by Fowler CJ, Elsevier, Boston, 229-243

[49] Sakakibara R, Hattori T, Kita K, Arai K, Yamanishi T, Yasuda K : Stress-induced urinary incontinence in patients with spinocerebellar degeneration J Neurol Neurosurg Psychiatry 64: 3; 389-391 1998

[50] Sakakibara R, Hattori T, Tojo M, Yamanishi T, Yasuda K, Hirayama K (1993). Micturitional disturbance in progressive supranuclear palsy. J Auton Nerv Syst. 45: 101-106.

[51] Sakakibara R, Hattori T, Uchiyama T, Asahina M, Yamanishi T (2000). Micturitional disturbance in pure autonomic failure. Neurology. 54: 499-501.

[52] Sakakibara R, Hattori T, Uchiyama T, Kita K, Asahina M, Suzuki A, Yamanishi T (2000) Urinary dysfunction and orthostatic hypotension in multiple system atrophy: which is the more common and earlier manifestation? Neurol Neurosurg Psychiatry 68: 65–69.

[53] Sakakibara R, Hattori T, Uchiyama T, Yamanishi T (2001) Videourodynamic and sphincter motor unit potential analyses in Parkinson's disease and multiple system atrophy. J Neurol Neurosurg Psychiatry 71: 600-606.

[54] Sakakibara R, Hattori T, Yasuda K, Yamanishi T (1996) Micturitional disturbance and pontine tegmental lesion; urodynamic and MRI analyses of the vascular cases. J Neurol Sci 141: 105-110

[55] Sakakibara R, Ito T, Uchiyama T, Asahina M, Liu Z, Yamamoto T, Yamanaka Y, Hattori T (2005) Lower urinary tract function in dementia of Lewy body type (DLB). J Neurol Neurosurg Psychiatry 76: 729-732.

[56] Sakakibara R, Mori M, Fukutake T, Kita K (1997) Orthostatic hypotension in a case with multiple sclerosis. Clin Auton Res 7: 163-165

[57] Sakakibara R, Nakazawa K, Shiba K, Nakajima Y, Uchiyama T, Yoshiyama M, Yamanishi T, Hattori T (2002) Firing patterns of micturition-related neurons in the pontine storage centre in cats. Auton Neurosci Basic Clin 99: 24-30

[58] Sakakibara R, Odaka T, Uchiyama T, Asahina M, Yamaguchi K, Yamaguchi T, Yamanishi T, Hattori T (2004) Colonic transit time, sphincter EMG and rectoanal videomanometry in multiple system atrophy. Mov Disord 19: 924-929

[59] Sakakibara R, Uchiyama T, Arai K, Yamanishi T, Hattori T (2004). Lower urinary tract dysfunction in Machado-Joseph disease: a study of 11 clinical-urodynamic observations. J Neurol Sci. 218: 67-72.

[60] Sakakibara R, Uchiyama T, Yamanishi T, Hattori T (2004). Urinary function in patients with corticobasal degeneration; comparison with normal subjects. Neurourol Urodyn. 23: 154-158.

[61] Sakakibara R, Uchiyama T, Yamanishi T, Shirai K, Hattori T. (2008) Bladder and bowel dysfunction in Parkinson's disease. J Neural Transm 115: 443-460

[62] Sakuta M, Nakanishi T, Toyokura Y (1978) Anal muscle electromyograms differ in amyotrophic lateral sclerosis and Shy-Drager syndrome. Neurology 28: 1289-1293.

[63] Sasaki M (2005) Role of Barrington's nucleus in micturition. J Comp Neurol 493: 21-26

[64] Schwarz J, Kornhuber M, Bischoff C, Straube A. (1997) Electromyography of the external anal sphincter in patients with Parkinson's disease and multiple system atrophy: frequency of abnormal spontaneous activity and polyphasic motor unit potentials. Muscle Nerve 20: 1167–1172.

[65] Singer C, Weiner WJ, Sanchez-Ramos JR, Ackerman M (1989). Sexual dysfunction in men with Parkinson's disease. J Neurol Rehab 3: 199-204.

[66] Steers WD (2002) Pathophysiology of overactive and urge urinary incontinence. Rev Urol 4 Suppl 4: S7-S18

[67] Stocchi F, Carbone A, Inghilteri M, Monge A, Ruggieri S, Berardelli A, Manfredi M (1997) Urodynamic and neurophysiological evaluation in Parkinson's disease and multiple system atrophy. J Neurol Neurosurg Psychiatry 62: 507–511.

[68] Thor KB (2003) Serotonin and norepinephrine involvement in efferent pathways to the urethral rhabdosphincter: implications for treating stress urinary incontinence. Urology 62: 3-9

[69] Tison F, Arne P, Sourgen C, Chrysostome V, Yeklef F (2000) The value of external anal sphincter electromyography for the diagnosis of multiple system atrophy. Mov Disord 15: 1148-1157

[70] Tsujimura A, Miyagawa Y, Fujita K, Matsuoka Y, Takahashi T, Takao T, Matsumiya K, Osaki Y, Takasawa M, Oku N, Hatazawa J, Shigeo Kaneko S, Okuyama A (2006). Brain processing of audiovisual sexual stimuli inducing penile erection: a positron emission tomography study. J Urol 176: 679-683.

[71] Valldeoriola F, Valls-Sole J, Tolosa E, Marti M (1995) Striated anal sphincter denervation in patients with progressive supranuclear palsy. Mov Disord 10: 550–555.

[72] van Furth WR, Wolterink G, van Ree JM (1995). Regulation of masculine sexual behavior; involvement of brain opioids and dopamine. Brain Research Reviews 21: 162-184.

[73] 74 Vaughan CJ, Aherne AM, Lane E, Power O, Carey RM, O'Connell DP (2000) Identification and regional distribution of the dopamine D1A receptor in the GI tract. Am J Physiol Regulatory Integrative Comp Physiol 279: R599–R609

[74] Vodusek DB (2001) Sphincter EMG and differential diagnosis of multiple system atrophy. Mov Disord 16: 600-607

[75] Wakabayashi K, Takahashi H (1997) Neuropathology of autonomic nervous system in Parkinson's disease. Eur Neurol. 38 Suppl 2: 2-7.

[76] Walker JK, Gainetdinov RR, Mangel AW, Caron MG, Shetzline MA (2000) Mice lacking the dopamine transporter display altered regulation of distal colonic motility. Am J Physiol Gastrointest Liver Physiol. 279: G311-318

[77] Wenning GK, Ben-Schlomo Y, Magalhaes M, Daniel S, Quinn N (1994) Clinical features and natural history of multiple system atrophy. Brain 117: 835-845.

[78] Yaguchi H, Soma H, Miyazaki Y, Tashiro J, Yabe I, Kikuchi S, Sasaki H, Kakizaki H, Moriwaka F, Tashiro K (2004) A case of acute urinary retention caused by periaqueductal grey lesion. J Neurol Neurosurg Psychiatry 75; 1202-1203

[79] Yamamoto T, Sakakibara R, Uchiyama T, Liu Z, Ito T, Awa Y, Yamanishi T, Hattori T (2006) Neurological diseases that cause detrusor hyperactivity with impaired contractile function. Neurourol Urodynam 25: 356-360

[80] Yamamoto T, Sakakibara R, Uchiyama T, Liu Z, Ito T, Awa Y, Yamanishi T, Hattori T (2005) When is Onuf's nucleus involved in multiple system atrophy? A sphincter electromyography study. J Neurol Neurosurg Psychiatry 76: 1645-1648.

[81] Yamanaka Y, Asahina M, Hiraga A, Sakakibara R, Oka H, Hattori T. (2007) Over 10 years of isolated autonomic failure preceding dementia and Parkinsonism in 2 patients with Lewy body disease. Mov Disord 22: 595-597.

[82] Yokoyama O, Yoshiyama M, Namiki M, de Groat WC (2002) Changes in dopaminergic and glutamatergic excitatory mechanisms of micturition reflex after middle cerebral artery occlusion in conscious rats. Exp Neurol 173, 129-135

[83] Yokoyama O, Yotsuyanagi S, Akino H, Moriyama H, Matsuta Y, Namiki M (2003) RNA synthesis in pons necessary for maintenance of bladder overactivity after cerebral infarction in rat. J Urol. 169: 1878-1884

Section 3

EMG Applications: Hand Gestures and Prosthetics

Chapter 13

Hand Sign Classification Employing Myoelectric Signals of Forearm

Takeshi Tsujimura, Sho Yamamoto and Kiyotaka Izumi

Additional information is available at the end of the chapter

http://dx.doi.org/10.5772/51080

1. Introduction

Electromyogram (EMG) signals are generated in muscles, when the muscles contract and a joint is flexed or extended. EMG signals can be measured from a skin surface with noninvasive electrodes, and they include some information on motions such as muscle torque or joint angles. Hence, it is possible to achieve more intuitive human-machine interface using EMG signals than conventional interfaces such as joysticks, data gloves, motion captures. Various interfaces using EMG signals have been proposed to control robot hands (Graupe et al.; Jacobson et al.; Yoshikawa et al., 2009; Ibe at al.). Some methods for hand motion identification have been reported since the 1990s based on soft-computing approaches, e. g. artificial neural networks (Fukuda et al.; Hudgins et al.), fuzzy logic (Karlik & Tokhi; Chan et al.), support vector machine (Yoshikawa et al., 2007; Oskoei & Huosheng), and so on (Chen et al.; Huang et al.). These approaches have improved accuracy of motion discrimination and the number of discriminated motions. However, they need complicated processes and huge amount of calculations.

The purpose of our study is to design an uncomplicated system to identify finger motion and to develop innovative human-machine interfaces. We began with the investigation of the forearm muscle EMG (Tsujimura et al.; Yamamoto et al.). We supposed that not only finger muscles but forearm ones work when the knuckles display hand signs. For this purpose, an EMG measurement system is constructed first to detect surface EMG signals of a forearm and to convert them to more manageable types of features. We next evaluate the correlation between the forearm EMG signals and finger motions. It discloses the activity pattern of each forearm muscle corresponding to specific hand sign. The identification algorithm of hand signs is then designed based on the optimized criterion of muscle activity. Finally, identification of finger gesture is experimented to demonstrate the effectiveness of our proposed method.

2. EMG measurement system

2.1. Measurement system design

Block diagram of our EMG measurement system is shown in Fig. 1. Surface EMG signals are measured with three electrodes placed on a forearm. The EMG signals are preprocessed and converted into integrated EMG (IEMG) signals through the EMG measurement instrument. An IEMG signal has been used as an index of a muscle activity level in exercise physiology (Milner-Brown & Stein). Both EMG and IEMG are introduced into a PC to evaluate the averaged IEMG (AIEMG) features. An estimation algorithm of finger gesture is installed in the PC. After determining criterions of muscle activity, the proposed system identifies motions of fingers.

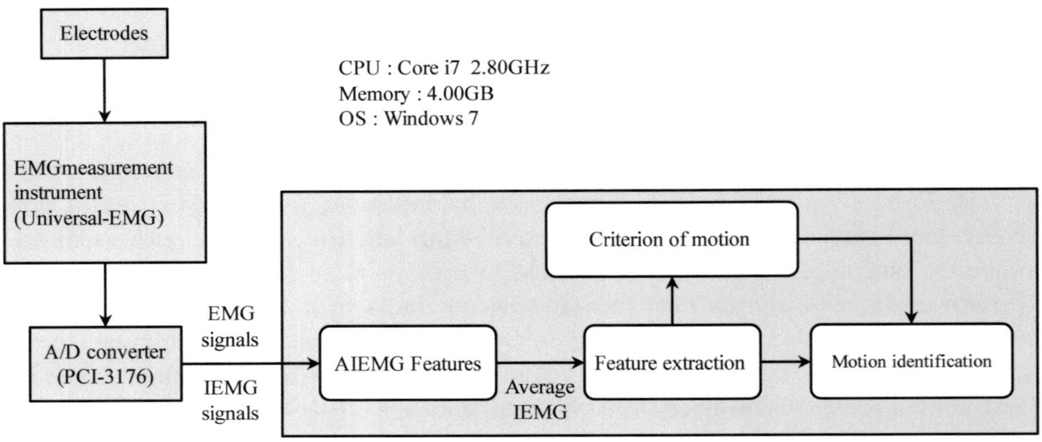

Figure 1. EMG measurement system

Figure 2 illustrates the forearm muscles whose EMG signals are measured by the instrument, and the positions of three electrodes placed on the forearm. The center figure shows forearm cross section of anatomical muscle placement.

Extensor pollicis brevis monitored with the electrode 1 (channel 1) is involved in finger extension. Extensor digitorum monitored with the electrode 2 (channel 2) is also involved in finger extension. Flexor digitorum profundus monitored with the electrode 3 (channel 3) is involved in finger flexion.

The EMG signals are measured with bipolar surface electrodes consisting of two parallel silver bars. These signals are amplified and converted into IEMG signals with rectification smoothing (the cutoff frequency 2.4 Hz) by means of a differential amplifier (Universal-EMG, Oisaka development Ltd.). The EMG signals are sampled at 10 kHz through a 16-bit A/D converter (PCI-3176, Interface Co.) and taken in a data-collection computer (Core i7 2.8 GHz, Windows 7).

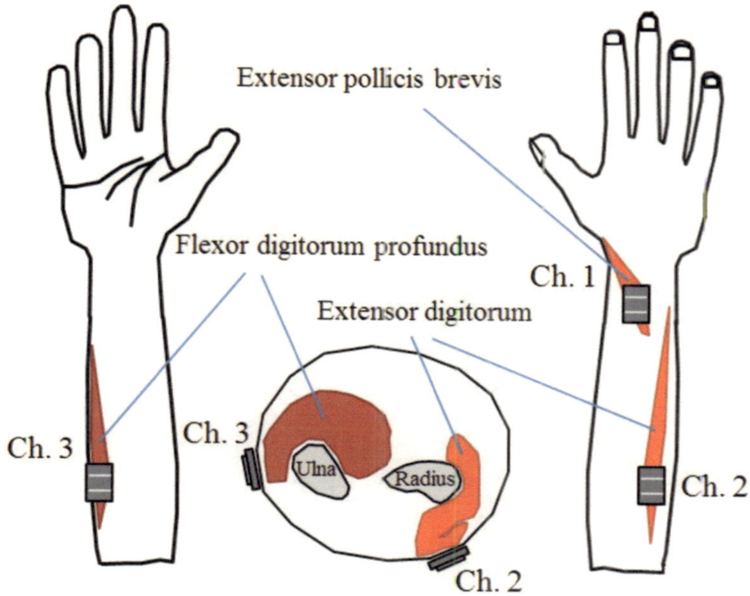

Figure 2. Measured muscles and electrodes placed on forearm

2.2. Electromyogram features

The AIEMG feature is a periodic average of EMG signals during a designated interval (Yoshikawa et al., 2007). It is extracted from the IEMG in the 100 ms frame, which is shifted for 12.5 ms (80 Hz). Hamming window functions are applied to the signals in each frame. Since the measured data is converted into digital quantity by the PC interface, the AIEMG is calculated in terms of the moving average of the IEMG magnitude as

$$AIEMG(k) = \frac{1}{N} \sum_{t=0}^{N-1} IEMG(t), \quad (1)$$

where AIEMG(k), and IEMG(t) represent the AIEMG feature of the k-th averaging frame and the IEMG magnitude of the t-th sample within the frame, respectively. Number of samples in a frame is denoted by N.

The AIEMG eliminates momentary noise such as a spike, because it is a kind of low-pass filters. The larger you take the sampling number, the smoother the AIEMG signal becomes. If you choose N=1, the AIEMG is the same as the IEMG signal.

3. Forearm EMG signals regarding finger motion

Not only muscles of fingers but of forearms work when you use your fingers. First of all, we have investigated the relationship between finger motion and the forearm EMG signals. Although we have obtained fundamental responses with regard to each single finger motion, this paper focuses only on typical gestures of composite finger configurations.

"Rock-paper-scissors" is a hand game played by two or more people. Each player changes his hand into one of three basic hand-signs representing rock, paper, or scissors as shown in Fig. 3. Each of the hand signs beats one of the other two, and loses to the other in the game.

Our purpose in this paper is to distinguish the hand-signs by analyzing the forearm EMG signals.

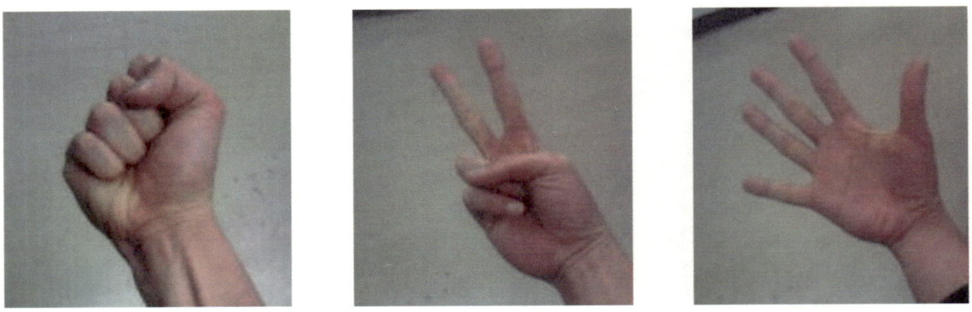

rock scissors paper

Figure 3. Hand signs to be distinguished

3.1. EMG and IEMG signals

We have evaluated the forearm EMG signals with our measurement system. When displaying "rock" by clenching fist, the EMG and IEMG signals were measured as shown in Figs. 4 and 5. Figure 4 (a1), (a2), and (a3) indicate the EMG signals measured with channels 1, 2, and 3, respectively, where the horizontal axis expresses time, and the vertical represents magnitude of the EMG signal. The IEMG signals are also evaluated as shown in Fig. 5. Figure 5 (b1), (b2), and (b3) indicate the IEMG signals measured with channels 1, 2, and 3, respectively, where the horizontal axis expresses time and the vertical represents magnitude of the IEMG signal. Those waveforms shown in Figs. 4 and 5 indicate that channel 1 is inactive, channel 2 is less active, and only channel 3 is active. It can be considered that flexor digitorum profundus is mainly working when you shape "rock" with your hand.

"Scissors" are represented by two fingers extended and separated. The EMG and IEMG signals were measured regarding "scissors" as shown in Figs. 6 and 7, respectively. These figures show that channel 2 is solely active and channels 1 and 3 are almost inactive. Results support that extensor digitorum contributes to showing "scissors."

An open hand signifies "paper." The EMG and IEMG signals are shown with regard to "paper" in Figs. 8 and 9, respectively. They indicate both channels 1 and 2 are active and channel 3 is less active. It is surmised that "paper" is formed owing to both extensor pollicis brevis and extensor digitorum.

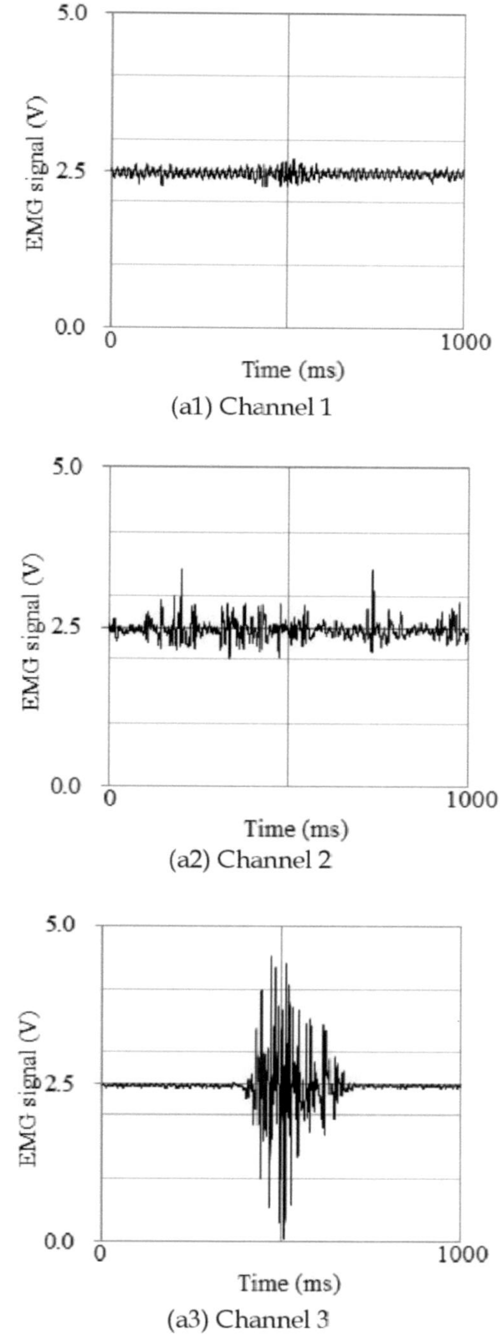

Figure 4. EMG signals regarding "rock"

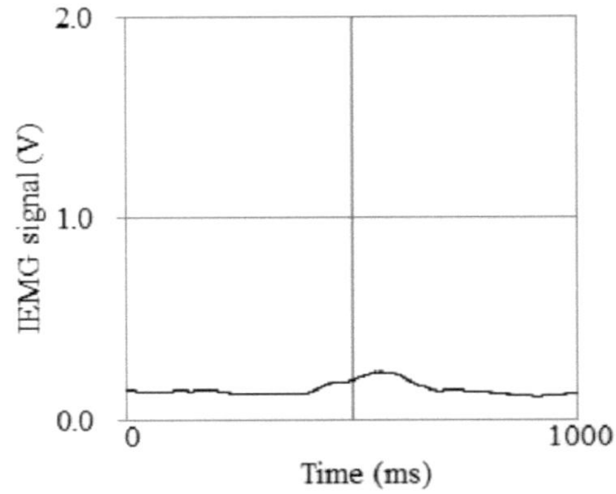

(b1) Channel 1

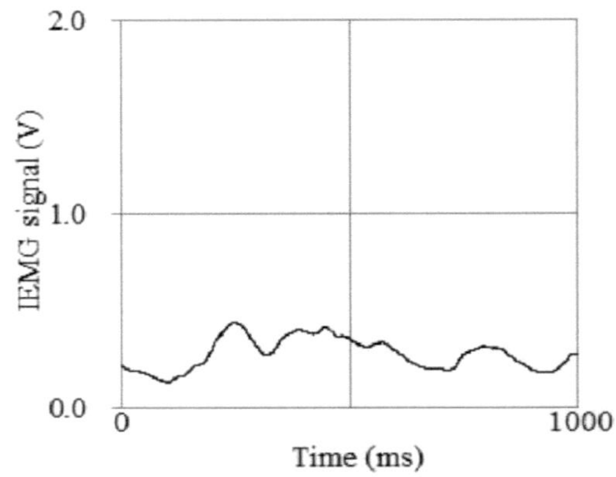

(b2) Channel 2

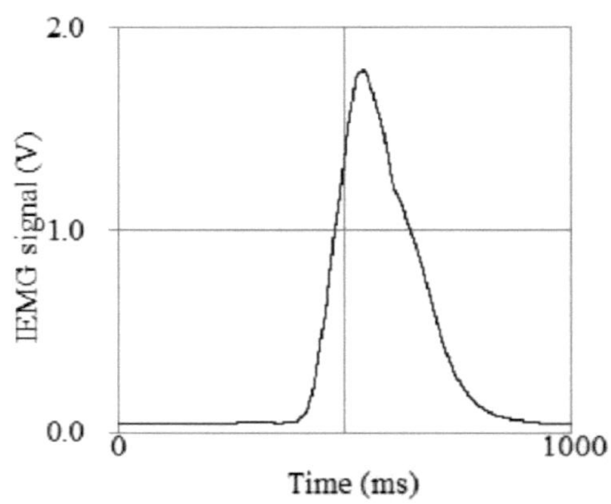

(b3) Channel 3

Figure 5. IEMG signals regarding "rock"

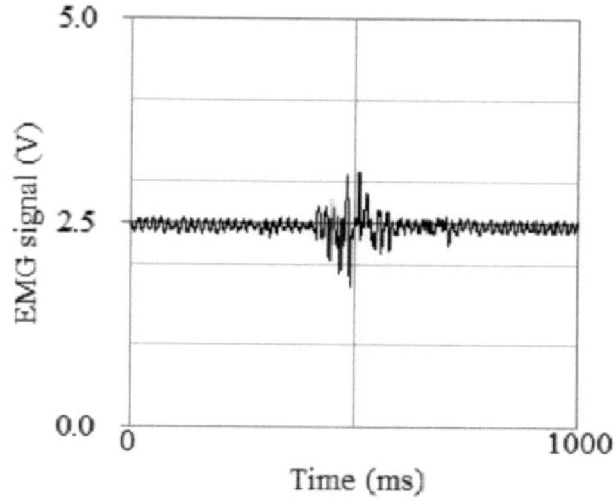

(a1) Channel 1

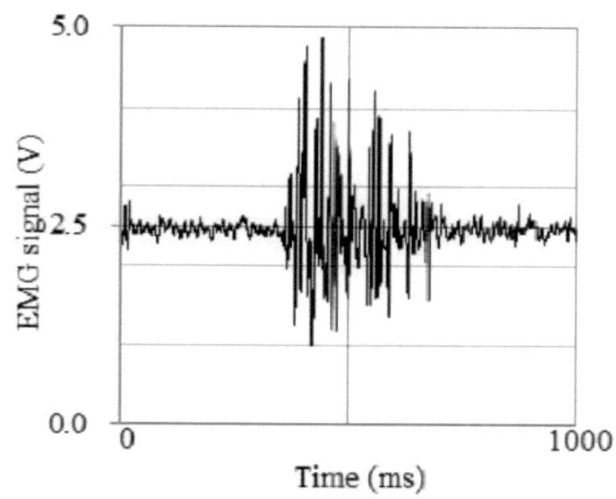

(a2) Channel 2

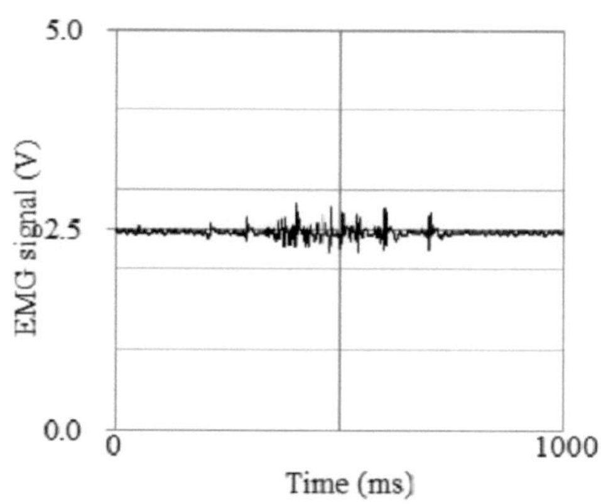

(a3) Channel 3

Figure 6. EMG signals regarding "scissors"

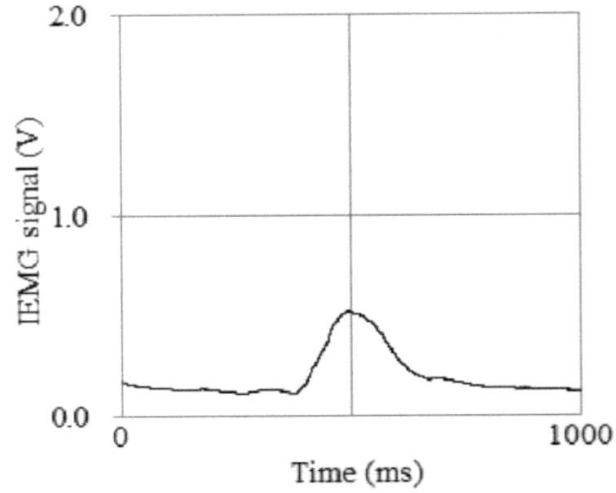

(b1) Channel 1

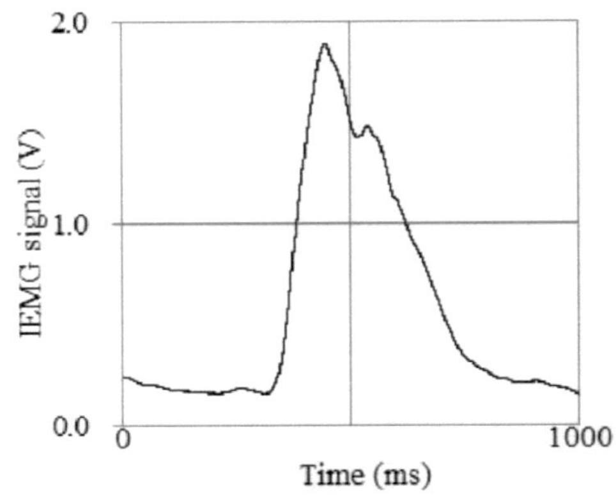

(b2) Channel 2

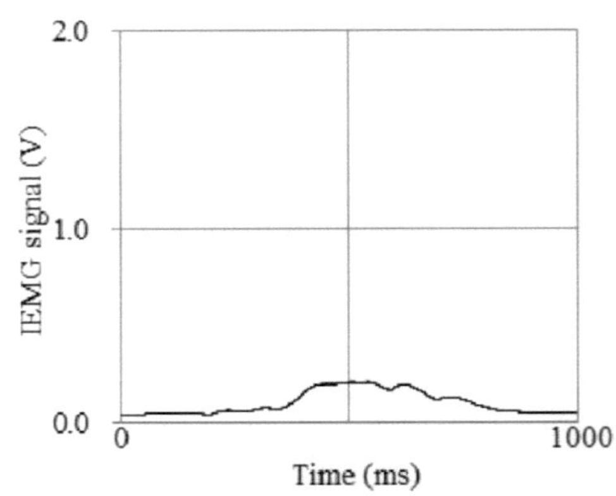

(b3) Channel 3

Figure 7. IEMG signals regarding "scissors"

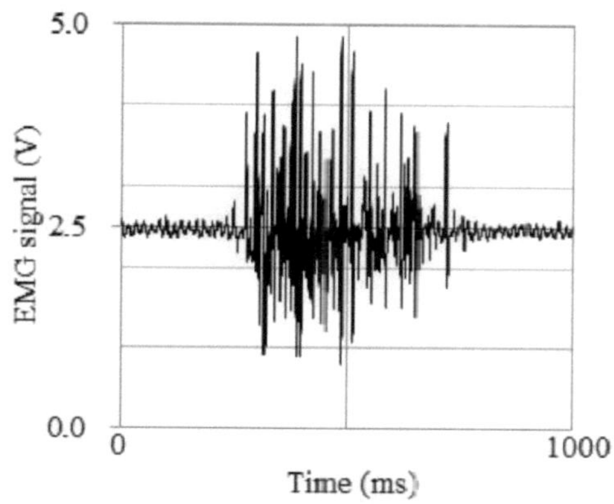

(a1) Channel 1

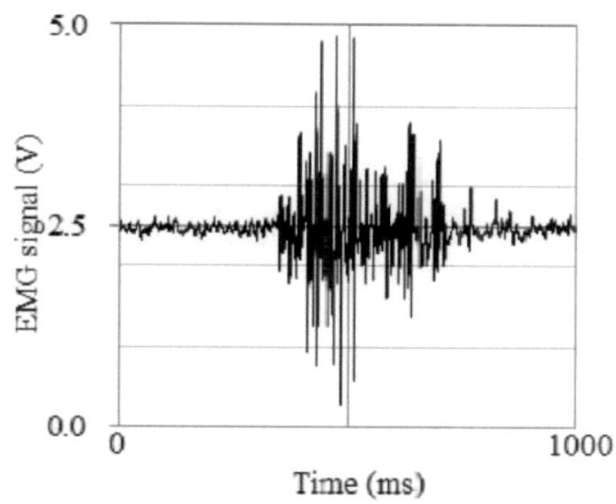

(a2) Channel 2

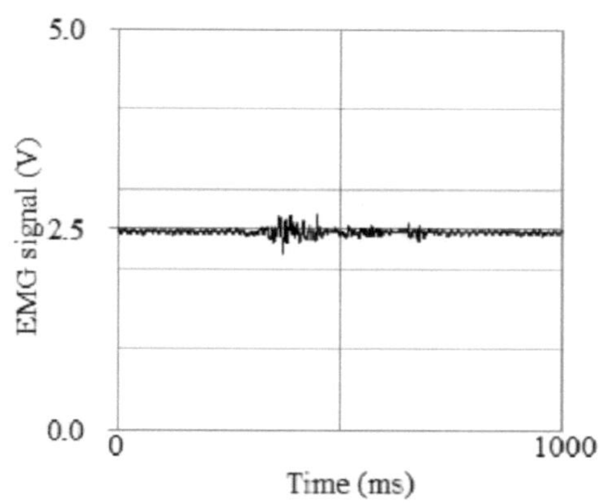

(a3) Channel 3

Figure 8. EMG signals regarding "paper"

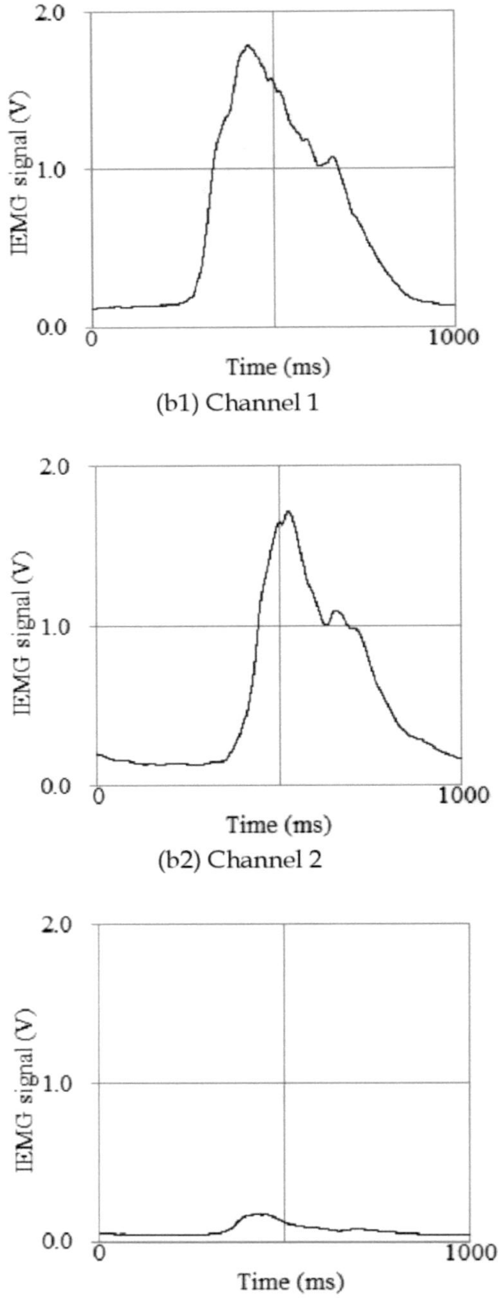

Figure 9. IEMG signals regarding "paper"

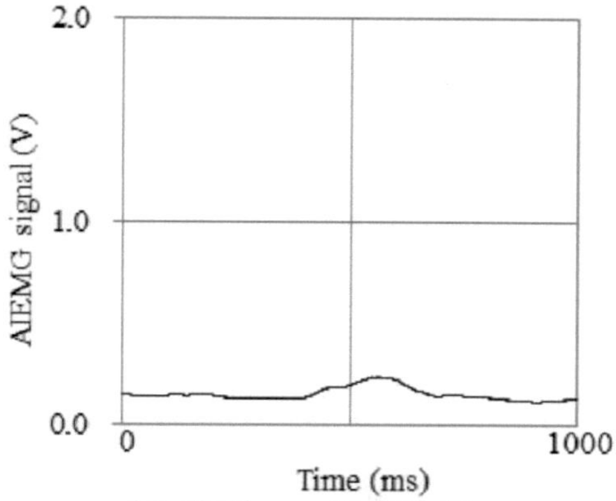

(c1_1) Channel 1 (N = 1)

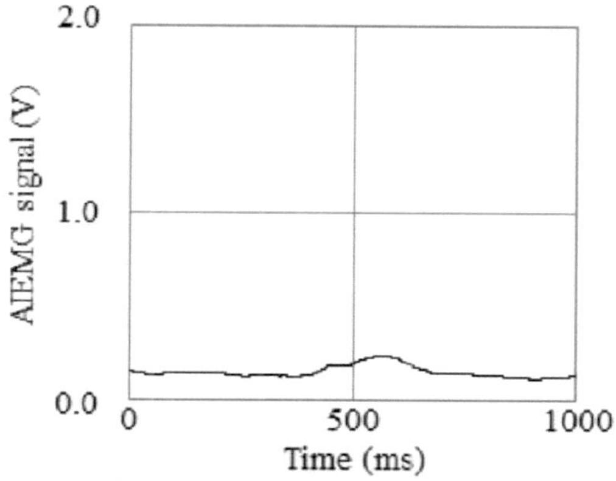

(c1_50) Channel 1 (N = 50)

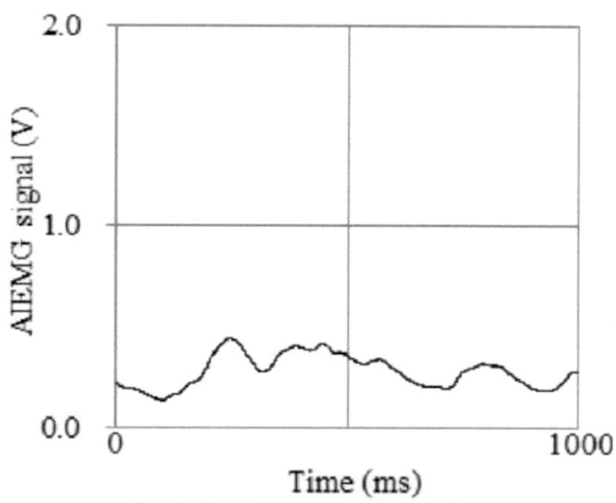

(c2_1) Channel 2 (N = 1)

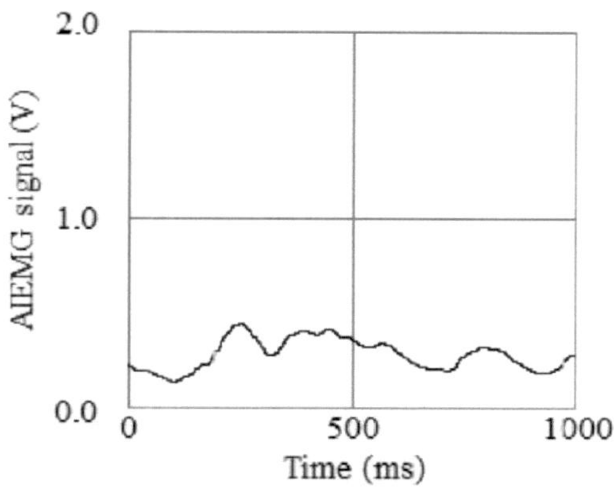

(c2_50) Channel 2 (N = 50)

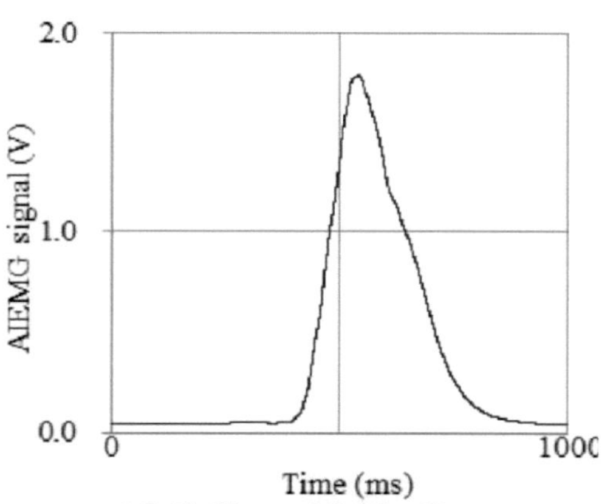

(c3_1) Channel 3 (N = 1)

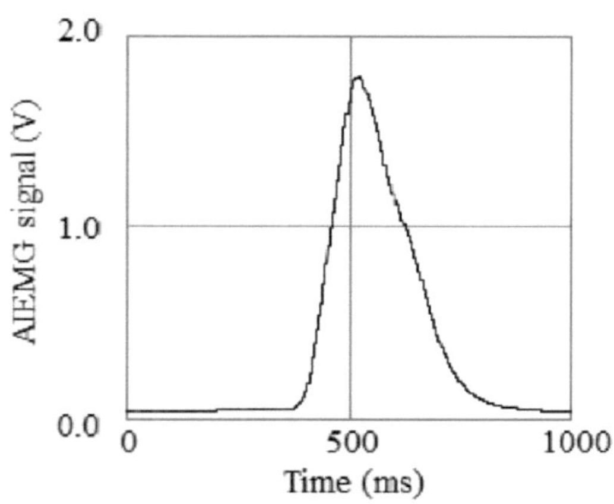

(c3_50) Channel 3 (N = 50)

(1)

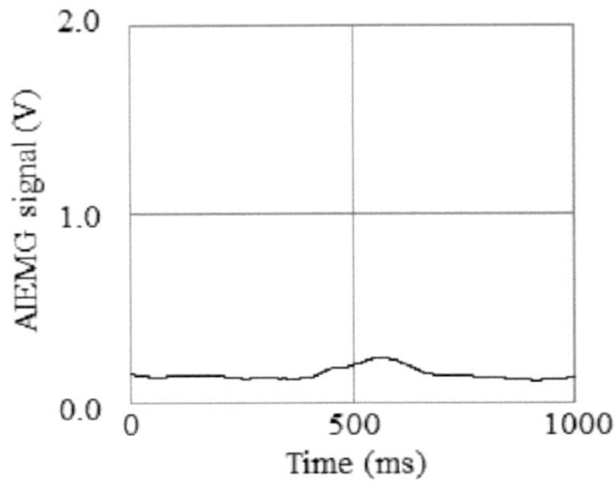

(c1_100) Channel 1 (N = 100)

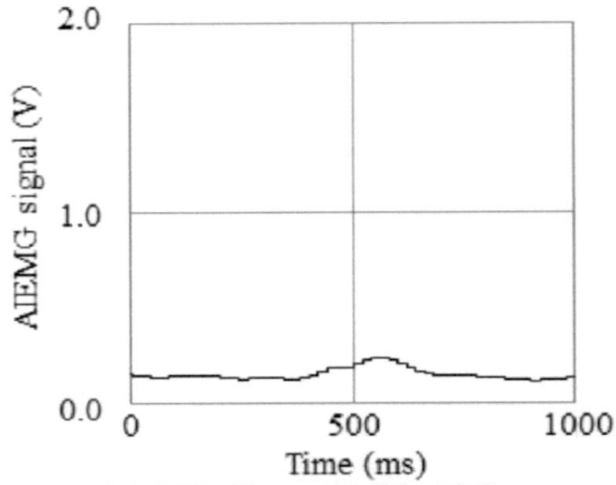

(c1_200) Channel 1 (N = 200)

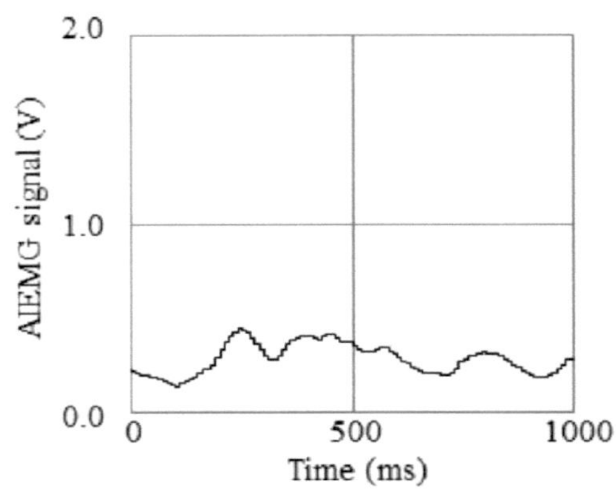

(c2_100) Channel 2 (N = 100)

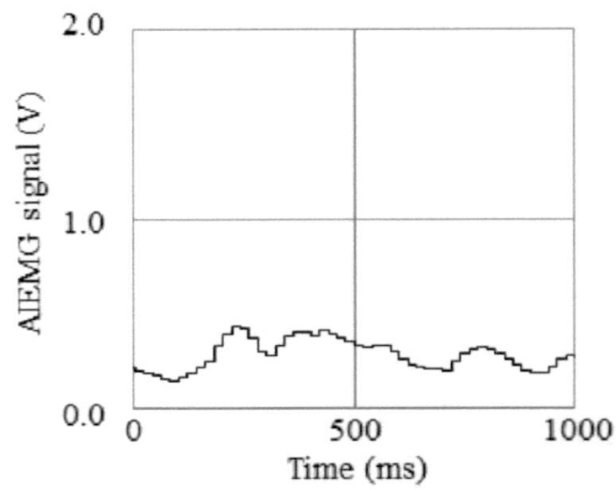

(c2_200) Channel 2 (N = 200)

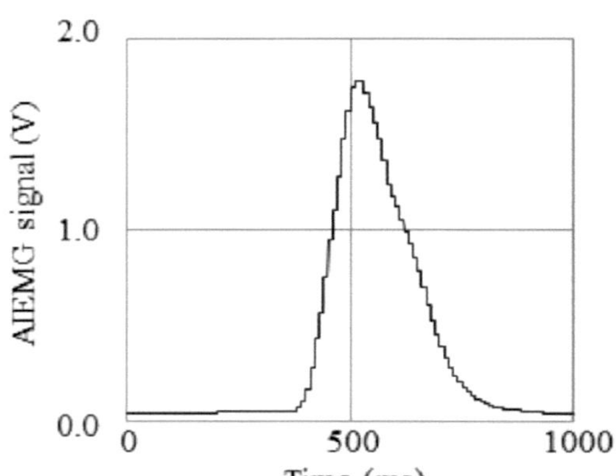

(c3_100) Channel 3 (N = 100)

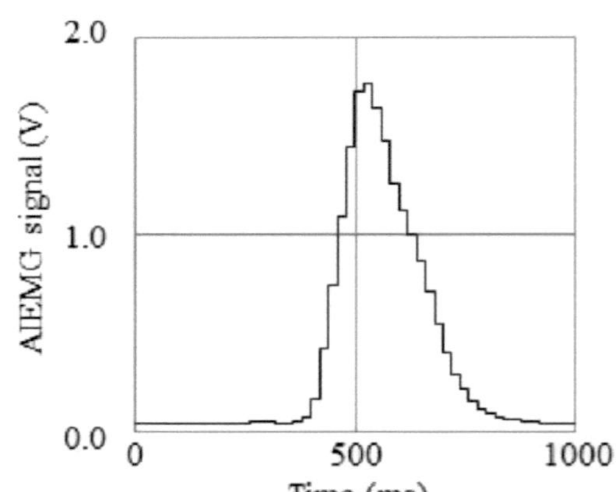

(c3_200) Channel 3 (N = 200)

(2)

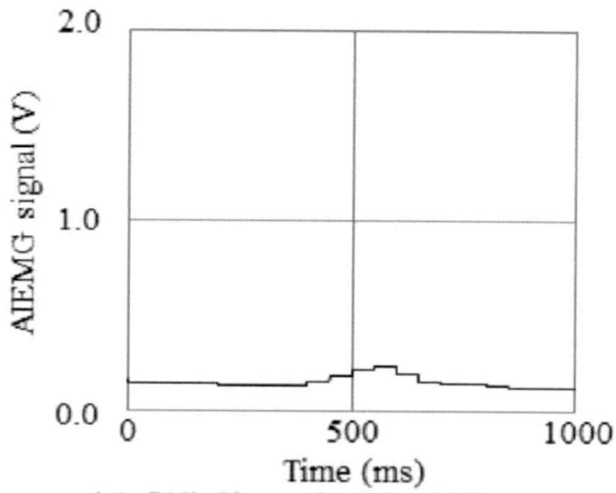

(c1_500) Channel 1 (N = 500)

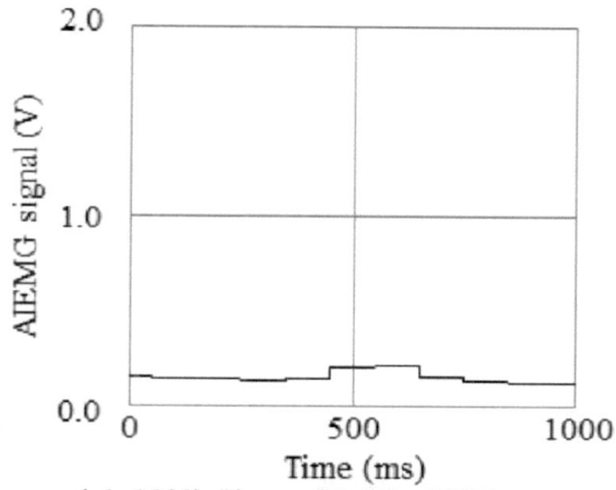

(c1_1000) Channel 1 (N = 1000)

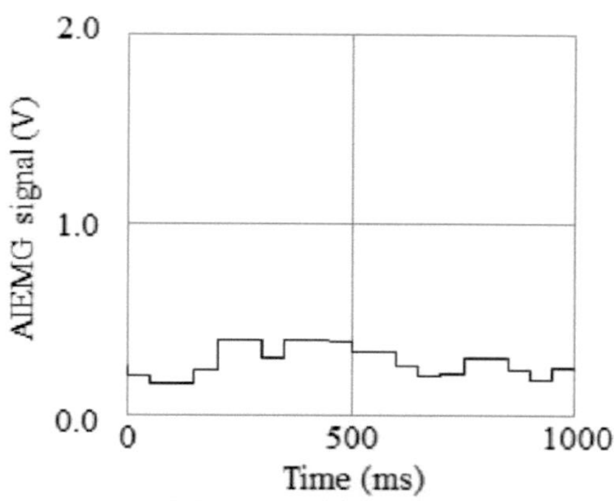

(c2_500) Channel 2 (N = 500)

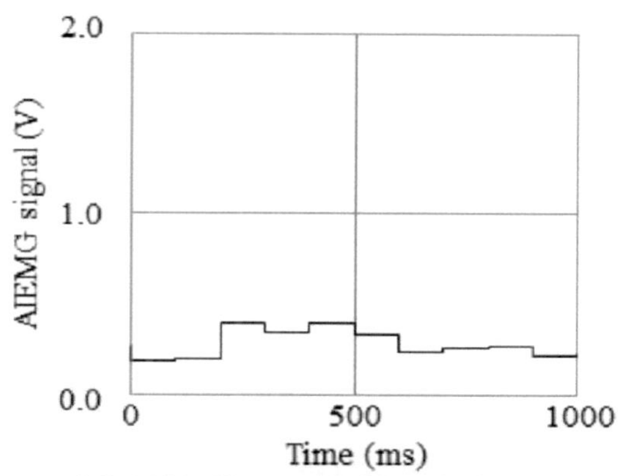

(c2_1000) Channel 2 (N = 1000)

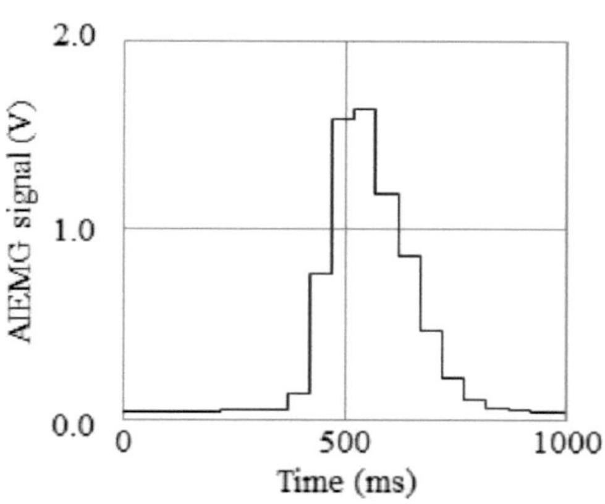

(c3_500) Channel 3 (N = 500)

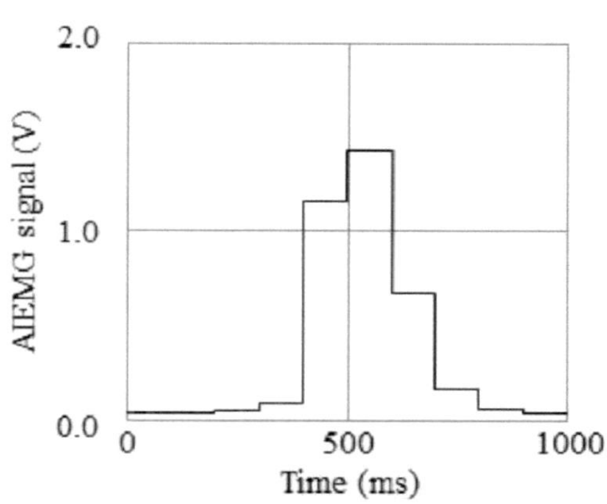

(c3_1000) Channel 3 (N = 1000)

(3)

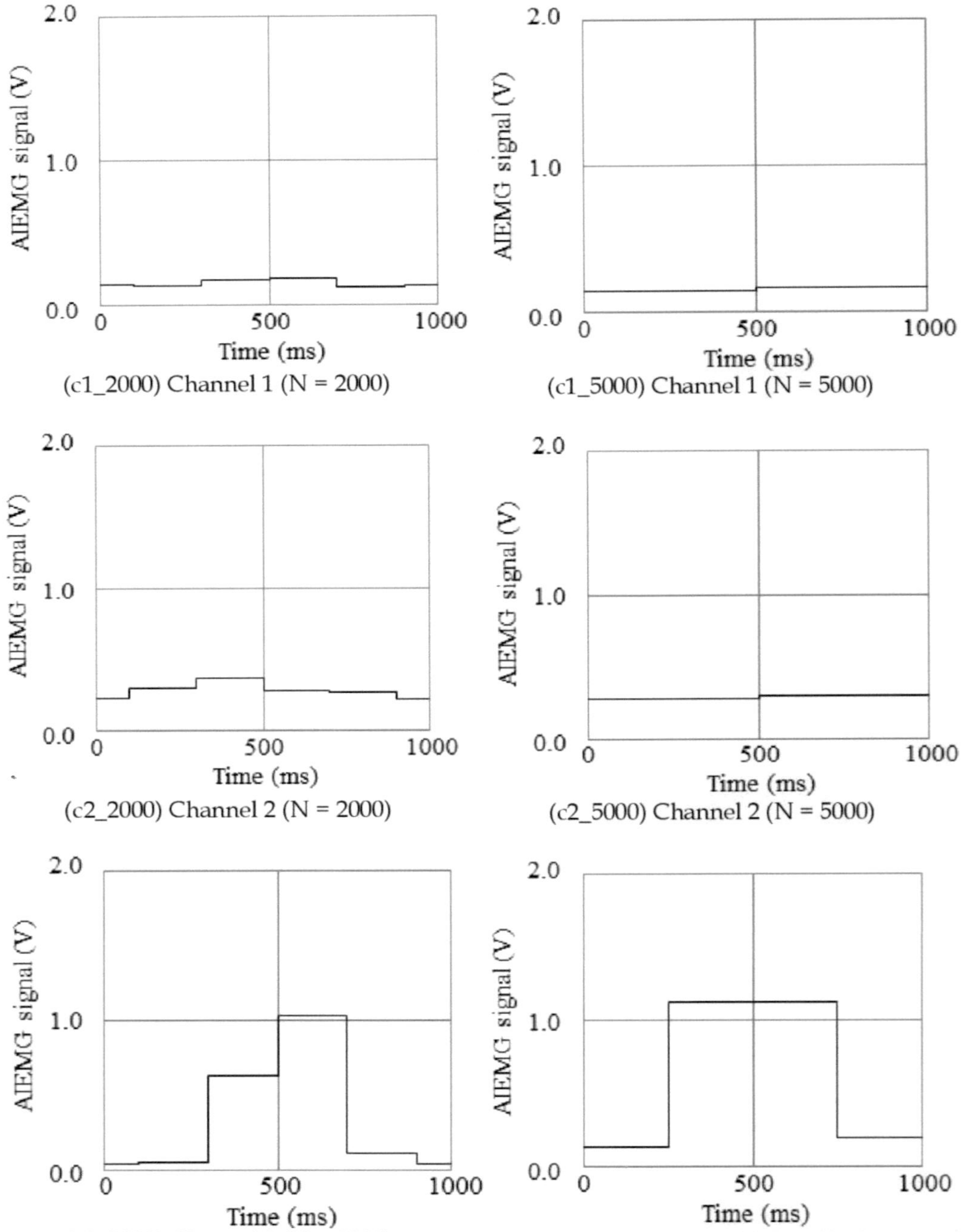

(c1_2000) Channel 1 (N = 2000)

(c1_5000) Channel 1 (N = 5000)

(c2_2000) Channel 2 (N = 2000)

(c2_5000) Channel 2 (N = 5000)

(c3_2000) Channel 3 (N = 2000)

(c3_5000) Channel 3 (N = 5000)

(4)

Figure 10. AIEMG signals regarding "rock"

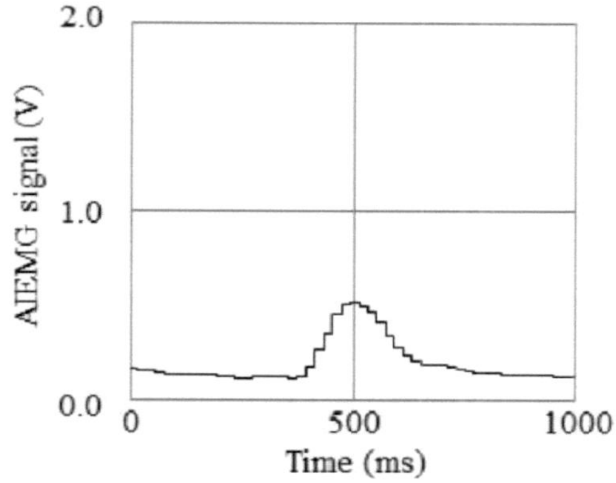

(c1_200) Channel 1

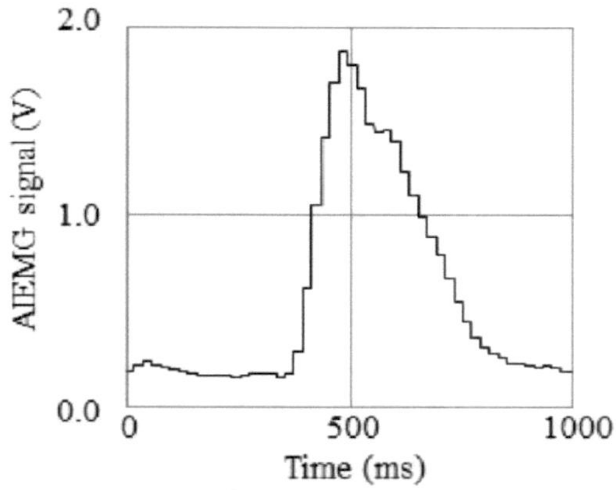

(c2_200) Channel 2

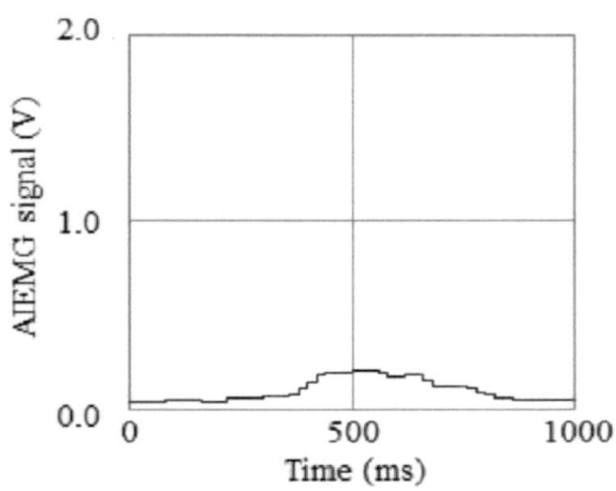

(c2_200) Channel 3

(N = 200)

Figure 11. AIEMG signals regarding "scissors"

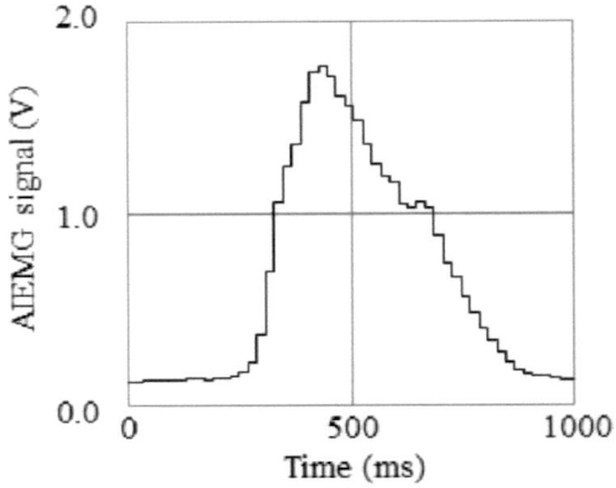

(c1_200) Channel 1

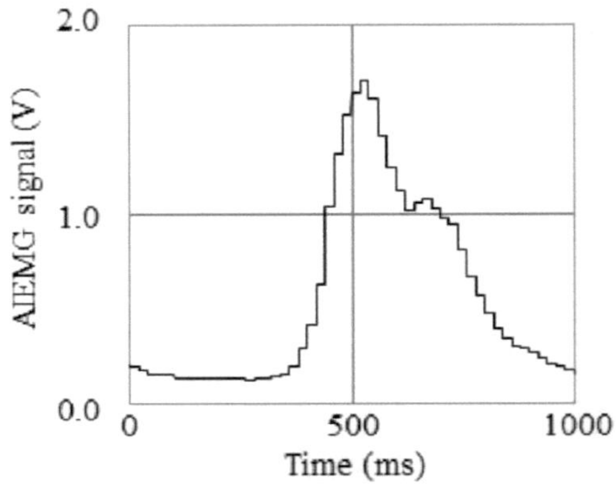

(c2_200) Channel 2

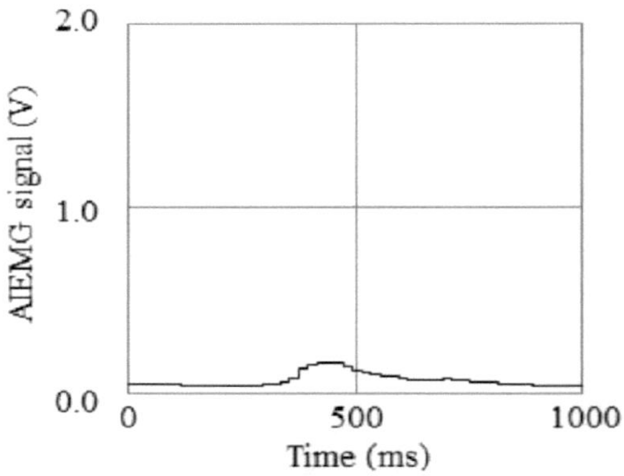

(c3_200) Channel 3

(N = 200)

Figure 12. AIEMG signals regarding "paper"

3.2. AIEMG signals

We next calculated the averaged IEMG (AIEMG) signals from IEMG according to eq. (1). They are stable and noiseless compared to the IEMG, because the feature prevents instantaneous noise of IEMG signals. It is important to adopt the optimum sampling number, N, to obtain the ideal AIEMG feature. When the number is too small, the signal intensity fluctuates and it is difficult to obtain consistent feature at every measurement. If it is too large, the AIEMG signal becomes blunt and thus its original waveform is lost.

Figure 10 shows the examples of AIEMG derived from IEMG signals indicated in Fig. 5, with regard to the number of sampling, N as 1, 50, 100, 200, 500, 1000, 2000, and 5000.

Figure 10(c1_1), for instance, displays the AIEMG signal measured by channels 1 with sampling number of 1, where the horizontal axis expresses time, and the vertical represents magnitude of the AIEMG signal.

Figures 11 and 12 are representations of the AIEMG signals regarding channels 2 and 3, respectively, whose sampling number is 200.

4. Finger sign identification based on forearm AIEMG signals

4.1. Muscle activity corresponding to finger sign

When evaluating the experimental results, we have Table 1 which indicates contribution of muscles to gesticulation by hands. Extensor pollicis brevis does its part only in displaying "paper" among three signs. Extensor digitorum works when forming "scissors" and "paper." Flexor digitorum profundus contributes only to indication of "rock."

This table helps us to classify displayed finger signs based only on the forearm surface EMG signals in real time. If obtaining any of the specific EMG signal combinations shown in the table, we can deduce one of the finger signs among three.

Note that an electrode does not necessarily catch signals only when the corresponding muscle works. Thus, it is necessary to differentiate active signals from inactive to identify muscle motion precisely.

Muscle		Rock	Scissors	Paper
Ch.1	Extensor pollicis brevis	×	×	○
Ch.2	Extensor digitorum	×	○	○
Ch.3	Flexor digitorum profundus	○	×	×

○: Active ×: Inactive

Table 1. Muscle activity pattern for finger sign

4.2. Criterion of muscle activity

We have next investigated an identification of finger signs by analyzing the AIEMG of a forearm. The EMG signals were detected by three electrodes put on the forearm skin of the subjects, and active signals were distinguished from inactive ones according to the following principle. An algorithm for identifying finger motion was designed to refer the active/inactive combination described above.

We have measured the forearm EMG signals in advance to determine the criterion for each muscle to discriminate between active and inactive signals. The criteria were separately settled with regard to several sampling numbers by observing activity of the muscles. The activity is evaluated by the peak voltage of each AIEMG signal.

Ten trials were conducted by gesturing each of the hand shapes for each sampling number.

Experimental results are arranged in Fig. 13.

Figure 13(d1_1), for example, indicates the magnitude of 30 AIEMG waveforms detected by channel 1 with the sampling number of 1. The vertical axis represents the peak voltage of the AIEMG signal when the subject made gestures of "rock," "scissors," and "paper." It implys the activity of extensor pollicis brevis. We determined the criterion index, CI_1 for channel 1 at N=1 as 0.58 V, which is illustrated by a bold line in the figure.

The activity of muscles can be estimated according to the criteria as follows. Provided that the magnitude of a measured signal is larger than the criterion, the corresponding muscle is presumed to be active. Otherwise it is considered to be inactive.

All the data regarding "rock" and "scissors" were smaller than the line, while those for "paper" were larger in this figure. That is why we could surmise that extensor pollicis brevis is active only for "paper."

In the same way, the output AIEMG signals of channels 2 and 3 are arranged as for N=1 in Figs. 11 (d2_1) and (d3_1), respectively. The criterion indices, CI_2 and CI_3 for channel 2 and 3 were determined as 0.76 and 0.61 V, respectively. By acquired AIEMG signals of extensor digitorum, channel 2 indicated the muscle is active for "scissors" and "paper." Channel 3, representing the activity of flexor digitorum profundus, confirmed that the muscle is active only in the case of "rock."

Note that these experimental data support the classification patterns of finger signs shown in Table 1.

With respect to other sampling numbers, similar features were observed as shown in Fig.11(d1_50) - (d3_5000). Their corresponding criteria were determined as shown in Table 2.

N	CI_1 (V)	CI_2 (V)	CI_3 (V)
1	0.58	0.76	0.61
50	0.54	0.76	0.58
100	0.53	0.76	0.58
200	0.53	0.76	0.59
500	0.48	0.73	0.56
1000	0.47	0.71	0.51
2000	0.38	0.54	0.33
5000	0.22	0.40	0.23

Table 2. Criterion of muscle activity

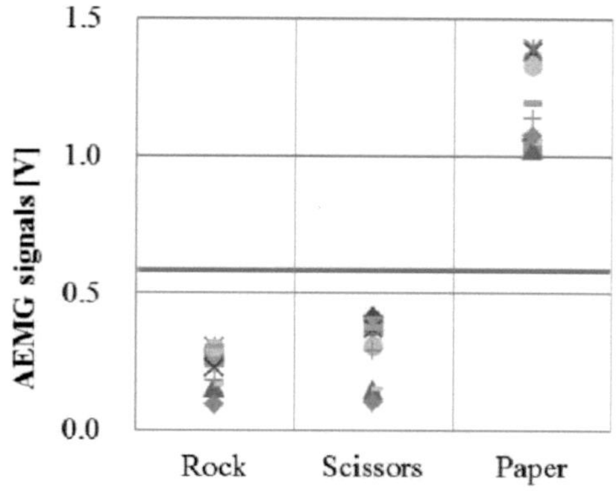

(d1_1) Channel 1 (N = 1)

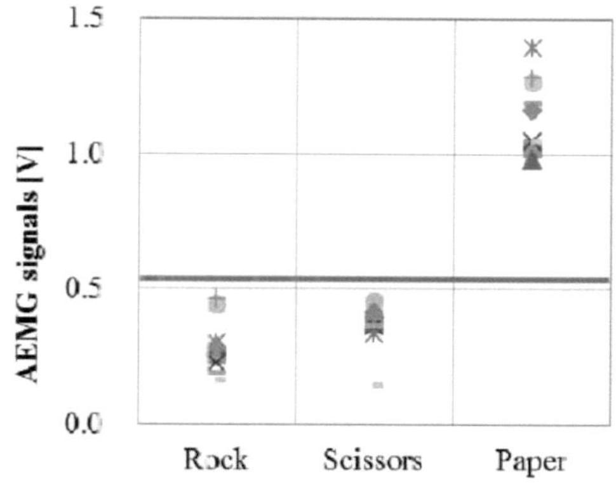

(d1_50) Channel 1 (N = 50)

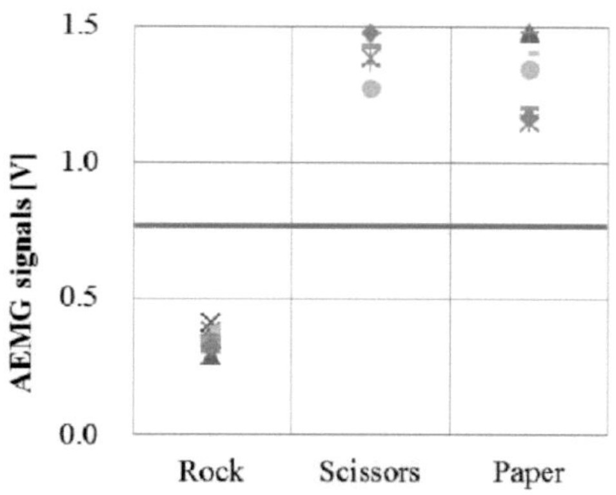

(d2_1) Channel 2 (N = 1)

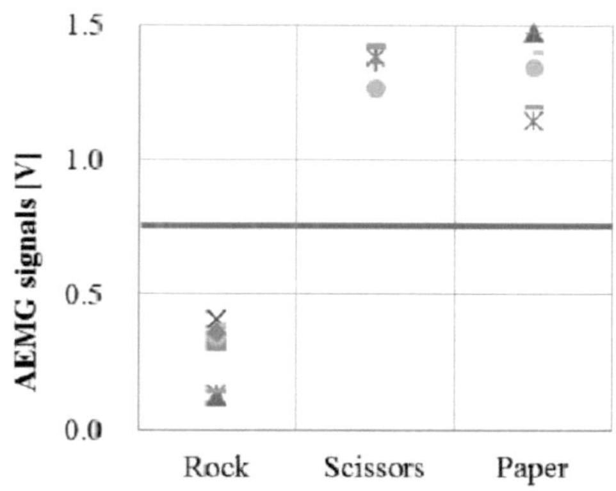

(d2_50) Channel 2 (N = 50)

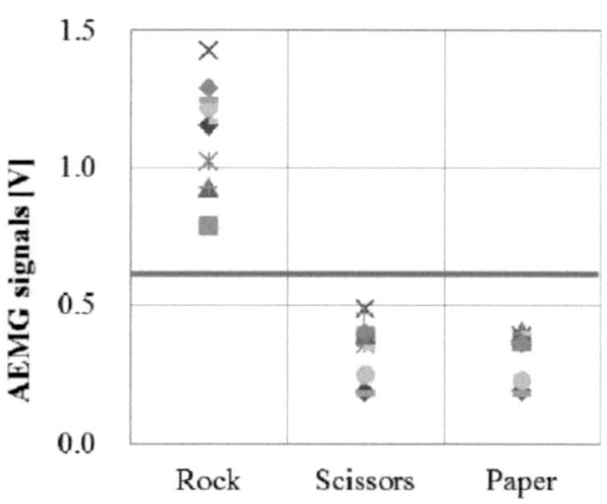

(d3_1) Channel 3 (N = 1)

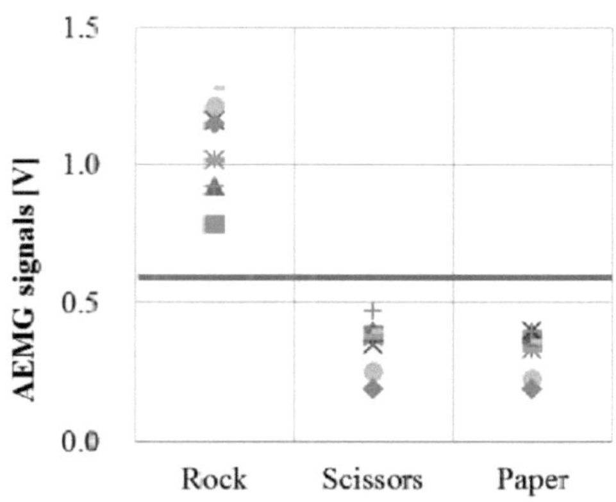

(d3_50) Channel 3 (N = 50)

(1)

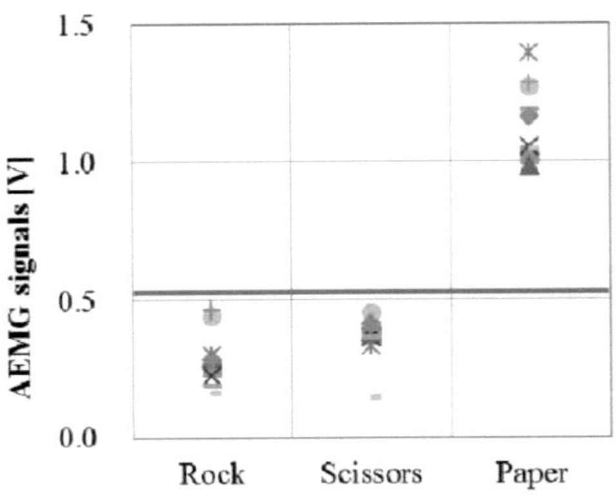

(d1_100) Channel 1 (N = 100)

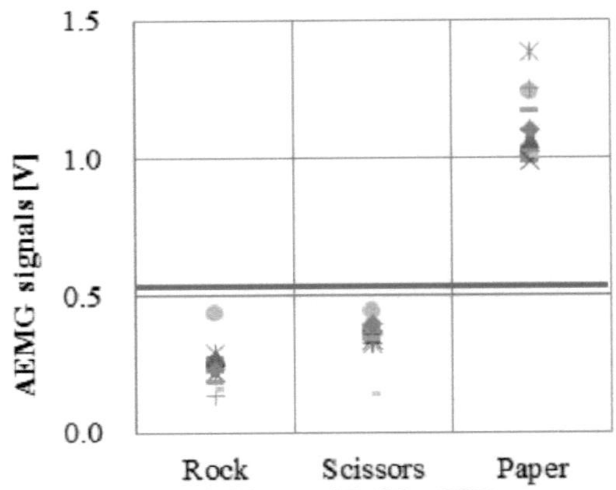

(d1_200) Channel 1 (N = 200)

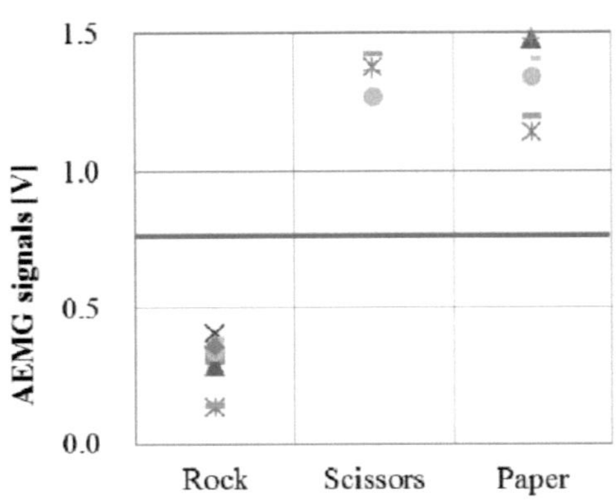

(d2_100) Channel 2 (N = 100)

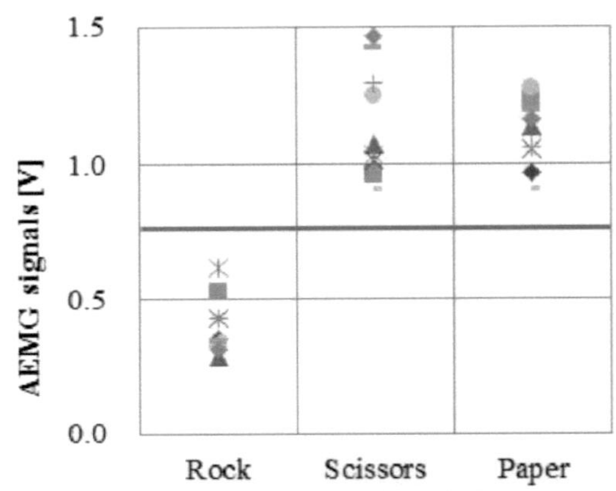

(d2_200) Channel 2 (N = 200)

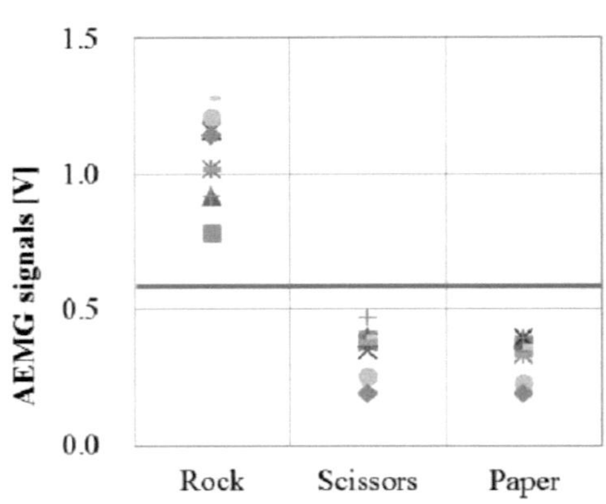

(d3_100) Channel 3 (N = 100)

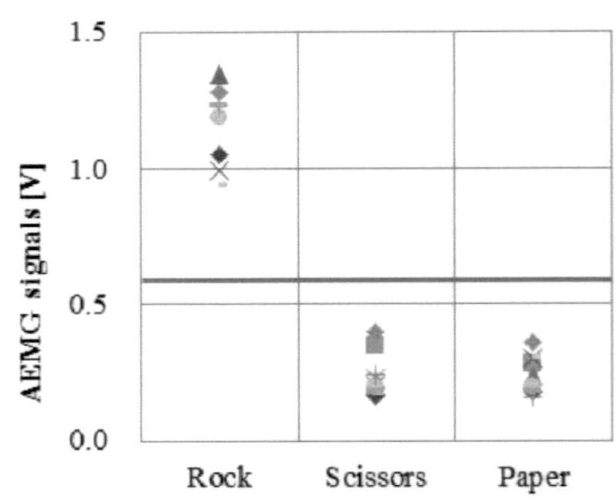

(d3_200) Channel 3 (N = 200)

(2)

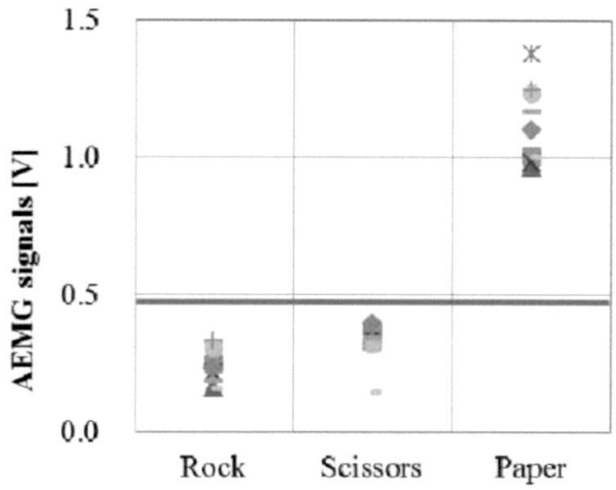

(d1_500) Channel 1 (N = 500)

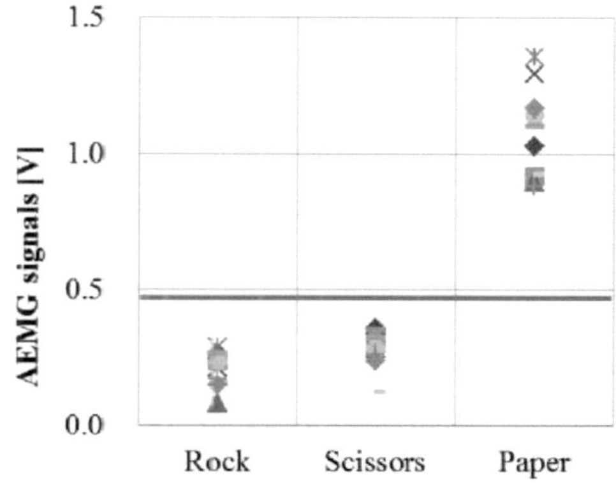

(d1_1000) Channel 1 (N = 1000)

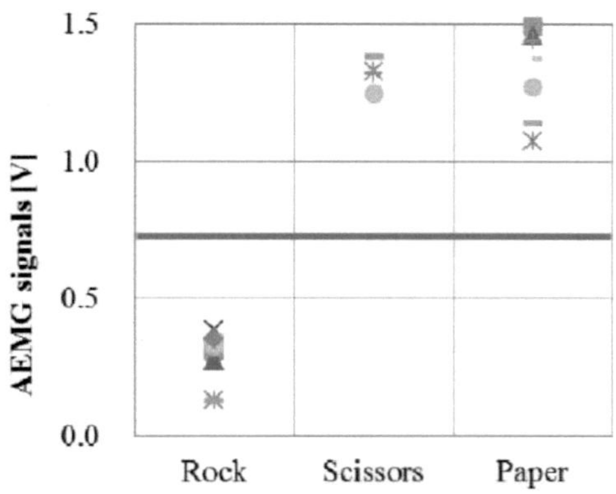

(d2_500) Channel 2 (N = 500)

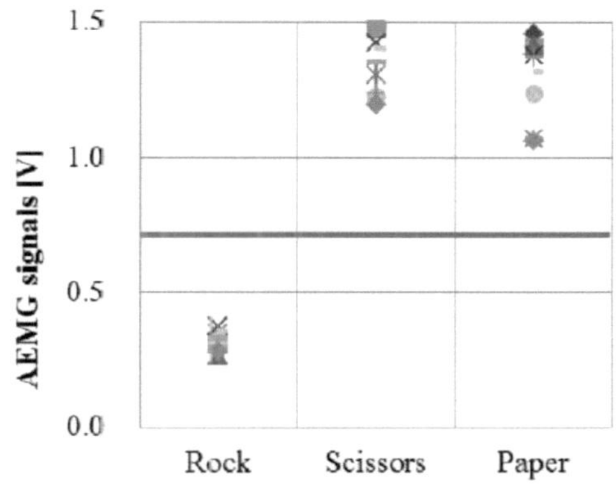

(d2_1000) Channel 2 (N = 1000)

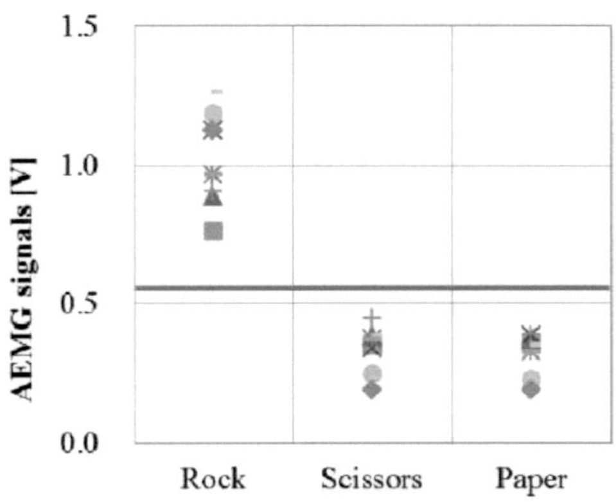

(d3_500) Channel 3 (N = 500)

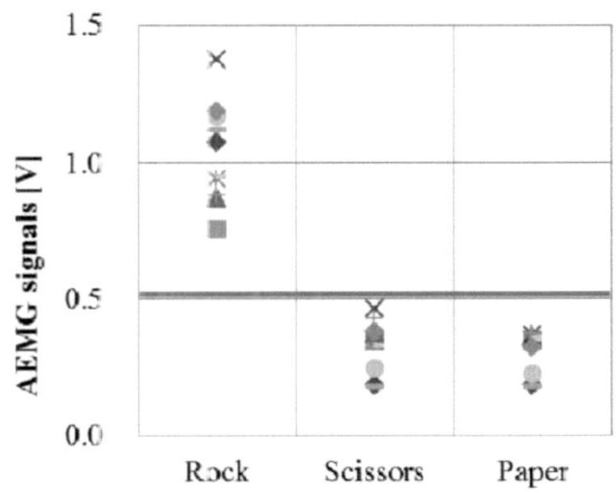

(d3_1000) Channel 3 (N = 1000)

(3)

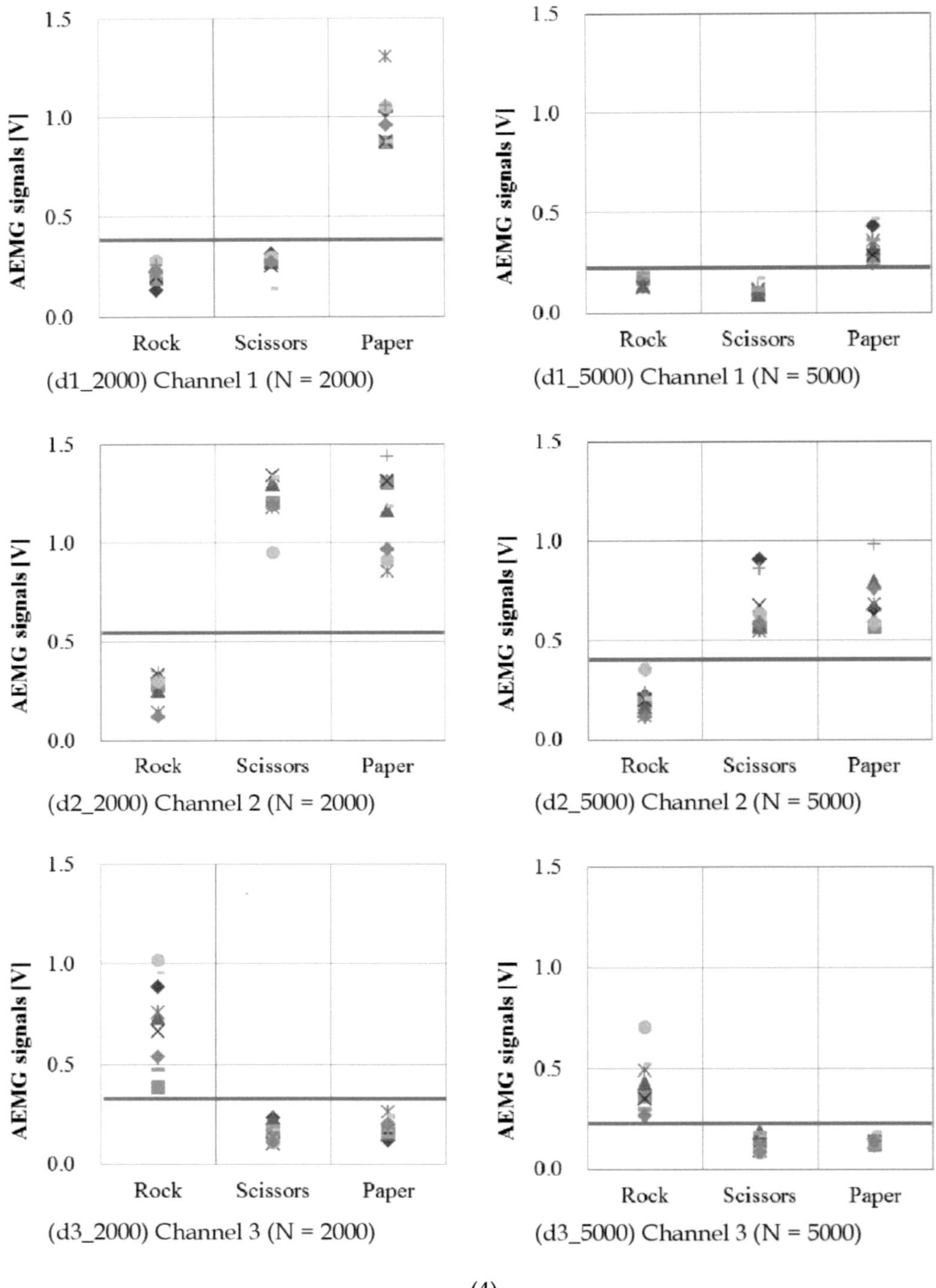

Figure 13. Discrimination between active and inactive muscle

4.3. Finger gesture estimation

A flowchart of the gesture estimation algorithm is shown in Fig. 14. First of all, the AIEMG features are calculated by eq. (1). Next, the peak intensity, $AIEMG_2$ of the AIEMG signal detected by channel 2 is compared with the criterion index, CI_2. Then, the intensities, $AIEMG_3$ and $AIEMG_1$ are weighed against the criterion indices, CI_3 and CI_1, respectively. This process checks the combination of the measured AIEMG signals against the activation patterns of muscles corresponding to the finger signs shown in Table 1.

We finally carried out the experiments of finger sign estimation based on the algorithm. Identification rate was evaluated after 40 trials were conducted for each finger sign. Several sampling numbers for AIEMG feature were investigated. Experimental results are indicated in Table 3 and Fig. 15, which show percentages of correct answers with regard to each sampling number. They suggest that N=200 is the optimum sampling number among our investigations after all. Detailed analysis clarified that larger sampling number, e. g. N=1000, deforms the signals into blunt waveforms and thus it occasionally prevents discriminating between active and inactive signals. On the other hand, the AIEMG signals contain some transient noise when the sampling number is too small. It caused misjudgment on discrimination of activity of extensor pollicis brevis, for instance, that is evaluated with electrode 1 (channel 1). It can be considered to be one of the reasons why the identification rate of "paper" is inferior to the others.

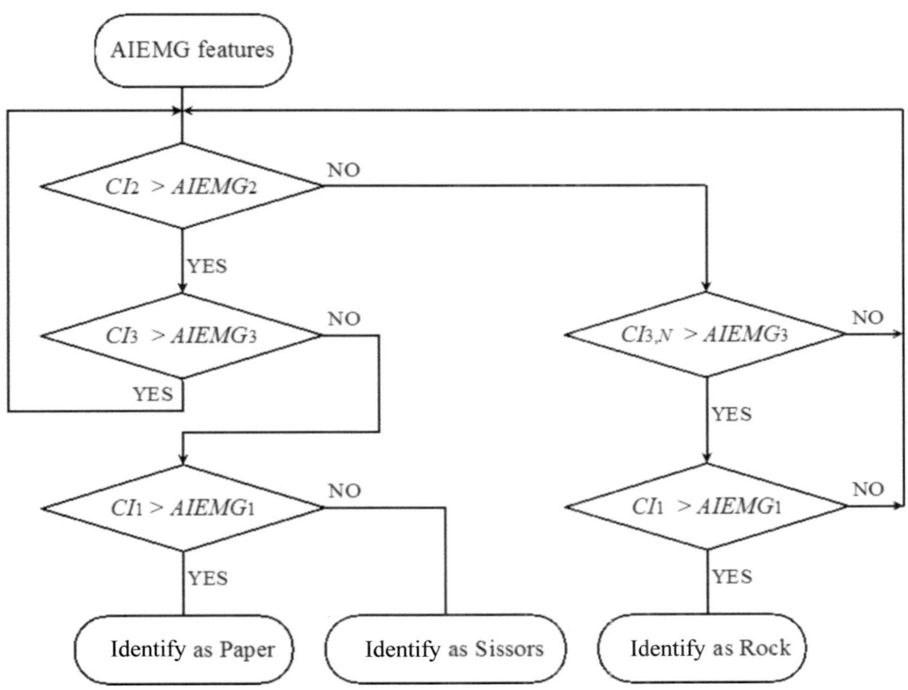

Figure 14. Finger sign estimation algorithm

N	Rock (%)	Scissors (%)	Paper (%)	Total(%)
1	97.5	87.5	57.5	80.8
50	97.5	97.5	65.0	86. 7
100	95.0	95.0	70.0	86. 7
200	97.5	97.5	97.5	97.5
500	95.0	85.0	70.0	83.3
1000	90.0	77.5	82.5	83.3
2000	80.0	62.5	57.5	66. 7
5000	37.5	27.5	20.0	28.3

Table 3. Accuracy rate of finger sign identification

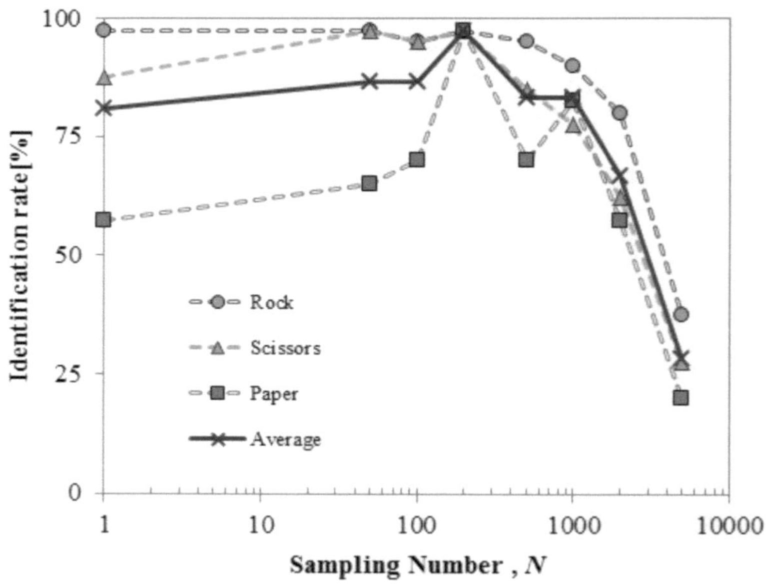

Figure 15. Experimental results of finger sign identification

5. Conclusion

We have studied the estimation method of hand signs employing the electromyogram. This paper focused on the forearm EMG signals caused by the finger motion. It relys on the proposition that the specific muscles of forearms work even if you only move your fingers.

First of all, the EMG measurement system was designed to detect signals from the surface skin of forearms. We constructed three-channel myoelectric signal processing system by assigning three forearm muscles; extensor pollicis brevis, extensor digitorum, and flexor digitorum profundus. It provided EMG and IEMG signals, and also calculated AIEMG features.

Fundamental experiments were carried out next to acquire data regarding the relationship between the finger motion and the forearm EMG signals. Investigation on myoelectric responses revealed that the specified forearm muscles were activated with respect to the corresponding finger motion.

The disclosed principles were applied to identification of typical hand signs such as "rock," "paper," and "scissors" in terms of the well-known hand game. We obtained correlative experimental data of hand signs and the myoelectric signals.

We found out the activity pattern of forearm muscles with regard to each hand sign as follows. If shaping "rock," flexor digitorum profundus is mainly working. When "scissors" are indicated, extensor digitorum is activated. Display of "paper" is owing to both extensor pollicis brevis and extensor digitorum.

We established the following principles in consequence to deduce the hand sign from the activities of forearm muscles. Extensor pollicis brevis is active in displaying "paper." Extensor digitorum operates when forming "scissors" and "paper." Flexor digitorum profundus contributes only to indication of "rock."

We then designed the classification algorithm based on the results. Because the myoelectric signals fluctuated and depended on the measurement conditions in reality, we determined the criterion of each muscle's activity by statistical treatment and we evaluated the averaged IEMG signals. The AIEMG functioned as a kind of low-pass filters, and its performance was dependent on the sampling number. We investigated the results of AIEMG features and determined the optimum sampling number was 200.

Finally, we conducted some experiments on real-time discrimination of three typical hand signs. The identification accuracy was no less than 97 % with respect to any hand sign when choosing the optimum sampling number.

Experimental results proved that the proper AIEMG feature was successful in inferring the shape of hands. We have confirmed the validity and effectiveness of our proposed estimation system at last. Thus, the method to estimate hand signs has been established based on the activity of forearm muscles instead of finger muscles.

6. Future directions

Our study was just started with myoelectrical analysis on the forearm muscles and finger motion. Proposed technique was applied to the hand game called "rock-paper-scissors." But it was configured so as to verify the validity of the method rather than to demonstrate its usefulness.

We are planning to improve the technique to human-robot interface system. The advanced input device for computers is one of the applications, which is more intuitive than the data-glove. Such versatile system is neccesary to distinguish many finger motions based on vague myoelectric information.

This paper evaluated the myoelectric signals processed simply by statistic evaluation for noise reduction or feature extraction. Higher performance may be expected by introducing some meta-heuristic method or intelligent method, e. g. neural networks, or suppot vector machine.

The muscle activity was determined on the basis of dualistic taxology according to the criterion established beforehand in this paper. It is necessary to determine the criterion adaptively to the measument conditions to apply to realtime robotic systems.

Practical systems will be realized by integrated measurement method combined with the other perceptual devices.

The proposed technique will be improved not only to the engineering applications but the medical ones, such as the bio-feedback system in rehabilitation or the phyisical support system for handicapped persons.

Author details

Takeshi Tsujimura
Department of Mechanical Engineering, Saga University, Japan

Sho Yamamoto
Department of Mechanical Engineering, Saga University, Japan

Kiyotaka Izumi
Department of Mechanical Engineering, Saga University, Japan

7. References

Chan, F. H., Lam, Y. Y., Zhang, Y., & Parker, P. A. (2000). Fuzzy EMG classification for prosthesis control, *IEEE Transactions on Rehabilitation Engineering*, Vol. 8, No. 3, (2000), pp. 305–311

Chen, X., Zhang, X., Zhao, Z., Yang, J., Lantz, V., & Wang, K. (2007). Multiple Hand Gesture Recognition based on Surface EMG Signal, *The 1st International Conference on Bioinformatics and Biomedical Engineering 2007*, (2007), pp.506-509

Fukuda, O., Tsuji, T., Kaneko, M., & Otsuka, A. (2003). A human-assisting manipulator teleoperated by EMG signals and arm motions, *IEEE Transactions on Robotics and Automation*, Vol. 19, No. 7, (2003), pp. 323–345

Graupe, D., Magnussen, J., & Beex, A. A. M. (1978). A micro-processor system for multifunctional control of upper limb prostheses via myoelectric signal identification, *IEEE Transactions on automatic control*, Vol. 23, No. 4, (1978), pp. 538–544

Huang, Y., Englehart, K.B., Hudgins, B., & Chan, A.D.C. (2005). A gaussian mixture model based classification scheme for myoelectric control of powered upper limb prostheses, *IEEE Transactions on Biomedical Engineering*, Vol. 52, No. 11, (2005), pp.1801-1810

Hudgins, B., Parker, P. A., & Scott, R. N. (1993). New strategy for multi-function myoelectric control, *IEEE Transactions on Biomedical Engineering*, Vol. 40, No. 1, (1993), pp. 82–94

Ibe, A., Gouko, M., & Ito K. (2009). Discrimination of Combined Motions for Prosthetic Hands Using Surface EMG Signals, *Transactions of the Society of Instrument and Control Engineers*, Vol. 45, No. 12, (2009), pp.717-723

Jacobson, S. C., Knutti, D. F., Johnson, R. T., & Sears, H. H. (1982). Development of the utah artificial arm, *IEEE Transactions on Biomedical Engineering*, Vol. 29, No. 4, (1982), pp. 249–169

Karlik, B., & Tokhi, M. O. (2003). A fuzzy clustering neural network architecture for multifunction upper-limb prosthesis, *IEEE Transactions on Biomedical Engineering*, Vol. 50, No. 11, (2003), pp. 1255–1261

Milner-Brown, H. S., & Stein, R. B. (1975). The relation between the surface electromyogram and muscular force, *Journal of Physiology*, Vol. 246, (1975), pp. 549–569

Oskoei, M.A., & Huosheng, H. (2008). Support Vector Machine-Based Classification Scheme for Myoelectric Control Applied to Upper Limb, *IEEE Transactions on Biomedical Engineering*, Vol. 55, Issue 8, (2008), pp.1956 - 1965

Tsujimura, T., Yamamoto, S., & Izumi K. (2011). Finger Gesture Estimation Based on Forearm Electromyogram Signals, *7th International Symposium on Image and Signal Processing and Analysis*, (2011), pp. 113-118

Yamamoto, S., Tsujimura, T., & Izumi K. (2012). Hand gesture identification using forearm surface EMG signals, *Proc. of 2012 JSME Conference on Robotics and Mechatronics*, (2012), A1A-V06

Yoshikawa, M., Mikawa, M., & Tanaka, K. (2007). A myoelectric interface for robotic hand control using support vector machine, *IEEE /RJS International Conference on Intelligent Robots and Systems*, San Diego, (2007), pp.2723-2728

Yoshikawa, M., Mikawa, M., & Tanaka, K. (2009). Real-Time Hand Motion Classification Using EMG Signals with Support Vector Machines, *The IEICE Transactions on information and systems (Japanese edition)*, Vol.J92-D, No.1, (2009), pp.93-103

Chapter 14

Proposal of a Neuro Fuzzy System for Myoelectric Signal Analysis from Hand-Arm Segment

Gabriela Winkler Favieiro and Alexandre Balbinot

Additional information is available at the end of the chapter

http://dx.doi.org/10.5772/48793

1. Introduction

Many with disabilities have some difficulties in integrating into society due to impossibility or to restriction in performing simple tasks of day-to-day. This situation is gradually changing by virtue of technological development in the biomedical instrumentation area in respect of human rehabilitation and especially with in the development of assistive technology managed by computational intelligence (computing algorithms and learning machines using techniques as fuzzy logic, artificial neural networks, genetic algorithms, support vector machines, among others). Scientific researches in this area are allowing the development of several mechanisms to improve the life quality of people with special needs, making them more independent and more likely to real social and economical integration.

It's possible to cite, for example, research related to robotic prosthesis. The development of system managed by myoelectric signals (MES) with the intention to mimic the human arm movement, is far from perfect, making the subject of many researches (Ajiboye & Weir, 2005; Chan et al., 2000; Englehart & Hudgins, 2003; Favieiro & Balbinot, 2011; Favieiro et al., 2011; Hincapie & Kirsch, 2009; Hudgins et al., 1991; Hudgins et al., 1994; Jacobsen et al., 1982; Katutoshi et al., 1992; Khushaba et al., 2010; Momen et al., 2007; Park & Meek, 1995). These researches are mainly being conducted in able-bodies subjects to verify the feasibility and performance of different algorithms for pattern recognition using EMG signals from the forearm muscles. In these studies are usually employed a high number of electrode pairs, ranging from 4 to 12. Using classification patterns techniques such as LDA, fuzzy logic, among others, was found high accuracies (>90%) for the classification of different moves ranging from four to ten. Develop a robotic prosthesis as similar as possible to the human arm is not a simple task. There are great difficulties both in the area of distinguish the various degrees of freedom that the arm can have as developing a robotic prosthesis that can accomplish or replicate all these movements.

Briefly, the myoelectric signal is the bio-signal muscle control of the human body which contains the information of the user's intent to contract a muscle and, therefore, perform a certain movement. Studies have shown that amputees are able to repeatedly generate certain standard myoelectric signals in front of intention to carry out a particular movement. It makes the use of such signal highly advantageous, because the control of a robotic prosthesis can be accomplished according to user's intention to perform a specified movement. Furthermore, detection of the myoelectric signal can be obtained noninvasively through surface electrodes. Although the distress signal has low amplitude (mV range) is sufficient for its analysis and surface electrodes are far more hygienic and convenient as the removal, insertion and sterilization can be accomplished by the user.

Therefore, it is possible to distinguish certain muscle movements while processing the electrical parameters of the myoelectric signal both in time domain and frequency domain. With the characterized movements is possible to control a robotic prosthesis that aims to replicate, the best possible, the movements of a human arm. Considering that premise, this research aims to study and develop a system that uses myoelectric signals, acquired by surface electrodes, to characterize certain movements of the human arm, allowing studies between man and machine with adequate precision for future enabling the actual replacement of an amputee limb with a robotic prosthesis suitable and intuitively controlled through the remaining muscle signals. To recognize certain hand-arm segment movements, was developed an algorithm for pattern recognition technique based on neuro-*fuzzy*, representing the core of this research. This algorithm has as input the preprocessed myoelectric signal, to disclosed specific characteristics of the signal, and as output the performed movement.

The present research was also preoccupy in not only distinguish certain simple movements of the human arm, but also characterize complex movements that combine several degrees of freedom, making this study more closely to the reality, in which more degrees of freedom represents an improve in the life quality of people with special needs, making them more likely to real integration in the society.

2. Soft computing

The understanding, processing or solving complex problems require intelligent systems that combine knowledge, techniques and methodologies from various sources (Zadeh, 1992). Thus, intelligent systems should aggregate human knowledge in a specific domain, adapt and learn the best way possible in environments that are constantly changing. For this reasons, it is very advantageous to use several computational techniques instead of just one, which is the essence of neuro-*fuzzy* technique: neural networks that recognize patterns and are able to adapt to changes and the *fuzzy* inference system that incorporates human knowledge for making decisions.

Typically a fuzzy system incorporates a rule base, membership functions and an inference procedure and has been presenting success in systems with applications in the presence of ambiguous elements (Begg et al., 2008; Zadeh et al., 2004). Systems combining neural networks with fuzzy systems usually have the following characteristics (Jang, 1997):

- human knowledge presented in the form of rules, for example, if-then;
- computational models based on biological models, such as the use of neural networks for pattern recognition;
- optimization techniques, such as the use of a hybrid technique;
- construction of a model with data sample;
- numerical computation instead of symbolic computation.

This chapter briefly presents the fuzzy techniques, adaptive algorithms, neuro-fuzzy and data clustering used in the present research.

2.1. Fuzzy logic

A fuzzy set is defined as a set or collection of elements with membership values between 0 and 1. Therefore, the transition between belonging or not belonging to the set is gradual and is characterized by its fuzzy Membership Function (MF) that is used to describe the fuzzy membership value given to fuzzy set elements (Begg et al., 2008) enabling the fuzzy set model linguist expression used in everyday life, such as, "the rms value of the masseter myoelectric signal is medium high". For these reasons, the fuzzy sets theory is very efficient when dealing with concepts of ambiguity (Zadeh, 1992) and allows its use in several applications.

Therefore, a fuzzy set not-empty Z in a given space **X** ($Z \subseteq \boldsymbol{X}$), is the set represented by equations (1) e (2):

$$Z = \{(x, \mu_Z(x)); x \epsilon \boldsymbol{X}\} \tag{1}$$

$$\mu_Z: \boldsymbol{X} \rightarrow [0,1] \tag{2}$$

since μ_Z a membership function of an specified fuzzy set. This function indicates for each element $x \epsilon \boldsymbol{X}$ its membership degree to the fuzzy set Z between three possibilities (Rutkowski, 2005):

- $\mu_Z(x) = 1$ means the full membership of element x to the fuzzy set Z, in others words, $x \epsilon Z$;
- $\mu_Z(x) = 0$ means the lack of membership of element x to the fuzzy set Z, in others words, $x \notin Z$;
- $0 < \mu_Z(x) < 1$ means a partial membership of element x to the fuzzy set Z.

2.1.1. Standard forms of membership functions

A membership function (MF) is a curve that defines how a point in the input space is mapped into a membership degree between 0 and 1 (Dubois, 1980). Typically a MF is defined by a mathematical expression. Following is a few membership functions ($\mu_Z(x)$) commonly used.

The triangular membership function or simply membership function of class t is defined by equation (3):

$$\mu_Z(x) = t(x; a, b, c) = \begin{cases} 0, & x \le a \\ \frac{x-a}{b-a}, & a \le x \le b \\ \frac{c-x}{c-b}, & b \le x \le c \\ 0, & c \le x \end{cases} \quad (3)$$

where b is the modal value ($a < b < c$) and a and b are the upper and lower bounds of $t(x;a,b,c)$, respectively.

The Gaussian-membership function é specified by equation (4):

$$\mu_Z(x) = g(x; \sigma) = exp\left(-\left(\frac{x-\bar{x}}{\sigma}\right)^2\right) \quad (4)$$

where $\bar{x}$ is the middle and σ defines the width of the Gaussian curve. It is the most common membership function (Rutkowski, 2005). While Bell membership function é specified by equation (5):

$$\mu_Z(x) = bell(x; a, b, c) = \frac{1}{1+\left|\frac{x-c}{a}\right|^{2b}} \quad (5)$$

where the parameter a defines its width, the parameter b its slopes, and the parameter c its center.

Other membership functions found in some applications are Γ-membership function, S-membership function, trapezoidal-membership function and exponential-membership functions. For more details, see (Rutkowski, 2005). As an example, Figure 1 shows the standard format of the MF Gaussian and MF Bell.

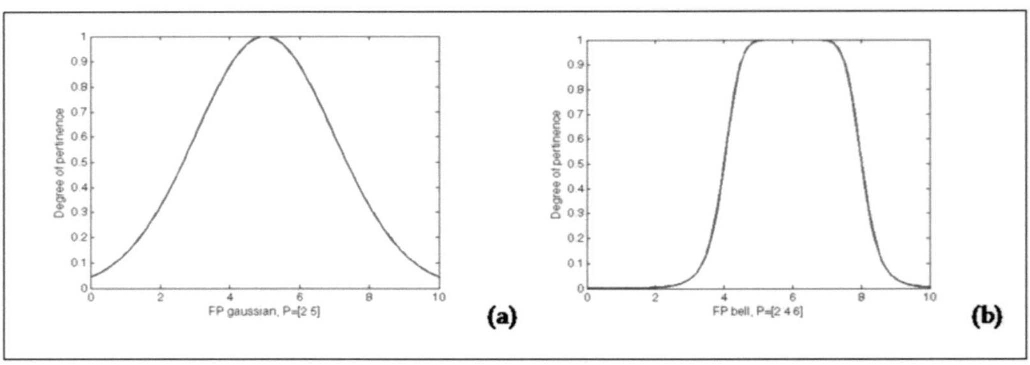

Figure 1. Membership function: (a) Gaussian and (b) bell.

The triangle and trapezoidal function are widely used in several applications because they are simple expressions and have suitable computational efficiency for real-time applications. However, these two membership functions are composed of straight line segments showing no soft edge at their ends. As a result, the Gaussian and Bell membership functions are increasingly used to specify fuzzy sets (Jang, 1997).

2.1.2. *Fuzzy reasoning and Sugeno fuzzy inference system*

In general, the fuzzy reasoning process can be divided into four main steps that are used in a fuzzy inference system (Dubois, 1980):

- comparison of the known facts to the fuzzy rules background facts to determine the compatibility degree for each of the antecedent membership function;
- combination of compatibility degrees in relation to the antecedents membership functions in a rule using fuzzy operators, for example, 'AND' or 'OR' to form the firing strength that indicates the degree whose part of the antecedent rule is satisfied;
- application of firing strength for the consequent membership function of a rule to generate a qualified consequent membership function that represents how the firing strength was propagated and utilized in a fuzzy implication statement;
- selection of all qualified consequent membership functions for the general output membership.

A fuzzy set is characterized by its membership function and operations on fuzzy sets manipulate these functions. For further details on fuzzy operations such as adding, subtracting, inverse operation, scaling operation, among others, just as, fuzzy relations and their properties consult the works indicated in the references of this chapter (Begg et al., 2008; Dubois, 1980; Rutkowski, 2005).

In recent years, different structures of neuro-fuzzy networks have been proposed combining the advantages of neural networks and fuzzy logic (Rutkowski, 2005). Several studies using the Mamdani type interference or the Takagi-Sugeno model. For this study the Sugeno fuzzy model proposed by Takagi, Sugeno and Kang (Sugeno, 1988; Takagi, 1985) had been used to generate fuzzy rules from a set of input and outputs. A typical fuzzy rule in the Sugeno fuzzy model is shown in (6):

$$\text{If x is equal to A and y is equal to B, then } z=f(x,y) \tag{6}$$

as A and B sets of fuzzy antecedents and $z= f(x,y)$ the crisp consecutive function. Considering the computational performance and the mathematical operations usually used (for instance, weighted sum) the Sugeno fuzzy model is the most popular inference system for fuzzy modeling based on input data (Jang, 1993)

2.2. Adaptive Neuro Fuzzy Inference System

Adaptive Neuro Fuzzy Inference System or ANFIS is a class of adaptive networks whose functionality is equivalent to a fuzzy inference system, proposed by Jang, which generates a fuzzy rule base and membership functions automatically (Jang, 1993).

Typically the ANFIS network topology consists of connected nodes that depend on parameters that change according to certain learning rules that minimize the error criteria. The learning technique most commonly used is the gradient method, however Jang proposed hybrid learning rule which includes the Least Square or simply LSE Estimator (Jang, 1993).

Considering a fuzzy system with three inputs x, y and z one output, v and a fuzzy inference Sugeno model. One possible set of rules is shown in equations (7) and (8):

Rule 1: If x is equal to A_1, y is equal to B_1, and z is equal to C_1, then $f_1 = p_1x + q_1y + r_1y + s_1$ (7)

Rule 2: If x is equal to A_2, y is equal to B_2, and z is equal to C_2, then $f_2 = p_2x + q_2y + r_2z + s_2$ (8)

as an example, Figure 2 illustrates the reasoning mechanism for the Sugeno inference model. The equivalent ANFIS architecture is presented in Figure 3 with nodes of same layer having similar functions. Following is an explanation for each of the network layers based on Jang's excellent text (Jang, 1997).

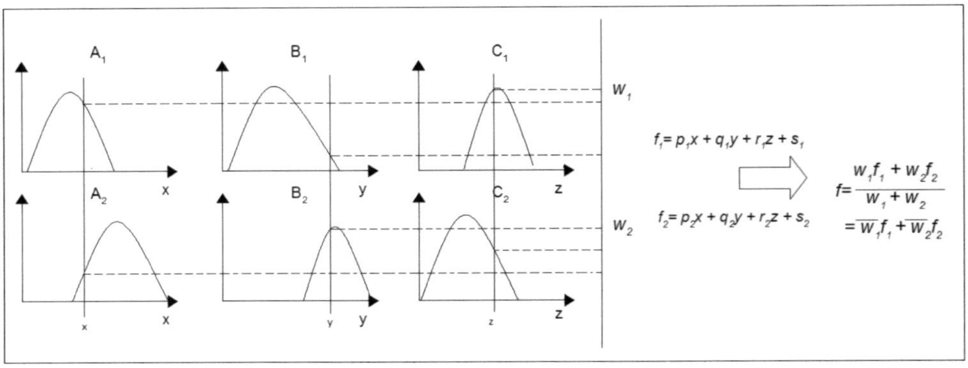

Figure 2. Example of a Sugeno inference model containing three inputs and two rules.

The first layer of Figure 3 is represented by adaptive nodes i whose functions are determined by equations (9), (10) and (11):

$$O_{1,i} = \mu_{A_i}(x), \quad para\ i = 1,2 \tag{9}$$

$$O_{1,i} = \mu_{B_{i-2}}(y), \quad para\ i = 3,4 \tag{10}$$

$$O_{1,i} = \mu_{C_{i-4}}(y), \quad para\ i = 5,6 \tag{11}$$

where x, y or z entries in node i and A_i B_{i-2} and C_{i-4} linguistic labels associated with that node. Thus, $O_{1,i}$ represents the pertinence degree to the fuzzy set A (A_1, A_2, B_1, B_2, C_1 or C_2) and specifies the degree to each input x, y or z satisfies the fuzzy set A. The membership function μ can be any of the membership functions presented in section 2.1.1. Importantly, when the values (called the premise parameters) of the membership function are changed, the function varies, i.e., display various types of MF to the fuzzy set A.

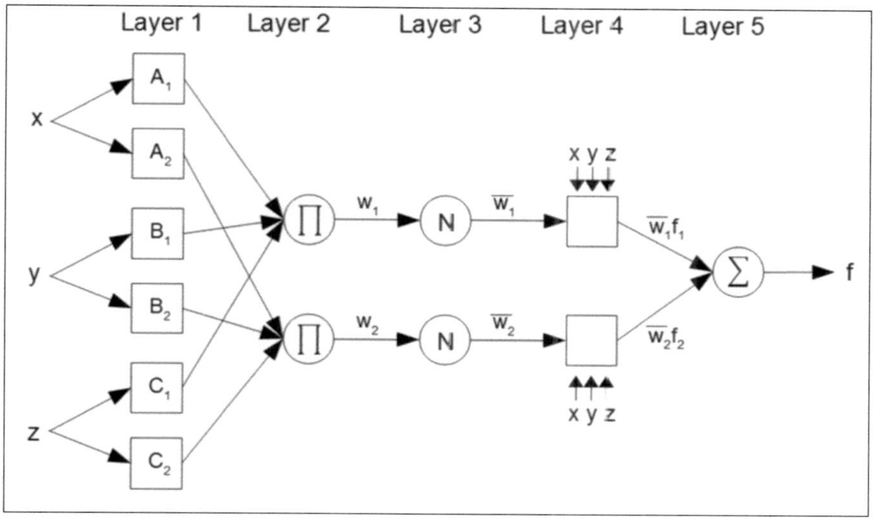

Figure 3. The equivalent ANFIS architecture of the Sugeno Fuzzy model represented in Figure 2.

The layer 2 has fixed nodes indicated by Π with outputs that represents the input signals product, as indicated in equation (12) – the output nodes represent the firing strength of a given rule:

$$O_{2,1} = \omega_i = \mu_{A_i}(x)\mu_{B_i}(y)\mu_{C_i}(z), \quad i = 1, 2. \tag{12}$$

In layer 3 the fixed nodes are referred to N. The i_{th} node calculates the firing strength rate of rule i_{th} to the sum of all firing strength of rules, given by equation (13) – the nodes in layer 3 are generally known as normalized firing strength:

$$O_{3,i} = \overline{\omega_i} = \frac{\omega_i}{\omega_1 + \omega_2}, \quad i = 1, 2. \tag{13}$$

Layer 4, for example, the nodes i are adaptive with the function given by equation (14):

$$O_{4,i} = \overline{\omega_i} f_i = \overline{\omega_i}(p_i x + q_i y + r_i z + s_i), \tag{14}$$

where $\overline{\omega_i}$ is a normalized firing strength from layer 3 and $\{p_i, q_i, r_i, s_i\}$ the set of parameters (called consequence parameters) of this node.

The last layer of the Figure 3 has only one fixed node called Σ that determines the final output as the sum of all signals represented by equation (15):

$$final\ output = O_{5,1} = \sum_i \overline{\omega_i} f_i = \frac{\sum_i \omega_i f_i}{\sum_i \omega_i} \tag{15}$$

Considering the architecture shown in Figure 3 it can be seen that while the values of the parameters of the premises is fixed, the final output can be expressed as a linear combination of consequence parameters. Therefore, the output can be rewritten, for example, by the linear equation with the following consequence parameters: p_1, q_1, r_1, s_1, p_2, q_2, r_2 and s_2 (see equation 16):

$$
\begin{aligned}
f &= \frac{\omega_1}{\omega_1+\omega_2} f_1 + \frac{\omega_2}{\omega_1+\omega_2} f_2 \\
&= \overline{\omega_\iota}(p_1 x + q_1 y + r_1 z + s_1) + \overline{\omega_2}(p_2 x + q_2 y + r_2 z + s_2) \\
&= (\overline{\omega_\iota} x)p_1 + (\overline{\omega_\iota} y)q_1 + (\overline{\omega_\iota} z)r_1 + (\overline{\omega_\iota})s_1 + (\overline{\omega_2} x)p_2 + (\overline{\omega_2} y)q_2 + (\overline{\omega_2} z)r_2 + (\overline{\omega_2})s_2
\end{aligned} \quad (16)
$$

The hybrid training algorithm is based on the following criteria: In the forward step of the hybrid algorithm, the outputs of the nodes will forward to the layer 4 and the consequence parameters are identified by the least squares method. In the backward step, the error signal is propagated backward and the premise parameters are updated by gradient descent method (Jang, 1993)

2.3. Subtractive clustering

The utilization of clustering algorithms allows characterization and organization of data, but also the construction of models from a database. Basically clustering divides data sets derived from a large group into similar groups. Clustering can be used to model an initial fuzzy network, in other words, to determine the fuzzy rules. For this purpose, the clustering technique is validated based on the following propositions:

- Similar entries in a target system should be modeled to produce similar outputs;
- These similar pairs input-output are packed in clusters of the training data set.

The technique subtractive clustering proposed by Chiu, considers any data points as candidates for the cluster centers (Chiu, 1994). Using this method, the processing is proportional to the number of data points, independent of the size of the problem under consideration.

For example, is a collection of n data points {x1,...,xn} in an M-dimensional space, whose points were normalized to a hypercube. Since each data point is candidate for the cluster center, the density measurement at each point xi is defined by equation (17):

$$\boldsymbol{D_i} = \sum_{j=1}^{n} \mathbf{exp}\left(-\frac{\|x_i - x_j\|^2}{(r_a/2)^2}\right) \quad (17)$$

where r_a is a positive constant. A point will have a great density it has many neighbor points. The radius r_a defines the neighborhood and the points outside of the neighborhood contribute very little to the density measurement.

After the density measurement (D_i) is calculated for all of the points, the point with highest density is selected to be the center of the first cluster. If x_{c1} is the selected point and D_{c1} your density value, the measured density for each point is revised according to the expression shown in (18):

$$\boldsymbol{D_i} = \boldsymbol{D_i} - \boldsymbol{D_{c1}} \mathbf{exp}\left(-\frac{\|x_i - x_{c1}\|^2}{(r_b/2)^2}\right) \quad (18)$$

After reviewing the density of each point, the next center x_{c2} is selected and all of the density measures of the points are revised again. This process is repeated until a sufficient number of clusters are created. When applied the *subtractive clustering* technique for a set of input-output data, each cluster center will represents a prototype that exhibits certain characteristics of the system being modeled. This cluster centers are used as centers of the premises of the fuzzy rules in a zero order Sugeno model.

3. Experimental methods

To help understanding, a block diagram of the proposed system is presented in the Figure 4. In the following sections are presented detailed discussions of the key elements that make up this block diagram.

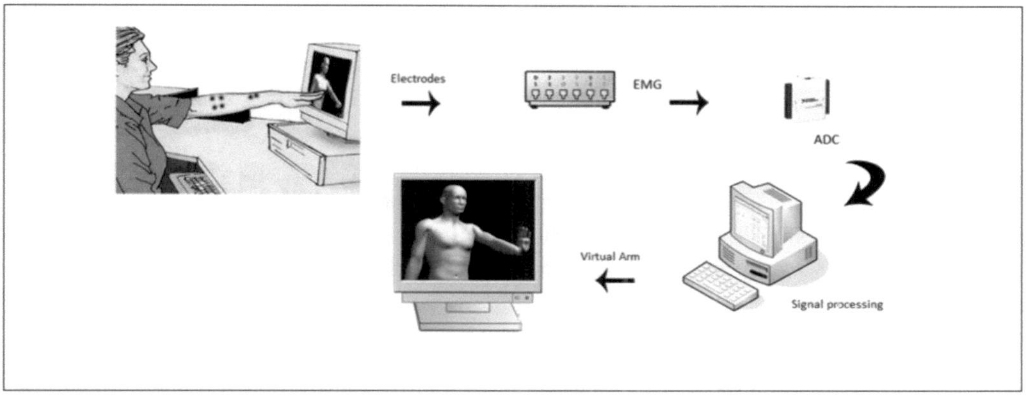

Figure 4. Block diagram of the purposed system.

The proposed experimental apparatus consists of an LCD screen that generates visual stimulus with animations of random movements of the hand-arm segment which should be replicated by the user An 8-channel electromyography is used with surface electrodes placed in strategic places and previously defined in the right arm to capture the myoelectric signal during displayed movements. Through a data acquisition board, the myoelectric signal is digitized and processed in a portable computer, where it is filtered and analyzed by software using the technique of pattern recognition, based on neuro fuzzy systems. Finally, the system has as output the characterization of the movement and also verifies if the executed movement was well recognized.

3.1. Electromyograph and data acquisition system

Electromyograph is a device used to capture the myoelectric signals with the help of electrodes. The electromyograph used in this work was developed in the research project coordinated by Balbinot (Balbinot, 2005).

The recording signal is performed using bipolar electrodes of passive configuration. Located near the electrodes, in each acquisition cable, was used an instrumentation amplifier with differential input, INA118, to minimize the noise as the amplitude of the acquired signal is in mV. The signal is amplified up to 1000 times

The frequency of the muscular signals captured by the surface electrodes has a range varying from 20 to 500 Hz. Due to this fact, the EMG designed consist of two cascaded second order low-pass filters with a cutoff frequency at 1000 Hz, and two cascaded second order high-pass filters with cutoff frequency at 20Hz.

To perform the data acquisition was chosen the National Instruments acquisition board NI USB 6008. This board features eight analog input channels with 10 bit resolution and sampling rate of 10 kS/s. In this study we used the eight analog input channels (one entry per channel) with an acquisition rate of 1 kHz per channel.

3.2. Virtual model

Virtual human body models are used in many applications that allow human-machine Interaction. The virtual model created in this work aims to help the standardization of tests for the acquisition of the myoelectric signal. With this virtual model is possible, for the Subject, visualize the movement to be performed during the tests, so that all Subjects perform as best as possible, the same movements at the same time base and at the same time, leaving the system more user-friendly. For the development of the virtual model we used the software MakeHuman Alpha5 and Blender 1.0 Beta 2:54.

Initially, MakeHuman software was used to define the parameters of the humanoid (height, weight, sex) that is subsequently exported to the software Blender. This virtual model is a skeleton whose manipulative joints are used to define the positions that it should take (Tale & Balbinot, 2011). For the development of the animation it was necessary to set the start and end position and movement timing of each of the respective movement. The software then builds an animation by connecting the two points during a defined duration. Also was established a rest position which was adopted for all movements. Importantly, all movements start from the rest position, run and return to it. It should be noted that after the generation of virtual models, a video of the animations are created using a standard rate of 24 fps Avi format.

To display the animations, a routine in Labview was developed enabling the reading of Avi files and reproduction of videos representing the virtual model through a window of Windows Media Player. This window opens in the auxiliary display (LCD screen in Figure 4) being viewed only by the user of the system. The operator sees only the Labview programming window on the laptop screen, where it is shown that the signal is being acquired during the tests.

The set of movements generated through the virtual model was divided into two groups: simple and complex movements (sequence of simple movements). There are seven simple movements represented in Figure 5, which are: wrist flexion; hand contraction, wrist extension, forearm flexion, forearm rotation, hand adduction and hand abduction. For the simple movements were adopted the following time sequence with a total duration of each animation of 8.3 s:

- Initial interval: 0,4 s in which the animation will be on rest position;

- forward movement: duration of 2,9 s;
- movement interval: 1,25 s, in which the animation keeps static at the end the going movement;
- backward movement: same duration of the forward movement (2,9 s);
- final interval: duration of 0,8 s, which the animation is again on rest position; .

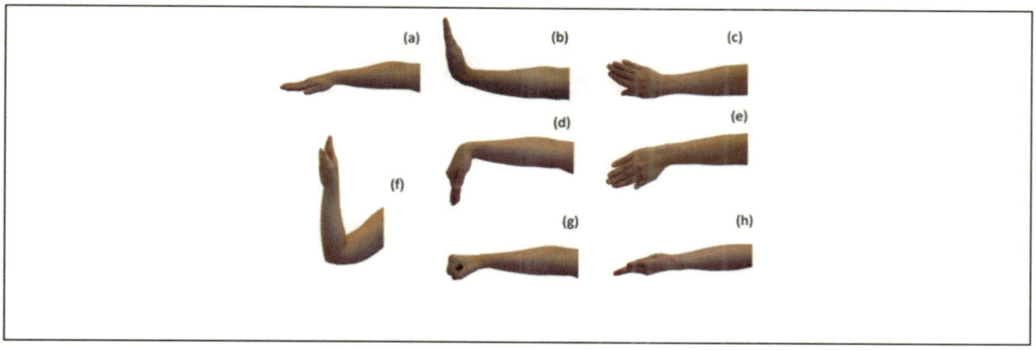

Figure 5. Pictures representing the simple movements created by the virtual model: (a) resting position, (b) wrist extension, (c) wrist adduction, (d) wrist flexion (e) wrist abduction, (f) forearm flexion, (g) hand contraction and (h) forearm rotation.

In the Figure 6 is shown a static representation of the simple movements presented in video format.

The movements that are called complex are characterized by a combination of determined basic movements defined above. For this study, five complex movements were selected as shown in Figure 7, that are: hand contraction with forearm rotation, forearm rotation with forearm flexion; forearm rotation with forearm flexion and wrist flexion, hand contraction with forearm flexion and wrist extension and flexion.

For the animations of the complex movements, the same parameters of the simple movement animations were been used, but with total duration of 17 second for each complex movement.

3.3. Experimental procedures

All the experiments were carried out with consent of the Subjects, according to the ethical precepts and respecting the bio signal acquisition techniques (in this case related to the myoelectric signal acquisition), like for instance the treatment of the skin, electrode positioning among other aspects.

For the data acquisition the NI USB 6008 board was used. Eight pairs of electrodes located in the main muscle groups of the Subject were been used, which are the main part of the movements that were chosen to characterize: Biceps (C0), palmaris longus (C1), flexor carpi ulnaris (C2), flexor carpi radialis (C3), pronator teres (C4), extensor digitorum (C5), brachioradialis (C6) and extensor carpi ulnaris (C7), as shown in Figure 8.

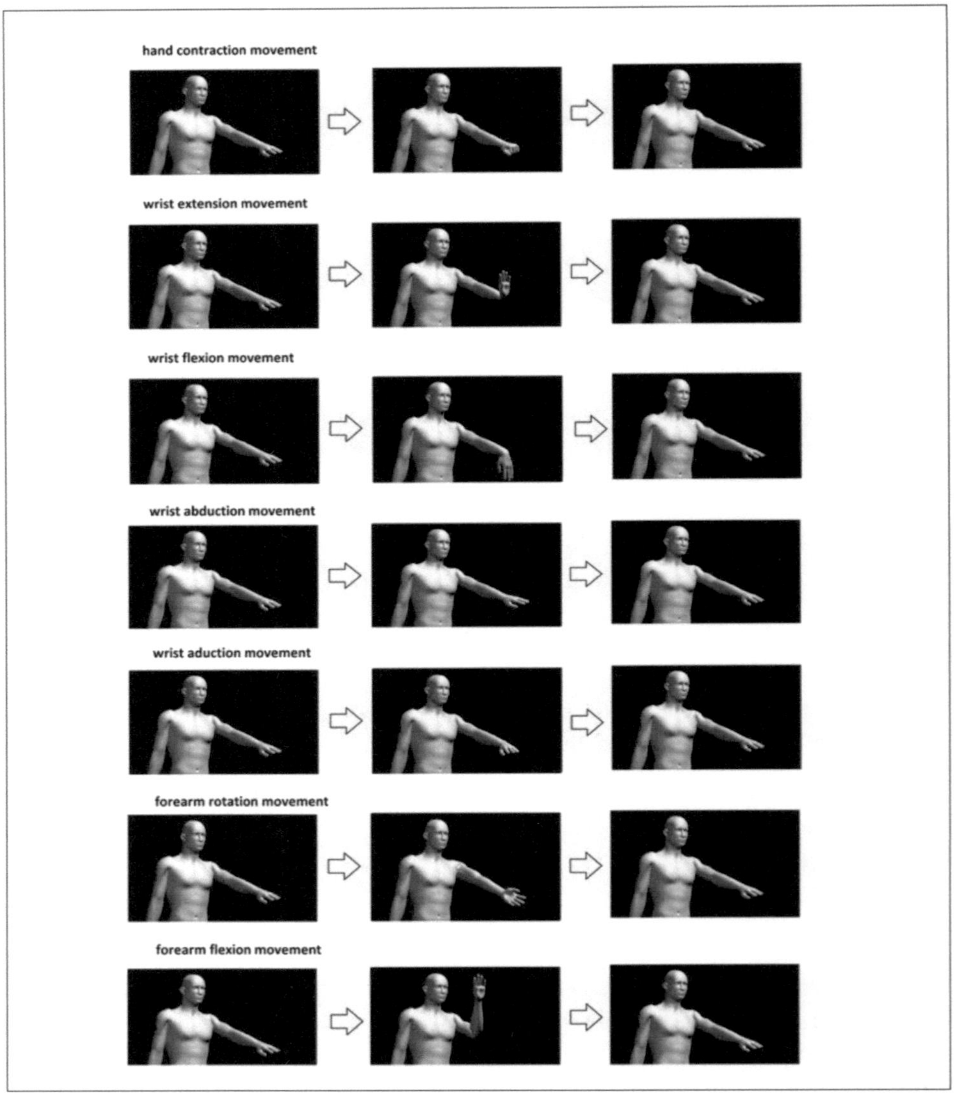

Figure 6. Diagram representing the videos of simple movements developed as a virtual model.

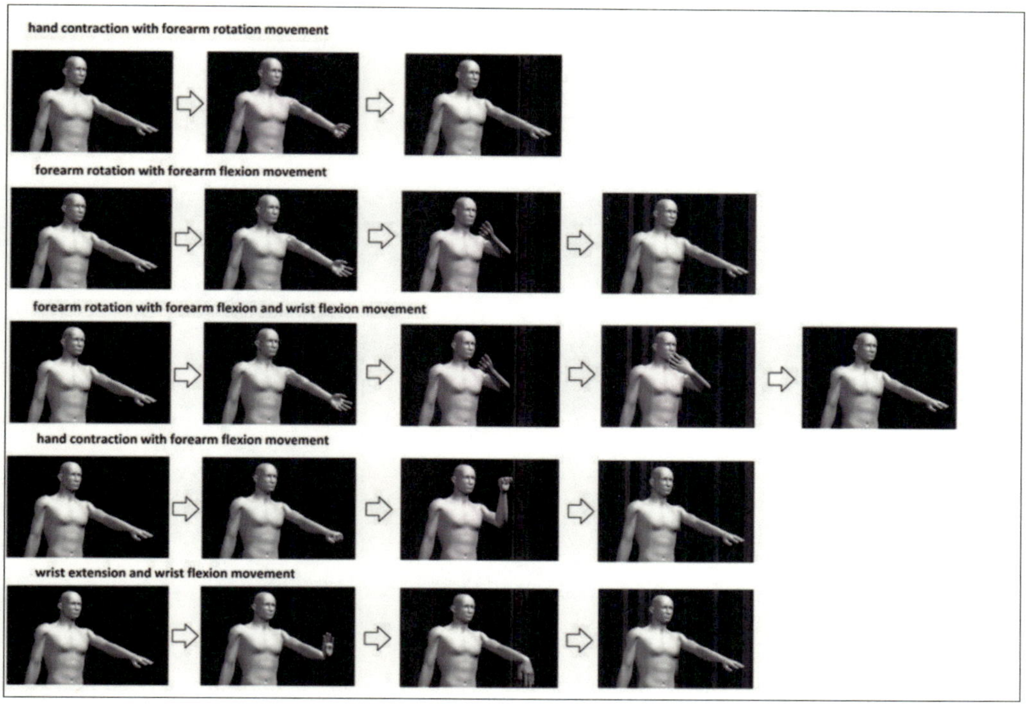

Figure 7. Diagram representing the videos of complex movements developed as a virtual model.

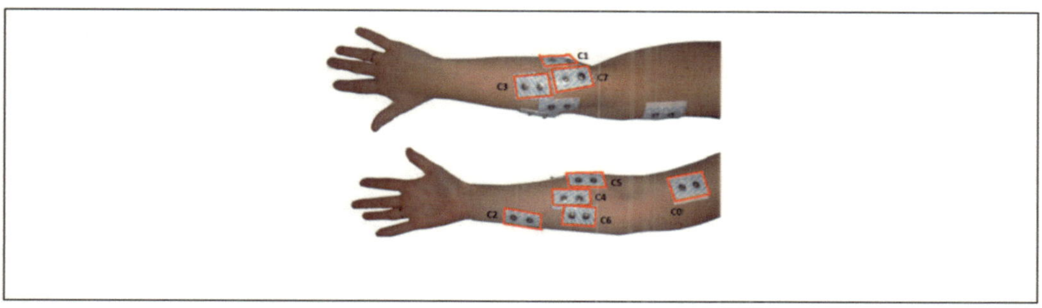

Figure 8. Picture showing the electrodes positions.

To start the acquisition, after correct positioning of the electrodes, the Subject is instructed to replicate the animations of the virtual model, which appear on the LCD screen, using a moderate strength. In order to standardize the testing of signal acquisition was adapted to the methodology proposed by Li (Li, 2010), considering the following aspects:

- each test consists of 5 sessions;
- is generated a random sequence of animations for each session of the test;
- each session is composed of 5 repetitions of each of the 12 selected movements;
- between movements, the Subject should rest for 3 seconds;

- each Subject participates in a single test.

In the figure 9 is shown a picture of one of the sessions.

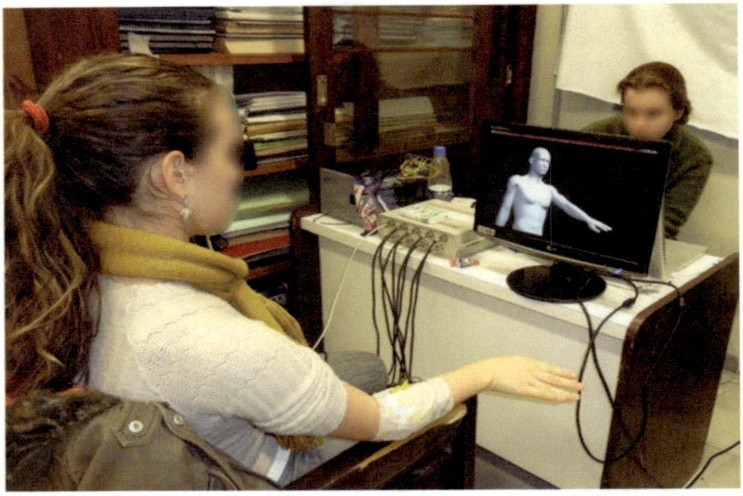

Figure 9. Picture of a session.

A Labview routine was developed to interface with Matlab to generate the sequence of movements (See figures 6 and 7) randomly. The output is a vector with a random order of the movements of the virtual model presented to the user.

3.4. Acquisition and signal pre processing

The programming language chosen for the development of the proposed system software is Labview (Laboratory Virtual Instrument Engineering Workbench) from National Instruments.

The acquisition and generation of the myoelectric signals database were obtained through a routine created in Labview software to read the input data acquired through the NI USB 6008 card and store them in a file.

To choose the sample rate was considered that the myoelectric signal of interest in this work is in the range 20-500 Hz, and most of the energy of this signal is in the frequency range 50-150 Hz based on this information, the sampling frequency used was 1 kHz which is suitable for the proposed system. For this specification, 1 ms was sufficient to identify the user movements.

The online acquisition is performed in a way that the signal is transferred to the computer in time windows of 50 ms, thought the acquisition board, and the signal is stored in a FIFO (First In First Out) queue, in which the stored time windows are being processed according to the acquisition order, ensuring no data loss. Figure 10 shows the corresponding flowchart of this stage.

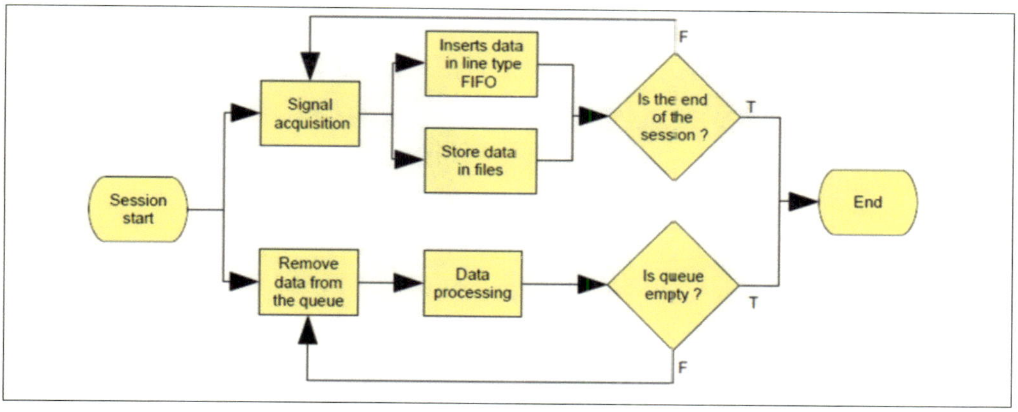

Figure 10. Flowchart of the online acquisition routine.

According to the flowchart shown in Figure 10, the data acquisition and processing are used simultaneously, since it is possible to perform parallel routines in Labview (note that the real parallelism is only supported from the Labview 2010 package).

3.4.1. *Calibration procedure*

The calibration of the system aims to achieve specific characteristics of the voluntary muscle signal, as each person may have a different muscle activity. Thus, the calibration allows that the system is generic and therefore adapts itself to different users. The calibration procedure of the system involves capturing the muscle signal in a time of relaxation and in a moment of maximum voluntary contraction (MVC).

Figure 11 shows a brief block diagram of the calibration procedure. This step involves eight Boolean variables (SNR (x), x = 1.2 .. 8) indicating that all channels of myoelectric signal acquisition were correctly calibrated. If a pair of electrodes is not properly positioned, the distress signal has low quality, and once again must be repositioned until the signal / noise ratio is at least greater than 2 - value established based on the signal acquisition trials previously conducted with this electromyograph (Favieiro, 2009).

For the calibration of each channel, initially an acquisition of the signal is performed with the muscle in rest position. Then the signal is processed to calculate the average peak values. Later on a MVC movement is performed and captured, and after this, again the average peak value is calculated. With this information is possible to evaluate the signal to noise ratio (SNR) that is given by dividing the value processed during the movement with MVC by the value found when captured a rest movement.

A percentage ranging from 30-50% of the average peak values of the acquired signal with the maximum voluntary contraction (MVC) is then used to determine, during processing of the signal, the threshold value which indicates whether or not a muscle contraction occurring during the process of windowing the signal.

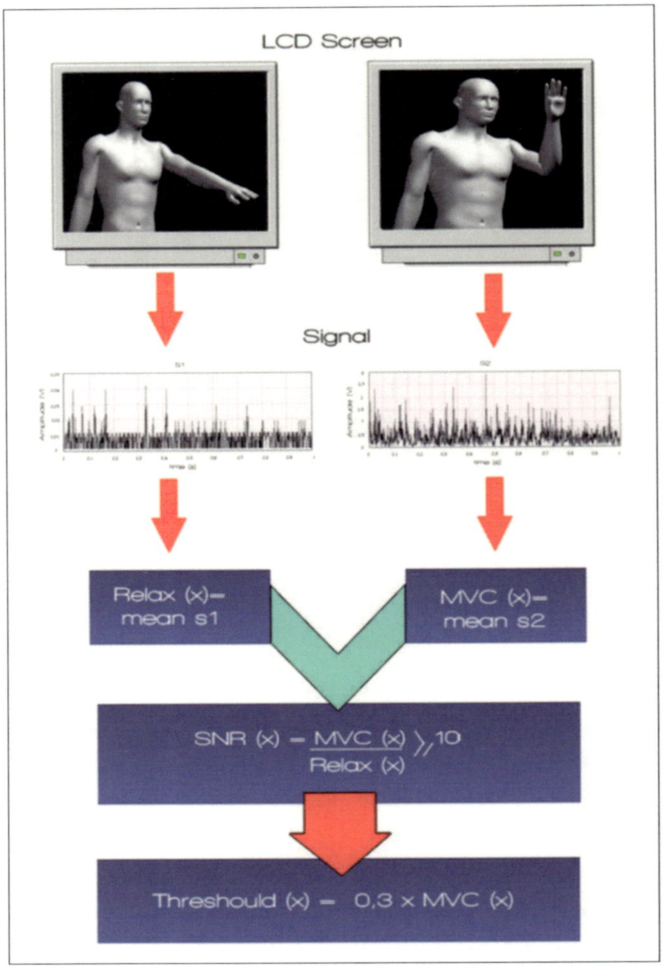

Figure 11. Block diagram of the calibration routine.

The movements with MVC used for the calibration of each channel are shown in the table 1.

Channel x	Muscle	Movement
0	Biceps	Forearm flexion
1	Flexor carpi ulnaris	Hand abduction
2	Flexor carpi radialis	Hand adduction
3	Extensor digitorum	Hand contraction
4	Pronator teres	Forearm rotation
5	Brachioradialis	Forearm rotation
6	Palmaris longus	Wrist flexion
7	Extensor carpi ulnaris	Wrist extension

Table 1. Representation of movement defined for each channel calibration.

3.4.2. Preprocessing procedures

Were used mathematical procedures typically used in the myoelectric signal analysis to preprocess the signal and generating one or more characteristics of interest to the classification stage.

The techniques used are this stage was (for further details consult Favieiro, 2011):

- removal of DC component (offset adjustment);
- full-wave rectification;
- windowing the signal of interest;
- determining the rms value of the signal of interest.

The signal is analyzed in periods of 50 ms, since it provides a comprehensive overview of the signal but, at the same time, specific, since it does not occur in tests muscle relaxation in period shorter than the determined, resulting in an efficient analysis of runtime system and results. To perform the windowing of the signal, the period in which a muscle contraction occurs were developed a routine in Labview which analyses the signal every 50 ms, where each channel is analyzed simultaneously, ensuring if in these data windows occurs a signal peak with value above the threshold. To consider that a movement is taking place is necessary to satisfy the following assumptions:

- is considered that the channel is active if, in the processed time window, there are any peaks above the threshold limit. Considering the threshold a variable that has a value ranging from 30-50% of the respective channel MVC. This percentage is defined empirically according to preliminary test conducted with a user;
- is necessary that at least three channels have a peak above the respective threshold, i.e., being active. This is done to ensure that any random noise introduced in at least one channel interfere with the signal windowing;
- the signal must be considered active, at least 80% of the last 20 windows, i.e., the last one second. The history of activation of the channels is taken into consideration to try to ensure that a movement is actually occurring.

With these assumptions satisfied, it is considered that a movement is occurring, and in turn, the signal is windowed in all channels simultaneously, considering the same time based for the beginning and end of the muscle contraction. Another assumption considered important is if two sequential movements were spaced in time by up to 3 seconds, they will be considered one single movement and the beginning time of the first movements and the end time of the second are used to define a new single window containing these two movements. Thus, ensuring that complex movements are not considered two or more distinct movements by the signal windowing.

The set time of 3 seconds has been based on in the resting time of the Subject, which is 3 seconds. Thus, the windowing of a movement is determined only after a time longer than 3 seconds without the occurrence of a movement, only then is possible to analyze the windows stored in each channel, calculating the rms value from each channel in the occurrence time of a muscle contraction.

3.5. Myoelectric signal preprocessing by the neuro fuzzy method

The step of characterizing the signal is achieved by a neuro fuzzy type ANFIS. The system takes as input the rms values of each pre-processed data acquisition channel. Presents as output the movements characterized that are being carried out by the human arm. The system ANFIS used in this research was implemented using the Matlab tool (Fuzzy Logic Toolbox). The fuzzy neural network is interfaced via Labview, where the routine developed in Matlab is called when needed, being processed in the background.

3.5.1. Neuro fuzzy network dimensioning

First was set the number of network inputs, which can vary from 2 to 8 depending on the number of channels which is intended to analyze. The channel that will be used on the network can be selected by the operator of the system which the developed routine performs reading of all channels and automatically separates the desired channels for processing. This function has as input the array of channels to be selected and as output only the desired channels. The output of the neuro-fuzzy networks is considered fixed, containing the 12 movements previously determined. The output values ranges from 0 to 1, and for each movement there is a corresponding fixed known value, as shown in Table 2.

He developed structure is a fuzzy network type Sugeno obtained in the generation of a initial structure adapted from a input-output set acquired in the systems tests. The structure contains eight inputs and one output.

Movement	Corresponded output
Hand contraction	0
Wrist extension	0.083
Wrist flexion	0.166
Forearm flexion	0.249
Forearm rotation	0.333
Hand abduction	0.416
Hand adduction	0.499
Complex 1	0.582
Complex 2	0.665
Complex 3	0.748
Complex 4	0.831
Complex 5	0.914

Table 2. Network output values associated with the recognized movements.

3.5.2. Fuzzy neural network structure definition

To adjust the system it is necessary first creates an initial fuzzy network, which should be representative of the Subject data. For this, was used the subtractive clustering technique, which can generate, from a input-output data, membership functions of input and output, and the fuzzy rules structure for type Sugeno. This technique was chosen because it obtained good results in preliminary studies cases, its routine is represented in Figure 12. This routine is performed using the MatlabScript node that defines a script to be run in Matlab.

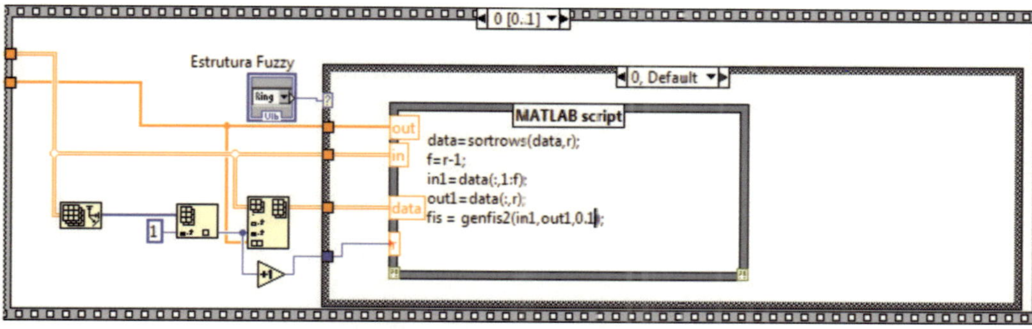

Figure 12. Routine developed for definition of the fuzzy network structure.

While creating the initial fuzzy structure was necessary to define the following parameters in Matlab:

- input data: array with fuzzy inputs of the network;
- output data: array with the expected output for the input data set;
- membership function: the Gaussian function was selected because it is a smooth function on the edges, have shown better results in these trials;
- radius: was selected the value of 0.1, which represents the influence radius of the cluster, when it is considered a unitary hypercube. The smaller the radius, more clusters are created and, consequentially, a greater number of rules.

In the first Subject assay, the expected input and output values are used to create the system initial structure representing the fuzzy network of 8 inputs, 60 clusters (i.e., 60 rules) e one output, generated for a system assay, and adjust it later to adapt to represent more faithfully a model that can characterize the Subject movements.

After creating the initial fuzzy structure is necessary to adapt the membership functions for the data acquired in the session, thus making a fine adjustment of the functions, leading to results more consistent with the ones expected. The adaptation step is very important, because it help to better define the limits and parameters of the membership functions, leaving the model best suited for the Subject. In this step were used a hybrid training function. The hybrid training is a combination of the gradient method with the LSE method to optimize the time convergence of the model, since it reduces the demand on the dimensional space. This function used the following parameters, according to the routine which utilized the MatlabScript function represented in Figure 13:

- initial fuzzy network, created from the subtractive clustering technique;
- input data: array with the network fuzzy inputs;
- output data: vector with the expected output for the input data set;

- number of training epochs: the value 10 was selected , which defines the number of training cycles, i.e., the maximum number of times the training set is presented to the network. An excessive number of cycles can lead to loss of power to the network generalization (over fitting). On the other hand, with a small number of cycles, the network cannot reach its best performance (under fitting);
- target error: the value 0 was selected, which consists in terminate the training after the mean square error falls below a predetermined value α.

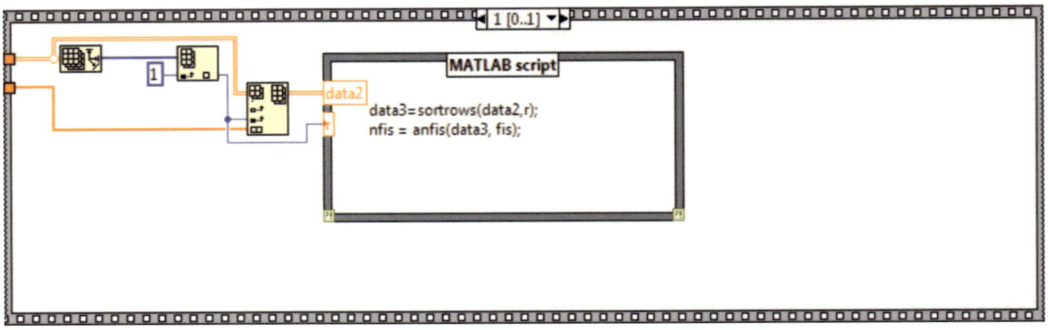

Figure 13. Training routine of the neuro-fuzzy network.

As output of the training step, is generated a fuzzy network with adapted membership functions to a particular Subject, causing the limits of each functions to be left according to the training data.

4. Results and discussion

This topic will discuss the test performed during system development, and the results obtained. It is important to note that the pre-processing routine and calibration have already been validated in previous studies (Favieiro, 2009; Favieiro & Balbinot, 2011).

Subjects participating in this research present an age range of 20±5 years old, of both sexes. Altogether were conducted trials with seven Subjects. The abbreviations of the characterized movements are presented in Table 3.

It is worth noting that the parameters of ANFIS training were the same for all Subjects. Figure 14 represents the result of section 2 for Subject 1 where is possible notice that for the movement M11 that is the hand contraction with the forearm flexion, 40% of the error was due to the fact that the network believed was dealing with movement M0 (hand contraction) which represents partially the movement performed. Another movement in which occurred the incorrect recognition was the M4 (forearm rotation) with M3 (forearm flexion), causing 60% of error, which may occur since these movements uses muscle in common, such as the biceps, and were used only surface electrodes.

As an example, Table 4 represents the average accuracy rate of the system for each movement per session, and the overall average of each movement per session for the Subject 1. The movements with lower hit rate are: hand contraction (M0), forearm rotation (M4) and hand contraction and forearm rotation (M11), with 65%, 57% and 50% hit rate, respectively. It happened by the similarity of M4 to M3 (forearm flexion) and by the similarity between M0 to M11.

Performed movement	Abbreviation
Hand contraction	M0
Wrist extension	M1
Wrist flexion	M2
Forearm flexion	M3
Forearm rotation	M4
Hand abduction	M5
Hand adduction	M6
Hand contraction with forearm rotation	M7
Forearm rotation and flexion	M8
Forearm rotation and flexion with wrist flexion	M9
Wrist extension followed by flexion	M10
Hand contraction with forearm flexion	M11

Table 3. Abbreviations representing the performed movements.

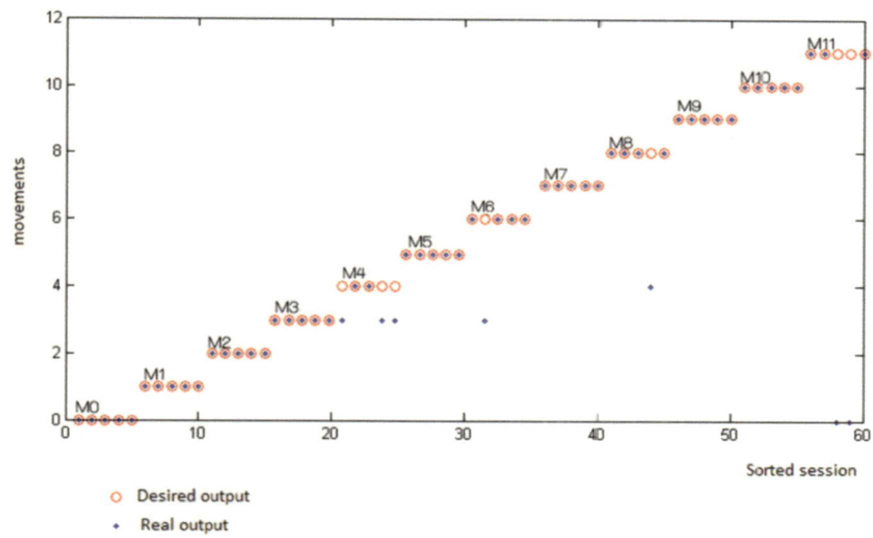

Figure 14. System output for Subject 1 – section 2 (5 repetitions).

Subject 1	M0	M1	M2	M3	M4	M5	M6	M7	M8	M9	M10	M11
Session 2 (%)	100	100	100	100	40	100	80	100	80	100	100	60
Session 3 (%)	40	100	80	80	60	60	100	80	100	100	80	80
Session 4 (%)	60	80	100	80	80	80	100	100	80	100	40	20
Session 5 (%)	60	100	100	100	50	100	20	100	40	60	60	40
Average (%)	65	95	95	90	57	85	75	95	75	90	70	50

Table 4. Summary of the system average accuracy rate to the subject 1.

4.1. Comparison between subjects

As an example, Figure 15 shows the average accuracy rate for movement M10 for all Subjects. The average score was higher than 70% in all cases. This happened mainly because of the simple movements that compose the M10 movement are easily detectable antagonistic movements. Like the movements M1 and M2 achieved accuracy rates above 75% in most cases.

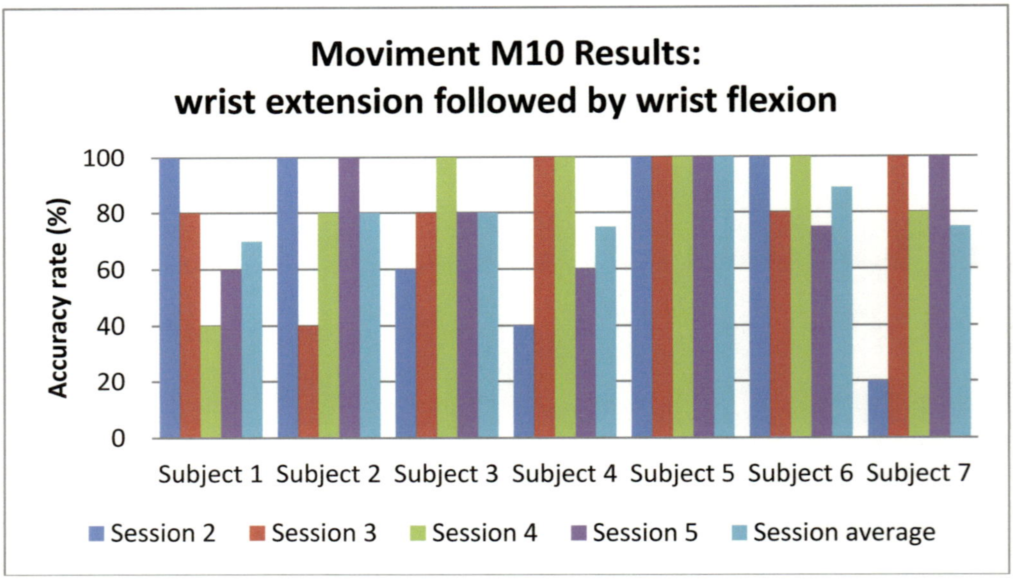

Figure 15. Results of movement M10.

Figure 16 represents the average of all tests performed for each movement. Analyzing the graph it is clear that the more accurate movements were M1, M2, M5 and M10 (combination of M1 and M2), with averages rates of approximately 80%. These movements are quite distinct, which increases the accuracy rate of the system. The worst case occurred with the movement M11, which had an average hit rate below 50%, it combines simple movements used in most of the complex movements performed, impairing the correct recognition. Overall the system achieved an average accuracy of 65%.

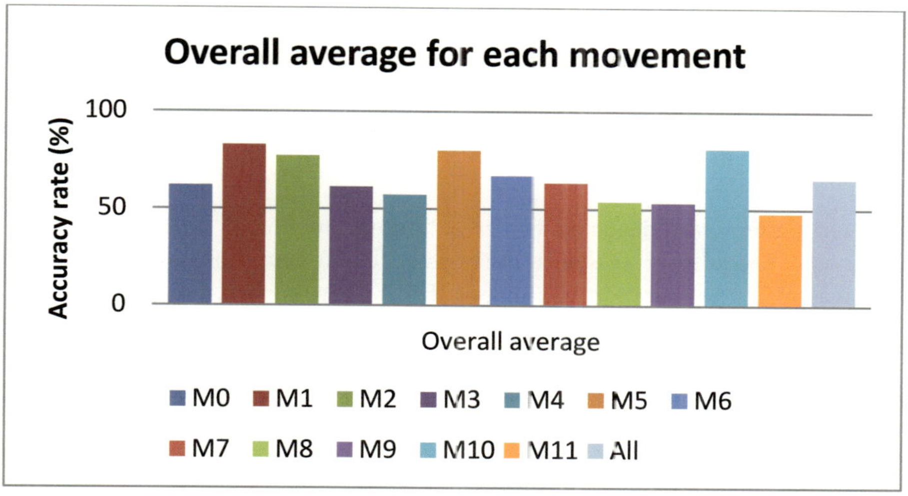

Figure 16. Overall result of the system for each movement.

4.2. Comparison between the researched results and other studies

The vast majority of studies in the area of recognition of hand-movements of the arm segment are based on the classification of simple movements, not taking into account combined movements, as was the aim of this study. As it was possible to see the results of this work, most of the errors were caused by similar movements, or the differentiation of compound movements with their simple movements. The human arm has many degrees of freedom and be able to develop a system that can characterize many different movements and combined is where the real challenge and for this reason is an active area of research (Favieiro et al., 2011; Favieiro & Balbinot, 2011).

Comparing the system developed by Chan using fuzzy techniques which were classified four simple movements using only two channels with an accuracy of 91% (Chan, 2000). Also a system was developed by Ajiboye to characterize four classes of movements using four channels, obtaining an accuracy of 86% (Ajiboye, 2005). These systems had similar results to those found in the preliminary study of this research in which the neuro fuzzy technique was used to classify five distinct movements using three channels of signal acquisition, obtaining an accuracy of 86% (Favieiro & Balbinot, 2011). Demonstrating the system using only simple movements and a limited number of channels achieved accuracy higher than that found to characterize the combined movements.

Compared with the research of Momen which categorize nine distinct movements, using only the rms characteristic of the window processed and four acquisition channels obtained an average accuracy of 48.9%. This study is very similar to the system developed, in the sense that uses the same characteristic of the signal and making a direct comparison of the average hit rate of the developed system is 30% higher than to 9 moves obtained per Momen (Momen, 2007).

Another difference that it is important to note is that the proposed study used only one feature extracted for each channel, unlike other studies that use up to 13 features per channel, whose average accuracy was 87% for the classification of 10 distinct movements (Khushaba, 2010).

5. Conclusions

The proposed system was designed to use a limited amount of up to 8 channels of the myoelectric signal acquisition and with the assistance of a more robust artificial intelligence technique was able to verify the validity of this system in terms of performance in the characterization of 11 distinct movements, including 5 complex movements. In tests, the mean peak signal with a maximum voluntary contraction (MVC) appeared at least four times greater than the average peak signal at a time of muscle relaxation. Thus, was possible determine a level ranging from 30 to 50% of MVC to differentiate a time of muscle contraction, representing a movement. With the windowing signal occurs at the instant when a movement occurs, is possible to obtain the rms value for each of the channels 8 and to use these values as input to a neuro fuzzy network with one output an up to 8 inputs. This network aims to characterize the movements that are being executed. The network is adapted in accordance with supervised training, to evaluate system performance over time. As can be seen on the results, some movements have achieved a lower hit rate, this may occur due to poor signal quality, user error, and the quantity of motion that was presented to the neuro fuzzy network, since most of the errors were caused by similar movements, or the differentiation of compound movements with their simple movements, which have a response very similar in rms value, causing the network to get confused. The average accuracy obtained was 65% of hit rate to 11 distinct movements in tests of long duration, about three hours.

Also, it's important to notice that the vast majority of studies in the area of recognition of hand-movements of the arm segment are based on the classification of simple movements, not taking into account combined movements, as was the aim of this study. The preliminary study of this research in which the neuro fuzzy technique was used to classify five distinct simple movements using three channels of signal acquisition, obtained an accuracy of 86% (Favieiro & Balbinot, 2011). Demonstrating the system using only simple movements and a limited number of channels achieved accuracy higher than that found to characterize the combined movements.

The human arm has many degrees of freedom and be able to develop a system that can characterize many different movements and combined is the real challenge of this kind of research, which will really improve the life quality of people with special needs, making them more independent and more likely to real social and economical integration.

6. Future studies

It would be very important in future studies performing the tests with a larger number of volunteers, to conduct a robust statistical analysis of results, and allow a more robust assessment of its results, its flaws and strengths. Is ongoing the use of the system with Volunteers with total and partial amputation of the upper limb. This is crucial for research to find out how the system would apply and adapt, it is possible to ascertain the validity of future control system for a prosthetic hand-arm segment by myoelectric signals. Another proposal for further work would find other characteristics that could be extracted from the signal to improve the performance of the fuzzy neural network, so that the system would be able to characterize a wide range of complex movements with a hit ratio above 90%, and a higher capacity to differentiate motion. One way to improve the hit rate of the system is to implement a feedback to the user, to the person performing the test whether they are doing it correctly, avoiding common errors of distraction, or applying excessive force.

Author details

Gabriela Winkler Favieiro and Alexandre Balbinot
Federal University of Rio Grande do Sul (UFRGS)
Graduate Program in Electrical Engineering (PPGEE), Department of Electrical Engineering, Instrumentation Laboratory, Porto Alegre, Rio Grande do Sul, Brazil

7. References

Ajiboye, A.B. & Weir, R.F. (2005). A heuristic fuzzy logic approach to EMG pattern recognition for multifunctional prosthesis control. *IEEE Transactions on Neural Systems and Rehabilitation Engineering*, Baltimore, V.13, No.3, pp. 280–291.

Balbinot, A. (2006). Desenvolvimento de uma Prótese experimental controlada por eletromiografia. *Proceedings of Congresso Ibero-Americano sobre Tecnologias de Apoio a Portadores de Dediciência*, Vitória, IBERDISCAP, 2006, V.1, MA-3–MA-6.

Begg R.K., Lai D. & Palaniswami M (2008). Computational Intelligence in Biomedical Engineering, Taylor & Francis Books Inc (CRC Press), Boca Raton, Florida, USA (392 pages), ISBN: 0-8493-4080-2.

Chan, F.H.Y (2000). Fuzzy EMG classification for prosthesis control. *IEEE Transactions on Neural Systems and Rehabilitation Engineering*, Baltimore, V.8, No. 3, pp. 305–311.

Chiu, S. L. (1994). Fuzzy model identification based on cluster estimation. *Journal of Intelligent and Fuzzy systems*, V.2, No. 3, pp. 267-278.

DeConto, E. & Balbinot, A. (2011). Desenvolvimento de modelos virtuais para EMG. Relatório de Pesquisa, Porto Alegre, UFRGS.

Dubois, D. & Prade, H. (1980). *Fuzzy set and systems: theory and applications*. New York: Academic Press.

Englehart, K. & Hudgins, B. (2003). A robust, real-time control scheme for multifunction myoelectric control. *IEEE Transactions on Biomedical Engineering*, Gainesville, V. 50, No. 7, pp. 848–854.

Favieiro, G. & Balbinot, A. (2011). Adaptive Neuro-Fuzzy Logic Analysis Based on Myoelectric Signals for Multifunction Prosthesis Control, *Proceedings of Annual International Conference of the IEEE Engineering in Medicine and Biology Society 2011*, pp. 7888-7891, Boston, EMBS, 2011.

Favieiro, G. (2009). *Controle de uma prótese experimental do segmento mão-braço por sinais mioelétricos e redes neurais artificiais*. 2009. 111 f. Trabalho de conclusão de curso. Engenharia de computação, Universidade Federal do Rio Grande do Sul, Porto Alegre.

Favieiro, G.; Balbinot, A. & Barreto, M.M.G. (2011). Decoding arm movements by myoeletric signals and artificial neural networks. *Proceedings of Biosignals and Biorobotics Conferecene (BRC) 2011*, pp. 1-6, Vitória, ISSNIP, 2011.

Hincapie, J.G. & Kirsch, R.F. (2009). Feasibility of EMG-Based neural network controller for an upper extremity neuroprosthesis. *IEEE Transactions on Biomedical Engineering*, Gainesville, V.17, No. 1, pp. 80–90.

Hudgins, B.; Parker, p. & Scott, R. (1994). Control of artificial limbs using myoelectric pattern recognition. *Medical and Life Sciences Engineering*, pp. 21-38.

Hudgins, B.; Parker, P. & Scott, R.N. (1991). A neural network classifier for multifunction myoelectric control. *Proceedings of International Confercence IEEE-EMBS*, Orlando, EMBS, 1991, V.13, No..3, pp. 1454-1455.

Jacobsen, S; Knutti, D.; Johnson R & Sears, H. (1982). Development of the Utah artificial arm. *IEEE Transactions on Biomedical Engineering*, No. 29, pp. 249-269.

Jang, J.R. (1993). ANFIS: adaptive-network-based fuzzy inference systems. *IEEE Transactions on systems, Man, and Cybernetics*, V. 23, No. 3, pp. 665-685.

Jang, J.R.; Sun, C. & Mizutani, E. (1997). *Neuro-fuzzy and soft computing: a computational approach to learning and machine intelligence*. New York: Prentice Hall.

Katutoshi, K.; Koji, O. & Takao, T. (1992). A discrimination system using neural network for EMG-controlled prosthesies. *Proceedings of the IEEE International Workshop on Robot Human Communication*, No. 1, pp. 63-68.

Khushaba, R.N.; Al-Ani, A. & Al-Jumaily, A. (2010). Orthogonal Fuzzy Neighborhood discriminant analysis for multifunction myoeletric hand control. *IEEE Transactions on Biomedical Engineering*, Gainesville, V.57, No. .6, pp. 1410–1419.

Li, G.; Schultz, A.E. & Kuizen, T. A. (2010). Quantifying pattern recognition: based myoeletric control of multifunctional transradial prosthesis. *IEEE Transactions on Neural Systems and Rehabilitation Engineering*, V. 18, No.. 2, pp. 185–192.

Momen, K.; Krishnan, S. & Chau, T. (2007). Real-time classification of forearm electromyographic signals corresponding to user-selected intentional movements for multifunction prosthesis control. *IEEE Transactions on Neural Systems and Rehabilitation Engineering*, Baltimore, V.15, No. .4, pp. 535–542.

Park, E. & Meek, S. (1995). Adaptive filtering of the electromyographic signal for prosthetic control and force estimation. *IEEE Transactions on Biomedical Engineering*, Vol. 42, No. 10, pp. 1048-1052.

Rutkowski, L & Cpalka, K. (2005). Designing and learning of adjustable quasi-triangular norms with applications to neuro-fuzzy systems. *IEEE Trans. on Fuzzy Systems*, V. 14, No. 1, pp. 140-151.

Sugeno, M. & Kang, G. T. (1988). Structure identification of fuzzy model. *Fuzzy Sets and Systems*, North Holland, V.28, N.3, pp. 15-33.

Takagi, T. & Sugeno, M. (1985). Fuzzy identification of systems and its applications to modeling and control. *IEEE Transactions on Systems, Man, and Cybertnetics*, New York, V.15, No. 1, pp. 116-132.

Zadeh, L., M. Nikravesh, & Loia V. (2004). *Fuzzy logic and the Internet. Studies in fuzziness and soft computing*, Vol. 137. Berlin, Springer.

Chapter 15

Design and Control of an EMG Driven IPMC Based Artificial Muscle Finger

R.K. Jain, S. Datta and S. Majumder

Additional information is available at the end of the chapter

http://dx.doi.org/10.5772/48814

1. Introduction

The medical, rehabilitation and bio-mimetic technology demands human actuated devices which can support in the daily life activities such as functional assistance or functional substitution of human organs. These devices can be used in the form of prosthetic, skeletal and artificial muscles devices (Andreasen et al., 2005; Bitzer & Smagt, 2006; DoNascimento et al., 2008). However, we still have some difficulties in the practical use of these devices. The major challenges to overcome are the acquisition of the user's intention from his or her bionic signals and to provide with an appropriate control signal for the device. Also, we need to consider the mechanical design issues such as lightweight and small size with flexible behavior etc (Arieta et al., 2006; Shenoy et al., 2008). For the bionic signals, the electromyography (EMG) signal can be used to control these devices, which reflect the muscles motion, and can be acquired from the body surface. We are familiar with the fact that ionic polymer metal composite (IPMC) has tremendous potential as an artificial muscle. This can be stimulated by supplying a small voltage of ±3V and shows evidence of a large bending behavior (Shahinpoor & Kim, 2001; 2002; 2004; Bar-Cohen, 2002). In place of the supply voltage from external source for actuating an IPMC, EMG signal can be used where EMG electrodes show a reliable approach to extract voltage signal from body (Jain et al. 2010a; 2010b; 2011). Using this voltage signal via EMG sensor, IPMC can illustrate the bio-mimetic behavior through the movement of human muscles. Therefore, an IPMC is used as an artificial muscle finger for the bio-mimetic/micro robot.

The main objective of this chapter is to discuss the design and control of an IPMC based artificial muscle finger where this finger is actuated by EMG signal via movement of human finger. The movement is sensed by EMG sensor which provides signal for actuating the IPMC. When designing IPMC artificial muscle finger based micro gripper for handling the light weight components in an assembly, IPMC bending behaviour is utilized to hold the object. During holding the object, stable EMG signal is required. For this purpose, stable EMG signal is sent through proportional–integral–derivative (PID) controller to the system. Experimentally, it is found that IPMC based artificial muscle finger achieves similar movement like human index finger. This IPMC based artificial muscle finger attains deflection upto 12 mm. By developing a prototype of IPMC artificial muscle finger based micro gripper, it is demonstrated that EMG driven system like IPMC artificial muscle finger based micro gripper can be applicable in handling of light weight components. The major advantages of such system are that IPMC based artificial muscle finger tip shows the compliant behavior and consumes less energy for actuation. Therefore, EMG driven system shows enough potential to substitute for conventional mechanism in micro manipulation and rehabilitation technology.

This chapter is organized as follows: Section 2 describes the prior research related to EMG applications in robotics and bio-mimetics. Section 3.1 explains the basic design of IPMC artificial muscle finger based micro gripper which is driven by EMG signal. The basic tendon of index finger is studied in section 3.2 where muscles are identified for actuation of IPMC based artificial muscle finger. In section 3.3, a model for controlling the EMG signal is highlighted. Different types of control system are implemented for achieving stable data from EMG signal via index finger which is sent to IPMC based artificial muscle finger. Section 4 discusses experimental testing setup for activation of IPMC based artificial muscle finger by human finger through EMG. In section 5, the results are discussed and the conclusions are drawn in section 6. The future work is recommended in section 7.

2. Prior research related to EMG applications

In the past, some researchers have reported work related to shape memory alloy (SMA) and other similar actuators to develop the bio-mimetic fingers but IPMC artificial muscle based finger related work is limited. Pfeiffer et al. (1999) have designed artificial limbs and robot prostheses that are lightweight, compact and dexterous. This mimics the human anatomy and maintains a high lifting capability. EMG control is used for SMA actuated fingers in robot prostheses. DeLaurentis & Mavroidis (2002) have discussed the design of a 12 degree-of-freedom (DOF) SMA actuated artificial hand where the SMA wires are embedded intrinsically within the hand structure. Cocaud & Jnifene (2003) have investigated the use of artificial muscles as SMA actuators for robot manipulators. A solution is established in order to determine the optimal position of a muscle in various musculoskeletal configurations. Herrera et al. (2004) have also designed and constructed a prosthesis where linear actuators are used for designing the mechanical system and EMG sensors are introduced for designing the electrical control system. Bundhoo et al. (2005, 2008) have reported the design of artificially actuated finger by SMA towards development of bio-mimetic prosthetic hands. Different finger joints are actuated through SMA wires via EMG and the relationship between elongation/contraction of the SMA wires & the finger joints have been obtained. O'Toole & McGrath (2007) have also focused on mechanical design of a 12 DOF SMA actuated artificial hand. The SMA material is used for combination of high strength polymers such as polytetrafluoroethylene (PTFE), polyether ether ketone (PEEK) and low density metals such as titanium. Lau (2009) have carried out research work on a design and development of an intelligent prosthetic hand based on hybrid actuation through DC motor & SMA wires. These are controlled by myoelectric signal. Two novel features are introduced in the new prosthetic hand. Firstly, its hybrid actuation mechanism has the advantage of increasing the active degrees of freedom and secondly, using only two myoelectric sensors, has the potential for controlling more than three patterns of fingers movements. Pittaccio & Viscuso (2011) have developed a SMA wire device for the rehabilitation of the ankle joint where active orthosis powered by two rotary actuators like, NiTi wire are used to obtain ankle dorsiflexion and EMG signal is used to control the orthosis and trigger activation from muscle. Stirling et al. (2011) have shown the potential of SMA wire for an active, soft orthotic in the knee where NiTi based SMA wires is also used. A prototype is tested on a suspended, robotic leg to simulate the swing phase of a typical gait. Thayer & Priya (2011) have designed a biomimetic dexterous humanoid hand where the dexterity of the DART hand have been measured by quantifying functionality and typing speed on a standard keyboard. The hand consists of 16 servo motors dedicated to finger motion and three motors for wrist motion where some of joints are activated through SMA wires.

Some of the researchers have focused on the design of a biomechatronic robotic hand using EMG. Cheron et al. (1996) have found the relationship between EMG and the arm kinematics through dynamic recurrent neural networks (DRNN) method whereas Hudgins et al. (1997) have focused on a new control scheme, based on the recognition of naturally myoelectric signal patterns, transfers the burden of multifunction myoelectric control from the amputee to the control system. Rosen et al. (2001) have developed a myosignal-based exoskeleton system. This is implemented in an elbow joint, naturally controlled by the human. The human–machine interface is set at the neuromuscular level, by using the neuromuscular signal (EMG) as the primary command signal for the exoskeleton system. The EMG signals along with the joint kinematics are fed into a myoprocessor (Hill-based muscle model) which in turn predicts the muscle moments on the elbow joint. Banks (2001) has given remarkable effort towards design and control of an anthropomorphic robotic finger with multi-point tactile sensation whereas Light et al. (2002) have emphasized on intelligent multifunction myoelectric control of hand prostheses. Peleg et al. (2002) have extracted multiple features via EMG signal from hand amputees which is selected by help of a genetic algorithm. Fukuda et al. (2003) have developed a prosthetic hand where human-assisting manipulator system based on the EMG signals is utilized. Wheeler (2003) has presented a neuro-electric interface method for virtual device control. The sampled EMG data is taken from forearm and then is fed into pattern recognition software that has been trained to distinguish gestures from a given gesture set. Krysztoforski et al. (2004) have given remarkable effort towards recognition of palm finger movements on the basis of EMG signals with the application of wavelets.

Crawford et al. (2005) have used EMG signals for classifying in real-time with an extremely high degree of accuracy in a robotic arm-and-gripper. A linear support vector machines (SVM) based classifier and a sparse feature representation of the EMG signal are used.

Hidalgo et al. (2005) have proposed a design of robotic arm employing fuzzy algorithms to interpret EMG signals from the flexor carpi radialis, extensor carpi radialis and biceps brachii muscles. The control and acquisition systems are composed of a microprocessor, analog filtering, digital filtering & frequency analysis, and finally a fuzzy control system. Mobasser & Hashtrudi-Zaad (2005) have estimated rowing stroke force with EMG signal using artificial neural network method from upper arm muscles which is involved in elbow joint movement, sensed elbow angular position and velocity. Gao et al. (2006) have focused on acquiring the data from the upper limb of the body for robotic arm motion using EMG whereas Frigo et al. (2007) have detected EMG signal from voluntarily activated muscles which is controlled for functional neuromuscular by electrical stimulation. A comb filter (with and without a blanking window) is applied to remove the signal components synchronously correlated to the stimulus. Roy et al. (2007) have compared the performance of different sEMG signal at various conditions. These performances depend on the electro-mechanical stability between the sensor and its contact with skin. Zollo et al. (2007) have put a remarkable effort on the control system of biomechatronic robotic hand and on the optimization of the hand design in order to obtain human like kinematics and dynamics. By evaluating the simulated hand performance, the mechanical design is iteratively refined. The mechanical structure and the ratio between numbers of actuators to the number of DOF have been optimized. Yagiz et al. (2007) have developed a dynamic model of the prosthetic finger where a non chattering robust sliding mode control is applied to make the model follow a certain trajectory. Wege & Zimmermann (2007) have shown the potential of EMG control for a hand exoskeleton device. The device has been developed with focus on support of the rehabilitation process after hand injuries or strokes. Itoh et al. (2007) have studied the hand finger operation using sEMG during crookedness state of the finger. Two electrodes (Ag/AgCl electrodes) are sticked randomly on the forearm muscles and the intensity of EMG signals at different muscles is measured for each crooked finger.

Hao et al. (2008) have studied the design of pneumatic muscle actuator based robotic hand where its compliance and dexterity handling are attempted. A single finger is controlled by fuzzy & PID controller and comparative studies are discussed. Murphy et al. (2008) have explored the micro electro-mechanical systems based sensor for mechanomyography system whereas Saponas et al. (2008) have also explored the feasibility on muscle-computer interaction methodology that directly senses and decodes human muscular activity rather than relying on physical device actuation or user actions. Andrews (2008) has determined an effective approach to finger movement classification in typing tasks using myoelectric data which are collected from the forearm. Cesqui et al. (2008) have explored the use of EMG signals for post-stroke and robot-mediated therapy. In this work, a pilot study has been reported under young and healthy subjects where experiments are conducted to determine whether it is possible to build a static map to cluster EMG activation patterns for horizontal reaching movements. Chen et al. (2008) have implemented an EMG feedback control method with functional electrical stimulation cycling system (FESCS) for stroke patients. The stroke patients often suffer from low limbs paralysis. By designing the feedback control protocol of FESCS, the physiological signal is recorded with help of FPGA biomedical module, DAC and electrical stimulation circuit. Lee et al. (2009) have described a development procedure of bio-mimetic robot hand and its control scheme where each robot hand has four under-actuated fingers, which are driven by two linear actuators coupled together. Dalley et al. (2009) have given emphasis of an anthropomorphic hand prosthesis that is intended for use with a multiple-channel myoelectric interface. The hand contains 16 joints, which are differentially driven by a set of five independent actuators. Hu et al. (2009) have presented a comparison between electromyography-driven robot and passive motion device on wrist rehabilitation for chronic stroke patients. By comparative study, it was found that the EMG-driven interactive training had a better long-term effect than the continuous passive movement (CPM) treatment.

Blouin et al. (2010) have focused on control of arm movement during body motion as revealed by EMG whereas Luo & Chang (2010) have explored a feasibility study on EMG signal integrated with multi-finger robot hand control for massage therapy applications. The forearm EMG of a person massaged by the human hands is recorded and analyzed statistically. Khokhar et al. (2010) have showed the potential of EMG applications where SVM classification technique is suitable for real-time classification of sEMG signals. This technique is effectively implemented for controlling an exoskeleton device. Huang et al. (2010) have designed a robust EMG sensing interface for pattern classification. The aim of this study was to design sensor fault detection (SFD) module through the sensor interface to provide reliable EMG pattern classification. This module monitors the recorded signals from individual EMG electrodes and performs a self-recovery strategy to recover the classification performance when one or more sensors are disturbed. Naik et al. (2010) has studied the pattern classification of myo-electric signal during different maximum voluntary contractions using BSS techniques for a blind person whereas Artemiadis & Kyriakopoulos (2010 & 2011) have presented a switching regime model for the EMG-based control of a robot arm where decode the EMG activity of 11 muscles has a continuous representation of arm motion in the 3-D space. The switching regime model is used to overcome the main difficulties of the EMG-based control systems, i.e. the nonlinearity of the relationship between the EMG recordings and the arm motion, as well as the non-stationary of EMG signals with respect to time. Vogel et al. (2011) have demonstrated the robotic arm/hand system that is controlled in real time in 6 dimension Cartesian space through measured human muscular activity via EMG. DLR Light-weight Robot III is used during demonstration of impedance control. Li et al. (2011) have presented a robot control system using four different gestures from an arm. These are achieved by EMG signal using phase synchrony features. The phase synchrony analysis using the recent multivariate extensions of empirical mode decomposition (MEMD) is carried out. Joshi et al. (2011) have focused on brain-muscle-computer interface using a single sEMG signal. Initial results show that the human neuromuscular system can simultaneously manipulate partial power in two separate frequency bands of a sEMG power spectrum at a single muscle site. Matsubara et al. (2011) have proposed an interface to intuitively control robotic devices using myoelectric signals. Through learning procedure, a set of myoelectric signals is captured from multiple subjects in the system and it can be used as an adaptation procedure to a new user after only a few interactions.

Recently, Ahmad et al. (2012) have presented a review report on different techniques of EMG data recording where condition of an ideal pre-amplifier, signal conditioning and its amplification are discussed. Sun et al. (2012) have conducted an isokinetic exercise to realize the characteristics of femoral muscles in human knee movement through EMG where a mechanical model of muscle for human knee movement is established. Qi et al. (2012) have developed algorithms for muscle-fatigue detection and muscle-recruitment patterns in routine wheel chair propulsion scenarios, e.g., daily practice where for analysis purpose two speeds of muscular behavior are chosen. Gandole (2012) has developed an artificial intelligent model using focused time lagged recurrent neural network (FTLRNN) method with a single hidden layer. FTLRNN method reduces noise intelligently from the EMG signal. Chan et al. (2012) have developed an assessment platform for upper limb myoelectric prosthetic devices using EMG. The assessment platform consists of an acquisition module, a signal capture module, a programmable signal generation module and an activation & measurement module. The platform is designed to create a sequence of activation signals from EMG data captured from a patient.

An EAP actuator based design for IPMC fingers have been discussed by Biddiss & Chau (2006). This shows the potential of electroactive polymeric sensors within an operating range of voltage (±3V) whereas Kottke et al. (2007) have reported on how to stimulate and activate a non-biological muscle such as an IPMC. Lee et al. (2006, 2007) have also demonstrated the potential of an IPMC actuating system with a bio-mimetic function using EMG signals. A mean absolute method is used for achieving the filtered EMG signal. Aravinthan et al. (2010) have designed a multiple axis prosthetic hand using IPMC. EMG signal through programmable interface controller (PIC) is sent to the IPMC prosthetic material to perform the required actions. By doing experiments, the potential of prosthetic hand using IPMC is shown. After that, we have also demonstrated actuation of IPMC through EMG via forearm muscles where potential of IPMC based micro robotic arm has been shown for lifting the object (Jain et al., 2010a; 2010b; 2011; 2012). For further application of EMG driven system, we are discussing detailed analysis of EMG signal control point view of IPMC based artificial muscle finger for micro gripper in this chapter.

3. Design and control of IPMC based artificial finger driven by EMG signal

3.1. Basic design of IPMC artificial muscle finger based micro gripper using EMG

For designing an IPMC artificial muscle finger based micro gripper using EMG, an IPMC strip (Size 40 mm × 10 mm× 0.2 mm) that imitates human finger movement, is assumed to be artificial muscle finger. This is fixed with holder and another plastic based finger of similar size is made for supporting the micro object as shown in Fig. 1. When human index finger moves up and down, it creates potential difference by its movements. This potential difference is transferred through EMG electrodes into the artificial muscle finger so that this finger is able to move accordingly and hold the object. The main function of EMG electrode is to detect the voltage from human muscles since human muscles generate few milli-voltages when they are contracting or expanding during movement. For transferring this voltage signal to actuate the artificial muscle finger, it needs the amplification setup which is discussed in section 4. Therefore, IPMC based artificial muscle finger is activated using EMG and it allows holding an object for micro assembly operation.

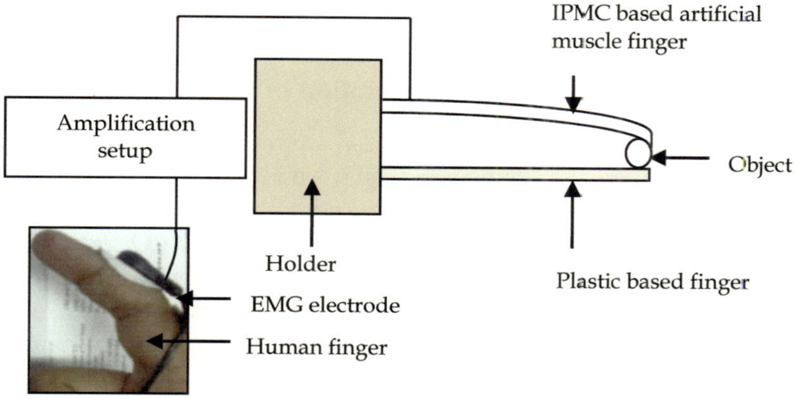

Figure 1. Schematic diagram of IPMC artificial muscle finger based micro gripper driven by EMG

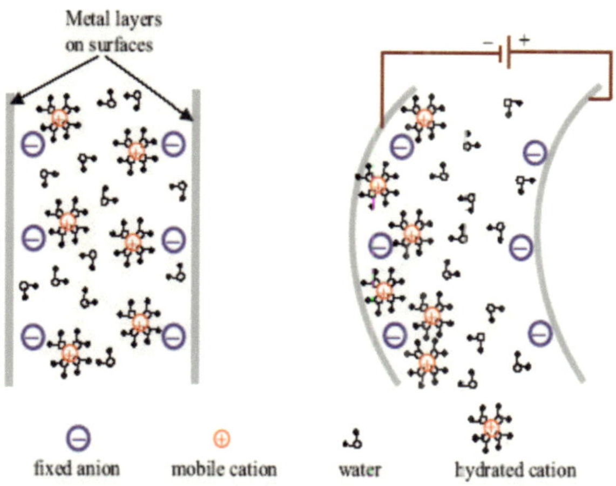

Figure 2. Schematic diagram of the actuation mechanism of IPMC (Chen et al., 2011)

During development of an EMG driven IPMC based artificial muscle finger, a typical IPMC strip (Procured custom made from Environmental Robots Inc., USA) is used which has a thin (approximately 200 μm) perfluorinated ion exchange base polymer membrane (Nafion-117) with metal electrodes of platinum (5–10 μm) fused on either side. As a part of the manufacturing process, this base polymer is further chemically coated with metal ions that comprise the metallic composites. It responds in wet/dry condition. An IPMC is usually kept in a hydrated state to ensure proper dynamic operation. When the material is hydrated, the cations will diffuse toward an electrode on the material surface under an applied electric field. Inside the polymer structure, anions are interconnected as clusters providing channels for the cations to flow towards the electrode (Chen et al., 2011). This motion of ions causes the structure to bend toward the anode as shown in Fig. 2. An applied electric field affects the cation distribution within the membrane, forcing the cations to migrate towards the cathode. This change in the cation distribution produces two thin layers, one near the anode and another near the cathode boundaries. The potential is generated by changing the potential electric field on cluster of ionic strips that provides the actuation of the strip.

3.2. Basic tendon of index finger for identification of EMG signal

To examine the bio-mimetic behavior of IPMC based artificial muscle finger, it is important to study the physiological structure of human finger. An internal structure of human index finger is shown in Fig. 3. The index finger is actuated by three intrinsic muscles and four extrinsic muscles. The intrinsic muscles consist of two interosseous (IO 1 and IO 2) muscles & one lumbrical (LU) muscle and four extrinsic muscles connected through long tendons i.e. extensor digitorum communis (EDC), extensor indicis proprius (EIP), flexor digitorum superficialis (FDS) and flexor digitorum profundus (FDP) (Bundhoo & Park, 2005). For heavy lifting & holding purpose, EDC and EIP are responsible in tendon network. Consequently, EMG electrodes are placed at these two positions on the human finger so that we can achieve direct actuation of IPMC based artificial muscle finger through said muscles.

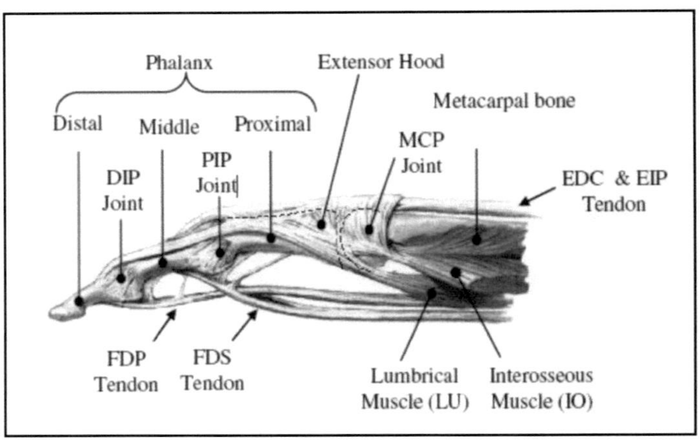

Figure 3. Basic tendons of the index finger (Bundhoo & Park, 2005)

3.3. Model for controlling the EMG signal for IPMC based artificial muscle finger

For acquiring the data from said muscles, EMG electrodes are placed for measuring the electric potential produced by voluntary contraction of muscle fiber on the human finger. The frequency range of the EMG signal is within 4 to 900 Hz. The dominant energy is concentrated in the range of 95 Hz and amplitude of voltage range is ±1.2 mV according to muscle contraction and the voltage function $V_{in}(t)$ in term of signal sample time (t) is given below,

$$V_{in}(t) = V_{ino} sin(2\pi ft) \quad (1)$$

Where, V_{ino} is amplitude of EMG voltage (±0.0012 V); f is frequency of EMG signal (95 Hz).

In Laplace domain, EMG input signal is written as

$$V_{in}(s) = \frac{2.96}{s^2 + 3.51e5} \quad (2)$$

Using these parameters, the circuit for filtered EMG signal is designed using MATLAB SIMULINK software as shown in Fig. 4.

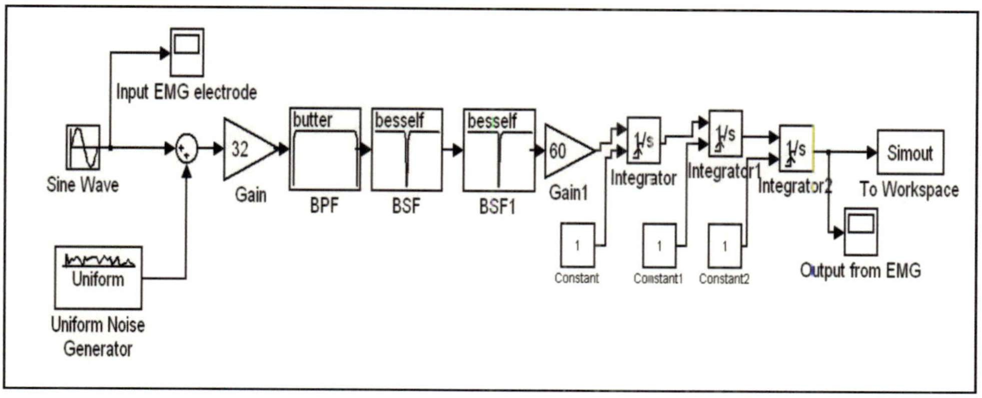

Figure 4. Block diagram of EMG signal behaviour from human index finger

In block diagram, the active EMG signal is taken from index finger muscle and uniform noise is considered. The electric potential is first amplified with gain 32 dB and then band pass filter (BPF) is used within specified frequency range (4 to 900 Hz). Using two band stop filters (BSF and BSF1), noise signal (60 Hz) that arises due to AC coupled power is eliminated. The signal is then passed through an amplifier with gain 60 dB. Subsequently, three integrators (Integrator, Integrator1 and Integrator2) are used for achieving better damped signal. The output of EMG signal with sampling time of 10^{-4} seconds after filtering is shown in Fig. 5.

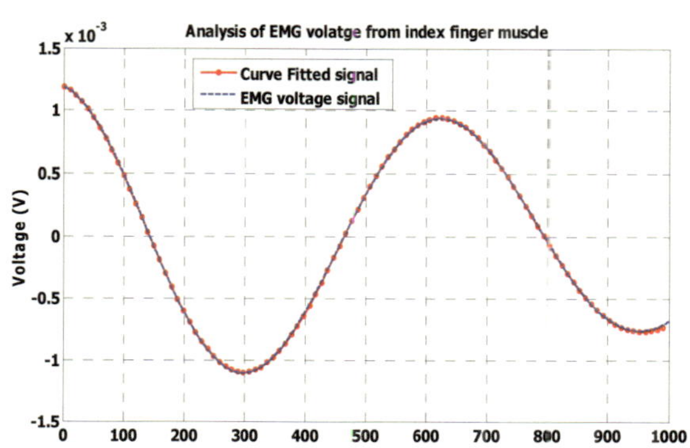

Figure 5. Acquired data from finger muscles via EMG signal

Thus, the total output duration of EMG signal for sampled data is 0.1 second. The general solution of acquired EMG voltage (V_{EMG}) through curve fitting method is obtained as given below,

$$V_{EMG}(t) = \sum V_0 sin(2\pi f_0 t + \delta_0), \quad 0 \le t \le 0.1 \tag{3}$$

where, V_0 is the amplitude of EMG voltage of sine function (±0.0012 V); f_0 is average frequency of sine function (4.7 Hz); δ_0 is initial phase difference of sine function (1.66 rad); t is signal sample time in second.

After adjustment of root mean square (RMS) value of this sine function, the EMG voltage $V_{EMGrms}(s)$ after filtering is written as

$$V_{EMG_{rms}}(s) = \frac{1.16e^{-5}(s^2 + 1.17e^{-4})}{\left(s^2 - 0.014s + 1.07e^{-4}\right)\left(s^2 + 0.014s + 1.07e^{-4}\right)} \tag{4}$$

For controlling purpose, single input single output (SISO) control system tool in MATLAB is used and the output $V_{EMG}(s)$ data is obtained. The initial overall transfer function of EMG voltage $V_{EMGinitial}(s)$ is obtained through output signal from (4) to input signal from (2) and is given as

$$V_{EMGinitial}(s) = \frac{3.92e^{-6}\left(s^2 + 1.17e^{-4}\right)\left(s^2 + 3.5e^{5}\right)}{\left(s^2 - 0.0146s + 1.07e^{-4}\right)\left(s^2 + 0.0146s + 1.07e^{-4}\right)} \tag{5}$$

After that, Nyquist criterion is applied to check the stability of EMG signal. The root-locus and bode scheme are plotted as shown in Fig. 6.

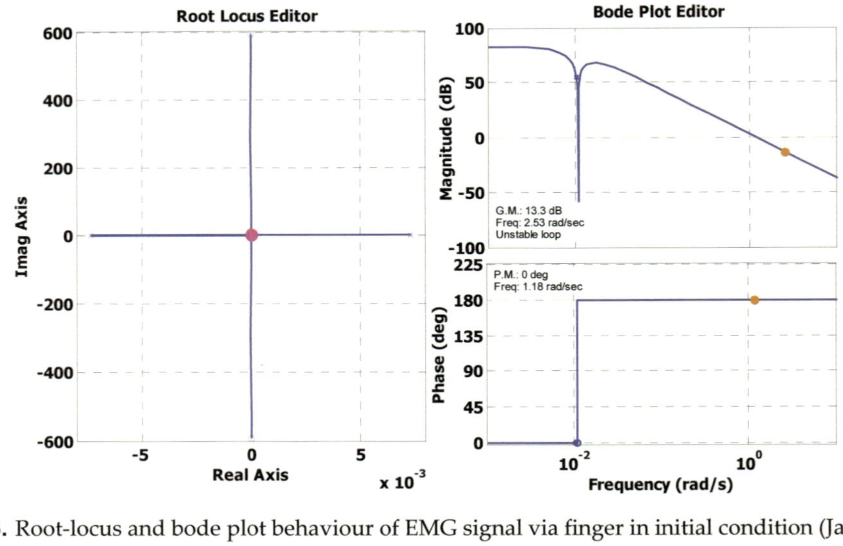

Figure 6. Root-locus and bode plot behaviour of EMG signal via finger in initial condition (Jain et al., 2011)

It is found that the zero-poles have real value on both sides of the real axis which does not meet the Nyquist stability criteria. Also from Fig. 6, gain cross-over frequency (GCF=2.53 rad/s) is greater than phase cross-over frequency (PCF=1.18 rad/s), indicating that this voltage obtained from EMG signal is unstable.

For achieving the stable EMG signal, different configurations of PID are analysed through SISO control tool of MATLAB software. By applying PD control with proportional control gain factor (K_p=1) and derivative control gain factor (K_d=1), EMG voltage $V_{EMGfinal\ 1}(s)$ is obtained as given below,

$$V_{EMGfinal1}(s) = \frac{(s^2+1.17e^{-4})(s^2+3.516e^5)}{(s+2.546e^5)(s^2-9.91e^{-9}s+1.17e^{-4})\,(s^2+1.38s+1.38)} \tag{6}$$

The root locus and bode plot are shown in Fig. 7. This indicates that the obtained data from EMG signal is unstable but through this control system the data is converging towards stability from initial condition.

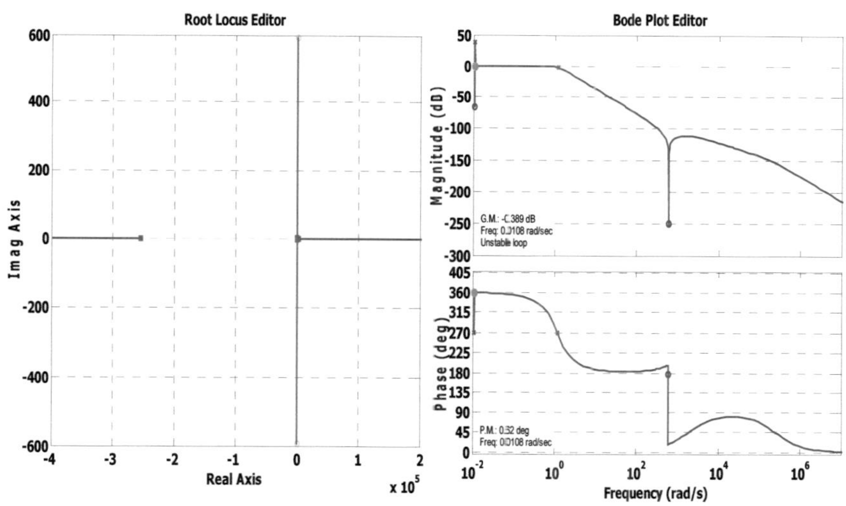

Figure 7. Root-locus and bode plot behaviour of human finger through PD controller

In case of PI controller, the unit proportional control gain factor (K_p=1) and integrator control gain factor (K_i=1) parameters are used. After applying this control system, EMG voltage $V_{EMGfinal\ 2}(s)$ is obtained as given below,

$$V_{EMGfinal2}(s) = \frac{3.92e^{-6}\ s\,(s^2+1.17e^{-4})\,(s^2+3.51e^5)}{(s+0.724)(s^2+9.91e^{-9}s+1.17e^{-4})(s^2-0.724s+1.90)} \tag{7}$$

The bode plot and root locus for this system are plotted as shown in Fig. 8. From this figure, it shows that the data from EMG signal is again unstable but the response has a better prospect of converging towards stability than previous configuration.

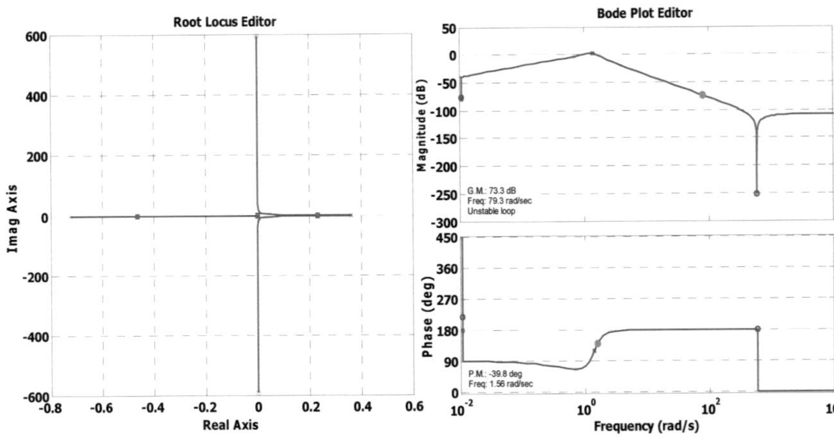

Figure 8. Root-locus and bode plot behaviour of EMG signal via finger through PI controller

After that, PID controller is used where proportional control gain factor (K_p= 0.5), integrator control gain factor (K_i= 1) and derivative control gain factor (K_d=1) are given in compensator to attain the stability of EMG voltage. For applying the PID control system, the SIMULINK block diagram is modified as shown in Fig. 9.

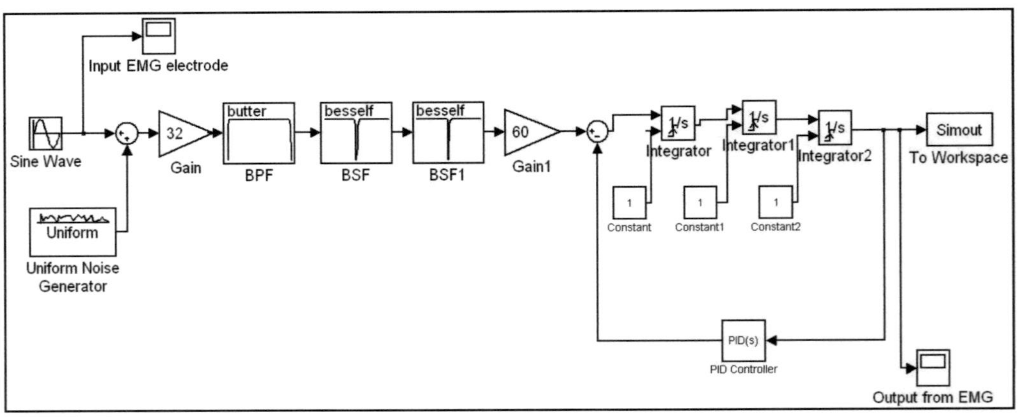

Figure 9. Block diagram of EMG signal via human finger after applying PID control system

Thereafter, the model is again simulated in MATLAB software, upon which, the data from finger muscles shows the all zero-poles in left hand side of real axis which satisfies the Nyquist criteria shown in Fig. 10. The final EMG voltage $V_{EMGfinal}(s)$ is acquired as given below,

$$V_{EMGfinal}(s) = \frac{s\left(s^2 + 1.17e^{-4}\right)\left(s^2 + 3.51e^5\right)}{\left(s + 2.54e^5\right)\left(s + 1.52\right)\left(s^2 + 1.83e^{-8}s + 1.17e^{-4}\right)\left(s^2 - 0.14s + 0.90\right)} \tag{8}$$

Also, GCF (1rad/s) is less than PCF (1.34 rad/s). Hence, a stable EMG voltage data is achieved. This filtered EMG signal is stable enough to provide necessary voltage signal across the IPMC for proper functioning during operation. The major advantage of this control system is that it is stable with least amount of noise. This signal is sent to artificial muscle finger for holding the object.

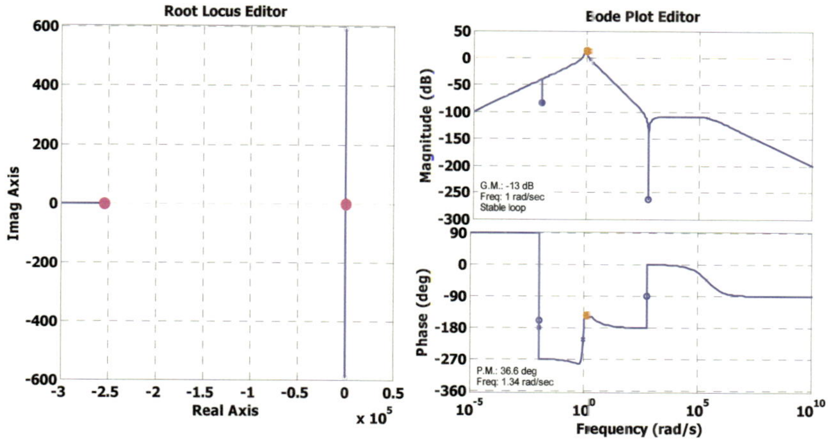

Figure 10. Root-locus and bode plot behaviour of EMG signal via finger through PID controller (Jain et al., 2011)

4. Experimental testing setup

In order to examine the bio-mimetic behaviour of IPMC based artificial muscle finger through EMG signal, EMG electrodes (Ag/Agcl based) are positioned at EDC and EIP muscles on the index finger. The input EMG signal from the muscle movement varies in the range of ±1.2mV (which is observed through oscilloscope). But activation of IPMC based artificial muscle finger needs the voltage of ±3V and current rating of 50-200 mA which is only possible by amplification of voltage and current. For desired output voltage to the artificial muscle finger, EMG signal is transferred through analog-digital convertor (ADC) card and PXI system (PXI-1031 along with NI-6289) in real time environment. EMG signal through electrodes are sent to an input channel at specified ports of the ADC card. Then this signal is amplified through amplification factor of 2550 using express VI of Labview 8.5 and sent to DAC output. But DAC output signal cannot provide enough current (50-200 mA) to drive an IPMC based artificial muscle finger. For achieving this current rating, the current amplification is done using customized IPMC control circuit by combining operational amplifier (Model: LM-324), transistor (Model: TIP 122) and resistances (1kΩ and 10Ω). Noise interference is eliminated by enabling low-pass filtering with PID control system to achieve the stability during operation of the artificial muscle finger as shown in Fig. 11. The IPMC size 40mm × 10 mm × 0.2 mm is used for testing purpose.

Now, in order to prevent the abrupt physio-chemical change of the IPMC nature and subsequent shortening of the actuation operating time of the IPMC material due to irreversible electrolysis (caused when the voltage applied across the two faces of an IPMC exceeds a maximum limit), two warning flags are used. One warning flag is placed at input EMG signal and another warning flag is placed at output voltage of DAC card where IPMC control circuit is connected. This limited voltage imposed on the IPMC based artificial muscle finger aborts the execution of the program when the warning flag has a high output. The flow chart for actuation of IPMC based artificial muscle finger is shown in Fig. 12. During operation, artificial muscle finger bends in a similar manner as that of the index finger. For generating force, this finger is held in cantilever configuration on the fabricated work bench. A load cell is used to collect the data at different angles of the index finger. The current and voltage analysis of the human muscles are also done through oscilloscope. Thus an IPMC artificial muscle finger based micro gripper driven by EMG is developed and the holding behaviour is demonstrated.

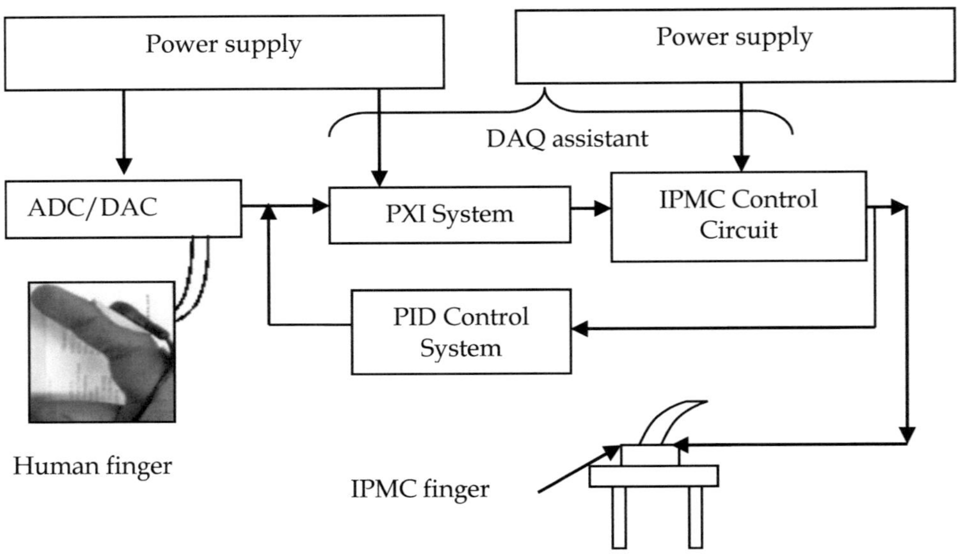

Figure 11. Basic testing layout for actuation of IPMC based artificial muscle finger

5. Results and discussion

During experimentation, the input parameter from muscle ranging from ±1.2 mV is taken through referenced single-ended (RSE) signal along with continuous sampled pulses. These pulses are amplified with the help of a PXI system (amplification factor 2550). The desired output voltage range is generated through a DAC output port. The output signal is connected to IPMC based artificial muscle finger. Due to amplified output voltage from the DAC, an IPMC strip bends in one direction for holding the object. By changing the movement of human finger in an opposite direction, reverse behaviour of IPMC is obtained. The characteristics of IPMC based artificial muscle finger are traced on a graph paper and plotted as shown in Fig. 13. It shows that IPMC based artificial muscle finger gives similar bending behaviour as a human finger (Fig. 14). It is also observed that the deflection of IPMC based artificial muscle finger changes with voltage upto 12 mm in one direction. When this finger moves reverse direction, the characteristic of artificial finger does not attempt the same behaviour. It shows the error between two paths is 0.5 mm. The deflection characteristic of IPMC based artificial muscle finger (δ) in term of voltage *(V)* with cubic behaviour for holding is given below,

$$\delta(V) = 0.67 \times V^3 - 1.9 \times V^2 + 3.7 \times V - 0.17 \ (\text{in mm}) \tag{9}$$

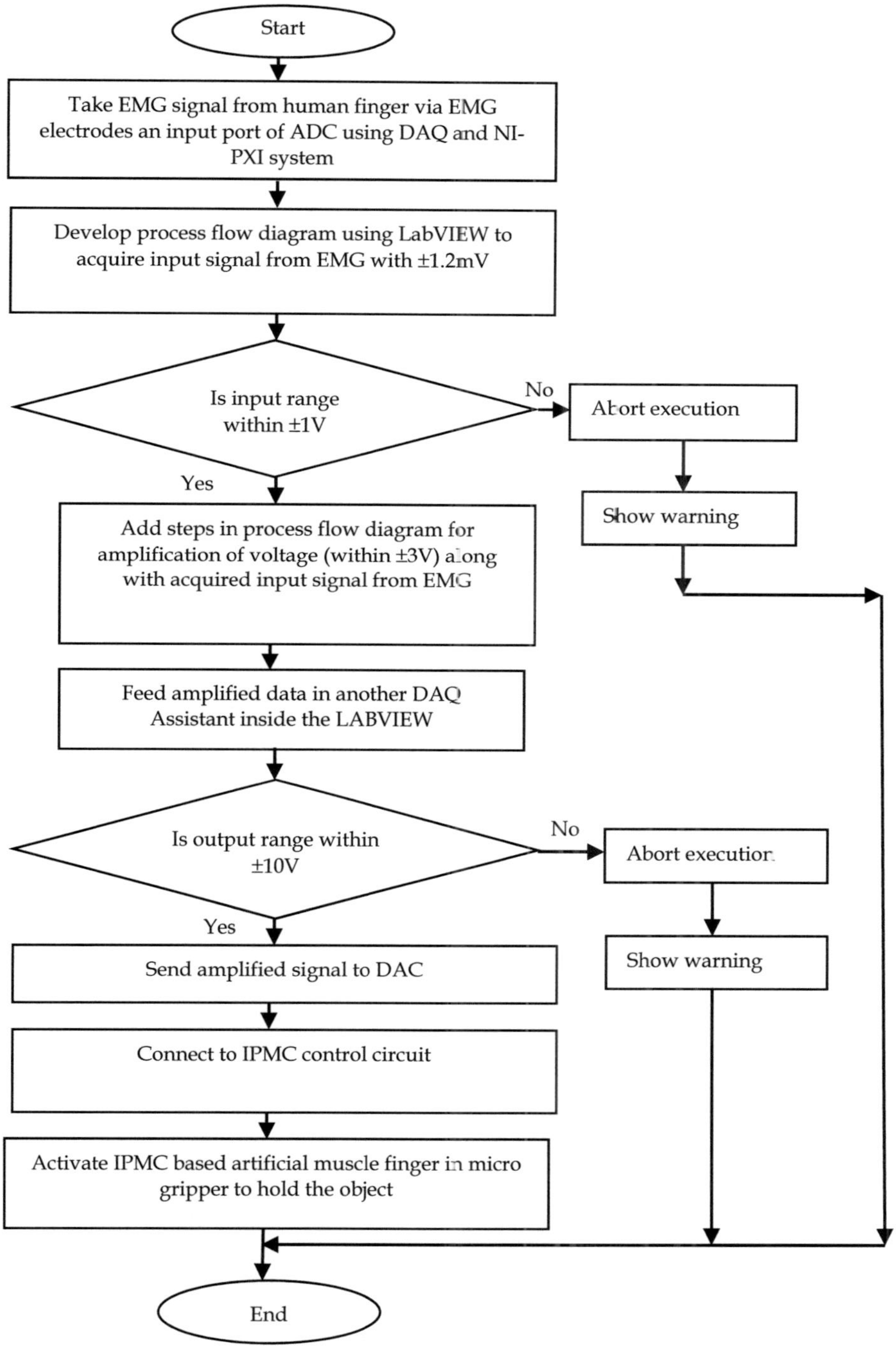

Figure 12. Flow chart of for actuation IPMC based artificial muscle finger using EMG signal

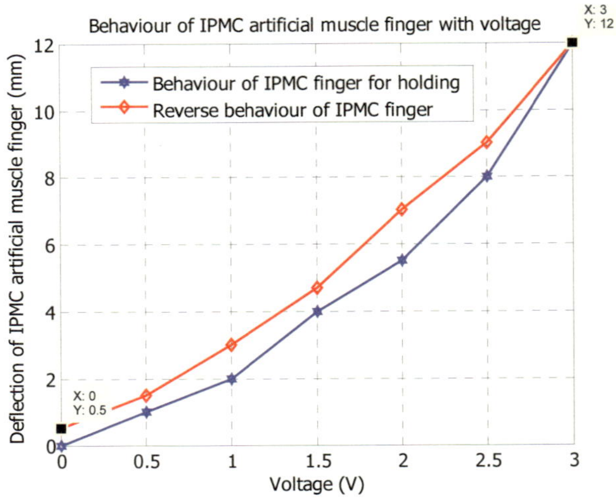

Figure 13. Deflection behaviour of IPMC based artificial muscle finger with different voltages

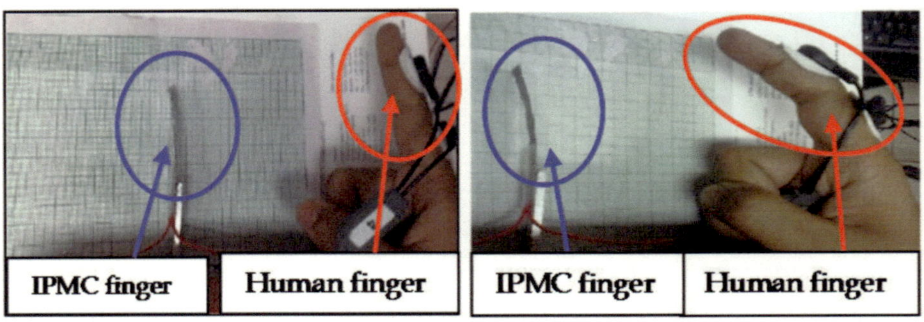

(a) Initial state (b) Activated state in ACW direction

Figure 14. Control of IPMC based article muscle finger through EMG signal (Jain et al., 2011)

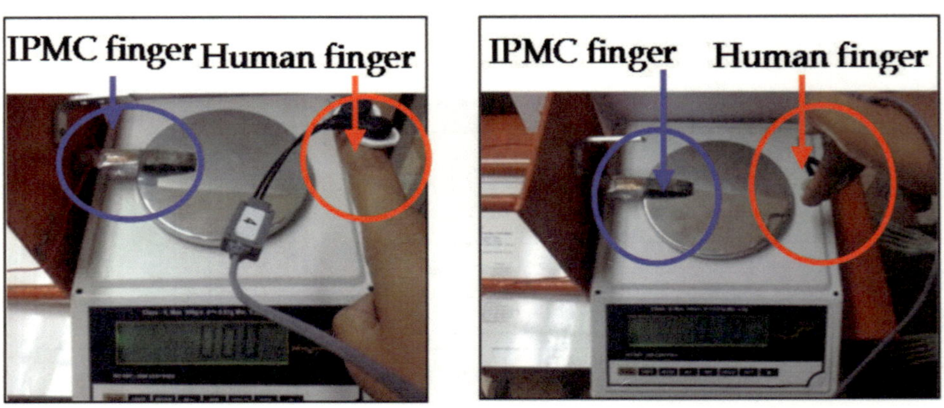

(a) Initial state (b) Activated state

Figure 15. Load test setup for IPMC based artificial muscle finger using load cell

For generating force by the artificial muscle finger, a testing setup with load cell is used. The IPMC based artificial muscle finger is placed in cantilever mode, and a load cell is placed under the tip of the IPMC which produces the reactive force. When human finger moves downward, the generated force by IPMC artificial muscle finger increases accordingly in the load cell as shown in Fig. 15.

By controlling the movement of human finger, the generated force varies accordingly. The generated force characteristic with voltage shows a cubic polynomial behaviour as shown in Fig. 16 when IPMC artificial muscle finger touches the load cell. This happens due to compliant behaviour of IPMC. The generated force *(F)* by IPMC based artificial muscle finger in term of voltage *(V)* is given below,

$$F(V) = 0.11 \times V^3 + 0.25 \times V^2 + 1.6 \times V - 0.11 \quad (\text{in mN}) \tag{10}$$

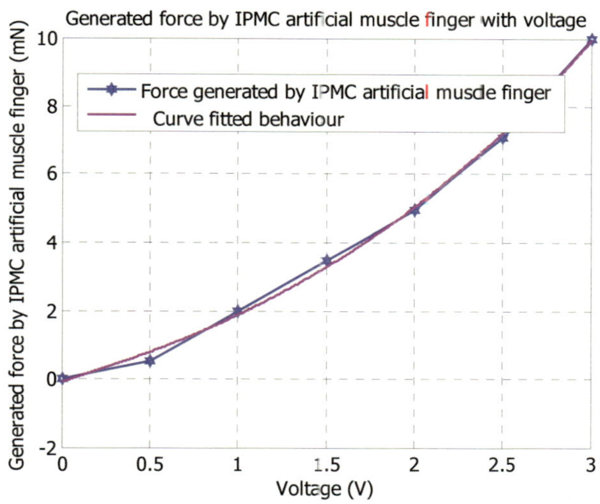

Figure 16. Generated force by IPMC based artificial muscle finger at tip with voltage

The maximum generated force of 10 mN is achieved by IPMC based artificial muscle finger at 45^0 angle of index finger with cubic polynomial behaviour as shown in Fig. 17. This happens due to human finger behaviour where EIP and EDC muscles are connected with DIP and PIP joints. The generated force *(F)* by IPMC based artificial muscle finger at tip in term of human finger angle *(θ)* is also obtained as under

$$F(\theta) = -\,0.000083 \times \theta^3 + 0.01 \times \theta^2 - 0.063 \times \theta + 0.045 \quad (\text{in mN}) \tag{11}$$

For observing the real time IPMC based artificial muscle finger behaviour with moving human finger angle, experiments are conducted and data are plotted as shown in Fig. 18 and it shows almost proportional behaviour with quadratic relationship. This occurs due to human finger behaviour where EIP and EDC are connected with IO and LU muscles (Fig. 3).

The relationship between IPMC based artificial muscle finger displacement (δ) and human finger angle (θ) is given below,

$$\delta(\theta) = -\,0.0016 \times \theta^2 + 0.34 \times \theta - 0.15 \quad (\text{in mm}) \tag{12}$$

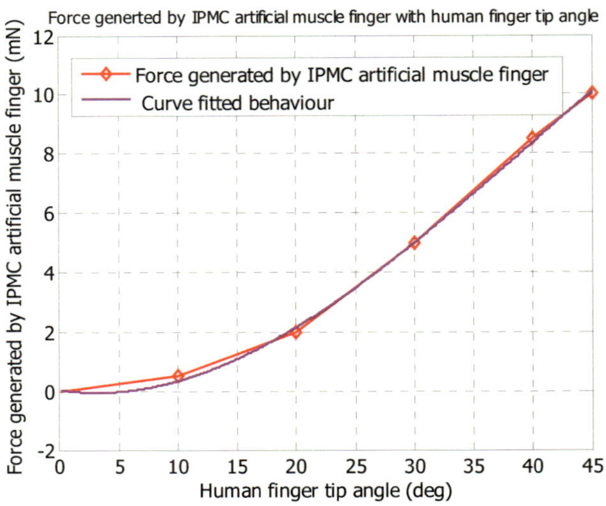

Figure 17. Generated force by IPMC based artificial muscle finger with human finger angle

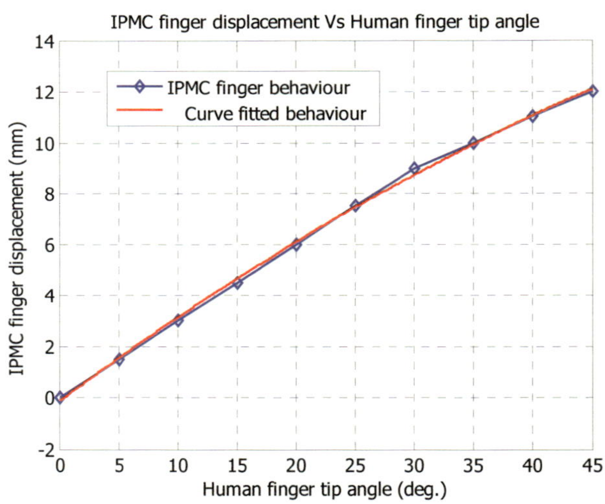

Figure 18. Relationship between IPMC based artificial muscle finger and human finger angle

For actuation of IPMC based artificial muscle finger, the analysis of activated muscles is carried out as given in Table 1. We have analysed different conditions during contraction of different muscles of index finger like intrinsic and extrinsic which are responsible for actuation of IPMC based artificial muscle finger so that they can be used to hold an object.

Cases	Intrinsic muscles			Extrinsic muscles				State	Polarity	
	IO 1	IO 2	LU	EDC	EIP	FDS	FDP		Side A	Side B
1	OFF	OFF	OFF	OFF	OFF	OFF	OFF	None	None	None
2	ON	OFF	ON	OFF	OFF	ON	ON	Adduction	+ive	-ive
3	OFF	ON	ON	ON	ON	OFF	OFF	Abduction	-ive	+ive
4	ON	ON	ON	ON	ON	ON	ON	None	None	None

Table 1. Analysis of different condition of muscles

The two surfaces of IPMC are denoted as side A and side B. In case of intrinsic muscles, the adduction is possible. When IO 1 or IO 2 are in either "on" or "off" condition along with LU muscle in "on" condition then it shows the abduction state. In case of extrinsic muscles, EDC and EIP muscles both are in "off" condition to achieve the adduction state when FDS and FDP muscles both are in "on" condition and for attaining the abduction state EDC and EIP both are in "on" condition when FDS and FDP both are in "off" condition. In rest cases, no power is achieved. Therefore, IPMC based artificial muscle finger is activated in above mentioned conditions from muscles.

The voltage characteristic behavior is taken from EMG and fed to IPMC based artificial muscle finger for actuation in real time environment as shown in Fig. 19. It is found that the trend of IPMC actuation voltage is similar to EMG voltage with amplification factor.

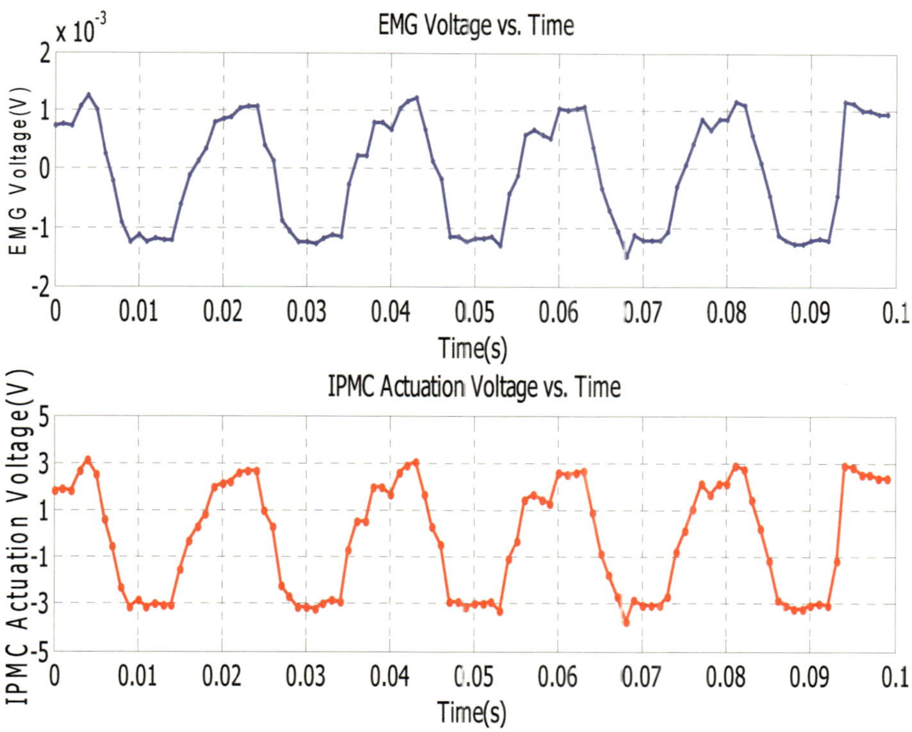

Figure 19. Different voltage responses in real time environment

The EMG voltage $V_{EMG}\ (t)$ and IPMC actuation voltage $V_{IPMC\ actuation}\ (t)$ equations are respectively given below,

$$V_{EMG}(t) = \sum V_{0E} sin(2\pi f_{0E} t + \delta_{0E}), \qquad 0 \le t \le 0.1 \tag{13}$$

and

$$V_{IPMCactuation}(t) = \sum V_{0I} sin(2\pi f_{0I} t + \delta_{0I}), \qquad 0 \le t \le 0.1 \tag{14}$$

Where, V_{0E} is average value of EMG voltage (V); f_{0E} is EMG frequency range (Hz) ; t is signal sample time (s) ; δ_{0E} is phase difference when signal is taken through EMG (rad); V_{0I} is average value of IPMC actuation voltage (V); f_{0I} is IPMC actuation frequency range (Hz); δ_{0I} is phase difference when signal is given to IPMC (rad). For finding the frequency range of each signal, the experimental data are taken and solved through MATLAB curve fitting tool. The numerical values are V_{0E}= 0.001451±0.0002707 V, f_{0E}= 4.7±0.006201 Hz, δ_{0E}= -1.736±0.036 rad, V_{0I}= 2.493±0.208, f_{0I}= 48.5±0.65 and δ_{0I}= -10.5732±0.6556 rad. From these data, it is found that EMG frequency range (f_{0I}) is similar to simulated data and IPMC actuation frequency range is 48.5±0.65 Hz which is in between human muscle frequency range (48-52Hz).

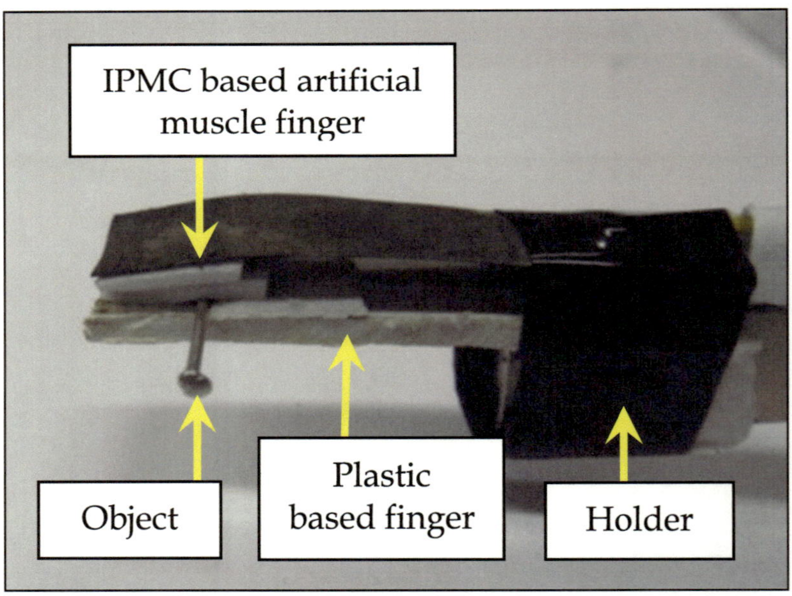

Figure 20. IPMC based artificial muscle finger based micro gripper driven by EMG

After these analyses, an IPMC artificial muscle finger based micro gripper is developed which is driven by EMG as shown in Fig. 20 where one IPMC based artificial muscle finger and other plastic based finger are fixed with double sided tape within one holder. The IPMC based artificial muscle finger is connected through copper tape and wire with EMG sensor so that an IPMC based artificial muscle finger is activated by EMG signal via human finger. The packing tape is also placed on the tip of IPMC based artificial muscle finger so that this finger perfectly holds the object like micro pin for assembly. After these observations, it is understood that IPMC finger behaves as an artificial muscle and this characteristic is implemented in the development of IPMC artificial muscle finger based micro gripper for holding the object through EMG. The major advantages of EMG-driven IPMC based artificial muscle finger are low voltage in man-machine interface, large bending amplitude and simple control that are applied in development of micro/bio robot.

6. Conclusion

In order to develop the micro/bio-mimetic robot for micro assembly, the potential of an EMG driven artificial finger is discussed in this chapter. An artificial finger for micro assembly is designed using IPMC where IPMC is used as an active artificial finger for holding the object. An IPMC has several advantages such as actuating through a small voltage (±3 V), light in weight, flexible in nature and does not involve sophisticated controllers for operation. For activating the IPMC based artificial finger, voltage is taken from human index finger through EMG sensor instead of battery source as this is used as a man-machine interface device. Principally, EMG sensor acquires the signal from body during expansion or contraction of muscles. These movements are transferred into an IPMC based artificial muscle finger. For achieving the stable data from EMG, different configurations of control methods are analysed. A PID control system is implemented for attaining the noiseless and stable signal from the user's myoelectric signal. While acquiring the data, a differential amplification technique is applied where data is filtered through a band pass filter and noise is eliminated through three band stop filters. For sending this signal to the IPMC, an algorithm has been developed in Labview software which gives emphasis on following points:

- Acquire voltage data (±1.2mV) from human index finger using EMG sensor through data acquisition system
- Amplify the continuous EMG signal through DAQ assistant enabling the filter and domain frequency range options
- Activate IPMC finger through amplified data (±3V) using interface device for functioning as artificial muscle finger

Experimentally, it is demonstrated that IPMC based artificial muscle finger is capable of adopting this voltage from EMG signal and mimics as a human finger. From application point of view, an IPMC artificial finger based micro gripper is developed and its capability is also verified. Through this demonstration, it is proved that IPMC can be activated through EMG signal and is applicable as flexible and compliant finger for holding the object in the fields of micro manipulation. IPMC based artificial muscle could also be a replacement of an electro-mechanical system like electric motors in the application field of rehabilitation technology.

7. Future direction

In future, we will focus on developing well equipped EMG driven micro robotic system where IPMC based micro robotic arm along with multiple IPMC artificial fingers will be used. IPMC based micro robotic arm will be operated through human fore arm movement for lifting and manipulation. Multiple IPMC fingers will be used for robust application like grasping, holding and mimicking of a human hand. Therefore, this new generation of robotic system can be really operated in real world through humans using EMG signals.

Author details

R.K. Jain*, S. Datta and S. Majumder
Design of Mechanical System Group/Micro Robotics Laboratory,
CSIR-Central Mechanical Engineering Research Institute (CMERI),
Durgapur, West Bengal, India

Acknowledgement

The authors are grateful to the Director, Central Mechanical Engineering Research Institute (CMERI), Durgapur, West Bengal, India for providing the permission to publish this book chapter. This work is financially supported by the Council of Scientific and Industrial Research (CSIR), New Delhi, India under eleventh five year plan on "Modular Re-configurable Micro Manufacturing System (NWP-30)".

8. References

Ahmad I., Ansari F. & Dey U. K. (2012). A review of EMG recording technique, *International Journal of Engineering Science and Technology*, Vol. 4, No. 2, pp. 530-539.

Andreasen D. S., Allen S. K. & Backus D. A. (2005). Exoskeleton with EMG based active assistance for rehabilitation, *Proceedings of the 2005 IEEE 9th International Conference on Rehabilitation Robotics,* Chicago, IL, USA, June 28 - July 1, pp. 333-336.

Andrews J. (2008). Finger movement classification using forearm EMG signals, *MS Thesis,* Queen's University, Kingston Ontario, Canada.

Aravinthan P., GopalaKrishnan N., Srinivas P. A. & Vigneswaran N. (2010). Design, development and implementation of neurologically controlled prosthetic limb capable of performing rotational movement, *IEEE International Conference RFID 2010,* Orlando, USA, 14-16April, pp. 241-244.

Arieta H., Katoh R., Yokoi H. & Wenwei Y. (2006). Development of a multi-DOF electromyography prosthetic system using the adaptive joint mechanism, *ABBI 2006,* Vol. 3, No. 2, pp. 1-10.

* Corresponding Author

Artemiadis P. K. & Kyriakopoulos K. J. (2010). EMG-based control of a robot arm using low-dimensional embeddings, *IEEE Transactions on Robotics*, Vol. 26, No. 2, pp. 393-398.

Artemiadis P. K. & Kyriakopoulos K. J. (2011). A switching regime model for the EMG-based control of a robot arm, *IEEE Transactions on Systems, Man and Cybernetics—Part B: Cybernetics*, Vol. 41, No. 1, pp. 53-63.

Banks J. L. (2001). Design and control of an anthropomorphic robotic finger with multi-point tactile sensation, *MS Thesis*, Artificial Intelligence Laboratory Massachusetts Institute of Technology.

Bar-Cohen Y. (2002). Electro-active polymers: current capabilities and challenges, *Proceedings of the SPIE Smart Structures and Materials Symposium EAPAD Conference* San Diego CA, 18-21 March, paper no 4695-02.

Biddiss E. & Chau T. (2006). Electroactive polymeric sensors in hand prostheses: bending response of an ionic polymer metal composite, *J. of Medical Engineering & Physics*, Vol. 28, pp. 568-578.

Bitzer S. & Smagt P. V. (2006). Learning EMG control of a robotic hand: towards active prostheses, *Proceedings of the 2006 IEEE International Conference on Robotics and Automation*, Orlando, Florida.

Blouin J., Guillaud E., Bresciani J. P., Guerraz M. & Simoneau M. (2010). Insights into the control of arm movement during body motion as revealed by EMG analyses, *J. of Brain Research*, Vol. 1309, pp. 40-52. Available: http:// www.sciencedirect.com

Bundhoo V. & Park E. J. (2005). Design of an artificial muscle actuated finger towards biomimetic prosthetic hands, *IEEE 12th International Conference on Advanced Robotics (ICAR)* Seattle WA, 18-20 July, pp. 368-370.

Bundhoo V., Haslam E., Birch B. & Park E. J. (2008). A shape memory alloy-based tendon-driven actuation system for biomimetic artificial fingers part I: design and evaluation, *J. of Robotica*, pp. 1-16.

Cesqui B., Krebs H. I. & Micera S. (2008). On the development of a new EMG–controlled robot-mediated protocol for post-stroke neurorehabilitation, *Proceeding ISG 08*. http://www.gerontechnology.info/Journal/Proceedings/ISG08/papers/130.pdf

Chan A., Kwok E. & Bhuanantanondh P. (2012). Performance assessment of upper limb myoelectric prostheses using a programmable assessment platform, *J. Med. Biol. Eng.*, (In press)

Chen C. C., Hsueh Y. H. & He Z. C. (2008). A Novel EMG Feedback Control Method in Functional Electrical Stimulation Cycling System for Stroke Patients, *World Academy of Science, Engineering and Technology*, Vol. 42, pp. 186-189.

Chen Z., Um T. I. & Smith H. B. (2011). A novel fabrication of ionic polymer–metal composite membrane actuator capable of 3-dimensional kinematic motions, *Sensors and Actuators*, Vol. A 168, pp. 131–139.

Cheron G., Draye J. P., Bourgeiosas M. & Libert G. (1996). A dynamic neural network identification of electromyography and arm trajectory relationship during complex movements, *IEEE Transactions on Biomedical Engineering*, Vol. 43, No. 5, pp. 552-558.

Cocaud C. & Jnifene A. (2003). Analysis of a two DOF anthropomorphic arm driven by artificial muscles, *Proceedings of the IEEE International Workshop on Haptic, Audio and Visual Environments and Their Applications (HAVE 2003),* Ottawa, Ontario, Canada, September 21-22, pp. 37-42.

Crawford B., Miller K., Shenoy P. & Rao R. P. N. (2005). Real-time classification of electromyographic signals for robotic control, *Proceedings of AAAI,* pp. 523-528.

Dalley S. A., Wiste T. E., Withrow T. J. & Goldfarb M. (2009). Design of a multifunctional anthropomorphic prosthetic hand with extrinsic actuation, *IEEE/ASME Transactions on Mechatronics,* pp. 1-8.

DeLaurentis K. J. & Mavroidis C. (2002). Mechanical design of a shape memory alloy actuated prosthetic hand, *Technology and Health Care,* Vol. 10, pp. 91–106.

DoNascimento B. G., Vimieiro C. B. S., Nagem D. A. P. & Pinotti M. (2008). Hip orthosis powered by pneumatic artificial muscle voluntary activation in absence of myoelectrical signal, *Artificial Organs,* Vol. 32, No. 4, pp. 317–322, Blackwell Publishing, Inc. © 2008.

Frigo C., Ferrarin M., Frasson W., Pavan E. & Thorsen R. (2007). EMG signals detection and processing for on-line control of functional electrical stimulation, *J. of Electromyography and Kinesiology,* Vol. 10, pp. 351–360.

Fukuda O., Tsuji T., Kaneko M. & Otsuka A. (2003). A human-assisting manipulator teleoperated by EMG signals and arm motions, *IEEE Transactions on Robotics and Automation,* Vol. 19, No. 2, pp. 210-222.

Gandole Y. B. (2012). Noise reduction of biomedical signal using artificial neural network model, *International Journal of Engineering and Technology,* Vol. 2, No. 1.

Gao Z., Lei J., Song Q., Yu Y. & Ge Y. J. (2006). Research on the surface EMG signal for human body motion recognizing based on arm wrestling robot, *Proceedings of the 2006 IEEE International Conference on Information Acquisition,* Weihai Shandong China, 20-23 August, pp. 1269-1273.

Hao L., Wei F., Lin Y., Zheng P. & Tao W. (2008). Study on a new dexterous hand actuated by pneumatic muscle actuators, *Proceedings of the 7th JFPS International Symposium on Fluid Power* ,Toyama, 15-18 September, pp. 521-526.

Herrera A., Bernal A., Isaza D. & Adjouadi M. (2004). Design of an electrical prosthetic gripper using EMG and linear motion approach, *Florida Conference on Recent Advances in Robotics,* University of Central Florida.

Hidalgo M., Tene G. & Sánchez A. (2005). Fuzzy control of a robotic arm using EMG signals, *International Conference on Industrial Electronics and Control Applications,* pp. 1-6.

Hu X. L., Tong K. Y., Song R., Zheng X. J. & Leung W. F. W. (2009). A comparison between electromyography-driven robot and passive motion device on wrist rehabilitation for chronic stroke, *Neuro rehabilitation and Neural Repair,* Vol. 23, No. 8, pp. 837-846, http://nnr.sagepub.com.

Huang H., Zhang F., Sun Y. L. & H. Haibo (2010). Design of a robust EMG sensing interface for pattern classification, *J. Neural Eng.,* Vol. 7, 056005 (10pp).

Hudgins B., Englehart K., Parker P. & Scott R. N. (1997). A microprocessor-based multifunction myoelectric control system, *CMBE*, Institute of Biomedical Engineering University of New Brunswick Fredericton NB Canada. Available: http://www.ee.unb.ca/kengleha/papers/ CMBES97.

Itoh Y., Uematsu H., Nogata F., Nemoto T., Inamori A., Koide K. & Matsuura H. (2007). Finger curvature movement recognition interface technique using SEMG signals, J. *of Achievements in Materials and Manufacturing Engineering (JAMME)*, Vol. 23, No. 2, pp. 43-46.

Jain R. K., Datta S., Majumder S., A Paul & Banerjee P. (2012). Bio-mimetic behavior of IPMC using EMG signal for micro robot, *International Conference on Micro Actuators and Micro Mechanisms MAMM-2012*, CSIR-CMERI India, January 19-20.

Jain R. K., Datta S., Majumder S., Chowdhury S. & Banerjee P. (2011). IPMC artificial muscle finger activated through EMG. *Worldwide EAP newsletter on http://www.EAPnewsletter*. Vol. 13, No 01, June (The 25th issue), pp.10-12.

Jain R. K., Datta S., Majumder S., Mukherjee S., Sadhu D., Samanta S. & Benerjee K. (2010b). Bio-mimetic behaviour of IPMC artificial muscles using EMG signal, *ACEEE International Conference in Recent Technologies in Communication and Computing*, Kottyam India, 16-17 October, pp. 186-189.

Jain R. K., Dutta S. & Majumdar S. (2010a). Control of IPMC-based artificial muscle using EMG signal for hand prosthesis, *Worldwide EAP newsletter on http://www.EAPnewsletter*, Vol. 12, No 01, June (The 23th issue), pp.11-13.

Joshi S. S., Wexler A. S., Maldonado C. P. & Vernon S. (2011). Brain-muscle-computer interface using a single surface electromyographic signal: initial results, *Proceedings of the 5th International IEEE EMBS Conference on Neural Engineering*, Cancun, Mexico, 27April – 1 May, pp. 342-347.

Khokhar Z. O., Xiao Z. G. & Menon C. (2010). Surface EMG pattern recognition for real-time control of a wrist exoskeleton, *J. of Bio. Med. Eng.*, Vol. 9, No. 41, pp. 1-17.

Kim K. J. & Shahinpoor M. (2002). A novel method of manufacturing three dimensional ionic polymer metal composites (IPMCs) bio mimetic sensors actuators and artificial muscles, *Polymer*, Vol. 43, pp. 797-802.

Kottke E. A., Partridge L. D. & Shahinpoor M. (2007). Bio-potential activation of artificial muscles, *J. of Intelligent Material Systems and Structures*, Vol. 18, No. 2, pp. 103-109.

Krysztoforski K., Wolczowski A., Bedzinski R. & Helt K. (2004). Recognition of palm finger movements on the basis of EMG signals with the application of wavelets, *Task Quarterly*, Vol. 8, No. 2, pp. 269-280.

Lau B. G. (2009). An intelligent prosthetic hand using hybrid actuation and myoelectric control, *Ph D Thesis*, The School of Mechanical Engineering, University of Leeds.

Lee M. J., Jung S. H., Kim G. S., Moon I., Lee S. & Mun M. S. (2007). Actuation of the artificial muscle based on ionic polymer metal composite by electromyography (EMG) signals, *J. of Intelligent Material Systems and Structures*, Vol. 18, pp. 165-170. doi: 10.1177/1045389X06063463.

Lee M. J., Jung S. H., Lee S., Mun M. S. & Moon I. (2006). Control of IPMC-based artificial muscle for myoelectric hand prosthesis, *The First IEEE/RAS-EMBS International Conference on Biomedical Robotics and Biomechatronics BioRob 2006,* 20-22 February, pp. 1172-1177.

Lee S., Noh S., Lee Y. & Park J. H. (2009). Development of bio-mimetic robot hand using parallel mechanisms, *Proceedings of the 2009 IEEE International Conference on Robotics and Biomimetics,* Guilin China, 19 -23 December, pp. 550-555.

Li L., Looney D., Park C., Rehman N. U., & Mandic D. P. (2011). Power independent EMG based gesture recognition for robotics, *IEEE Engineering in Medicine and Biology Magazine,* pp. 793-796.

Light C. M., Chappell P. H., Hudgins B. & Englehart K. (2002). Intelligent multifunction myoelectric control of hand prostheses, *J. of Medical Engineering & Technology,* Vol. 26, No. 4, July/August, pp. 139-146.

Luo R. C. & Chang C. C. (2010). Electromyographic signal integrated robot hand control for massage therapy applications, *IEEE/RSJ International Conference on Intelligent Robots and Systems,* Taipei, Taiwan, October 18-22, pp. 3881-3886.

Matsubara T., Hyon S. H. & Morimoto J. (2011). Learning and adaptation of a stylistic myoelectric interface: EMG-based robotic control with individual user differences, *IEEE International Conference on Robotics and Biomimetics* (ROBIO), Phauket Island, Thailand, 7-11 December, pp. 390-395.

Mobasser F. & Hashtrudi-Zaad K. (2005). Rowing stroke force estimation with EMG signals using artificial neural networks, *IEEE International Conference on Control Application (CCA-2005),* 28-31 August, pp. 825-830.

Murphy C., Campbell N., Caulfield B., Ward T. & Deegan C. (2008). Micro electro mechanical systems based sensor for mechanomyography, *19th International Conference on Bio-Signal,* Brno, Czech Republic.

Naik G. R., Kumar D. K. & Arjunan S. P. (2010). Pattern classification of myo-electrical signal during different maximum voluntary contractions: a study using BSS techniques, *Measurement Science Review,* Vol. 10, No. 1, pp. 1-6.

O'Toole K. T. & McGrath M. M. (2007). Mechanical design and theoretical analysis of a four fingered prosthetic hand incorporating embedded SMA bundle actuators, *World Academy of Science Engineering and Technology,* Vol. 31, pp. 142-149.

Peleg D., Braiman E., Yom-Tov E. & Inbar G. F. (2002). Classification of finger activation for use in a robotic prosthesis arm, IEEE *Transactions on Neural Systems and Rehabilitation Engineering,* Vol. 10, No. 4, pp. 290-293.

Pfeiffer C., DeLaurentis K. & Mavroidis C. (1999). Shape memory alloy actuated robot prostheses: initial Experiments, *Proceedings of IEEE International Conference on Robotics and Automation,* Vol. 3, pp. 2385-2391.

Pittaccio S. & Viscuso S. (2011). An EMG-controlled SMA device for the rehabilitation of the ankle joint in post-acute stroke, *Journal of Materials Engineering and Performance,* Vol. 20, No.4–5, pp. 666-670.

Qi L., Wakeling J., Grange S. & Ferguson-Pell M. (2012). Changes in surface electromyography signals and kinetics associated with progression of fatigue at two speeds during wheelchair propulsion, *JRRD*, Vol. 49, No. 1, pp. 23–34.

Rosen J., Brand M., Fuchs M. B. & Arcan M. (2001). A myosignal-based powered exoskeleton system, *IEEE Transaction on Systems, Man and Cybernetics—Part A: Systems and Humans*, Vol. 31, No. 3, pp. 210-222.

Roy S. H., Luca G. D., Cheng M. S., Johansson A., Gilmore L. D. & Luca C. J. D. (2007). Electro-mechanical stability of surface EMG sensors, *J. of Med. Bio. Eng. Comput.*, Vol. 45, pp. 447-457

Saponas T. S., Tan D. S., Morris D. & Balakrishnan R. (2008). Demonstrating the feasibility of using forearm electromyography for muscle-computer Interfaces, *CHI 2008*, Florence Italy, 5-10 April.

Shahinpoor M. & Kim K. J. (2001). Ionic polymer–metal composites: I. Fundamental, *Smart Materials Structure*, Vol. 10, pp. 819–833.

Shahinpoor M. & Kim K. J. (2004). Ionic polymer–metal composites: III. Modeling and simulation as biomimetic sensors actuator transducer and artificial muscles, *Smart Materials Structure*, Vol. 13, pp. 1362-1388.

Shenoy P., Miller K. J., Crawford B. & Rao R. P. N. (2008). Online electromyographic control of a robotic prosthesis, *IEEE Transactions on Biomedical Engineering*, Vol. 55, No. 3, pp. 1128-1135.

Stirling L., Yu C. H., Miller J., Hawkes E., Wood R., Goldfield E. & Nagpal R. (2011). Applicability of shape memory alloy wire for an active soft orthotic, *Journal of Materials Engineering and Performance*, Vol. 20, Issue 4-5, pp. 658-662.

Sun Y. P., Yen K. T., Kung H. K., Tsai Y. C., Lu K. C., Du C. M. & Liang Y. C. (2012). The muscular function for human knee movement revealed from electromyography: a preliminary study, *Life Science Journal*, Vol. 9, No. 1, pp. 453-456.

Thayer N. & Priya S. (2011). Design and implementation of a dexterous anthropomorphic robotic typing (DART) hand, *Smart Mater. Struct.*, Vol. 20, pp. 035010 (12pp).

Vogel J., Castellini C., & Smagt P. V. (2011). EMG-based teleoperation and manipulation with the DLR LWR-III, *IEEE/RSJ International Conference on Intelligent Robots and Systems*, San Francisco, CA, USA, September 25-30, pp. 672-678.

Wege A. & Zimmermann A. (2007). Electromyography (EMG) sensor based control for a hand exoskeleton, *Proceedings of the 2007 IEEE International Conference on Robotics and Bio-mimetics*, Sanya China, 15 -18 December, pp. 1470-1475.

Wheeler K. R. (2003). Device control using gestures sensed from EMG, *IEEE International Workshop on Soft Computing in Industrial Applications*, Binghamton University, Binghamton, New York, June 23-25, 2003.

Yagiz N., Arslan Y. Z. & Hacioglu Y. (2007). Sliding mode control of a finger for a prosthetic hand, *J. of Vibration and Control*, Vol. 13, No. 6, pp. 733–749, doi: 10.1177/1077546307072352.

Zollo L., Roccella S., Guglielmelli E., Carrozza M. C. & Dario P. (2007). Biomechatronic design and control of an anthropomorphic artificial hand for prosthetic and robotic applications, *IEEE/ASME Transactions on Mechatronics*, Vol. 12, No. 4, pp. 418-429.

Chapter 16

Application of Surface Electromyography in the Dynamics of Human Movement

César Ferreira Amorim and Runer Augusto Marson

Additional information is available at the end of the chapter

http://dx.doi.org/10.5772/52463

1. Introduction

Surface electromyography (sEMG) is a generic term for a method of recording electrical muscle activity. Numerous applications for this method have been developed in clinical practice, such as diagnosing neuromuscular diseases, analyzing and determining abnormalities or disorders and muscular rehabilitation (biofeedback) [3, 12, 27, 28].

sEMG is mainly used in the fields of physiotherapy, dentistry, physical education and biomechanics [12].

The duration of sEMG activity corresponds to the duration of muscle activation. The amplitude is the level of signal activity and varies with the amount of electrical activity detected in the muscle; it provides information about intensity of muscle activation. The observed sEMG frequency is due to a wide range of factors: muscle composition, characteristics of the action potential of the active muscles fibers, the intramuscular coordination process and electrode properties [22, 23, 28].

sEMG signals are also affected by the anatomical and physiological properties of the muscles, neuromuscular control of the peripheral nervous system and the instrumentation used to collect the signal.

The electronic EMG device amplifies, isolates and filters the electrical signal of muscles that occurs during muscle contraction. This signal must undergo conditioning to be captured [12].

A differential amplifier is, ideally, insensitive to noise and amplifies only the EMG signal, although in practice this is not the case. This situation occurs, first of all, because the noise that reaches the electrodes (inputs) doesn't necessarily have the same magnitude. Moreover, due to technological limitations, differential amplifiers cannot perfectly separate two-signal input.

The measurement that indicates the success of this separation is the common mode rejection ratio (CMRR), which is usually expressed in decibels (dB). The CMRR value of the differential amplifiers used in sEMG is on the order of 80 to 100 dB [3, 22, 24].

The sEMG equipment should be calibrated before recording signals. Calibration is important for fidelity, accuracy and reliability when reading the signal. The amplification factor is critical during the calibration process, since it is the ratio between the input voltage and that which comes out of the amplifier. The gain is selected according to the requirements of the type of experiment, the studied muscles, the type of electrodes involved and the planned use of the amplified signal. Whereas an sEMG signal has a maximum voluntary contraction amplitude not exceeding 5 millivolts (mV) peak-to-peak, the gain should be adjusted to 500-1000x [2,3,5].

During the mathematical processing of the sEMG signal, filters can be used to remove components that don't belong to the signal or components that are irrelevant for a given analysis.

The useful information in the sEMG signal is located in a particular frequency band (20-500 Hz), and is reduced by a filtering effect from the tissue located between the muscle fibers and the active sensing surface. The filter band corresponds to the frequency between the low- and high-cut filter frequencies [28].

Time-based signal processing can be carried out using a set of processing procedures intended to characterize the signal's curve and measure signal strength during the contraction. Signal processing applications in the time domain are widely used in areas such as neuromuscular coordination, motor control, the relationship between EMG and strength and muscular coordination in the dynamics of human movement.

This chapter will report, therefore, on the importance of sEMG with respect the dynamics of human movement [27].

2. Electromyography

The hypothesis that muscles generate electricity was by Francesco Redi in 1666 due to the suspicion that the discharges of electric fish were of muscular origin.

Along with other scientific developments during the Renaissance, interest in the muscles also began to increase. Leonardo da Vinci (1452 - 1519), for example, devoted careful attention to muscles and their anatomical function by conducting dissections of cadavers [12]

The main objectives of the first scientific experiments on muscles were to understand their structure and function [12]. A number of scientists since studied muscle dynamics. Luigi Galvani presented the first study on the electrical properties of muscles and nerves in 1791. He termed this neuromuscular potential "Animal Electricity". This discovery was recognized as the starting point for neurophysiology. Thereafter, a growing number of studies have been developed in this field [11]. sEMG is a technique for recording and monitoring the electrical signals from muscle contractions. A major methodological problem for EMG is the frequent presence of artifacts or noise. Artifacts or noise are defined as information whose origin is distinct from the neuroelectrical muscle activity signal. Some examples of this include interference, heart rate, poor contact between the electrode and the skin, etc.[12].

The presence of artifacts is difficult to avoid with this type of signal acquisition, since in order to amplify the signal, which is received in microvolts (μV), unwanted signals are also amplified and can compromise interpretation of the EMG signal. Thus, the signal-to-noise ratio has been a problem, and numerous studies have been undertaken to resolve EMG signal interpretation problems. After several attempts, a solution was found in the development of the differential amplifier [3] (ACIERNO, BARATTA & SOLOMONOW, 1995).

The signal amplifier is an electronic device that filters, amplifies and records bands of signals.

The initial problem with the amplifiers was that signal acquisition was dependent on the electrical resistance of the skin. Thus, in many studies skin resistance and temperature were initially monitored when the test was performed, conditions that made it difficult or impossible to reproduce and some EMG experiments [1].

Over time, corrections have been made to this system so that the amplifiers currently have high input impedance and attenuate noise levels, which allows the reproduction of experiments without interference with the results.

A main feature of this new generation of amplifiers is that they can amplify a particular type of biological signal independent of skin resistance [28]. The evolution of cables and connectors must also be considered in the development process of EMG acquisition equipment, since the type of conductive material and insulation system help minimize noise.

The main purpose of these developments is to help investigate and analyze human movement. The field of biomechanics is a practical example of the use of technological resources to interpret human movement [28].

Biomechanics can be defined generally as the study of the mechanics of living beings, or more specifically, the science that examines forces acting upon and within a structure and the biological effects produced by these forces [17]. Given the complex approach involved in biomechanics and human movement analysis [17], it is important to discuss the concepts, criteria and methods involved, focusing on the use of EMG for reliable interpretations.

EMG can be defined as the study of muscle function by analyzing the electrical signal generated during muscle contraction. Studying muscle function by means of EMG can be carried out under both normal and pathological conditions [12]. EMG has been used in important studies on muscle activity that have both qualitatively and quantitatively addressed the function of human movement. New information about muscle activity has been discovered as developments in processing and instrumentation have been applied to EMG [3,12, 15, 28] .

However, the purpose of this study is to present and discuss the use of sEMG as a quantification tool for studying motor and functional rehabilitation and neurophysiological abnormalities in the nervous system in comparison with peripheral stimuli.

Many authors have used different procedures to analyze EMG signals, which impedes both the comparison and reproducibility of results obtained in laboratory experiments, although their experiments have been described in internationally recognized scientific journals.

Thus, although there is diversity in the procedures for both applying EMG and analyzing the signals, this technique for investigating myoelectrical activity can be used in many different areas of study for different research purposes.

It is important, therefore, to demonstrate some of the applications of EMG as a research tool as well as different methods of analyzing EMG signals to facilitate the design of future and to foster appropriate analysis methods for signal data.

3. Kinesiological electromyography

The numerous applications of EMG include the diagnosis of neuromuscular disease or trauma in clinical practice, rehabilitation and the study of kinesiological muscle function in specific activities [2].

In one study [13] the EMG behavior of some of the major muscles of mastication was compared while subjects chewed different materials (two brands of chewing gum, cotton and parafilm) in order to identify the best material based on performance during bilateral chewing.

The EMG signal serves as an indicator of the initiation of muscle activity and can provide the firing sequence of one or more muscles involved in a specific task [12]. Information from the EMG signal is used to indicate the strength contributed by individual muscles and muscle groups.

In EMG, potentials are produced as a direct result of voluntary effort [18].

The electrodes used in EMG convert the electrical signal resulting from muscle depolarization into an electrical potential that can be amplified, and the difference in electrical potential can be processed. The potential amplitude depends on the difference in potential between the electrodes, such that the greater the potential difference, the greater the amplitude of the electrical potential or voltage [24].

The instrumentation used during the collection of EMG signals includes electrodes, amplifiers, filters, registers, decoders and sound equipment [27]. The choice of the electrode will depend on the muscle being studied.

The factors that influence the EMG signal can be divided into three categories: causes, determinants and intermediate factors [14].

Causative factors have an effect on the basic or elementary signal and are divided into extrinsic and intrinsic factors. Among the extrinsic factors are electrode configuration, the distance between the electrodes, the location of the electrodes over the motor point and the myotendonous junction, the location of the electrodes in relationship to the lateral border of the muscle and the orientation of the electrode in relation to muscle fibers. Intrinsic factors are the physiological, anatomical and biochemical characteristics of the muscle, such as the number of active motor units at the time a particular contraction occurs, the muscle fiber type, blood flow in the muscle, the fiber diameter, depth and location of the active fibers of the muscles in relation to the detection electrodes, the amount of tissue between the electrode and the muscle surface, as well as other factors such as the length of the depolarization zone and the ion flux across the membrane.

The intermediate factors are the physical and physiological phenomena that are influenced by one or more causative factors and, in turn, influence the determinants. Among this type are the detection electrode volume, the overlap of the action potential in the EMG signal, "cross-talk" with neighboring muscles, the conduction velocity of the action potential and the effect of spatial filtering. Since the determinant factors have a direct effect on the EMG signal and include the number of active motor units, the mechanical interaction between muscle fibers, the firing rate and the number of motor units detected, the amplitude, duration and shape of action potentials of motor units, as well as the recruitment and the stability of these units.

Soderberg and Cook described the limitations, collection methods and interpretation of electrical activity. Regarding the type of electrode, they believe that the sEMG can be used to analyze superficial muscles without causing discomfort to the volunteer [25].

The normalization procedure is usually considered necessary for recording, quantifying and comparing the EMG data obtained from different individuals or the same individual on different days [27].

Concern about the establishment of common standards for the collection, recording, analysis and interpretation of EMG signals has been expressed by a number of authors [12,27,28,], and more recently a practical guide for standardizing procedures to be used in EMG studies has been presented [1]. Thus, there is a tendency toward consensus among researchers on the use of appropriate instrumentation for collecting, recording and processing EMG signals.

Several studies [3, 5, 16, 27] have described the need to normalize the EMG signal amplitude when trying to make comparisons between different muscles, subjects, materials and days. This is due to the great variability observed in EMG tracings obtained from both different individuals and different muscles.

The EMG signal can be rectified by mathematical processing or by the root mean square (RMS) of squared instantaneous values . This signal can be passed through a low-pass filter for a presentation wrap the curve. Signal processing can then be carried out in accordance with the specific aim of the work [2]. In general, it is necessary to normalize the EMG signal in order to minimize the differences between individuals [15], when not comparing pre-and post-treatment.

4. Type and placement of electrodes

The electrodes available for kinesiological EMG are the passive and active surface type and the intramuscular type, each with its distinct characteristics, recommendations for use, advantages and disadvantages. The choice of electrode for capturing the EMG signal depends on the characteristics of the evaluated muscles. Thus, when analyzing certain muscles, size and location should be considered in the selection and application of electrodes [27].

The placement of surface electrodes is also another factor that influences the reliability of EMG recordings. The size, orientation and topography of electrodes influence EMG recordings [25].

Since the amplitude of the electrical potential is derived from the difference in potential observed between the electrodes, the inter-electrode distance should be controlled. Due to changes in distance, the same levels of contraction can result in different EMG signal amplitudes [24]. A major concern in sEMG is signal interference (cross-talk) from muscles surrounding the electrode. In one study [12], the surface electrodes were positioned on the midline of the muscle venter between the motor and the myotendonous junction with the detection surface towards the oriented fibers. However, this study was limited in that the electrodes were positioned between the motor and the myotendonous junction without electrically stimulating the motor points.

The surface area and shape of the electrode's contact surface as well as its location affect the signal amplitude, and the distance between the contact surfaces of the electrode affects the signal frequency. Figure 1 shows the characteristics of the EMG signal relative to the electrode position over the fibers. The most suitable location for electrode placement is in the direction of muscle fibers (Figure 2) and near the point of greatest electrical activity.

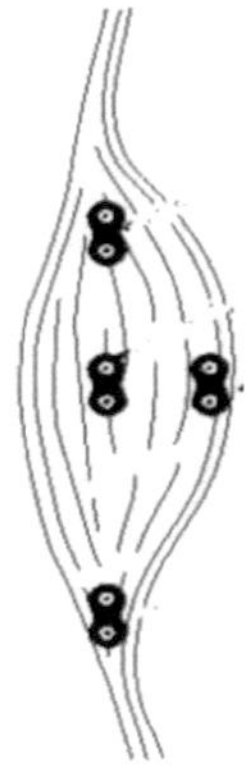

Figure 1. Representative signal results from different points in the muscle [3].

The electrodes must be carefully placed with regard to the adjacent muscles, since if the electrodes are too close to the other muscles then cross-talk may occur. Another important factor is the placement of the ground or reference electrode, which must have a good contact area.

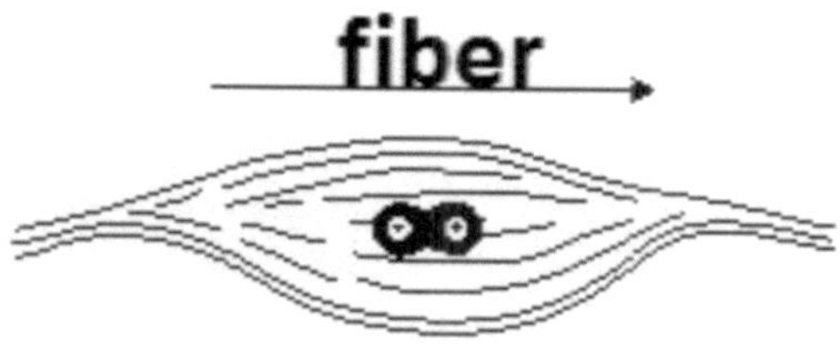

Figure 2. Diagram representing the placement of surface electrodes the direction of muscle fibers [3].

4.1. Considerations on the acquisition of EMG signals

EMG is a generic term for a method of recording the electrical activity of a muscle contraction. The numerous applications of electromyography (EMG) include diagnosing neuromuscular disease and determining the presence of dysfunctions or abnormalities in clinical practice, the rehabilitation of muscle action via EMG biofeedback, demonstrating kinesiology in anatomical studies, use in ergonomics as a tool for studying kinesiological muscle function related to posture and other biomechanical stress indicators, as well as a movement pattern identifier and a nervous system control parameter of the nervous system [28].

When interpreting the EMG signal for quantitative analysis, three fundamental characteristics can be distinguished: duration, amplitude and frequency, each of which is briefly described below [12].

The duration of EMG activity corresponds to the activation time of the selected muscle. The amplitude expresses the level of signal activity and varies with the amount of electrical activity detected in the muscle. It provides information on the intensity of muscle activation. RMS, average value, peak value and peak-to-peak value are ways of evaluating the amplitude of the signal. The frequency can be understood as the rate of excitation of the muscle cell. The frequency distribution of the EMG signal is due to a wide range of factors: muscle composition, the characteristics of the action potential of the active muscle fibers, the intramuscular coordination processes, the properties of the electrodes and their placement.

It can be said that signal processing begins, indirectly, as soon as the electrodes are placed. Electrode placement involves several factors that are decisive for the level and purity of the EMG signal to be collected, including: cleaning the skin, the amount and temperature of the conductive gel, the position of the electrodes and the signal-to-noise ratio, which expresses the balance between the energy of the signal generated during muscle contraction and the energy of noise from various undesirable sources [27].

The EMG signals are affected by anatomical and physiological muscle properties, peripheral nervous system control and the instrumentation used to collect the signal. Thus it is important to understand the basic muscle functions to correctly record EMG signals [12].

5. Biological amplifiers

In signal acquisition, analyzable information is obtained by studying the physical quantities involved in the activation process. These physical quantities can be measured by sensors that convert them into electrical signals and then record them using a data acquisition system (Figure 3). Computers make data acquisition more efficient and reliable and have the advantage of combining data storage with analysis and processing capability [21].

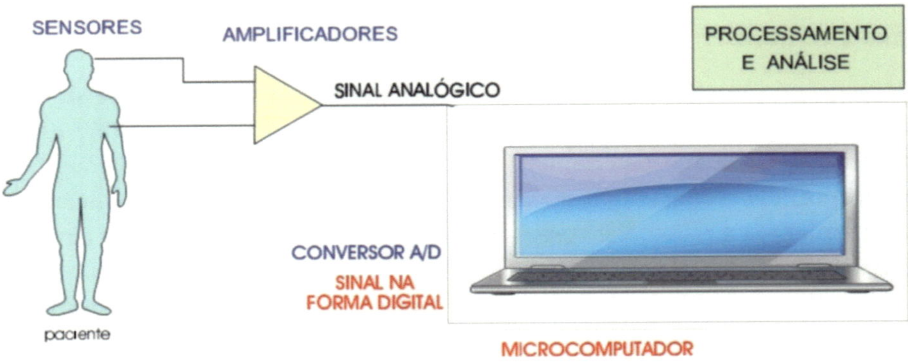

Figure 3. Diagram of a biological signal acquisition system [3].

Sensors and transducers are devices that convert physical quantities into electrical signals or current. Signal conditioners are electronic devices that modify the input signal in some way, whether by amplification, attenuation, filtering or isolation. The EMG signal, for example, enters at an amplitude of μV and must be amplified and filtered [3].

There are basically two techniques capturing an EMG signal: either monopolar or bipolar electrodes. In the monopolar configuration, only one electrode is placed on the skin over the muscle in question (Figure 4). This electrode detects the electrical potential relative to a reference electrode, which is placed in a location unaffected by the electrical activity generated by the analyzed muscle. In the bipolar configuration, two electrodes are used on the muscle as well as a reference (or ground) electrode placed in a neutral location (Figure 5). The human body is actually a good antenna for electromagnetic energy [3].

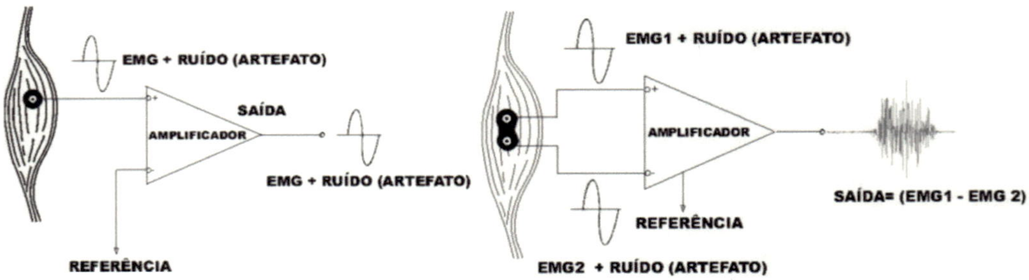

Figure 4. A) Schematic representation of a unipolar amplifier. B) Schematic representation of a bipolar amplifier [3].

6. Signal amplification

Gain is defined as the ratio between the voltage that enters and exits the amplifier. Gain should be selected to suit the characteristics of the experiment, the studied muscle, the electrode type and the use planned for the amplified signal. Considering that a sEMG signal has a maximum voluntary contraction amplitude not exceeding 5 mV peak-to-peak (Figure 6), the gain can be adjusted between 10 and 1000x. It is important to choose a gain that does not exceed at any stage the voltage expected from the system, or there will be a risk of either losing part of information or damaging the system itself [1].

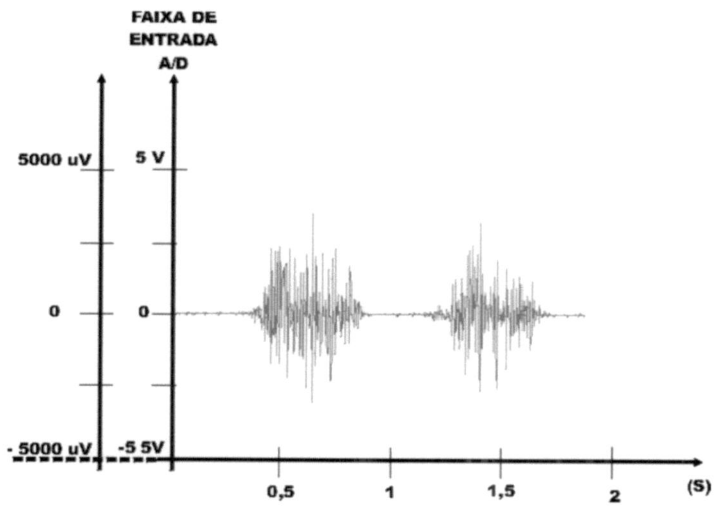

Figure 5. Appropriate gain range [3].

7. Signal filtering

Filters can be used to remove frequency components that do not belong to the signal or components that are irrelevant for a given analysis.

The captured signal can be filtered by hardware or software. Signal-filtering hardware can be used in the amplification step, while signal filtering by means of software can be performed during processing.

When using surface electrodes to measure EMG signals, interference from various sources can be mixed with the EMG signal. Each type of interference has its own characteristics that must be understood in order to remove it during the measurement phase or during processing. The useful information in the sEMG signal, which is a sum of the waves of varying frequency, is located between 20 and 500 Hz [12]. The signal is reduced due to the filtering effect of tissue located between the muscle fibers and the active sensing surface. The band pass filter corresponds to the frequency between the low frequency (high pass) and high frequency (low pass) cut-offs. Specific frequencies can also be filtered out with what are called "notch filters" [5, 11, 3, 23].

8. Analog-digital converter

An analog-digital (A/D) converter converts analog signals (EMG goniometry, force transducer) into digital data. The digitized signal can then be processed by the computer.

8.1. Input range and resolution of the A/D converter

The input range is a parameter associated with resolution and indicates the range of voltage that the A/D converter board can represent numerically. This band can be ± 5 V, ± 2.5 V, 0 to 5V, ± 10V etc.

When the input signals do not fall within the A/D card's range, it is necessary to condition them (amplify or attenuate) before inputting them into the A/D converter. Figure 6 shows an example in which the A/D converter or the conditioning gain is misaligned with the signal. Figure 7 depicts a gain adequate for visualizing the EMG signal.

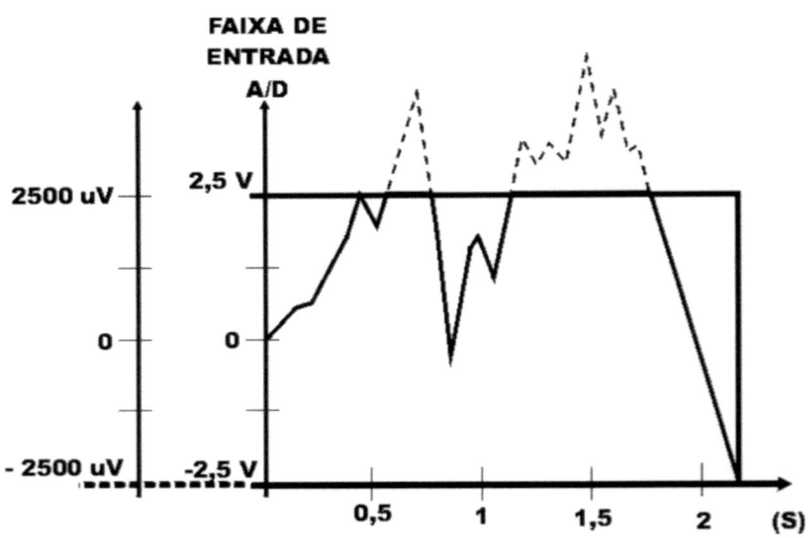

Figure 6. A/D converter range at odds with the amplification gain [3].

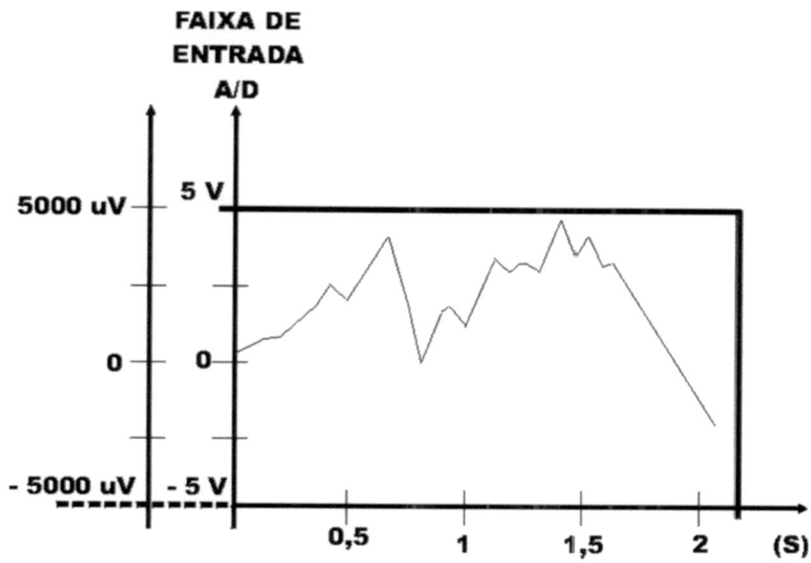

Figure 7. Properly aligned A/D converter range and amplification gain [3].

The resolution of an A/D converter indicates the lowest variation in analog signal that the converter can detect, which is generally presented in bits. Thus, converter resolutions can be 10, 12, 14 or 16 bits, etc., with the most common being 12- and 16-bit.

A converter with a 5V input range and a resolution of ± 12 bits can represent the input signal in 4096 (212) divisions and levels or detect changes of 2.4 mV (10 V divided by 4096 levels). A 16-bit converter may represent the same signal in 65536 (216) divisions and detect changes at levels of 153 μV. (10 V divided by 65,536 levels), [4].

8.2. Sampling rate

In practice, the input signal to the A/D converter varies over time; the goal is to record this variation. Since a computer's storage capacity is finite, the recording can only continue for a limited time.

The discretization of time is carried out by sampling the signal at regular intervals. The reverse of this interval is the sampling rate. For example, at a sampling rate of 100 samples per second (i.e., 100 Hz), the interval between samples is 10 ms. The sampling rate is equivalent to the resolution of the A/D conversion but applied to time.

However, due to the limited space available for data storage, there is a compromise between the sampling rate and the duration of acquisition. For example, for sampling rate of 100 samples per second, the maximum acquisition will be 166 minutes and 40 seconds. By increasing the rate to 1000 samples per second, the maximum is 16 minutes and 40 seconds.

The sampling rate must also be very low compared to the frequency of signal variation due to the effects of sub-sampling (aliasing).

An aliasing effect occurs whenever the sampling frequency is less than twice the highest frequency component of signal frequency, according to the Nyquist theorem [12].

EMG recording is usually done at a maximum frequency of 500 Hz, and the sample should be at least 1000 Hz. To analyze muscle activity in the most comprehensive way possible, it is advisable to work with a sampling rate on the order of 2000 Hz, with the highest frequency component of the signal always limited by the low-pass filter [4, 12, 28].

8.3. Calibration

The measured physical magnitude is converted to voltage using a sensor or transducer, which is then applied to the A/D converter. Knowing the input range and resolution of the A/D converter, one can calculate the voltage of the converter input value from the digitized value, as shown in Figure 8.

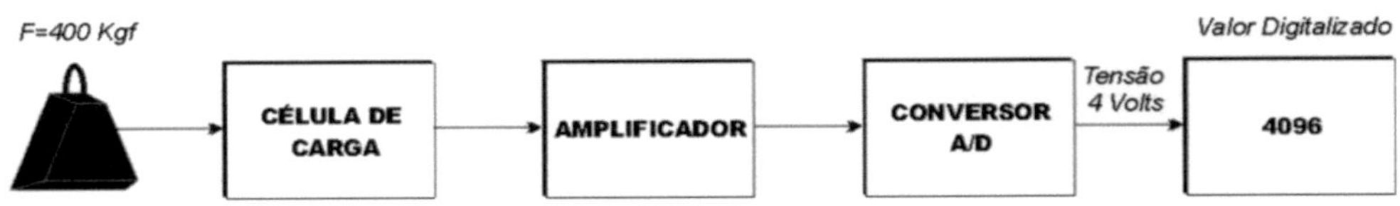
F=400 Kgf
CÉLULA DE CARGA
AMPLIFICADOR
CONVERSOR A/D
Tensão 4 Volts
Valor Digitalizado
4096

Figure 8. Relationship of physical quantity to a digital signal [3].

9. Mathematical processing

Two types of processing are usually used in research: time domain processing, used when one is interested in the temporal analysis of EMG amplitude, and frequency domain processing [1, 26, 28].

9.1. Processing in the time domain

In order to process EMG signals in the time domain, there is a set of processing procedures for characterizing the curve and measuring the signal strength during muscle contraction. Having several kinesiological applications, EMG time domain analysis is often used in areas such as neuromuscular coordination, motor control, the relationship between EMG and muscle force or human movement [25].

9.1.1. Removing the slow-drift (or DC) component present in the signal

Sometimes the signal involves a DC component that causes displacement of the baseline signal. This component is a common signal that has no relation with myoelectric activity. It can be the result of electrochemical phenomena between the electrodes and skin or the limitations of the amplifiers. An easy way to remove it is to calculate the average of all sampling points and shift the curve of the EMG result (high-pass filter) [12, 28].

9.1.2. Signal rectification

Correcting the curve is an operation normally used to enable the subsequent integration of the signal, since it transforms a curve containing both positive and negative values (Figure 10) and a zero mean to a curve of only positive absolute values (Figure 11).

There are two ways to rectify the curve: eliminating the negative values (half-wave rectification), or reversing the negative values and adding them to the positive values (full wave rectification). Full-wave rectification has the advantage of maintaining all of the information contained in the signal, unlike half-wave rectification [5, 28].

9.1.3. Root-mean-square value of the signal

The RMS is the amount of continuous signal able to contain the same amount of energy. It is mathematically defined as the square root of the mean of the squares of the instantaneous values of the signal [4, 12, 22, 23].

9.1.4. Normalization of the signal in the time domain

One problem when comparing different EMG signals has to do with differences in the duration of the various signals to be compared.

Normalizing means transforming, without changing the signal's structure, the duration differences into signals with the same number of samples. This can be done, for example, by taking the signal containing the lowest number of samples as a reference. An algorithm can be applied that determines, depending on the duration of each signal, the number of samples to be removed at certain intervals, reducing all signals to the same number of samples contained in the shorter of the two signals, and thus retaining the original forms [16].

9.1.5. Amplitude normalization

The EMG signal varies greatly upon comparison with recordings from the same individual or different individuals. The absolute value of the EMG signal thus provides little information, especially when dealing with signals from different individuals or the same individual at different times. One way to compensate for this limitation is to normaliz EMG amplitude curves. This technique consists of transforming the absolute amplitude values of the different curves to be compared into values relative to a reference EMG taken as 100% [4, 7, 15].

9.1.6. Integral of the EMG signal

The mathematical interpretation of the integral concept consists of determining the area enclosed by curve, whether an EMG or any other signal. In the case of the EMG, so that the result of integration is not zero, a rectified signal must be used. By integrating the EMG signal, a result that is proportional to the number of electrical impulses is obtained [3].

9.1.7. Filtering of the rectified signal

The signals collected in real time in the original format are stored in files. After this phase certain mathematical processes are applied. The purpose of this processing is to make correction, i.e., to transform negative signals into positive signals. This is necessary to allow averaging of the analyzed signal, since if such correction is not performed, the average of the signals will be near zero. This is because the negative and positive are symmetrical. In the post-rectification, a 5 Hz low-pass filter can be run in order to have a signal wrap. The lower the value of this filter, the smoother the curve will be [27, 28].

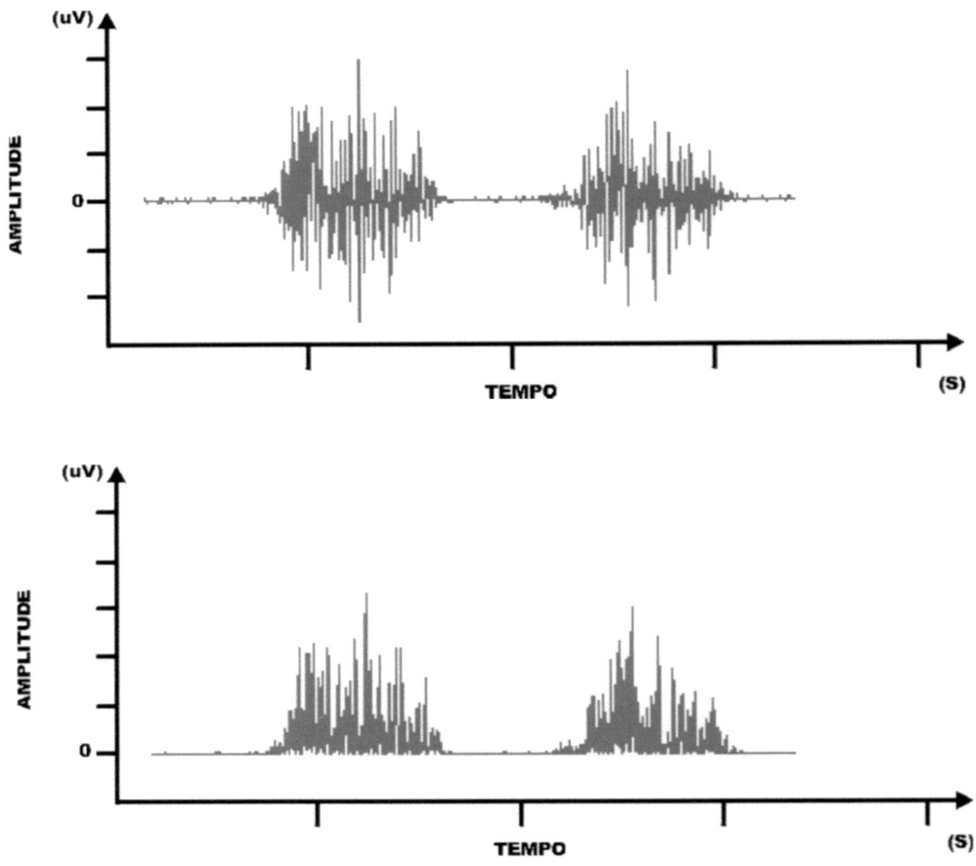

Figure 9. A) original signal interference. B) rectified original signal [3].

9.2. Processing the frequency domain – Spectral analysis

The EMG signal's frequencies are distributed between 1 and 500 Hz, with a great concentration between 20 and 250 Hz in the case of simple muscular activity. The distribution of energy at different frequencies (power spectral density) reflects the predominance of the low or high frequency components in the signal and has been used in kinesiological research. Factors that influence the spectral profile of the EMG signal have been listed by various authors.

EMG can be considered an overlapping of the action potentials of all the active motor units. The spectrum of EMG frequencies thus contains information about the characteristics of different fibers that contribute to the signal. Spectral analysis can provide information about the mean duration of the active fiber potentials, which in turn can be used to determine the mean velocity of muscle fiber conduction [3,4].

10. Conclusion

For dynamic sampling, active electrodes (with preamps) are less susceptible to artifacts or ambient noise, which can be observed when comparing them with signals collected during isometric contractions in volunteers with dysfunctions.

EMG signals are affected by the anatomical and physiological properties of muscles, the peripheral nervous system and the instrumentation used to collect the signal. Thus it is important to understand basic muscle functions to correctly record EMG signals [12].

It can be said that signal processing begins, indirectly, as soon as the electrodes are placed. Electrode placement involves several factors that are decisive for the level and purity of the EMG signal to be collected, including: cleaning the skin, the amount and temperature of the conductive gel, the position of the electrodes and the signal-to-noise ratio, which expresses the balance between the energy of the signal generated during muscle contraction and the energy of noise from various undesirable sources [27].

Therefore, sEMG can be recommended as a tool for analyzing and interpreting electrical signals emanated during muscular contractions in both normal and pathological situations and can be applied in the study of motor function and functional rehabilitation [4].

11. Future directions

Studies in the field of signal processing, especially, surface electromyography signals, have been widely used for understanding the dynamic motions by the fact that most human movements happening dynamically. Thus, processing in the field of time and frequency should be increasingly directed to this specificity.

Understanding the phenomena of depolarization of motor units, future research should be related to the physiological, mechanophysiological and functional human movement.

Applications in the area of functional biomechanics, ergonomics, rehabilitation, sports and physical activity must be analyzed dynamically so that the signal processing, fairly represent the specific characteristics of human movement-environment relationship. Thus, these factors provide parameters for understanding the non-stationary signals, the variation components of the muscle fiber in relation to the positioning of the electrodes and in the bioelectrical conductivity.

Author details

César Ferreira Amorim
University of City of São Paulo- UNICID, São Paulo - SP, Brazil

Runer Augusto Marson
Laboratory of Biomechanics, Brazilian Army Physical Capacitation Research Institute, Rio de Janeiro, Brazil
Laboratory of Biomechanics and Kinesiology, Sport Center, Federal University of Ouro Preto, Minas Gerais, Brazil

12. References

[1] Acierno, S.P. Baratta, R.V., Solomonow, M. A pratical guide to electromyography for biomechanists. Lousiana: State University, 1995.

[2] Amadio, A.C. ; Duarte, M. Fundamentos Biomecânicos para análise do movimento. São Paulo: Editora Laboratório de Biomecânica EEFUSP, 162p. 1996.

[3] Amorim, C.F; Hirata,Tamotsu. Behavior analysis of electromyographic activity of the masseter muscle in sleep bruxers, Journal of Bodywork & Movement Therapies (2009), doi:10.1016/j.jbmt.2008.12.002

[4] Amorim, C.F. Sistema de Aquisição de Sinais Eletromiográficos com Eletrodos Bipolares com Pré-Amplificação. In: 3c Biomédica,18., Setembro de 2002. Anais... São José dos Campos: Univap, 2002.

[5] Andrade, A.D.; Silva,T.N.S.;Vasconcelos, H.; Marcelino, M.; Rodrigues-Machado, M.G.; Filho, G.; Moraes, M.; Marinho, P.E.M.; Amorim, C.F. Inspiratory muscular activation during threshold therapy in elderly healthy and patients with COPD, Journal of Electromyography and Kinesiology (2005), doi:10.1016/j.jelekin.2005.06.002

[6] Araujo, R.C.;Amadio, A .C.; Furlani, J. Contribuição para a interpretação da relação força e atividade EMG. In: Congresso Nacional De Biomecânica, 4.,1992, São Paulo. Anais... São Paulo: Escola de Educação Física da Universidade de São Paulo, 1992. p. 146-153.

[7] Araujo, R.C.; Duarte, M.; Amadio, A .C. Evaluation of increase in force and EMG Activity´s Cirves. In: Congress Of The International Society Of Biomechanics, 15., Jyvaskyla, 1995. Abstract… Jyvaskyla, University Of Jyvaskyla, 1995. p.64-65.

[8] Baba, K.; Akishige, S.; Yaka, T.; Ai, M. Influence of alteration of occlusal relationship on activity of jaw closing muscles and mandibular movement during submaximal clenching. Journal of Oral Rehabilitation. v.27, p.783-801 2000.

[9] Bardsley, P.A., Bentley, S., Hall, H.S., Singh, S.J., Evans, D.H., Morgan, M.D., 1993. Measurement of inspiratory muscle performance with incremental threshold loading: a comparison of two techniques. Thorax 48, 354-359.

[10] Basmajian, J.V. Muscle Alive. 4 ed. Baltimore: Willians & Wilkins, 1978.

[11] Basmajian, J.V. Muscles alive: their function revealed by electromyography. Baltimore: Williams e Wilkins, 1962.

[12] Basmajian, J.V.; De Luca, C.J. Muscle alive: their function revealed by electromyography. 5a ed. Baltimore, Williams e Wiikins, 1985. p.501-561

[13] Biasotto, D. A. Estudo eletromiográfico de músculos do sistema estomatognático durante a mastigação de diferentes materiais. Dissertação(Mestrado) - Faculdade de Odontolocia de Piracicaba da UNICAMP, 2000. 134p.

[14] Blanksma, N.G ;Van Eijden, T.M.G.J. Electromyographic Heterogeneity in the Humam Temporalis and Masseter Muscles during Static Biting. Open Close Excursion, and Chewi. Journal of Dental Research. v.74, n.6,p. 1318- 1327. June 1995.

[15] Dainty, D.A.; Norman, R.W. Standarding biomechanical testing in sport. Champaign, Human Kinetics, 1987.

[16] Ervilha, U.F., Duarte, M Amadio, A.C. Estudo sobre procedimento de normalização do sinal eletromiográfico durante o movimento humano. Rev. Bras. Fisiot., p.15-20,1998

[17] Hatze, H. The meaning of the term"Biomechanics". Journal of Biomechanics, v.7,p.189-190,1974.

[18] Landulpho, A.B. et al. The effect of the oclusal splints on the treatment of temporomandibular disorders – a computerized electromyographic study of masseter and anterior temporalis muscles. Electomyogr. Clin. Neurophysiol. v.42, p.187-191.2002.

[19] M.A. Mananas, R. Jane, J.A. Fiz, J. Morera, P. Caminal, Study of myographic signals from sternomastoid muscle in patients with chronics obstructive pulmonary disease, IEEE Trans. Biomed. Eng. V.47, p. 674-681. 2000.

[20] Mclean L. The effect of postural correction on muscle activation amplitudes recorded from the cervicobrachial region. J Electromyogr Kinesiol., v.15,p.527–535. 2005.

[21] Nascimento, L.N.; Amorim, C.F.; Giannasi, L.C.; Oliveira, C.S.;Nacif, S.R.; Silva, A.M.; Nascimento,D.F.F.; Marchini, Daniela; Oliveira,L.V.F., Occlusal splint for sleep bruxism: na electromyographic associated to Helkimo Index evoluation, Sleep Breath,v.12, p.275–280, 2008.DOI 10.1007/s11325-007-0152-8

[22] Nobre, M.E.P.N.; Lopes, F.; Cordeiro, L.; Marinho, P.E.M.; Silva, T.N.S.S.; Amorim, C.F.; Cahalin, L.P.; Andrade, A.D., Inspiratory muscle endurance testing: pulmonary ventilation and electromyographic analysis, Respiratory Physiology & Neurobiology, (2006), doi:10.1016/j.resp.2006.04.005

[23] Politti, F., Amorim C.F., Calili L., Andrade, A.O., Palomari, E.T., The use of surface electromyography for the study of auricular acupuncture, Journal of Bodywork & Movement Therapies (2009), doi:10.1016/j.jbmt.2008.11.006

[24] Portney, L. Eletromiografia e testes de velocidade de condução nervosa. In: O'sullivan, S.B.; Schmitz, T.J. Fisioterapia: avaliação e tratamento. 2 ed. São Paulo- Manole, 1993. Cap. 10, p. 183-223.

[25] Soderberg, G.L. & Cook, T.M. Electromyography in Biomechanics. Physical Therapy, v.64, p.: 1813-20,1984.

[26] Suda, E.Y; Amorim, C.F.; Sacco, I.C.N. Influence of ankle functional instability on the ankle electromyography during landin after volleyball blocking, Journal of Electromyography and Kinesiology (2007), doi:10.1016/j.jelekin.2007.10.007

[27] Turker, K.S. Electromyographyc: Some methodological problems and issues. Physical .Therapy. v.73, n.10,p. 698-710, 1993.

[28] Winter, D.A. Biomechanics and Motor Control of Human Movement. New York: John Wiley & Sons Inc.,1990.

Chapter 17

Virtual and Augmented Reality: A New Approach to Aid Users of Myoelectric Prostheses

Alcimar Barbosa Soares, Edgard Afonso Lamounier Júnior,
Adriano de Oliveira Andrade and Alexandre Cardoso

Additional information is available at the end of the chapter

http://dx.doi.org/10.5772/50600

1. Introduction

During the past decades, great effort has been devoted to devise new strategies for the control of artificial limbs fitted to patients with congenital defects or who have lost their limbs in accidents or surgery [1-6]. Most of that work was dedicated to minimize the great mental effort needed to control the prosthetic limb, especially during the first stages of training. When working with myoelectric prosthesis, that effort increases dramatically. These devices use EMG signals (the electrical manifestation of the neuromuscular activation associated with a contracting muscle) collected from remnant muscles to generate control inputs for the artificial limb. As these devices use a biological signal to control their movements, it is expected that they should be much easier to control. However, the prosthesis control is very unnatural and requires a great mental effort, especially during the first months after fitting [2, 7, 8]. As a result, a number of patients give up the use of those devices very soon. To overcome those problems, different techniques have been tried as an attempt to devise better strategies for myoelectric control.

This chapter describes the advent of Virtual Reality (VR) systems to create training environments dedicated to users of prosthetic devices. Those VR systems generally simulate a prosthesis that can react to commands issued by the users. A sophisticated system proposed by the authors is also described. Known as *"The Virtual Myoelectric Prosthesis"*, the system is based on the use of EMG to control a virtual prosthesis in an Augmented Reality (AR) environment, in real time, providing the user with a more natural and intuitive training environment. The overall aim is to reproduce the operation of a real prosthesis, in an immersive AR environment, using a virtual device that operates in similar fashion to the real one. Also, the research team believes that, since real upper limb prostheses are relatively heavy and can become uncomfortable and cumbersome, especially during the first stages of fitting, the use of a virtually weightless and fully controllable device can help reducing the great physical and metal effort usually necessary, especially in the first trials.

2. Myoelectric prostheses

The human body has been considered a perfect machine, in which all parts work in harmony one with each other. Most of us can control this "machine" without much effort, until some disturbance caused by disease or injury results in loss of some of its functionality.

The absence of limbs caused by trauma or congenital disorders, can affect our lives profoundly. Simple tasks such as walking or dressing can become extremely difficult or even impossible to execute. There is no doubt that the best solution for the loss of a limb might be the development of some kind of genetic manipulation that stimulates the regeneration of tissue. However, while this is not possible, the best we can do is to restore some of the lost functionality by means of artificial limbs.

For centuries, mankind seek ways to replace lost limbs by mechanical devices. Several ancient designs can be found in museums and libraries. However, the first artifact to be formally named artificial limb was a Roman prosthesis, made of wood and bronze, which appeared around 300 BC [9]. During the Middle Ages, while the poor wore "wooden legs", which were simple, inexpensive and stable, the rich nobles used devices made of iron, which were more decorative than functional. In 1818 Peter Ballif designed the first prosthesis actuated by movements of healthy parts of the body. Before this, the upper limb prostheses were heavy and depended on an able hand for operation [10]. Thereafter, a number of experiments have been carried out seeking the "perfect prosthesis", a device that could be similar to what Wolfe had visualized in 1952 in his book *"New York: Random House"* [11]:

> *"They had perfected an artificial limb superior in many ways to the real thing, integrated into the nerves and muscles of the stump, powered by a built-in atomic energy plant, equipped with sensory as well as motor functions"*

As we know, to date, this prediction has yet to be completely materialized, but much has been done since then. Due to the great number of casualties of World War II, the government of the United States created in 1945 a program of research and development from which scientists and engineers were deeply involved in projects aimed at the development of artificial limbs for amputees [10].

Another fact that lead to the acceleration of the researches in the area, was the large number of congenital defects caused by the use of a drug called Thalidomide. As describe by Soares [10], it was synthesized by the German laboratory Chemie Grünenthal in 1957 and marketed worldwide between 1958 and 1962. This drug was prescribed to minimize sickness during pregnancy. The Thalidomide consumers were not warned that the drug could exceed the placenta affecting the fetus. This oversight had a catastrophic effect: drug abuse, especially during the first trimester of pregnancy, has killed thousands of babies. Those who survived experienced birth defects such as deafness, blindness, disfigurement, and especially the shortening or absence of members. Responding to this tragedy, several research centers intensified the efforts towards the design of artificial limbs as an attempt to improve the lives of those children.

Also, during that period, russian scientists had introduced a prosthetic hand controlled by a signal generated by the activity of remaining muscles from amputated limbs [8]. That type of control has been described as "myoelectric control" and the prosthesis, by extension, has been described as "myoelectric prosthesis".

2.1. Controlling strategies

The control of prostheses can be considered one of the most interesting challenges related to prosthetics. Ideally, a prosthetic limb should be controlled without any effort from the user, similar to the subconscious control of a natural limb.

Currently, there are two main strategies for controlling artificial limbs: biomechanical and bioelectrical. In the first, the motion of parts of the body results in the activation of the limb, whereas, in the latter, biosignals, generated from the electrical activity of muscles, are detected and interpreted in order to generate commands for controlling the prosthesis. Nevertheless, there is ongoing research seeking other forms of control based on more natural strategies, such as those that employ brain or neuronal activity together with sensory feedback [5-7, 12-14].

As described earlier, the first prostheses were generally passive devices that relied on intact parts of the body for their positioning and controlling. This extremely successful design allowed the user to control the device so that the movement of a part of the body was reflected in movements of parts of the prosthesis. Despite some modifications, this design remains basically the same nowadays, being the most popular control mechanism among users [10]. The reasons for such success are not well established, but according to Doeringer and Hogan [15] some of the key factors are: it results in a relatively inexpensive prosthesis; the final prosthesis is not too heavy; after training, the user begins to use the prosthesis as a natural extension of his body, having, for example, the notion of weight and size of the prosthetic limb. Kruit and Cool [16] described the main drawbacks: the mechanism of harnesses used to propagate the movements of the body is usually uncomfortable; the movement of the prosthesis requires significantly large forces; the number of control inputs is limited and thus the number of degrees of freedom of the prosthesis is also limited.

An alternative to the Body-Powered control is to employ the myoelectric control, which uses the electrical activity of muscle contraction (electromyographic signal) as a primary source of control. The prostheses that use this type of control typically do not require cables and, in some situations, there is no need for suspension straps. The operation of a myoelectric device can be summarized as follows: the brain sends commands, i.e., neuronal impulses that travel through nerves and reach the endplate of a given muscle, which, in turn, causes muscle contraction; The electrical muscle activity is then captured by electrodes (normally in a socket attached to the stump), interpreted by customized programs in a microcontroller, and used to activate the actuator of the prosthesis.

Many myoelectric prostheses employed a type of control called "two-site two-states", from which a pair of electrodes is placed on two distinct muscles. The contraction of one of these muscles produces the opening of the hand. The antagonist muscle is used in the same way to control the closing of the hand. As pointed out by Scott and Parker [8], this approach works in a manner analogous to the human body, i.e., two antagonistic muscles (or group of muscles) control the movement of a joint. However, as patients must learn to generate independent contractions of the muscles, which requires a high degree of concentration, the training can be lengthy and demand a lot of mental effort. There are also some situations in which it is not possible to find two available groups of muscles, or there might be more than one joint to be controlled. For these situations other controlling approaches have been developed [17]. For instance, the "one-site three-states", from which a little contraction of a muscle produces the closing of the hand, a strong contraction open it, and the lack muscle activity stops the hand. Figure 1 shows an example of a hand prosthesis controlled by electromyographic signals captured by four pairs of dome electrodes, distributed around the residual limb ([18]).

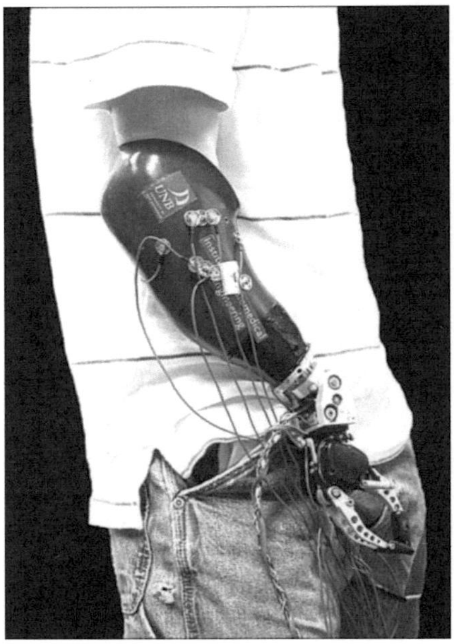

Figure 1. An experimental setup for a myoelectric prosthesis, developed at the University of New Bruswick, Canada (extracted from [18]).

Currently there are a number of methods using proportional control based on the electrical activity of muscles to control the speed, torque and position of prosthetic joints. However, due to the nature of the myoelectric signal, errors and inaccuracies may occur [19]. Myoelectric signals can be detected using basically two types of electrodes: surface electrodes positioned on the skin surface, and needle electrodes inserted in relevant positions of the muscle. In both cases the electrodes produce a difference of potential relative to a reference (typically another electrode located elsewhere on the body). This voltage is the result of an asynchronous activation of hundreds of muscle fibers. The signal is similar to a random noise whose amplitude is modulated by a voluntary input. Its shape depends on variables such as strength and speed of activation, positioning and types of electrodes used in its detection, electronic circuits used for acquisition, amplification and processing [20]. These factors make the translation of myoelectric activity into commands for a prosthetic limb a challenge. Moreover, the generation of myoelectric patterns must be learned by the user, and this is a task which requires concentration, regular training and a great amount of physical effort.

A common way of training an individual to generate myoelectric patterns is by using feedback software, which provides the user with visual feedback about the relation between the forces associated to the contraction with the amplitude of the generated myoelectric signal. The main drawback of this strategy is that it does not give the user feedback information or sense of proprioception. Recent studies have suggested that virtual and augmented reality [21] may be a relevant tool to address the limitations of conventional training techniques. The main advantage of this technique is that it can simulate the physical presence of the artificial limb in the real world, as well as in imaginary worlds. Moreover, some simulations may include additional sensory information, such as sound through speakers or headphones. It is also possible to include tactile information, generally known as force feedback, for the individual.

3. Virtual and augmented reality

Virtual Reality (VR) can be defined as an advanced computer interface where the user can, in real time, navigate within a tridimensional environment interacting with its virtual objects. Such interaction is achieved in a very intuitive and natural way. To do so, multisensory devices are supplied [22].

In order to illustrate this concept, consider Figure 2, in which a user is shown standing inside a research laboratory. However, since she is equipped with multisensory devices (Head Mounted Display – HMD and hand (glove) sensors), a computer-based system provides her the feeling of being steeped into a different environment.

The system, known as BioSimMER© (from Sandia National Laboratories) [23], is used to train rescue personnel to respond to terrorist attacks. The screen on the top shows the working environment displayed only for the eyes of the health professional and the virtual patient exhibits realistic symptoms. Such facilities are not supported by traditional computer interfaces.

Therefore, to achieve the high level of natural interface required by VR systems, it is important to provide the user with the feeling of immersion and the ability for interaction. To reach such requirements, VR developers must guarantee: 1) Real life 3D object images from the user´s perspective; 2) The aptitude to track the user's motions, particularly his head and eye movements, and correspondingly adjust the images on the output device to reflect the change in perspective.

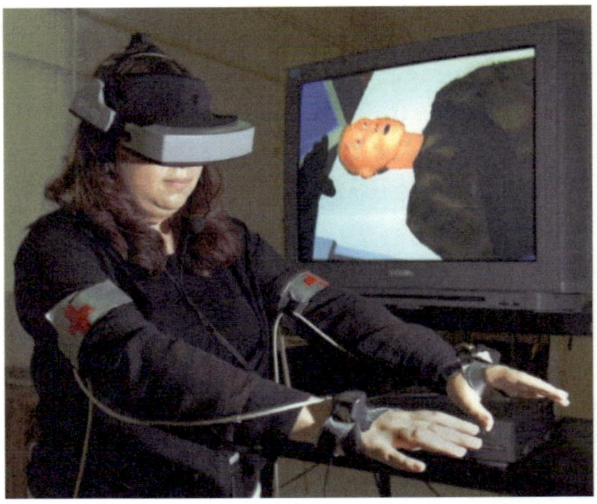

Figure 2. Experiment with virtual reality techniques and devices (extracted from [23]).

Augmented Reality (AR) is a technique that allows the integration of virtual objects within a real physical environment. Interaction is again supported by multisensory equipment. Essentially, a real scene, captured by a digital camera, is "augmented" with the insertion of virtual objects [24]. Figure 3 illustrates this concept.

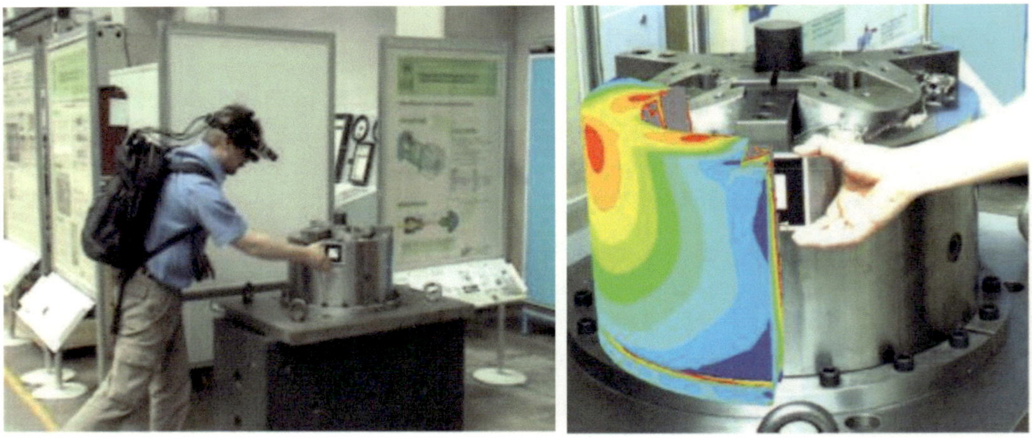

(a) (b)

Figure 3. An example of Augmented Reality extracted from [25]: (a) Positioning a fiduciary marker in mechanical part; (b) Heating distribution visualization through user´s glasses.

In Figure 3(a), an engineer uses a fiduciary square marker to identify the heating distribution throughout a mechanical part, as shown in Figure 3(b). However, this "virtual" information can only be seen by him, through the equipment and glasses he carries.

A very well-known framework to support AR is the ARToolKit ([26]). It provides Computer Vision techniques to calculate position and orientation of a digital camera in relation to fiduciary markers. The augmentation is produced after a series of transformations, as shown in Figure 4. First, the real video image is transformed into a binary one. Then, this image is processed in order to determine square black regions (fiduciary markers – regions whose outline contour can be fitted by four line segments) containing an image pattern that is compared to patterns stored in a database. Next, the algorithm uses size-known squares and the pattern orientation as the base for the coordinates frame and to calculate the real position of the digital camera in relation to the physical marker. After that, the 3D objects are placed over the fiduciary markers, and the final image is sent to the display.

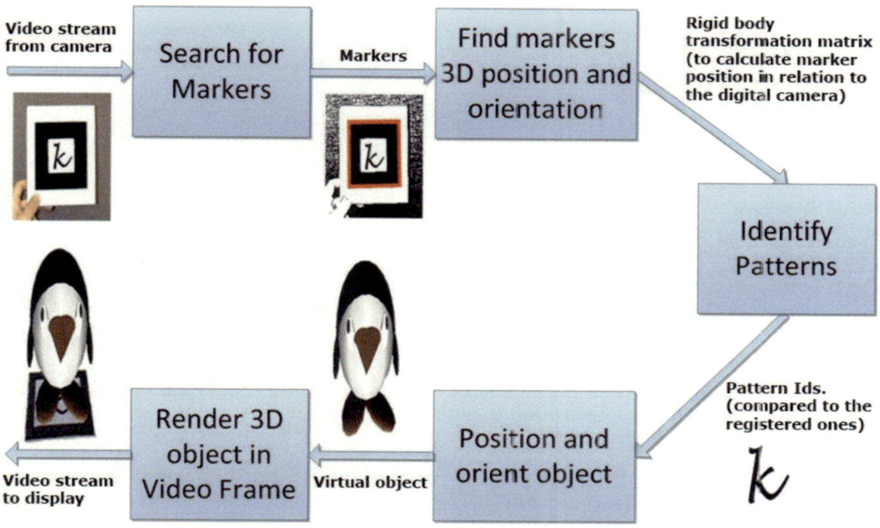

Figure 4. ARToolKit workflow.

Nowadays, VR and AR systems have been intensively used for training and simulation. According to [27] and [28], the main reasons for that are:

- It provides "Learning by doing" - according to pedagogical studies, the learning curve and the amount of knowledge acquired are intensified when the apprentice plays an active role during the process;
- It supports virtual and interactive experiments/simulations - replacing physical counterparts that could pose health hazard or even be too expensive in real life;
- It allows training to be executed outside classes and clinics; and
- It inspires creativity.

The strategies adopted by systems like the ARToolKit are promising and relatively simple to be incorporated into final applications. However, the need for physical markers can limit their application in many areas. Hence, an interface that is able to represent the real environment, capture movements and sounds and transforming them into actions to interact with virtual objects, have been the focus of many recent researches seeking a human-computer dialogue closer to natural. That's why the expression "natural user interface" has emerged as new computer interaction technology. It focuses on human abilities such as touch, vision, voice and higher cognitive functions, such as expression, perception and recall [29]. The main objective here is to give a physical meaning for the digital information. In so doing, data manipulation with the use of bare hands, gestures, voice commands and pattern recognition are supported.

Recently, Santos et al. [30] presented an application that uses gestures to interact with virtual objects in an Augmented Reality, based on Kinect© (a motion sensing input device developed by Microsoft Inc.). The application is not limited by environment, lighting or skin color and doesn´t require fiduciary markers. The system allows the user to perform operations on menus and interact with virtual objects solely by hand gestures (Figure 5).

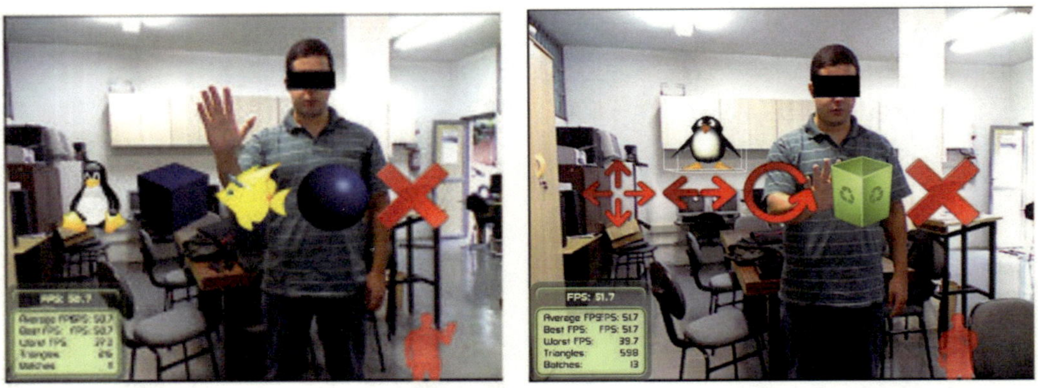

(a) (b)

Figure 5. Natural User Interface with Augmented Reality: (a) User selecting menu options; and (b) User manipulating a virtual object (extracted from [30]).

In recent past years, it has been observed a steady growth in the use of Virtual and Augmented Reality in health care [31, 32]. There a number of examples in the literature. However, to ilustrate the technique, let´s take two examples into account.

Payandeh and Shi [33] presented a mechanics-based interactive multi-modal environment designed to teach basic suturing and knotting techniques for simple skin or soft tissue wound closure. Two haptic devices are used for force-feedback, simulating the experience of suturing a real tissue (Figure 6).

That realist feeling was provided by a number computer-based techniques, such as mass-spring system, to simulate the deformable tissue (skin), mechanics-based techniques to simulate the deformations of a linear object (the suturing material) and collision detection for the interactions between the soft tissue and the needle. Figure 7 shows a pre-wound scene (a) and the result after the virtual suture (b).

Virtual and Augmented Reality have also been studied as a tool for phobia treatment [34]. As an example, consider the system describe in [35]. The project, which is accompanied by a psychologist, aims to design a system to gradually confrontate the patient with his object phobia. Clinical studies have shown that some patients cannot handle, or even do not evolve in the treatment, if exposed to a real arachnid in the initial sessions. Thus, AR is used to present the patient with virtual objects that reminds a spider (like a cartoon) and this object, gradually, becomes a very 'realistic' virtual one (with photorealism modeling techniques). Figure 8(a) shows a potential user wearing the system apparatus and Figure 8(b) shows the image seen by the user.

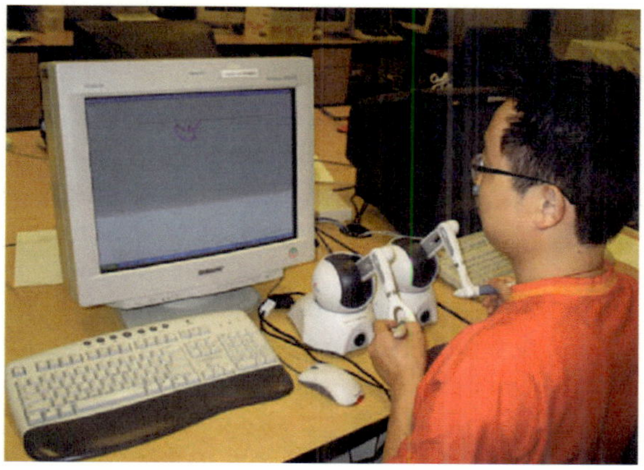

Figure 6. VR multi-modal experimental setup for simulating surgical sutures (extracted from [33]).

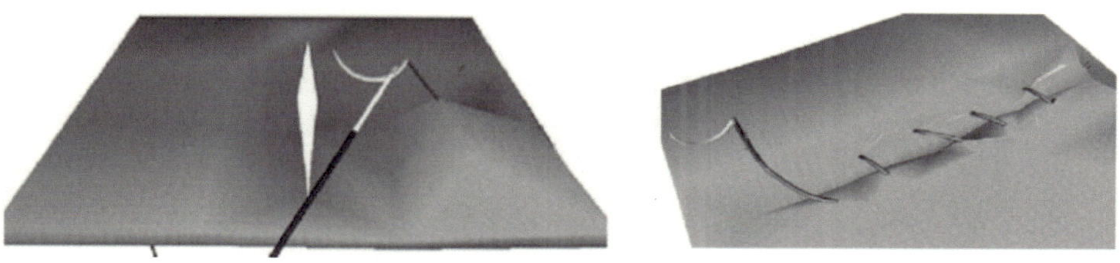

(a) (b)

Figure 7. (a) Virtual pre-wound tissue for suturing; (b) Virtual wound closed (extracted from [33]).

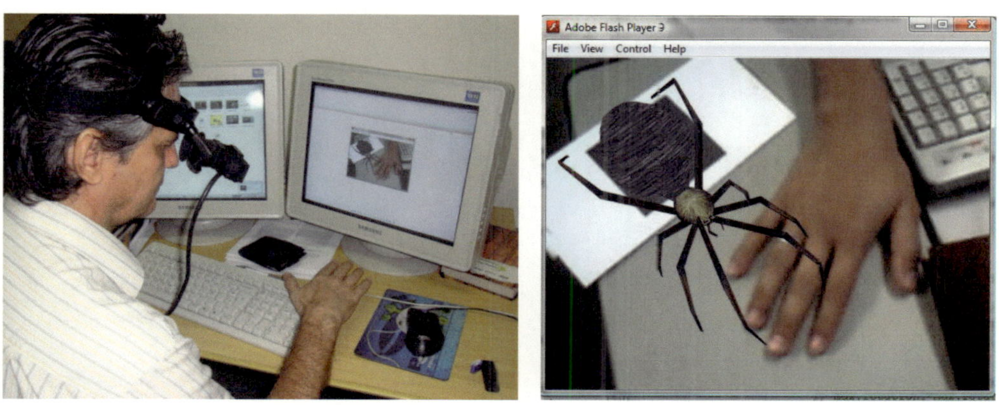

(a) (b)

Figure 8. (a) User wearing HMD for arachnophobia treatment; (b) The AR image, as seen by the user.

Based on the discussions above, we can infer that VR and AR incorporate a number of features with great potential to overcome some of the difficulties associated with the training of prosthetic users.

4. Virtual prostheses

As described earlier, great effort has been devoted to devise new strategies for the control of artificial limbs fitted to patients with congenital defects or who have lost their limbs in accidents or surgery. In general, the devices do not properly resemble the real counterpart, do not react in the same manner, do not provide proper feedback and cannot be controlled using the "natural" interfaces, i.e., signals emanated from the central nervous system. Therefore, a number of difficulties arise when a new user tries to control an artificial limb, since he/she will have to devise a completely new strategy to generate input signals for the prostheses, so that it will act according to his/her wishes. This leads to a lengthy, tiring, and sometimes frustrating, training period. That is true for the great majority of the strategies for prosthesis control that have been designed to date.

Recently, a number of research groups turned their attention to VR and AR, in an attempt to overcome some of those problems. Although many works can be found in the literature, we have chosen just a few to illustrate the concept.

Pons *et al.* [36] describe the use of VR to support the training process for a multifunctional myoelectric hand prosthesis (MANUS) capable of generating up to four grasping modes (cylindrical, precision, lateral and hook grasps, in addition to wrist pronation-supination).

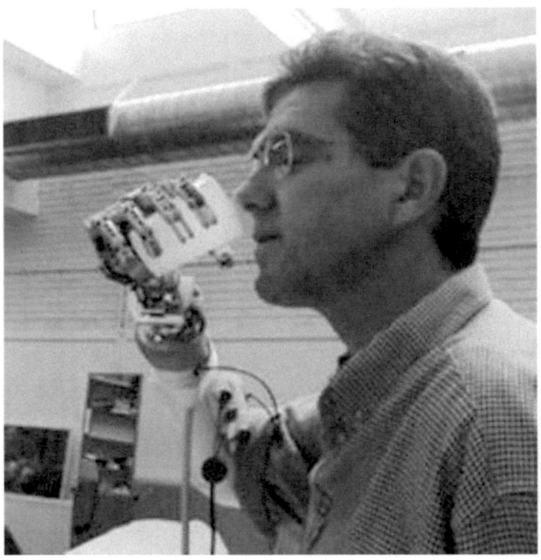

Figure 9. One of the MANUS users performing a combined cylindrical grasp and wrist rotation (extracted from [36]).

As expected, multifunctional prostheses pose an additional problem for users: the more dexterous the device, the higher the number of command channels required to control it. As a result, a large number of different EMG commands, generally obtained by extra EMG channels, are required for successful management of the prosthesis. To minimize the number of channels, the authors proposed a three-bit ternary EMG command strategy. The users were asked to produce EMG bursts (by sudden contraction of a single muscle) and, if proper EMG thresholds could be defined, each burst was classified in three different levels. Each of those three levels were then given the digital values "0", "1" or "2" (no signal, low, high), corresponding to one ternary bit. In so doing, if the user generates three bits, he/she could generate up to 27 different combinations (commands) from a single muscle. However, since the commands starting with "0" (i.e., "0XY") were not valid, the three-bit ternary strategy allowed the generation of 18 effective commands. This means that, from a single muscle, the user could control up to 18 different functions/actions of the prosthesis. However, that is no easy task to learn. Hence, a special training device, based on VR simulation of the multifunctional prosthesis, was created to enable the learning of that "EMG command language". Only after the training process was finished, the prosthesis was fitted and real manipulative operation started. The authors report that all of the volunteers were able to successfully perform basic commands after about 45 minutes.

In similar fashion, Resnik *et al.* [37] show the use of VR as an aiding tool for training users of advanced upper-limb prostheses. The device known as DEKA Arm (DEKA Research & Development Corporation) allows users 10 powered degrees of movement (Figure 10a). A VR environment program (Figure 10b) was created to allow users to practice controlling an avatar, using the controls designed to operate the DEKA Arm in the real world.

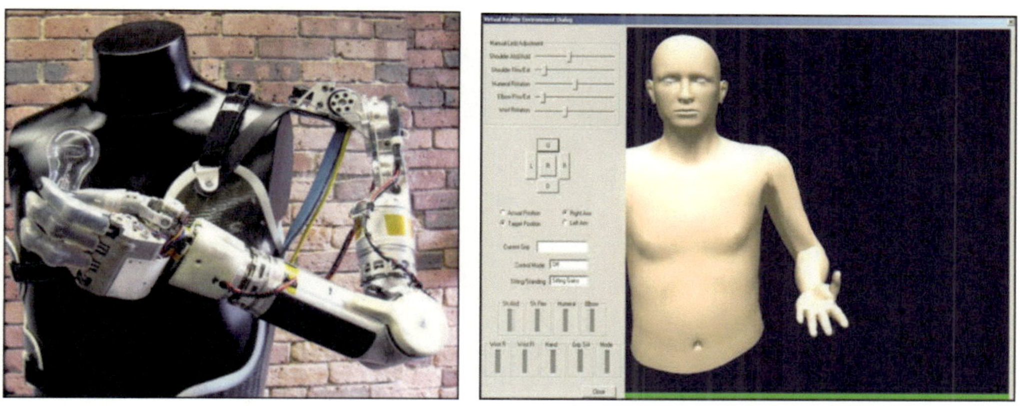

(a) (b)

Figure 10. (a) DEKA Arm displayed on manikin; (b) VR avatar (extracted from [37]).

The authors report that the VR environment allows a gradual acclimatization to the arm, as the experience with the arm-control scheme prior to use of the physical arm allows a staged introduction of the new elements of the system. However, the system did not allow for interaction with virtual objects, i.e., it was not possible, for instance, the manipulation of an object with the virtual hand. Nevertheless, the system proved to be an important asset for upper-limb users who must master a large number of controls and for those who need a structured learning environment, due to cognitive deficits.

4.1. The virtual myoelectric prosthesis

Although VR has been extensively used as an aiding tool for users of prosthetic devices, the interaction with the virtual world still needs to be improved, in order to provide a real immersive training environment. To do so, the research group headed by the authors, have developed new techniques for VR interaction and for detection and processing of EMG signals, in order to extract the correct commands issued by the user which, in turn, could be used to control the movements of a device in a VR environment [21, 28, 30, 38]. However, although a purely non-immersive VR environment showed some good results, it was thought that an Augmented Reality (AR) environment would provide a more realistic experience. Hence, an AR environment was designed so that images of the virtual device (the prosthesis) are combined with images of the real world, providing a realistic environment for training upper limb prosthetic users [39]. A simplified block diagram of the system is shown in Figure 11.

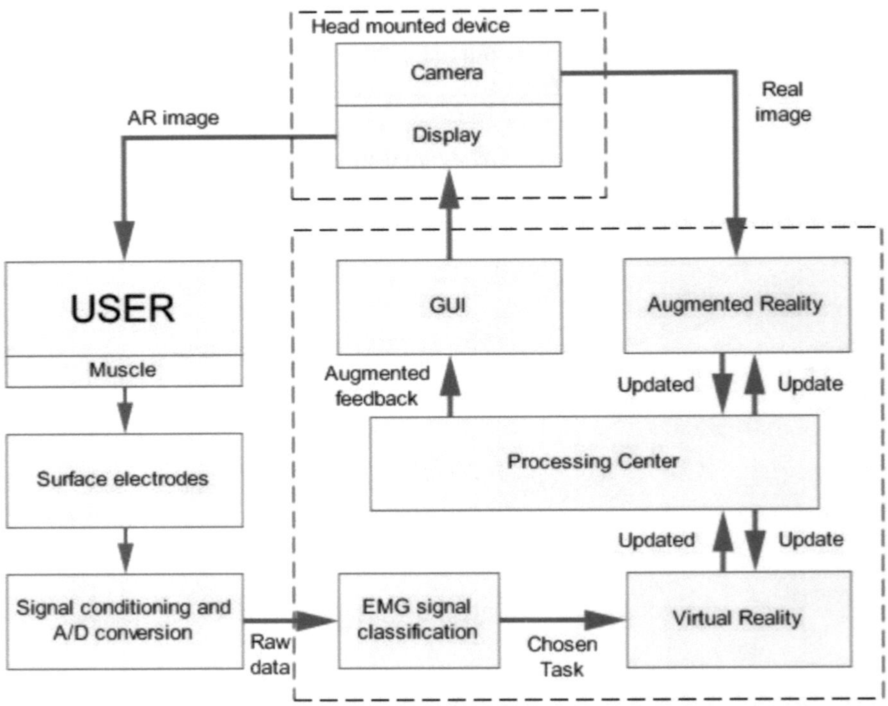

Figure 11. The authors' approach for a Virtual Myoelectric Prosthesis (extracted from [39]).

In the system, the user is fitted with a head mounted device that includes a camera, for capturing the real images of the user´s view point, and a display to show the mixed images (augmented: real and virtual). The EMG signals are collected and processed to generate inputs to the VR unit [21]. A processing center decides when to update both the virtual arm (Figure 12) and the augmented reality image, to further send them to the graphics user interface (the head mounted display).

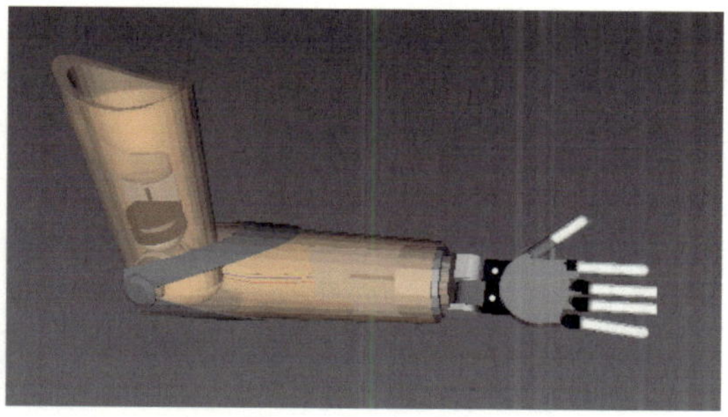

Figure 12. A Virtual Prosthesis designed by the authors.

During operation, the camera captures the image and locates a marker at the user's shoulder. The algorithm then searches for a virtual object that corresponds to such marker (Figure 13) and inserts it into the real world, captured by a camera.

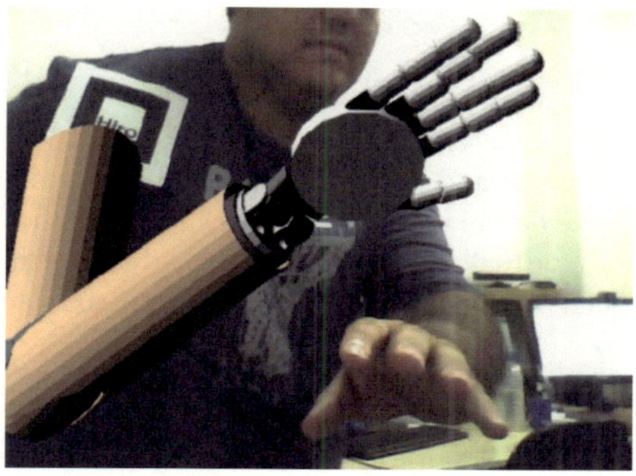

Figure 13. Image of a virtual object combined with the real world scene – an outsider point of view (extracted from [39]).

As described in [39], the control inputs for the AR environment are generated by EMG signals, collected from remnant muscles. The raw EMG signal, detected by surface electrodes is conditioned and processed to find out which movement the user wants to perform. To do so, the areas of activity in the EMG data were detected (windowing) and the resulting signal was then processed to generate a set of features used by an artificial neural network classifier. Basically, each EMG contraction was represented by a set of Auto-Regressive (AR) coefficients calculated according to a modified algorithm described in [38]. According to the authors, the choice of a neural network as a classifier was due to its ability to learn and later recognize signals as being part of the same class of movement in real time. Also, depending on the level of amputation, different users may generate different levels of contractions of the remaining part of the limb, for the same class movement. Besides, even if a single user performs only isometric or isotonic contractions, there will not be two identical contractions for the same movement. The neural network was trained with four classes of movements (elbow flexion, elbow extension, wrist pronation and wrist supination). The results showed a near perfect performance of the classifier (95% to 100% rate of success). The output of the neural network is then used as control input (position and motion) to the virtual device, which can be rendered and mixed with the real world scene, as shown in Figure 14.

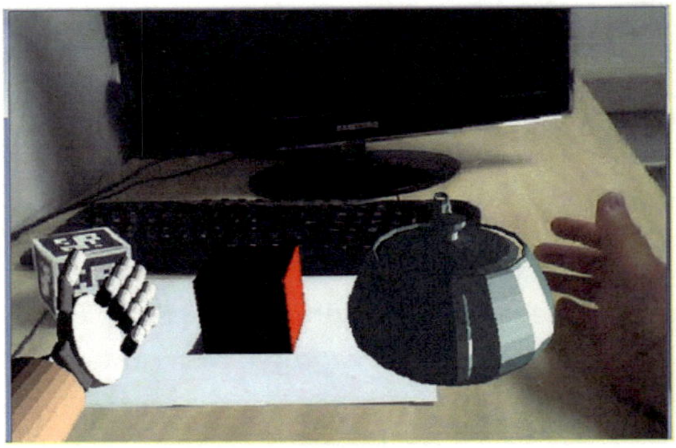

Figure 14. User´s point of view within the AR environment (extracted from [39]).

Note that this system allows the user to interact within the virtual environment - the virtual myoelectric prosthesis can touch and grab other virtual objects embedded in the real scene (such as the cube and the kettle in Figure 14). Also, a strong cognitive feedback is provided by this real time mixture of virtual objects with the real environment, given the feeling that it is almost possible to touch the virtual arm with the real one, and vice-versa.

5. Conclusion

This chapter presented an overview on the search of human beings for artificial devices capable of restoring, if not all, at least part of the functionality lost when we are affected by diseases, congenital disorders or trauma that results in the loss of a limb. Focusing on upper limb prosthesis, a series of sophisticated technical solutions have been proposed during the past decade to design devices whose behavior and control approach that of their healthy natural counterparts. However, as described along this chapter, operating a highly complex artificial limb is not a simple task. This is especially true for myoelectric multifunctional prostheses with many degrees of freedom. Since the necessary control commands, in most instances, can be very different from the "natural" commands, learning how to produce them is extremely difficult and time consuming. With the advent of Virtual and Augmented Reality, those technologies have been proposed as relevant tools to address some of the limitations of conventional training techniques. It is possible to design a virtual device very similar, in shape and behavior, to a real one. Also, it is even possible to collect commands from the real world (EMG signals generated by remnant muscles) and use them as inputs to control the actions of a virtual prosthesis in an Augment Reality Environment, according to the training stage of the user, or any other setup defined by the therapist. In so doing, those techniques allow for a considerable reduction of physical and metal efforts usually necessary to master the control of a prosthetic device.

6. Future directions

Despite the progress achieved so far, the authors believe that, as technology advances, the use of virtual and augmented reality for controlling myoelectric prostheses should also undergo continuous improvements. These future developments should be focused on issues such as: (i) improving the modeling of the virtual devices, in order to increase the sense of realism when compared to actual prostheses; (ii) new adaptive protocols for controlling the virtual prosthesis, so that it could emulated different strategies and different joint actuators; and (iii) the design of new devices to provide physiological feedback, allowing the user to "feel" what the virtual prosthesis is actually doing, thus, increasing the feeling of a complete mix between the real and virtual worlds.

Author details

Alcimar Barbosa Soares* and Adriano de Oliveira Andrade
Laboratory of Biomedical Engineering, Faculty of Electrical Engineering,
Federal University of Uberlândia, Brazil

Edgard Afonso Lamounier Júnior and Alexandre Cardoso
Laboratory of Computer Graphics and Virtual Reality, Faculty of Electrical Engineering,
Federal University of Uberlândia, Brazil

Acknowledgement

The authors would like to express their gratitude to "Coordenação de Aperfeiçoamento de Pessoal de Nível Superior" (CAPES - Brazil), "Conselho Nacional de Desenvolvimento Científico e Tecnológico" (CNPq – Brazil) and "Fundação de Amparo à Pesquisa do Estado de Minas Gerais" (FAPEMIG – MG – Brazil) for the financial support.

7. References

[1] Davoodi R, Loeb GE. Real-Time Animation Software for Customized Training to Use Motor Prosthetic Systems. IEEE Transactions on Neural Systems and Rehabilitation Engineering 2012; 20(2) 134-142.

[2] Scheme E, Englehart K. Electromyogram Pattern Recognition for Control of Powered Upper-Limb Prostheses: State of the Art and Challenges for Clinical Use. Journal of Rehabilitation Research & Development 2011; 48(6) 643–660.

[3] Simon AM, Hargrove LJ, Lock BA, Kuiken TA. Target Achievement Control Test: Evaluating Real-time Myoelectric Pattern-recognition Control of Multifunctional Upper-limb Prostheses. Journal of Rehabilitation Research & Development 2011; 48(6) 619–628.

* Corresponding Author

[4] Su Y, Fisher MH, Wolczowski A, Bell GD, Burn DJ, Gao RX. Towards an EMG-Controlled Prosthetic Hand Using a 3-D Electromagnetic Positioning System. IEEE Transactions on Instrumentation and Measurement 2007; 56(1) 178-186.

[5] GEAKE TH. An Advanced Feedback System for Myoelectrically Controlled Prostheses. MPhil Thesis. School of Computer Science and Electronic Systems, Kingston University, UK, 1994.

[6] Patterson PE, Katz JA. Design and Evaluation of a Sensory Feedback System that Provides Grasping Pressure in a Myoletric Hand. Journal of Rehabilitation Research and Development 1992; 29(1), 1-8.

[7] Paciga JE, Richard PD, Scott RN. Error rate in five-state myoelectric control systems. Medical and Biological Engineering and Computing 1980; 18(3) 287-90.

[8] Scott RN, Parker PA. Myoeletric Prosthesis: State of the Art. Journal of Medical Engineering & Technology 1988; 12 143-151.

[9] Lamb DH, Law H. Upper-Limb Deficiencies in Children – Prosthetic, Orthotic and Surgical Management. Boston, USA: Little, Brown and Company, 1987.

[10] Soares AB. *Shape Memory Alloy Actuators for Upper Limb Prostheses*. PhD Thesis. University of Edinburgh; 1997.

[11] Childress DS. Powered Limb Prostheses: Their Clinical Significance. IEEE transactions on biomedical engineering 1973; BME-20(May) 200-207.

[12] Cram JR. The history of surface electromyography. Applied Psychophysiology and Biofeedback 2003; 28 81-91.

[13] Horowitz S. Biofeedback Applications: A Survey of Clinical Research. Alternative and Complementary Therapies 2006; 12(6) 275-281.

[14] Oskoei MA, Hu H. Support vector machine-based classification scheme for myoelectric control applied to upper limb. IEEE Transactions on Biomedical Engineering 2008; 55(Aug) 1956-1965.

[15] Doringer JA, Hogan N. Performance of Above Elbow Body-Powered Prostheses in Visually Guided Unconstrained Motion Tasks. IEEE Transactions on Biomedical Engineering 1995; 42(6) 621-631.

[16] Kruit J, Cool JC. Body-powered Hand Prosthesis with Low Operating Power for Children. Journal of Medical Engineering & Technology 1989; 13 129-133.

[17] Andrade AO. Methodology for EMG Signal Classification for the Control of Artificial Members. MSc Dissertation. Federal University of Uberlândia, Brazil; 2000.

[18] Kyberd PJ, Lemaire ED, Scheme E, MacPhail C, Goudreau L, Bush G, Brookeshaw M. Two-degree-of-freedom Powered Prosthetic Wrist. Journal of Rehabilitation Research & Development 2011; 48(6) 609–618.

[19] Hoff LA. Errors in Frequency Parameters of EMG Power Spectra. IEEE transactions on biomedical engineering 1991; 38 1077-1088.

[20] O'Neill PA, Morin EL, Scott RN. Myoletric Signal Characteristics from Muscles in Residual Upper Limbs. IEEE Transactions on Rehabilitation Engineering 1994; 2 266-270.

[21] Soares AB, Andrade AO, Lamounier Jr EA, Carrijo R. The Development of a Virtual Myoelectric Prosthesis Controlled by an EMG Pattern Recognition System Based on Neural Networks. Journal of Intelligent Information Systems 2003; 21(2):127-41.

[22] Cardoso A, Kirner C, Lamounier Jr EA, Kelner J. Technologies to the development of virtual and augmented reality systems; Editora Universitária da UFPE, Portuguese version, 2007.

[23] Sandia National Laboratories. BioSimMER - Virtual Life-saver. http://www.sandia.gov/media/NewsRel/NR1999/biosim.htm (accessed 25 April 2012).

[24] Kirner C, Kirner TG. Virtual Reality and Augmented Reality Applied to Simulation Visualization. In: El Sheikh, A.A.R.; Al Ajeeli, A.; Abu-Taieh, E.M.O. (Org.). Simulation and Modelling: Current Technologies and Applications. 1st ed. Hershey-NY: IGI Publishing, 2007; 1 391-419.

[25] Weidlich D, Scherer S, Wabner M. Analyses Using VR/AR Visualization. IEEE Computer Graphics and Visualization 2008; Sept/Oct 84-86.

[26] GNU General Public License. http://www.gnu.org/licenses/gpl.html (accessed 5 February 2007).

[27] Azuma R, Bailot Y, Behringer R, Feiner S, Julier S, MacIntyre B. Recent Advances in Augmented Reality. IEEE Computer Graphics and Applications 2001. 21(6) 34-47.

[28] Soares AB, Lamounier Jr EA, Lopes K, Andrade AO. Augmented Reality: A Tool for Myoelectric Prostheses. In: ISEK 2008: XVIIth Congress of the International Society of Electrophysiology and Kinesiology, ISEK2008, 18-21 June 2008, Niagara Falls, Canada.

[29] Liu W. Natural User Interface - Next Mainstream Product User Interface. In: 2010 IEEE 11th International Conference on Computer-Aided Industrial Design & Conceptual Design (CAIDCD), 17-19 November 2010; 1 203 - 205.

[30] Santos E, Lamounier Jr EA, Cardoso A. Augmented Reality Interaction with Kinect Device. In: Proceedings of the XIII Brazilian Symposium on Virtual and Augmented Reality, SVR2011, 23-26 May 2011.

[31] Riva G. Virtual Reality for Health Care: The Status of Research. CyberPsychology & Behavior 2002; 5(3) 219-225.

[32] Marescaux J, Rubino F, Arenas M, Mutter D, Soler L. Augmented-Reality–Assisted Laparoscopic Adrenalectomy. The Journal of the American Medical Association 2004; 292(18) 2214-2215.

[33] Payandeh S, Shi. F. Interactive Multi-Modal Suturing. Virtual Reality 2010; 14(4) 241–253.

[34] Juan MC, Alcaniz M, Monserrat C, Botella C, Banos R, Guerrero B. Using Augmented Reality to Threat Phobias. IEEE Computer Graphics and Aplications 2005; 25(6) 31-37.

[35] Lima L, Cardoso A, Nakamoto P, Lopes E, Lamounier Jr EA. Development of a Computer Tool to Aid Arachnophobia Treatment with Augmented Reality. In: Proceedings of the XIII Brazilian Symposium on Virtual and Augmented Reality, SVR2011, 23-26 May 2011.

[36] Pons JL, Ceres R, Rocon E, Levin S, Markovitz I, Saro B, Reynaerts D, Van Moorleghem W, Bueno L. Virtual reality training and EMG control of the MANUS hand prosthesis. Robotica 2005; 23 311-317. doi:10.1017/S026357470400133X

[37] Resnik L, Etter K, Klinger SL, Kambe C. Using Virtual Reality Environment to Facilitate Training with Advanced Upper-Limb Prosthesis. Journal of Rehabilitation Research & Development 2011; 48(6) 707–718.

[38] Soares AB, Veiga ACP, Andrade AO, Pereira AC, Barbar JS. Functional Languages in Signal Processing Applied to Prosthetic Limb Control. Systems Analysis Modelling Simulation 2002; 42 1377-1389.

[39] Lamounier Jr EA, Lopes K, Cardoso A, Soares AB. Using Augmented Reality Techniques to Simulate Myoelectric Upper Limb Prostheses. Journal of Bioengineering & Biomedical Science 2012; S1:010. doi:10.4172/2155-9538.S1-010

Chapter 18

Signal Acquisition Using Surface EMG and Circuit Design Considerations for Robotic Prosthesis

Muhammad Zahak Jamal

Additional information is available at the end of the chapter

http://dx.doi.org/10.5772/52556

1. Introduction

Electromyography (EMG) is the subject which deals with the detection, analysis and utilization of electrical signals emanating from skeletal muscles. The field of electromyography is studied in Biomedical Engineering. And prosthesis using electromyography is achieved under Biomechatronics [1]. The electric signal produced during muscle activation, known as the myoelectric signal, is produced from small electrical currents generated by the exchange of ions across the muscle membranes and detected with the help of electrodes. Electromyography is used to evaluate and record the electrical activity produced by muscles of a human body. The instrument from which we obtain the EMG signal is known as electromyograph and the resultant record obtained is known as electromyogram [2].

The human body is a wonder of nature. The functioning of human body is an intriguing and fascinating activity. Motion of the human body is a perfect integration of the brain, nervous system and muscles. It is altogether a well-organized effort of the brain with 28 major muscles to control the trunk and limb joints to produce forces needed to counter gravity and propel the body forward with minimum amount of energy expenditure [3]. The movement of the human body is possible through muscles in coordination with the brain. Whenever the muscles of the body are to be recruited for a certain activity, the brain sends excitation signals through the Central Nervous System (CNS). Muscles are innervated in groups called 'Motor Units'. A motor unit is the junction point where the motor neuron and the muscle fibers meet. A depiction of the Motor Unit is given in Figure 1. When the motor unit is activated, it produces a 'Motor Unit Action Potential' (MUAP) [4]. The activation from the Central Nervous System is repeated continuously for as long as the muscle is required to generate force. This continued activation produces motor unit action potential trains. The trains from concurrently active motor units superimpose to produce the resultant EMG signal. A group of muscles are involved in a certain movement of the human body. The number of muscles recruited depends upon the activity in which the body is involved. E.g. in lifting a small weight such as a tiny pebble, fewer amount of muscles will be involved as compared to lifting a heavy mass like a 6 kg weight, where the muscles employed will be greater. In technical terms, whenever it is required to generate greater force, the excitation from the Central Nervous System increases, more motor units are activated and the firing rate of all the motor units increase resulting in high EMG signal amplitudes [4,5].

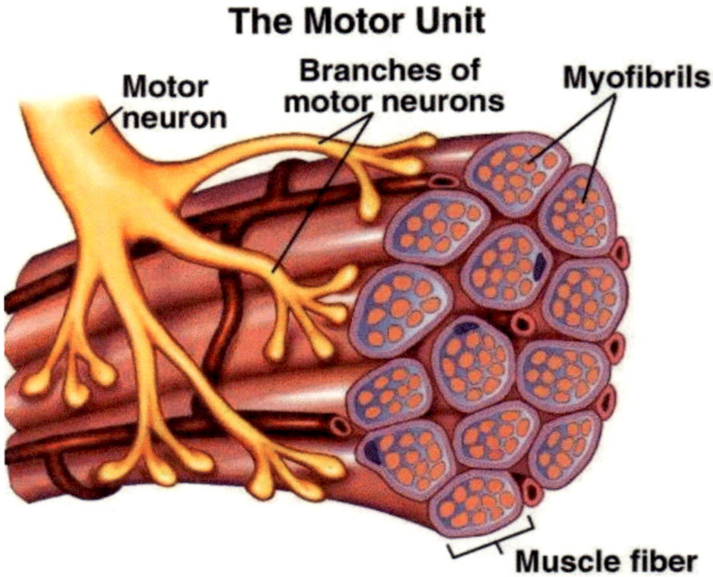

Figure 1. A Motor Unit consists of one motor neuron and all the muscle fibers it stimulates [6]

Electromyography enables us to generate force, create movements and allow us to do countless other functions through which we can interact with the world around us. The electromyograph is a bioelectric signal which has, over the years, developed a vast range of applications. Clinically, electromyography is being used as diagnostic tool for neurological disorders. It is frequently being used for assessment of patients with neuromuscular diseases, low back pain and disorders of motor control [7]. Other than physiological and biomechanical research, EMG has been developed as an evaluation tool in applied research, physiotherapy, rehabilitation, sports medicine and training, biofeedback and ergonomics research.

In the recent past, EMG has also found its use in rehabilitation of patients with amputations in the form of robotic prosthesis. EMG proves to be a valuable tool as it provides a natural way of sensing and classifying different movements of the body. A multi-degree of freedom robotic mechanism can effectively imitate the motion of the human limb. Recent advances in electronics and microcontroller technology have allowed improved control options for robotic mechanisms. One of the most vital advantages of microprocessor technology in robotic prosthetics is the advanced EMG filtering algorithms. Nowadays, control options are even available to those who were not at one time qualified for such prosthetic management.

This chapter will discuss in detail, the effective use of surface electromyography (SEMG) as a tool for achieving robotic prosthesis. An elaborate account of SEMG electrode types, signal acquisition technique, electronics circuit design considerations and the control procedure to drive electric motors in a robotic mechanism is provided in this chapter.

2. EMG electrodes and its types

The bioelectrical activity inside the muscle of a human body is detected with the help of EMG electrodes. There are two main types of EMG electrodes: surface (or skin electrodes) and inserted electrodes. Inserted electrodes have further two types: needle and fine wire electrodes. The three electrodes (needle, fine wire and surface) are explained as follows. Among these three electrodes, surface EMG electrodes will be specifically discussed in detail as it pertains to the topic of this chapter.

2.1. Needle electrodes

Needle electrodes are widely used in clinical procedures in neuromuscular evaluations. The tip of the needle electrode is bare and used as a detection surface. It contains an insulated wire in the cannula. The signal quality from the needle electrodes is comparatively improved from other available types. Needle electrodes have two main advantages. One is that its relatively small pickup area enables the electrode to detect individual MUAPs during relatively low force contractions. The other is that the electrodes may be conveniently repositioned within the muscle (after insertion) so that new tissue territories may be explored [5]. A needle electrode is shown in Figure 2.

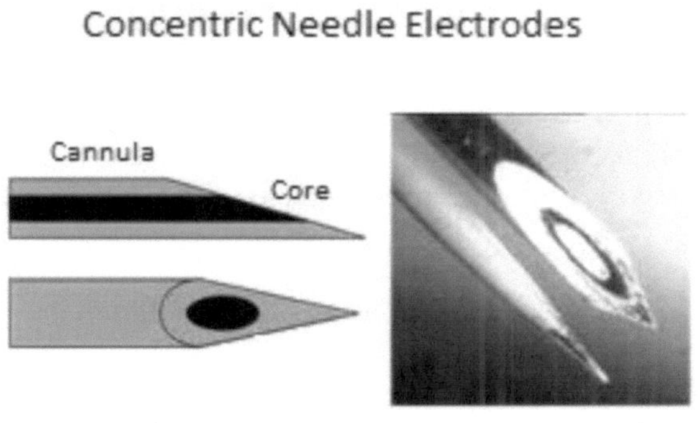

Figure 2. A Needle EMG Electrode [8]

2.2. Fine wire electrodes

Wire electrodes are made from any small diameter, highly non-oxidizing, stiff wire with insulation. Alloys of platinum, silver, nickel, and chromium are typically used. Wire electrodes are extremely fine, they are easily implanted and withdrawn from skeletal muscles, and they are generally less painful than needle electrodes whose cannula remains inserted in the muscle throughout the duration of the test [5]. A fine wire electrode is shown in Figure 3.

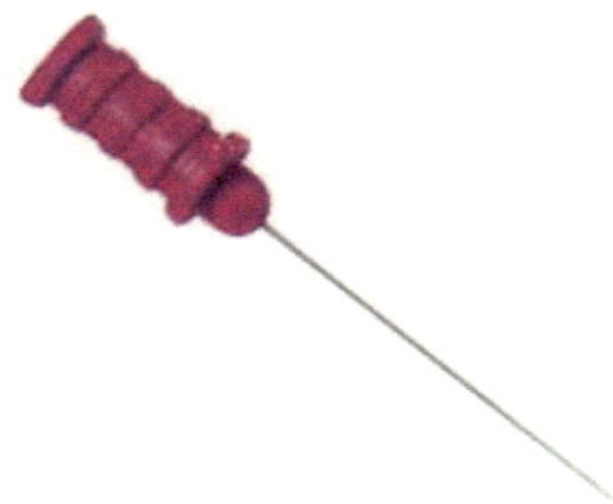

Figure 3. Fine Wire EMG Electrode

2.3. Surface EMG electrode

Surface EMG electrodes provide a non-invasive technique for measurement and detection of EMG signal. The theory behind these electrodes is that they form a chemical equilibrium between the detecting surface and the skin of the body through electrolytic conduction, so that current can flow into the electrode.

These electrodes are simple and very easy to implement. Application of needle and fine wire electrodes require strict medical supervision and certification. Surface EMG electrodes require no such formalities. Surface EMG electrodes have found their use in motor behavior studies, neuromuscular recordings, sports medical evaluations [9] and for subjects who object to needle insertions such as children. Apart from all this, surface EMG is being increasingly used to detect muscle activity in order to control device extensions to achieve prosthesis for physically disabled and amputated population.

Surface EMG has some limitations as well. Since these electrodes are applied on the skin, hence, they are generally used for superficial muscles only. Crosstalk from other muscles is a major problem. Their position must be kept stable with the skin; otherwise, the signal is distorted.

2.3.1. Types of EMG Electrodes

There are two types of surface EMG electrodes: Gelled and Dry EMG electrodes [10].

2.3.1.1. Gelled EMG Electrodes

Gelled EMG electrodes contain a gelled electrolytic substance as an interface between skin and electrodes. Oxidation and reduction reactions take place at the metal electrode junction. Silver – silver chloride (Ag-AgCl) is the most common composite for the metallic part of gelled electrodes. The AgCl layer allows current from the muscle to pass more freely across the junction between the electrolyte and the electrode. This introduces less electrical noise into the measurement, as compared with equivalent metallic electrodes (e.g. Ag). Due to this fact, Ag-AgCl electrodes are used in over 80% of surface EMG applications [10].

Disposable gelled EMG electrodes are most common; however, reusable gelled electrodes are also available. Special skin preparations and precautions such as (hair removal, proper gel concentration, prevention of sweat accumulation etc.) are required for gelled electrodes in order to acquire the best possible signal. Gelled EMG electrodes are shown in Figure 4.

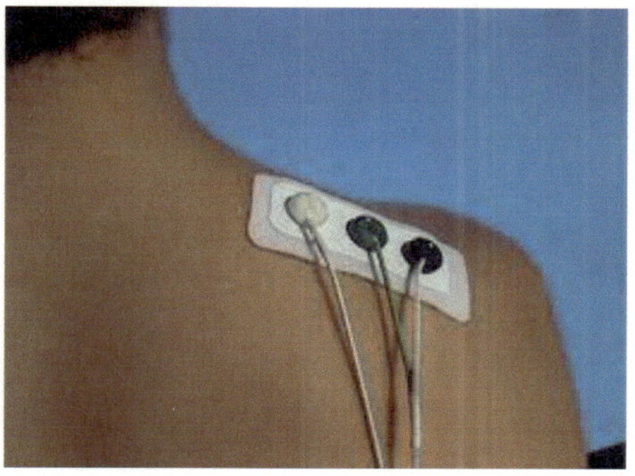

Figure 4. Gelled EMG Electrodes

2.3.1.2. Dry EMG electrodes

Dry EMG electrodes do not require a gel interface between skin and the detecting surface. Bar electrodes and array electrodes are examples of dry electrodes. These electrodes may contain more than one detecting surface. In many examples, an in-house pre-amplification circuitry may also be employed in these electrodes. A reusable bar electrode is shown in Figure 5. Dry electrodes are usually heavier (>20g) as compared to gelled electrodes (<1g). This increased inertial mass can cause problems for electrode fixation; therefore, a material for stability of the electrode with the skin is required [10].

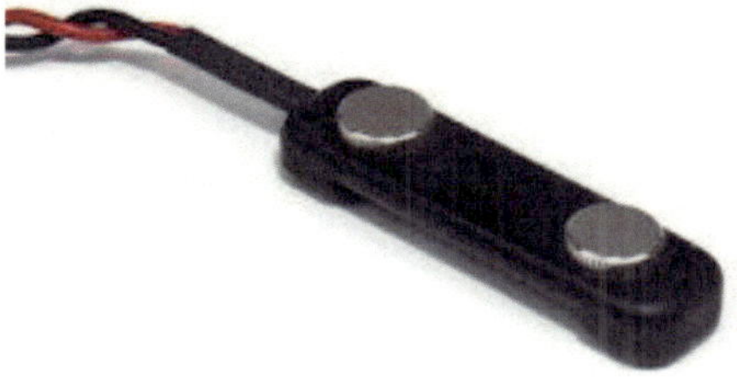

Figure 5. A Reusable Bar Electrode (an Example of Dry EMG Electrode)

2.3.2. Categories of Surface EMG Electrodes

There are two categories of surface EMG electrodes [5]: Passive and Active EMG electrodes. They are briefly explained as follows:-

2.3.2.1. Passive EMG electrodes

These electrodes should be connected to an external amplification circuitry with the help of connecting wires for the proper acquisition of the EMG signal. Passive EMG electrodes can be disposable or reusable.

Electrodes shown in Figure 4 and Figure 5 both fall under passive surface EMG electrodes.

2.3.2.2. Active EMG electrodes

Active EMG electrodes contain a pre-amplifier attachment for surface electrodes. Needle and fine wire surface electrodes are also available. These electrodes usually fall under the dry surface EMG electrodes type. The in-house high impedance amplifier in these electrodes transfers the pre-amplified signal to the rest of the circuitry. Figure 6 shows an active EMG electrode.

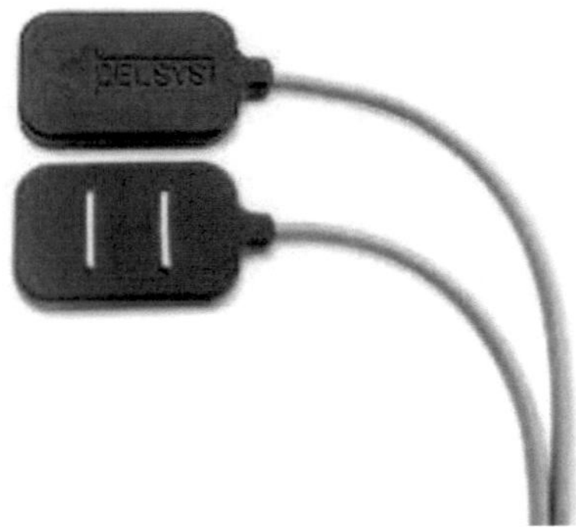

Figure 6. The Delsys 2.1 Active EMG Electrode [11]

3. EMG electrode placement and signal acquisition technique

Surface EMG is relatively easy to use as compared to other EMG electrodes. This is the reason why it is being extensively used in the control of robotic mechanisms to achieve prosthesis. It is also widely used in latest EMG researches by engineers as no medical certification or expertise is required for its application. Its use in rehabilitation prosthesis is favorable as it does not cause any kind of discomfort to the subject on whom it is applied. Other kinds of EMG electrodes (needle and fine wire), when inserted into the skin of the subject, may effect a twitching sensation and cause him or her to make movements.

In order to get the best results from SEMG, it is really important to have a proper understanding of the muscles from which the EMG signal is being extracted. The placement on skin also requires adequate study and requires skin preparation beforehand as well.

The EMG electrodes, their types, sub-types and categories have already been explained in detail in the previous section. Since, our concern is only with Surface EMG (SEMG), hence, we will only deal with the placement and signal acquisition technique using surface EMG electrodes.

3.1. Overview of muscle architecture

Skeletal muscle architecture is defined in terms of "the arrangement of muscle fibers relative to the axis of force generation." The skeletal muscle arrangement as well as their activity reveals striking organization at the macroscopic level. The functional properties of the skeletal muscle depend strongly on their architecture [12].

There are various kinds of muscle fiber arrangements, which are discussed as follows:-

i. Muscles with fibers that extend parallel to the muscle force-generating axis are termed **parallel, fusiform** or **longitudinally** arranged muscles. Examples of such types of muscles are Biceps Brachii (bicep muscle) and Sartorius (groin muscle).
ii. Muscles with fibers that are oriented at a single angle relative to the force generating axis are termed **unipennate** muscles. Example of unipennate muscle is Extensor Digitorum Longus.
iii. The angle between the fiber and the force-generating axis generally varies from 0° to 30°. The muscles are oriented at more than one angle. Most muscles fall into this category and they are called as **multipennate** muscles. Examples are Rectus Femoris which is bipennate and Deltoid which is multipennate.
iv. The muscles which surround an opening so as to form a closed shape are known as **circular** muscles. Example of such kind of muscle is Orbicularis Oris (mouth muscle).
v. The muscles in which their fibers converge on the insertion to maximize force of contraction are known as **Convergent** muscles. E.g. Pectoralis Major.

A detailed depiction of these muscle arrangements is provided in Figure 7.

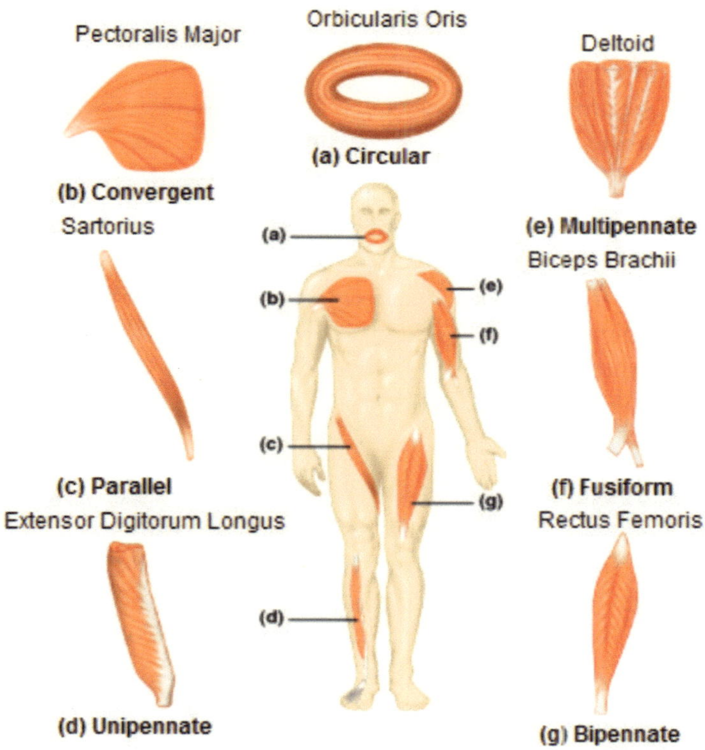

Figure 7. Muscles and their Architecture [13]

3.2. Skin preparation

Application of surface EMG electrodes requires proper skin preparation beforehand. In order to obtain a good quality EMG signal, the skin's impedance must be considerably reduced. For this purpose, the dead cells on the skin e.g. hair must be completely removed from the location where the EMG electrodes are to be placed. It is advisable to use an abrasive gel to reduce the dry layer of the skin [9]. There should be no moisture on the skin. The skin should be cleaned with alcohol in order to eliminate any wetness or sweat on the skin.

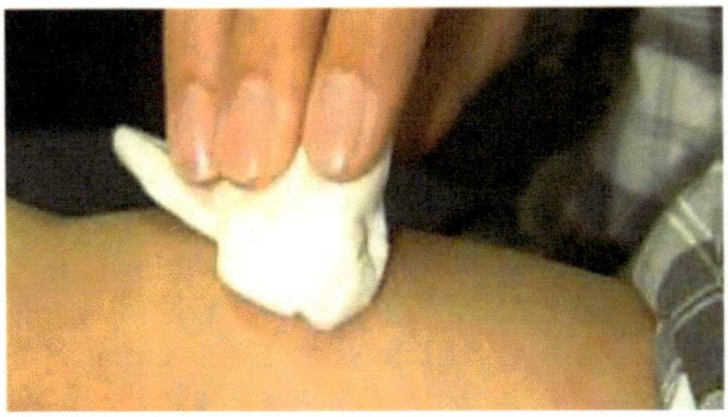

Figure 8. Skin Preparation prior to application of EMG electrodes

3.3. EMG electrode placement

The application of EMG electrodes requires adequate know how of the skeletal muscles. The EMG electrode placement will be discussed in detail under this section.

In most cases, two detecting surfaces (or EMG electrodes) are placed on the skin in bipolar configuration [14, 15]. In order to acquire the best possible signal, the EMG electrode should be placed at a proper location and its orientation across the muscle is important. The surface EMG electrodes should be placed between the motor unit and the tendinous insertion of the muscle, along the longitudinal midline of the muscle [15]. The distance between the center of the electrodes or detecting surfaces should only be 1-2 cm. The longitudinal axis of the electrodes (which passes through both detecting surfaces) should be parallel to the length of the muscle fibers.

As mentioned previously, the EMG detecting surfaces should be placed in between the motor unit and the tendon insertion of the muscle. Detecting surfaces placed on the belly of the muscle has proved to be a more than acceptable location. Here, the target muscle fiber density is the highest [15]. Figure 9 shows the proper EMG electrode placement. When the electrodes are arranged in this way, the detecting surfaces intersect most of the same muscle fibers, and as a result, an improved superimposed signal is observed.

The electrodes should not be placed elsewhere. In the past, a misconception prevailed that the EMG detecting surfaces should be placed on the motor unit. But, as a matter of fact, the electrode location on the motor point serves as the worst location for signal detection [15].

Similarly, the electrodes should neither be placed at or near the tendon nor at the edge of the muscle. The muscle fibers become thinner and smaller in number when they approach the tendon of the muscle resulting in a weak EMG signal, proving the fact that electrode placement near the tendon is not feasible. If the electrode is placed at the edge of the muscle, the chances of crosstalk from other muscles will considerably increase, and the resultant signal will be disturbed by those of other muscles [15].

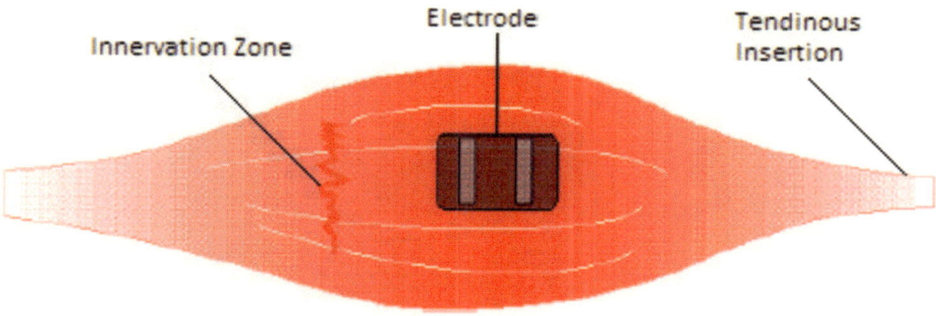

Figure 9. The ideal position of the electrode (two detecting surfaces) is between the innervation zone (or motor unit) and the tendinous insertion (or belly of the muscle) [15]

3.4. General concerns

Before we move on to the signal acquisition phase, it is very important to get acquainted with the EMG signal and the various concerns and factors affecting the qualitative properties of the signal.

The EMG signal's amplitude lies in between 1-10 mV, making it a considerably weak signal. The signal lies in the frequency range from 0-500 Hz and most dominant in between 50-150 Hz [15].

The EMG signal is highly influenced by noise [16], as shown in Figure 10. The characteristics of electrical noise can be caused from various sources. Ambient noise can be caused by electromagnetic radiation sources e.g. radio transmission devices, fluorescent lights and power line interference from electrical wires. These interferences are almost impossible to avoid from external means. This particular noise exists in the frequency range of 50-60 Hz. Noise can also be generated from motion artifact. The two main sources of this noise are instability of electrode skin interface and movement of the electrode cable and lies mostly in the range of 0-20 Hz. It can be eliminated by proper set of EMG equipment and circuitry. The maximum fidelity of the signal is determined by the acquired EMG signal-to-noise ratio [5, 14].

3.5. Reference electrode placement

The signal from the EMG detecting surfaces is gathered with respect to a reference. An EMG reference electrode acts as a ground for this signal. It should be placed far from the EMG detecting surfaces, on an electrically neutral tissue [15].

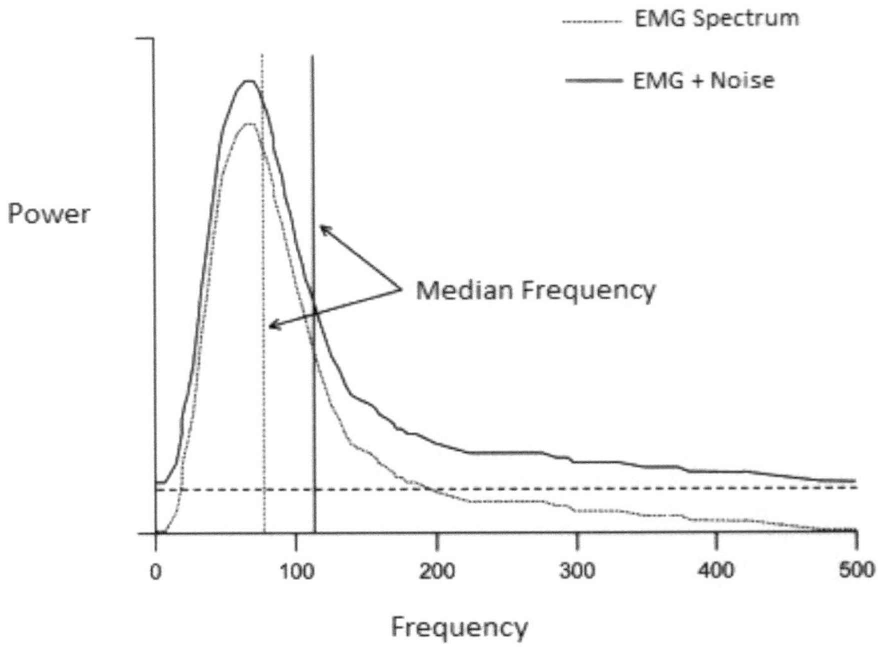

Figure 10. EMG Spectrum and noise influence on this spectrum [16]

3.6. EMG signal acquisition circuitry and configurations

The EMG electrode placement has been elaborately explained under the previous heading. So, after properly understanding the target muscle profile, preparing the skin and positioning the EMG detecting surfaces, comes the EMG signal acquisition step.

EMG signal is acquired through differential amplification technique. The differential amplifier should have high input impedance and very low output impedance. Ideally, a differential amplifier has infinite input and zero output impedance [17].

Differential amplification is achieved with the help of an instrumentation amplifier for high input impedance. A classic three amplifier instrumentation amplifier is shown in Figure 11.

The instrumentation amplifier carries out differential amplification by subtracting the voltages V_1 and V_2. This way, the noise signal which is common at V_1 and V_2 (electrode inputs) e.g. power line interference etc. are eliminated. The tendency of a differential amplification to reject signals common to both inputs is determined by common mode rejection ratio (CMRR). A CMRR of 90 dB is enough for elimination of common signals for instrumentation amplifiers, but latest technology, even though expensive, provides us with a CMRR of 120 dB. But there are reasons for not pushing the CMRR to the limit, as the electrical noise detected by the electrodes may not be in phase [15]. The gain for the instrumentation amplifier can be set using a single resistor (R_{gain}). The gain equation and output equation of the instrumentation amplifier is given in Eq. 1 and 2.

$$Gain = \left(1 + \frac{2R1}{Rgain}\right)\frac{R3}{R2} \tag{1}$$

$$Vout = (V2 - V1) \times Gain \tag{2}$$

A small gain of 5 or 6 is recommended for signal acquisition. Extensive amplification will be carried out in further steps. The placement of the EMG detecting surfaces can be done through three different configurations: monopolar, bipolar and multipolar.

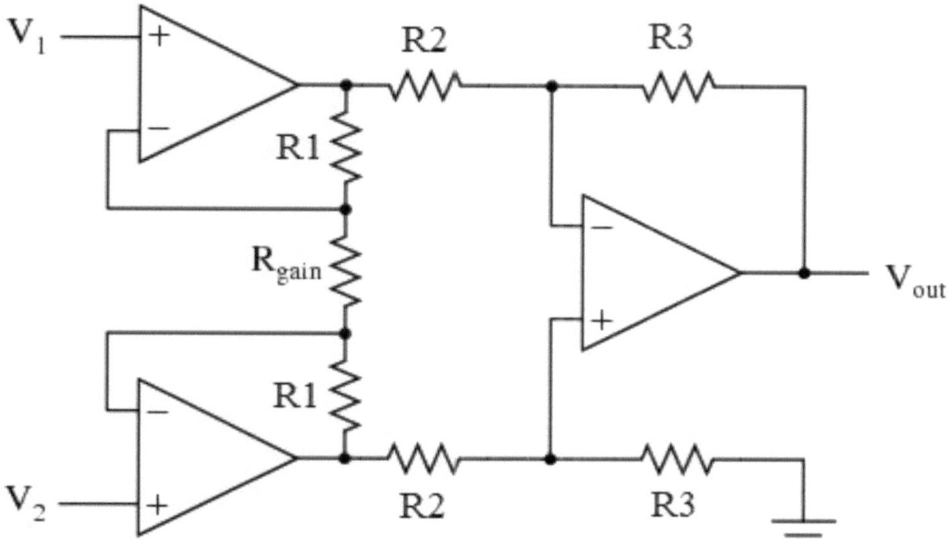

Figure 11. A Three Amplifier Instrumentation Amplifier

3.6.1. Monopolar configuration

The monopolar configuration is implemented using only a single electrode on the skin with respect to a reference electrode as shown in Figure 12. This method is used because of its simplicity, but is strictly not recommended as it detects all the electrical signals in the vicinity of the detecting surface [5, 14].

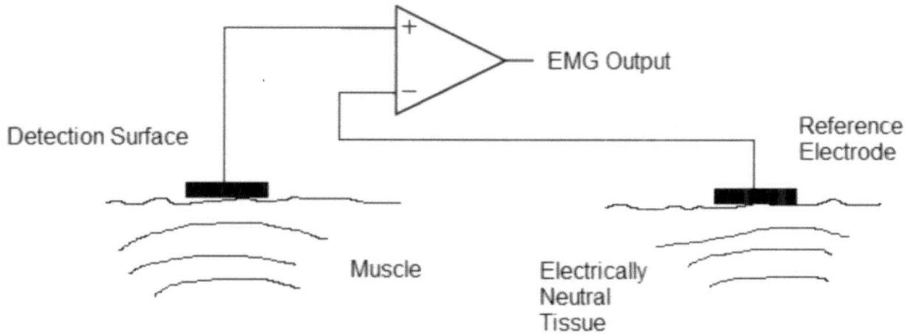

Figure 12. Monopolar signal acquisition technique

3.6.2. *Bipolar configuration*

Bipolar configuration is used to acquire EMG signal using two EMG detecting surfaces with the help of a reference electrode. The signals from the two EMG surfaces are connected to a differential amplifier. The two detecting surfaces are placed only 1-2 cm from each other. The differential amplifier suppresses the common noise signals to both inputs and then amplifies the difference [5, 14]. The limitations of the monopolar configuration are catered for by this configuration. This is the most commonly used electrode configuration. The bipolar EMG electrode configuration is shown is Figure 13.

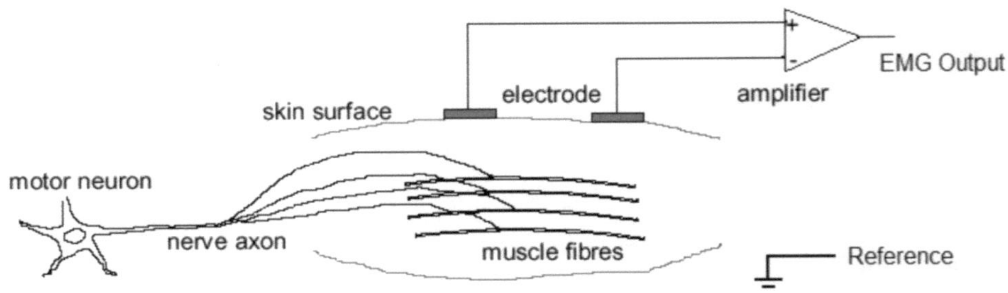

Figure 13. Bipolar Configuration

3.6.3. *Multipolar configurations*

This configuration uses more than two detecting surfaces to acquire the EMG signal with the help of a reference electrode. This configuration further reduces crosstalk and noise concerns [14]. A much more enhanced EMG signal is acquired from this configuration. The signals from three or more EMG detecting surfaces, placed 1-2 cm from each other, are passed through more than two stages of differential amplification. For example if three detecting surfaces are used then double differential technique is employed.

This configuration is used in comprehensive researches carried out to study EMG muscle fiber orientation, conduction velocity and motor point localization.

4. Electrical design considerations

This section will discuss the electrical design considerations in order to synthesize the best possible EMG signal from the muscles of the human body in thorough detail. The basic circuitry for signal acquisition or preamplification circuitry is explained in due detail in the previous section. In this section we will discuss the circuitry implemented after the preamplification stage.

4.1. Filtering

As discussed earlier, there are many concerns regarding the proper detection of the EMG signal. Once the electrode is properly placed and the signal is extracted, noise plays a major role in hampering the recording of the EMG signal. For this purpose, the signal has to be properly filtered, even after differential amplification [18, 19].

The noise frequencies contaminating the raw EMG signal can be high as well as low. Low frequency noise can be caused from amplifier DC offsets, sensor drift on skin and temperature fluctuations and can be removed using a high pass filter. High frequency noise can be caused from nerve conduction and high frequency interference from radio broadcasts, computers, cellular phones etc. and can be deleted using a low pass filter.

In order to remove these high and low frequencies, high pass and low pass bio-filters will be discussed in adequate detail in this section.

4.1.1. High pass filter

A high pass filter is used to remove low frequency component from a particular electrical signal. A term 'cut-off frequency', denoted by 'f_c', is the frequency below which all frequencies are eliminated. All frequencies above f_c are carried forward. The frequency range where the filter response is '1' and the signals are transmitted is known as 'passband' region. On the contrary, the frequency range where the filter response is '0' and the signals are attenuated is known as 'stop band' region [18]. A high pass filter response is shown in Figure 14.

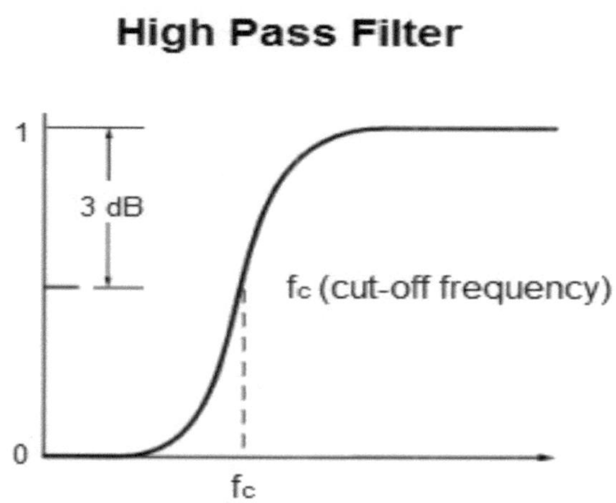

Figure 14. A high pass filter response

A high pass filter can be developed by using a resistor and a capacitor. This circuit will then be known as a CR circuit [20]. This circuit is a first order high pass filter. It is the simplest high pass filter possible. The high pass filtered signal is gathered across the resistor. The filter is shown in Figure 15.

The cut-off frequency of the high pass filter is given in Eq. 3.

$$fc = \frac{1}{2\pi RC} \tag{3}$$

A second order high pass filter can also be designed. An effective design can employ an active electronic component [20]. The design uses two first order filters in series and is facilitated by an operational amplifier. The circuit is given Figure 16.

For this circuit, if $R_1 = R_2$; $C_1 = C_2$ then f_c is given as:-

$$fc = \frac{1}{2\pi RC} \quad (4)$$

R_3 and R_4 are optional and are required for separate gain settings as:-

$$A_0 = 1 + R_4/R_3 \quad (5)$$

Using a 2nd order filter is recommended as they provide a roll-off of 40 dB/dec as compared to 20 dB/dec provided by 1st order filters [18]. The use of active components can isolate the filter from the rest of the circuitry.

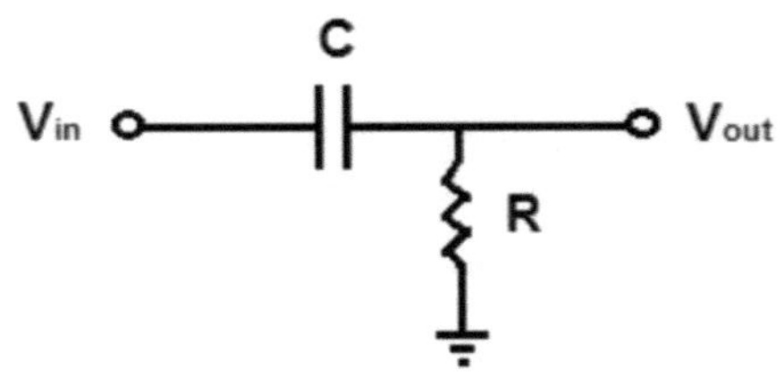

Figure 15. First order high pass filter

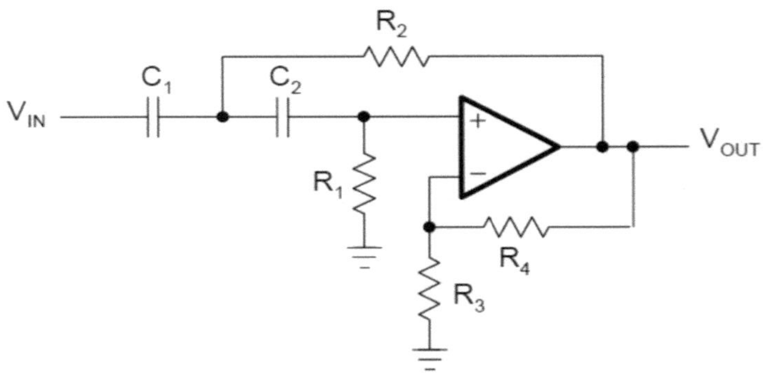

Figure 16. A 2nd Order High Pass Filter

4.1.2. Low pass filters

The concept of low pass filters is entirely opposite to that of high pass filters. In these filters, the frequencies less than the cut-off frequency are transmitted and above that are removed [18]. A low pass filter response is shown in Figure 17.

The simplest low pass filter can be designed with the help of a resistor and a capacitor called as a 1st order RC circuit [20]. The low pass filtered signal is detected across the capacitor. The 1st order low pass filter circuit is shown in Figure 18.

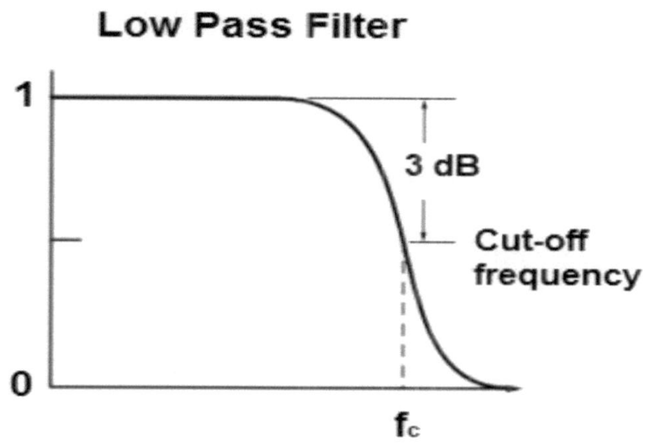

Figure 17. Low Pass Filter Response

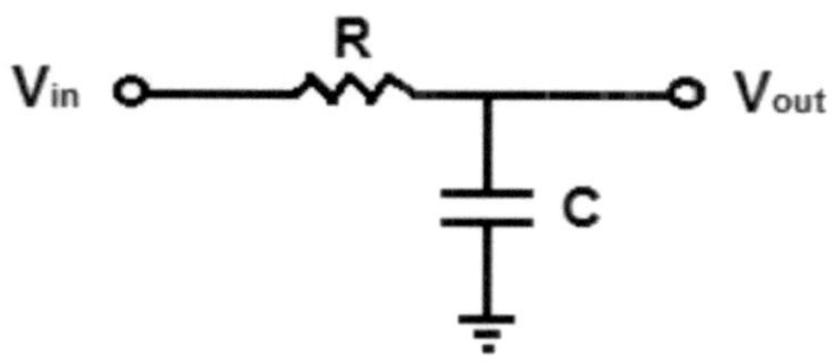

Figure 18. 1st Order Low Pass Filter

The cut-off frequency equation for the circuit in Figure 18 is the same as that of Eq. 3.

A 2nd order low pass filter can be more effective as compared to a 1st order one. It can be designed by cascading two 1st order filters attached to an operational amplifier. The circuit is given in Figure 19.

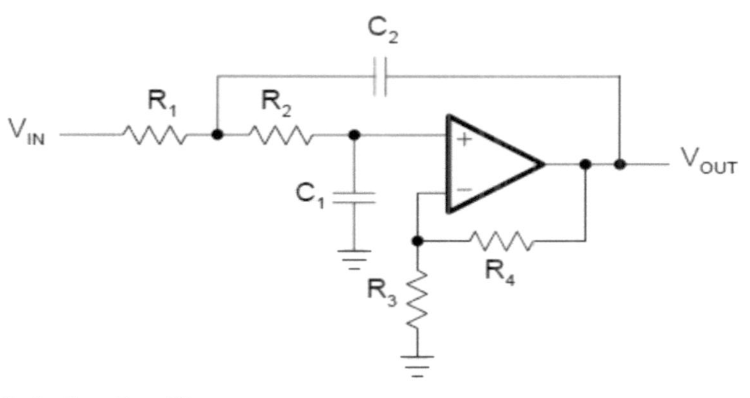

Figure 19. 2nd Order Low Pass Filter

For $R_1 = R_2$ and $C_1 = C_2$, the cut-off frequency of the circuit in Figure 19 is the same as that of Eq. 4. R_3 and R_4 are optional as they are required for separate gain settings as given in Eq. 5.

A 2nd order low pass filter is again recommended as compared to a 1st order one for the same reasons mentioned for a 2nd order high pass filter.

4.1.3. Band pass filtering for EMG

As mentioned previously, for the transmission of pure EMG, the high and low frequency noise should be deleted. For this purpose, only a specific band of frequency should be carried forward [20]. This can be made possible with the help of a band pass filter. A band pass filter response is shown in Figure 20.

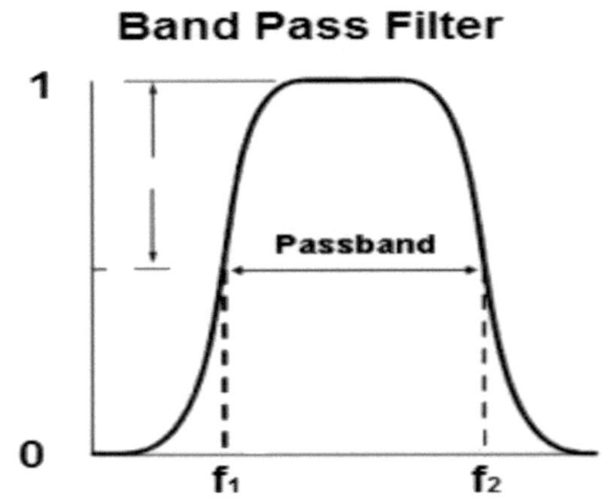

Figure 20. Band Pass Filter Response

The frequency region where the response of the EMG signal is '1' is called the 'passband' and in the case of band pass filter, it is between f_1 and f_2.

A band pass filter can be designed by connecting a low pass and a high pass filter in series. By selecting proper values of R and C, we can develop a band pass filter which can carry forward the most effective component of the EMG signal. It is recommended that for EMG, f_1 should be 65-70 Hz and f_2 be 150-180 Hz.

4.2. Amplification

After the signal has been filtered properly and a suitable band of EMG frequency is obtained, the next stage is amplification. The EMG signal obtained has to be powered up to a suitable level. The amplification of the EMG signal can be easily carried out with the help of a non-inverting amplifier, shown in Figure 21.

The gain of the amplifier is provided in the figure as 'A_v'. The non-inverting amplifier is only used when the signal is being received from a single wire referenced to ground. Amplification can be done in stages in order to cater for chip requirements, by cascading them in series.

The EMG signal, as mentioned before, is very weak i.e. only 1-10 mV. For certain muscles, for which the signal response is very strong e.g. Biceps Brachii, a gain of 500-1000 can be enough. But for muscles, whose EMG response is weak e.g. Flexor Palmaris Longus (ring finger muscle), the gain settings should be very high i.e. 10000.

The proper gain setting solely depends upon the signal response observed from the subject's target muscle. It is to be noted that every subject gives a separate signal response. Some subjects will give weak responses as compared to others. So, in that case, appropriate gain value should be set once the subject's EMG signal response is properly observed.

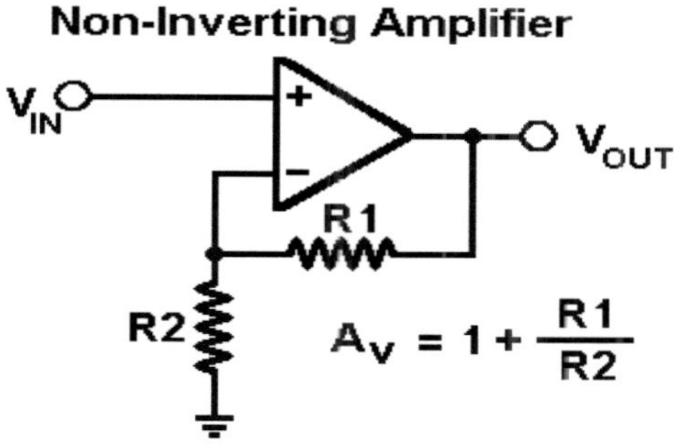

Figure 21. A Non-Inverting Amplifier

5. Control technique

In order to successfully achieve robotic prosthesis, an effective control technique is very important in order to drive the electric motors in the mechanism. With the advent of modern microcontroller technology, the control options available today have never been so effective.

For implementing the desired control to the motors, the amplified EMG signal in analog form has to be converted into digital format. After this, the motors are driven with the help of a microcontroller through the thresholding technique. These techniques will be discussed in detail in this section.

5.1. Analog to digital conversion

The digitization process of the analog signal is carried out with an Analog to Digital Converter (ADC). Nowadays, the ADC has become a common component of modern electronic devices. Their use has become highly varied and widespread. Before using the ADC, its specifications, advantages and limitations have to be analyzed in order to select the most appropriate one for the application. In the same way, important considerations have to be taken into account while converting EMG signals into digital format.

Control of the motor will be developed after the EMG signal is converted into digital format. A particular ADC has a specific range of conversion i.e. there are maximum and minimum levels defined for an ADC over which it can operate. An ADC can convert the analog signal over a certain number of bits. The number of bits which an ADC can convert is known as its "quantization scheme". If an ADC has a defined range and a quantization scheme of *'n-bits'*, then the resolution of the ADC can be given as:-

$$V_{resolution}= V_{range}/(2)^n \quad (6)$$

While converting an EMG signal into digital format, three specifications should be taken into account. 1) Quantization, 2) Range of conversion and 3) Sampling rate [21].

The number of bits, which an analog signal can be converted into digital format by an ADC, is known as quantization. The maximum amount of voltage an ADC can convert into digital quantized bits defines the range of an ADC. The sampling rate means the number of samples an ADC can convert in one second.

After the EMG signal has been amplified up to a suitable level, the range of an ADC should be selected so that it can comprehend a particular voltage level. The number of quantization bits is important, as they determine the resolution of the ADC. The more the number of quantization bits, the less will be resolution of the ADC; the more it will help in control purposes. The ADC sampling rate is also a key consideration. It should be kept as large as possible so that the data loss of EMG is kept at a minimum [21].

ADCs are now available as a peripheral with microcontroller chips and can give sampling rates greater than 1000 kSPS and quantization schemes of more than 24 bits.

5.2. Thresholding and motor drive

The control of robotic prosthesis is provided through the thresholding technique [21]. Once the signal is received in digital format, taking all necessary considerations as described before, a suitable threshold is applied to that particular quantized digital signal.

Before applying the threshold, the digital quantized signal is to be observed properly. A threshold value should then set be accordingly. It is recommended to set the threshold value to a point which is less than half the digital quantized output of the EMG signal. When the digital signal exceeds this threshold, the microcontroller should set an output pin to '1' and '0' otherwise [21]. E.g. if the maximum value of the digital quantized signal is 750 (decimal value) then we can set a threshold of 275. This signal is forwarded to an H-bridge or a motor driver in order to drive the respective electric motors of a robotic mechanism.

The motor driver should be designed or selected according to our requirements of electric motor. Usually a motor driver which can drive a 12V motor and handle up to 4A current can adequately meet requirements for a robotic arm.

6. Results and conclusions

A useful way of acquiring EMG signals and motor drive has been explained in this chapter. Modern microelectronics and controllers have enabled us to develop efficient control of prosthetic robotic mechanisms. To summarize the discussions made earlier, Figure 22 shows a block diagram depicting all the necessary steps required to achieve successful prosthesis.

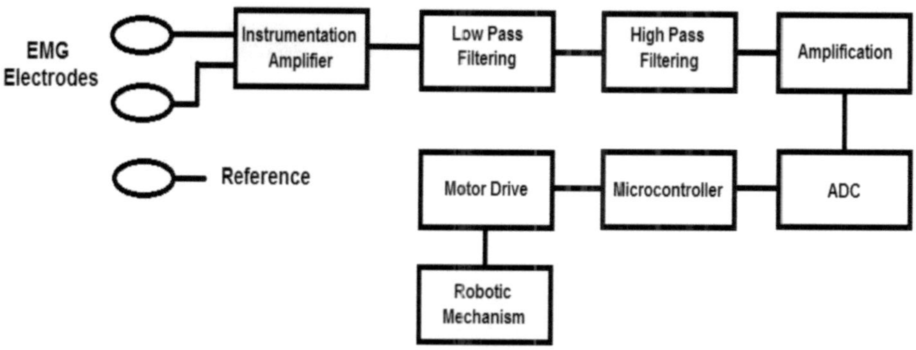

Figure 22. Block diagram indicating all steps for driving a robotic mechanism

As an example, we discuss the control of a robotic hand. There are two primary motions of the human hand, flexing and extending. For flexion, electrode should be placed on Flexor Digitorum Profundus and for extension; the electrode should be placed on Extensor Digitorum Communis [21]. As both muscles exhibit different signal patterns, therefore, a multi-channel input scheme should be employed, so that both signals are gathered independently. Both signals should be observed carefully and a suitable threshold should be set after filtering and amplification. The same procedure is to be followed in order to develop control of all the fingers of the robotic hand i.e. by placing EMG electrodes on specific muscles which control them, allowing us to classify different motions of the hand [22].

The signal observed from a subject with a moderate built is shown in Table 1. The amplification set for the detected EMG signals from the subject was 10,000. Table 1 provides the EMG signal response from each of the subject's fingers after amplification and threshold set for their control [21].

Size is a very important factor while designing an electronics circuit. A circuit occupying minimum space will be most appropriate in application. A size effective circuit will be easy to place and handle in a robotic mechanism. Advances in biomedical instrumentation have brought fruitful gains to robotic prosthetic technology. The ADS1298 is a 64 pin IC with 8 differential inputs with programmable gain amplifiers (PGAs) and a 24 bit ADC. The PGAs can provide a maximum gain of 12 but the 24 bit ADC quantization scheme is enough to process the EMG signal [23]. With all necessary peripherals attached to a single IC, the size of the whole circuitry can be reduced up to 95%.

Latest robotic researches have enabled us to design and create multi-degree of freedom robotic mechanisms [24]. A good mechanical design and apparatus is essential for efficient robotic prosthesis. Newer electronic components and materials have made robotic prosthesis more functional and adaptable. When we talk about materials, the perfect one should be lighter, durable, adjustable and comfortable for the user. Nowadays, carbon fiber frames are being employed as a solution to this matter. An example of a carbon fiber limb is the state of the art Ottoblock C-Leg. The C-Leg has a built in computer which analyzes data from various sensors and actuates the knee using a hydraulic cylinder.

When a human uses a robot, he desires to use his natural limb movements to control the mechanism. In order to achieve this, EMG provides the perfect assistance to allow a subject to make normal movements using a robotic apparatus, hence, efficient controllers and improved algorithms are essential for enhanced control of the device. Given the fact that EMG was introduced more than 30 years ago, the research community has a come a long way in coming up with innovative techniques, hardware solutions and advanced procedures to design, control and utilize these signals to produce resourceful prosthetic means to tackle disabilities and amputations effectively.

S. No.	Finger/ Hand	Peak Voltage Reading before Contracting (V)	Peak Voltage Reading after Contracting (V)	Threshold Set (V)
1	Thumb (flexing)	0.8	3.7	1.4
2	Index (flexing)	0.6	1.4	0.8
3	Ring (flexing)	0.2	2.5	0.7
4	Pinkie (flexing)	0.2	1	0.5
5	Hand (flexing)	0.2	5	1
6	Hand (extending)	0.15	4.5	0.8

Table 1. EMG signals observed and the threshold in terms of voltage [17]

7. Future challenges and directions

Scientists working on upper limb prosthesis define their goal in this field as to develop a 'simultaneous, independent, and proportional control of multiple degrees of freedom with acceptable performance and near "normal" control complexity and response time' [25]. The major challenges faced in prosthetics are: electromechanical implementation, use of EMG control signals and the interface between robotic and clinical communities [26]. Designing a robotic mechanism which is fully capable of integrating with human neuromuscular system is a tough proposition. The requirements can only be fulfilled if the apparatus is of light and flexible material with small but powerful actuators, size effective electronic components, sensors which can easily adapt with the skin and a long lasting battery life. Only then the machine will qualify to be used in everyday practical life [26].

The human hand has 20 degrees of freedom, and the body works in a unique variety of ways to tackle various hindrances placed in front of it. It is therefore, a great challenge to extract all of these motions from the body and utilize them in a resourceful way. Nowadays, two degree of freedom mechanisms are most common. To achieve further DOFs, sensors will be required to be placed at more sophisticated locations, which is a tough task.

The most important challenge of robotic prosthesis in rehabilitation is the feasibility of the mechanism. The apparatus should be comfortable, silent and aesthetically viable for the subject [26]. Our target should be the effective use of the robotic artificial limb on the physically disabled, not to waste our efforts in fruitless objects. Hence, for the reliability of the mechanism's implementation on the amputated population, clinician's approval should be made a part of the procedure.

Due to its practicality and noninvasiveness, SEMG proves to play a significant role in medical applications and rehabilitation prosthesis. However, the human machine interface will decide if the robotic mechanism will be used in everyday life application or not. It is very important to improve the Quality of Life (QOL) of elder and disabled population. It is believed that in the near future, "we will be able to replace entire limbs with prosthetics that can replicate one's own biological functions precisely, casting natural outward appearance and requiring minimum upkeep" [26].

Robotic researchers and biomedical engineers have been trying to combine their techniques to make the perfect biomechatronic mechanism. However, in order to ensure that challenges are met and to create a more smart and intelligent machine, communication between clinicians, users and engineers should be established on a greater scale.

Author details

Muhammad Zahak Jamal
National University of Sciences and Technology, Pakistan

Acknowledgement

The study was carried out at College of Electrical and Mechanical Engineering (CEME), NUST in collaboration with Armed Forces Institute of Rehabilitation Medicine (AFIRM). The author is highly indebted to Brig. Dr. Javaid Iqbal and Dr. Umer Shahbaz Khan for their help in the study and CEME for providing necessary funds to make this research possible. Special thanks to all colleagues and people who have willingly helped out with their abilities.

8. References

[1] Alan G. Outten, Stephen J. Roberts and Maria J. Stokes (1996) "Analysis of human muscle activity", Artificial Intelligence Methods for Biomedical Data Processing, IEE Colloquium, London
[2] Musslih LA. Harba and Goh Eng Chee (2002) "Muscle Mechanomyographic and Electromyographic Signals Compared with Reference to Action Potential Average Propagation Velocity", Engineering in Medicine and Biology Society, 19th Annual International Conference of the IEEE, Vol.3
[3] Nissan Kunju, Neelesh Kumar, Dinesh Pankaj, Aseem Dhawan, Amod Kumar (2009) "EMG Signal Analysis for Identifying Walking Patterns of Normal Healthy Individuals" Indian Journal of Biomechanics: Special Issue
[4] Carlo J. De Luca (1997) "Use of Surface Electromyography in Biomechanics" Journal of Applied Biomechanics, Vol.3
[5] Carlo J. De Luca (2006) "Electromyography: Encyclopedia of Medical Devices and Instrumentation" (John G. Webster Ed.), John Wiley Publisher
[6] Jarret Smith (2010) image title: "motor-unit-lg"

[7] S.L. Pullman, D.S. Goodin, A.I. Marquinez, S. Tabbal and M. Rubin (2000) "Clinical Utility of Surface EMG" Report of the Therapeutics and Technology Assessment, Subcommittee of the American Academy of Neurology, Neurologly Vol. 55:171–177
[8] Paul E. Barkhaus and Sanjeev D. Nandedkar (2000) "Electronic Atlas of Electromyographic Waveforms" Vol. 2, 2nd Edition
[9] Nuria Masso, Ferran Rey, Dani Romero, Gabriel Gual, Lluis Costa and Ana German (2010) "Surface Electromyography and Applications in Sport" Apunts Medicina De L'Esport, Vol. 45: 127-136
[10] Dr. Scott Day "Important Factors in Surface EMG Measurement", Bortec Biomedical Incorporated
[11] (2008) "Bagnoli EMG Systems Users Guide", Delsys Incorporated
[12] Netter FH (1997) "Atlas of Human Anatomy" East Hanover, New Jersey: Novartis.
[13] Elaine Marieb and Katja Hoehn (2007) "Human Anatomy and Physiology" 7th Edition, Pearson Education
[14] Björn Gerdle, Stefan Karlsson, Scott Day and Mats Djupsjöbacka (1999) "Acquisition, Processing and Analysis of the Surface Electromyogram". In: U. Windhorst, H. Johansson, editors. "Modern Techniques in Neuroscience Research", Springer
[15] Carlo J. De Luca (2002) "Surface Electromyography: Detection and Recording", Delsys Incorporated
[16] D.J. Hewson, J.Y. Hoqrel and J. Duchene (2003) "Evolution in impedance at the electrode-skin interface of two types of surface EMG electrodes during long-term recordings" Journal of Electromyography and Kinesiology, Vol. 13, Issue 3 , pp. 273-279
[17] (2009) "Instrumentation Amplifier Application Note", Intersil Incorporated
[18] Gianluca De Luca (2001) "Fundamental Concepts in EMG Signal Acquisition", Delsys Incorporated
[19] P.R.S. Sanches, A.F. Müller, L. Carro, A.A. Susin, P. Nohama (2007) "Analog Reconfigurable Technologies for EMG Signal Processing" Journal of Biomedical Engineering, Vol. 23, pp. 153-157
[20] M. E. Van Valkenburg (1982) "Analog Filter Design", Holt, Rinehart & Winston
[21] Zahak Jamal, Asim Waris, Shaheryar Nazir, Shahryar Khan, Javaid Iqbal, Adnan Masood and Umar Shahbaz (2011) "Motor Drive using Electromyography for Flexion and Extension of Finger and Hand Muscles" 4th International Conference on Biomedical Engineering and Informatics, Vol. 3 pp. 1287-1291
[22] Sebastian Maier and Patrick van der Smagt (2008) "Surface EMG suffices to classify motion of each finger independently" Proceedings of MOVIC 2008, 9th International Conference on Motion and Vibration Control
[23] Datasheet ADS1298 "Low-Power, 8-Channel, 24-Bit Analog Front-End for Biopotential Measurements" Texas Instruments Incorporated.
[24] A. H. Arieta, R. Katoh, H. Yokoi and Y. Wenwai (2006) "Development of a Multi D.O.F Electromyography Prosthetic System Using Adaptive Joint Mechanism", Applied Bionics and Biomechanics, Vol. 3, Woodheads Publishing
[25] D. Edeer and C.W. Martin (2011) "Upper Limb Prostheses – A Review of the Literature with a Focus on Myoelectric Hands", WorksafeBC Evidence-Based Practice Group
[26] Brian Dellon and Yoki Matsuoka (2007) "Prosthetics, Exoskeletons, and Rehabilitation-Now and the Future" IEEE Robotics & Automation Magazine, March, 2007